Anatomy Trains

Fourth Edition

DEDICATION

To Edward, for the gift of language.

To Julia, for the tenacity to see it through.

'Every act of the body is an act of the soul.'
(*William Alfred*[1])

'I don't know anything, but I do know that everything is interesting
if you go into it deeply enough.'
(*Richard Feynman*[2])

1. Alfred W. *The Curse of an Aching Heart.* Out of print.
2. Feynman R. *Six Easy Pieces.* New York: Addison Wesley; 1995.

Anatomy Trains

Myofascial Meridians for Manual Therapists and Movement Professionals

Fourth Edition

Thomas W. Myers

Licensed Massage Therapist (LMT)
Nationally Certified in Therapeutic
Massage and Bodywork (NCTMB)
Certified Rolfer® (ARP)
Practitioner and Lecturer
Director, Anatomy Trains LLC
Maine, USA

Color illustrations by

Graeme Chambers
Debbie Maizels
Philip Wilson

For additional online content visit ExpertConsult.com

ELSEVIER

First edition 2001
Second edition 2009
Third edition 2014

ISBN: 9780702078132

Content Strategist: Lauren Willis
Content Development Specialist: Kim Benson
Project Managers: Anne Collett, Julie Taylor
Design: Brian Salisbury
Illustration Manager: Muthukumaran Thangaraj
Marketing Manager: Ed Major

Printed in China by 1010 Printing International Ltd

Last digit is the print number: 9 8 7 6

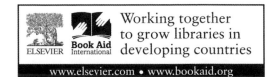

Contents

Preface

Since initial publication in 2001, the reach and application of the ideas in this book have far outstripped this author's expectations. We and our faculty have been invited to present these ideas and their application on every continent save Antarctica to a wide variety of professionals, including orthopedists, physiatrists, orofacial surgeons, physiotherapists, podiatrists, chiropractors, osteopaths, psychologists, athletic and personal trainers, performance coaches, midwives, yoga teachers, martial artists, massage therapists, dancers, musicians, and somatic educators of all stripes. The book is now available in 15 languages. A simple Google search of *Anatomy Trains* now yields over 13 million hits, as therapists and educators find useful applications beyond our original conception.

This fourth edition includes many small updates and corrections that arose out of our continuing teaching and practice, as well as preliminary evidence from fascial dissections and the few available studies in myofascial force transmission beyond muscles' origin and insertion. We have been able to include some recent discoveries made in the fascial and myofascial world since the third edition, as well as to fill in areas where our initial ignorance of the wider world has been rectified.

For ease of assimilation, the current understanding of fascia has been summarized in this edition as a substantial appendix at the end of the chapters. Those seeking a detailed picture of the workings of the fascial system can wander happily through this organized re-working of what was Chapter 1 in previous editions. This appendix is heavily referenced for those who wish to delve more deeply beyond what we had space to include.

Additionally, we are very pleased to include in this edition an exploration of the myofascial continuities in the quadruped form – specifically horses and dogs – as developed by Danish veterinarians.

The appendix that outlines our flagship protocol – the Anatomy Trains 12-series of Structural Integration – has been expanded to reflect our increasing experience with teaching this progression cross-culturally.

This edition benefits from updated and corrected artwork by Graeme Chambers, Debbie Maizels and Philip Wilson. We are also pleased to include some preliminary photographs from the nascent Fascial Net Plastination Project, which is using the techniques pioneered by Gunther von Hagens in *BodyWorlds* to produce images that convey the beauty, intricacy, and ubiquity of the fascial system. We look forward to further revealing images and models from this approach.

The book is designed to allow rapid comprehension of the relevant concepts for a casual reader, or a detailed analysis for the curious. Thumb through to get the overall concept. Follow the illustrations and read their captions to be led through the story at an easily graspable level. Delve into the text – which is coded with icons for the varying interests of readers – for the more complete story.

Like most textbooks these days, this edition makes increasing use of electronic media. The text is studded with website addresses for further study, and our own website, www.anatomytrains.com, is being constantly updated. There are also references to the dozens of video programs we have produced to support professional application of the Anatomy Trains concepts.

The eBook on the accompanying website (and app) – www.expertconsult.com – provides access to many hours of goodies not otherwise available in a book format, including video clips from our technique, dissection, and visual assessment video programs, computer graphic representations of the Anatomy Trains, webinars, extra client photos for visual assessment practice, and other incidental videos of interest.

Both the understanding of the role of fascia and the implications and applications of Anatomy Trains are developing rapidly. This new fourth edition, with its expanded connections to the web, ensures an up-to-date point of view on fascia, a largely missing element in movement study.

Thomas W. Myers
Clarks Cove, Maine, February 2020

Preface to the First Edition

I stand in absolute awe of the miracle of life. My wonder and curiosity have only increased during the more than three decades of immersion in the study of human movement. Whether our ever-evolving body was fashioned by an all-knowing if mischievous Creator, or by a purely selfish gene struggling blindly up Mount Improbable,[1-3] the ingenious variety and flexibility shown in somatic design and development leaves the observer shaking his head with a rueful grin of astonishment.

One looks in vain inside the fertilized ovum for the trillion-cell fetus that it will become. Even the most cursory examination of the complexities of embryology leaves us amazed that it works as often as it does to produce a healthy infant. Hold a helpless, squalling baby, and it seems almost unbelievable that so many escape all the possible debilitating pitfalls on the road to a healthy and productive adulthood.

Despite its biological success, the human experiment as a whole is showing some signs of strain. When I read the news, I confess to having feelings of ambivalence as to whether humankind can or even should continue on this planet, given our cumulative effect on its surface flora and fauna and our treatment of each other. When I hold that baby, however, my commitment to human potential is once again confirmed (Video 4.12).

This book (and the seminars and training courses from which it developed) is devoted to the slim chance that we as a species can move beyond our current dedication to collective greed – and the technocracy and alienation that proceed from it – into a more cooperative and humane relationship with ourselves, each other and our environs. One hopes the development of a 'holistic' view of anatomy such as the one outlined herein will be useful to manual and movement therapists in relieving pain and resolving difficulties in the clients who seek their help. The deeper premise underlying the book, however, is that a more thorough and sensitive contact with our 'felt sense' – that is, our kinesthetic, spatial sense of orientation and movement – is a vitally important front on which to fight the battle for a more human use of human beings, and a better integration with the world around us. The progressive deadening of this 'felt sense' in our children, whether through simple ignorance or by deliberate schooling, lends itself to a collective dissociation, which leads in turn to environmental and social decline. We have long been familiar with mental intelligence (IQ)

and more recently have recognized emotional intelligence (EQ). Only by re-contacting the full reach and educational potential of our kinesthetic intelligence (KQ) will we have any hope of finding a balanced relationship with the larger systems of the world around us, to fulfill what Thomas Berry called 'the Dream of the Earth'.[4,5]

The traditional mechanistic view of anatomy, as useful as it has been, has objectified rather than humanized our relationship to our insides. It is hoped that the relational view ventured in this book will go some little way toward connecting Descartes' view of the body as a 'soft machine' with the living experience of being in a body which grows, learns, matures and ultimately dies. Although the Anatomy Trains ideas form only one small detail of a larger picture of human development through movement, an appreciation of the fascial web and balance in the myofascial meridians can definitely contribute to our inner sense of ourselves as integrated beings. This, coupled with other concepts to be presented in future works, leads toward a physical education more appropriate to the needs of the 21st century.[6-9]

As such, Anatomy Trains is a work of art in a scientific metaphor. This book leaps ahead of the science to propose a point of view, one that is still being literally fleshed out and refined. I have frequently been taken to task by my students and my colleagues for stating my hypotheses baldly, with few of the qualifying adjectives which, though necessary to scientific accuracy, dampen the visceral force of an argument. As Evelyn Waugh wrote: 'Humility is not a virtue propitious to the artist. It is often pride, emulation, avarice, malice – all the odious qualities – which drive a man to complete, elaborate, refine, destroy, and renew his work until he has made something that gratifies his pride and envy and greed. And in so doing he enriches the world more than the generous and the good. That is the paradox of artistic achievement.'[10]

Being neither a scholar nor a researcher, I can only hope that this work of 'artifice' is useful in providing some new ideas for the good people who are.

Finally, I hope that I have honored Vesalius and all the other explorers before me by getting the anatomy about right.

Thomas W. Myers
Maine, 2001

References

1. Dawkins R. *The Selfish Gene*. Oxford: Oxford University Press; 1990.
2. Dawkins R. *The Blind Watchmaker*. New York: WB Norton; 1996.
3. Dawkins R. *Climbing Mount Improbable*. New York: WB Norton; 1997.
4. Csikszentimihalyi M. *Flow*. New York: Harper & Row; 1990.
5. Berry T. *The Dream of the Earth*. San Francisco: Sierra Club; 1990.
6. Myers T. Kinesthetic dystonia. *J Bodyw Mov Ther*. 1998;2(2): 101–114.
7. Myers T. Kinesthetic dystonia. *J Bodyw Mov Ther*. 1998;2(4): 231–247.
8. Myers T. Kinesthetic dystonia. *J Bodyw Mov Ther*. 1999;3(1):36–43.
9. Myers T. Kinesthetic dystonia. *J Bodyw Mov Ther*. 1999;3(2): 107–116.
10. Waugh E. *Private letter, quoted in the New Yorker*; 1999.

Acknowledgments

I would like to express my profound gratitude to a number of people who have guided my way and helped lead to the 'myofascial meridians' concept. To Buckminster Fuller, whose systems approach to design and wide appreciation for the way the world works have informed my work from the very beginning, who urged me not to reform people but to reform the environment around them.[1] To Dr Ida Rolf and Dr Moshe Feldenkrais, both of whom pointed the way to practical and literal ways of reforming the most immediate environment people have, their body and their perception of it;[2,3] I owe these pioneers a deep debt of gratitude for the gift of worthwhile work.

To Dr James Oschman and Raymond Dart, for giving me the original inspiration on fascially connected kinetic chains.[4] To the late Dr Louis Schultz, the original Chair of the Rolf Institute's Anatomy Faculty, whose ideas are much in evidence in this book.[5] Dr Schultz gave me the broadest of conceptual fields in which to play as he started me on my path of learning fascial anatomy. To my colleagues on the Rolf Institute's Life Sciences faculty, and particularly Robert Schleip, who continues to offer warm but firm critical feedback to these ideas and thus improve them.[6] To Deane Juhan, whose comprehensive view of human function, so elegantly put forth in *Job's Body*, has been an inspiration to me as to so many.[7] To Michael Frenchman, my old friend, who demonstrated early faith in our ideas by putting in many hours realizing them in video form. To the innovative Gil Hedley of Somanautics and Todd Garcia of the Laboratories of Anatomical Enlightenment, whose skills in dissection are on view in this book, through the medium of Averill Lehan's camera and Eric Root's microscope. I honor their dedication to exposing the actual experience of the human form for testing new ideas such as those in this book. We honor the many donors whose generosity makes these advances in knowledge possible.

Many other movement teachers, at slightly greater distance, also deserve credit for inspiring this work: the yoga of Iyengar as I learned it from his able students such as Arthur Kilmurray, Patricia Walden, and Francois Raoult; the highly original work in human movement of Judith Aston through Aston Patterning, the contributions of Emilie Conrad and Susan Harper with their Continuum work, and Bonnie Bainbridge-Cohen and her Body-Mind Centering school.[8–11] I owe a debt to Caryn McHose for bringing some of this work close enough to grasp, and also to Frank Hatch and the late Lenny Maietta for their developmental movement synthesis expressed in their unique Touch-in-Parenting program.[12,13]

From all these people and many more I have learned a great deal, although the more I learn, the farther the horizon of my ignorance extends. They say that stealing ideas from one person is plagiarism, stealing from ten is scholarship, and stealing from one hundred is original research. Thus, there is nothing completely original in this bit of grand larceny. Nevertheless, while these people are responsible for instilling exciting ideas, no one but myself is responsible for any errors, which I look forward to correcting in future iterations of this work.

To my many eager students, whose questions have goaded more learning than I would ever have undertaken on my own. To the late Annie Wyman, for early support and maritime contributions to my sanity. To my teachers in the Anatomy Trains school, especially the early support of Lou Benson and Michael Morrison, whose tenacity in dealing with both my eccentricities and my poetic treatment of fact (as well as my electronic challenges) contributed signally to the original edition. To the current members of my faculty: thank you to one and all for your work in traveling the world to inform a wide variety of practitioners of the practical benefits of working in terms of connected anatomy. The effective work of my staff – especially Mel Burns, Stephanie Stoy, Erin Sproul, and the indomitable Becky Eugley – allows our influence to be much more pervasive than it otherwise would be.

In this edition we celebrate the late and magnificent Dr Leon Chaitow, who bullied, cajoled, and otherwise effectively encouraged (as he did with so many) my initial exposition of these ideas in the *Journal of Bodywork & Movement Therapies* in 1996. The editorial staff at Churchill Livingstone, including my first editor, Mary Law and all who followed, bringing their patience to bear on my long-winded prose and desire to include everything. To Debbie Maizels, Philip Wilson, and Graeme Chambers, who so meticulously and artistically brought the concept to life via the illustrations. To my proofreaders Felicity Myers and Edward Myers, whose timely and tireless work has improved the sense and sensibility of this book.

To my daughter Mistral and her mother Giselle, who enthusiastically and good-naturedly tolerated my fascination with the world of human movement, which often led me far from home, and took up a great deal of time which might otherwise have been theirs. And finally to Nature herself, whose generous but unassailable rules have allowed the unfolding of the silent but potent currents of love, depth, and a connection to a greater reality that run below the surface of this and all my work.

References

1. Fuller B. *Utopia or oblivion*. New York: Bantam Books; 1969. www.bfi.com. Further information and publications can be obtained from the Buckminster Fuller Institute.
2. Rolf I. *Rolfing*. Rochester VT: Healing Arts Press; 1977.
3. Feldenkrais M. *The Case of Nora*. New York: Harper and Row; 1977.
4. Oschman J. *Energy Medicine*. Edinburgh: Churchill Livingstone; 2000.
5. Schultz L, Feitis R. *The Endless Web*. Berkeley: North Atlantic Books; 1996.
6. Schleip R. *Talking to Fascia, Changing the Brain*. Boulder, CO: Rolf Institute; 1992.
7. Juhan D. *Job's Body*. Tarrytown, NY: Station Hill Press; 1987.
8. Iyengar BKS. *Light on Yoga*. New York: Schocken Books; 1995.
9. Silva M, Mehta S. *Yoga the Iyengar Way*. New York: Alfred Knopf; 1990.
10. Cohen B. *Basic Neurocellular Patterns*. El Sobrnte VA: Burchfield Rose Pub.; 2018.
11. Aston J. *Aston Postural Assessment*. Edinburgh: Handspring; 2019.
12. McHose C, Frank K. *How Life Moves*. Berkeley: North Atlantic Books; 2006.
13. Hatch F, Maietta L. Role of kinesthesia in pre- and perinatal bonding. *Pre- Peri-Nat Psychol*. 1991;5(3).

How to Use This Book

*A*natomy Trains is designed to allow the reader to gather the general idea quickly or to allow a more detailed reading in any given area. The book includes frequent forays into several related areas, designated in the margins next to the headings by icons:

❖ Manual techniques or notes for the manual therapist

❖ Movement techniques or notes for the movement teacher

✿ Visual assessment tools

✿ Ideas and concepts related to kinesthetic education

▶ Video material integrated in the accompanying eBook at www.expertconsult.com (numbers indicate specific videos)

🌐 Video material available at www.anatomytrains.com

✿ Return to main text

The chapters are color-coded. The first two chapters explain the 'Anatomy Trains' approach to the body's anatomical structures. Chapters 3–9 elaborate on each of the 12 mapped 'lines' of the body commonly observed in postural and movement patterns. Each of the 'lines' chapters opens with summary illustrations, descriptions, diagrams and tables for the reader who wants to grasp the scope of the concept quickly. The final two chapters apply the 'Anatomy Trains' concept to some common types of movement and provide a method of analyzing posture.

Five appendices appear at the end. The new Appendix 1 examines fascia and the myofascial meridians concept, and the new Appendix 5 adds information about Anatomy Trains in quadrupeds. The others include a discussion of the latitudinal meridians of Dr Louis Schultz, an explanation of how the Anatomy Trains schema can be applied to Ida Rolf's Structural Integration protocol, and a correlation between the meridians of acupuncture and these myofascial meridians.

Because individual muscles and other structures can make an appearance in different lines, use the index to find all mentions of any particular structure. A glossary of 'Anatomy Trains' terms is also included. The full Bibliography is available in the eBook.

The accompanying eBook at www.expertconsult.com includes a large number of videos, podcasts, and animations useful to the interested reader, teacher, or presenter. While many of the videos are referred to in the book, readers will be pleased to find additional items present in the eBook, with overall video footage running into several hours.

Bonus content:
- Video B1: Introduction to fascia and biotensegrity
- Video B2: Anatomy Trains Lines overview
- Video B3: Feeling the Anatomy Trains Lines (palpation guide)
- Video B4: How fascia moves (fascial properties webinar)
- Video B5: Interview clips with Tom Myers discussing fascia

Videos

Introductory Concepts

Fascial Release Techniques

Evidence from Dissections and *in Vivo* Observation

Computer Graphics

Webinars

Acknowledgments

Elsevier would like to offer sincere thanks to the people below for graciously allowing them to use the following material in the eBook at www.expertconsult.com:

Dr Jean-Claude Guimberteau MD, Plastic and Hand Surgeon, and Endovivo Productions for providing videos 6-12 (Living fascia 1: surrounding tendon) and 6-13 (Living fascia 2: milieu of the body). The original sources are:

Guimberteau JC (ed). New ideas in hand flexor tendon surgery. Aquitaine Domaine Forestier; 2001 (www.livres-medicaux.com)

Guimberteau JC. Promenades sous la peau. Strolling under the skin. Elsevier Masson; 2004. Language: French.

Eric Root for providing videos 4-1 (Fascial microscopy 1: latissimus), 4-2 (Fascial microscopy 2: subscapularis), 6-19 (Fascial microscopy 3: plantar) and 6-20 (Fascial microscopy 4: erector).

Michael Frenchman and Videograf for providing the computer graphic imagery.

The Laboratories of Anatomical Enlightenment, Inc. & Singing Cowboy Productions for providing video 4-4 (Spiral Line). Excerpt from Anatomy Trains Revealed: Early dissective evidence.

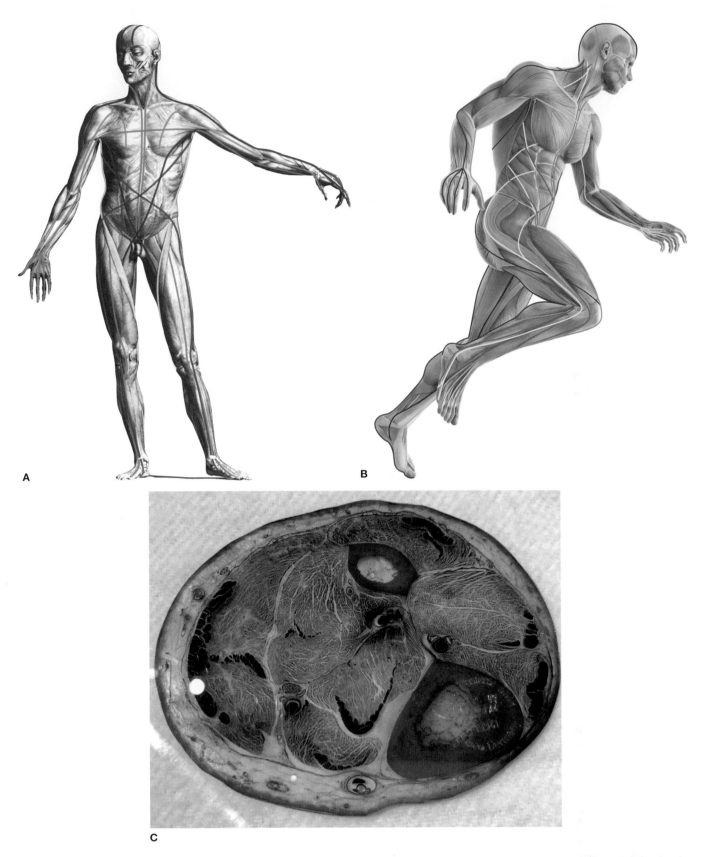

• **Fig. 1.1** (**A**) A general Anatomy Trains 'route map' laid out on the surface of a familiar figure from Albinus. This was our initial way of showing the trains. (**B**) More recent computerized versions allow for more diversity in portraying the lines in action. (**C**) This amazingly detailed plastination of a cross-section of the lower leg holds many treasures and rewards continued study. Start with the blue tibia and fibula and see the thin, strong interosseous membrane pulled between them. On either side of the membrane, vessels cluster between the muscles in their adventitial tunics. Look at the filigreed extent of the fascial fabric into the muscle, looking for all the world like the veins of a leaf – and indeed these are the paths of nutrition and draining for the hungry mitochondria in the muscle. The intermuscular septa between the muscle groups lead from the edges of the bones out to the surrounding fascia profundis, which surrounds the whole leg and holds the otherwise floppy muscles tightly together. The fascia of the profundis is continuous with the fascia that runs through the fat layer, hooding the visible vessels and the invisible nerves, right out to the skin and its thin, tough, elastic backing adherent to the fat. Imagine taking away all the red to see the fascial net alone, a three-dimensional wet spider web holding everything in place, yet allowing it to move, bend, and adapt.

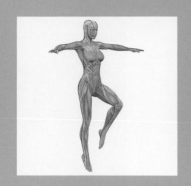

1

Laying the Railbed

The Philosophy

The heart of healing lies in our ability to listen, to see, to perceive, more than in our application of technique. That, at least, is the premise of this book (Video B1).

All therapeutic or training interventions of whatever sort are a conversation between two intelligent systems. It is not our job here to promote one technique over another, nor even to posit a mechanism for how any technique works. It matters not a whit to our argument whether the mechanism of myofascial change is due to simple muscle relaxation, release of a trigger point, a change in the sol/gel chemistry of ground substance, viscoelasticity among collagen fibers, resolution of central nervous system patterning, resetting of the muscle spindles or Golgi tendon organs, increase in stretch tolerance, a shift in energy, or a change in attitude (Fig. 1.1A). Use the Anatomy Trains map to comprehend the larger pattern of your client's structural relationships, then apply whatever techniques you have at your disposal toward shaping change (Fig. 1.1B–C). Pattern recognition is the key skill, not the technique employed.

Pattern recognition in posture and movement is a central skill to what we could call 'spatial medicine', the study of how we develop, how we stand, handle loads, move through our environment and occupy space – as well as how we perceive our bodily selves. A lot of what we think we 'know' about human movement is up for revision in the coming decades. All manual therapy and movement education approaches are part of building this larger coherent conceptual framework of spatial medicine whether we realize it or not. Spatial medicine (or whatever it comes to be called) will formulate the new principles to make movement training coupled with hands-on work into a very powerful arm of healing and education. (For more on spatial medicine, see Appendix 1, p. 289.)

Manual therapy techniques for pain reduction, performance enhancement, and overall wellness include the traditional fields of physiotherapy, physiatry, and orthopedics, as well as osteopathic and chiropractic manipulations (Video 1.5). More recently, we are offered a wide variety of soft-tissue approaches from Rolfing to Reiki.

Movement training is an essential aspect of spatial medicine, and training methods abound from the most meditative yoga across the perfect Pilates to the most scrappy martial arts. Personal trainers and athletic coaches of all stripes work to make movement 'functional'. Spatial medicine in a wider sense could include all of what is now called physical education, dance, developmental movement, acupuncture, and somatically based psychotherapies. All of these fields have something to contribute to our library of pattern recognition and using movement to build health and combat the evolutionary mismatch of an increasingly sedentary lifestyle.[1,2]

New brand names sprout daily in these fields, many newly christened 'fascial', though in truth there is very little that is actually new under the sun of manipulation or movement. Our observation is that any number of angles of approach can be beneficial, regardless of whether the explanation offered for their efficacy ultimately prevails.

The current requirement is less for new techniques, and more for new premises that lead to new strategies for application. Unfortunately, useful new premises are a lot harder to come by than seemingly new techniques. Significant developments are often opened by the point of view assumed, the lens through which the body is seen.

Anatomy Trains is one such lens – a global way of looking at musculoskeletal patterns that lead to bodywide interconnected protocols (Fig. 1.2). What can we learn from looking at synergetic relationships – stringing our parts together rather than dissecting them further (Fig. 1.3)?

Much of the manipulative therapy of the last 100 years, like most of our thinking in the West for at least half a millennium, has been based on a mechanistic and reductionistic model – the microscopic lens (Fig. 1.4). We keep examining things by breaking them down into smaller and smaller parts, to examine each part's role. Introduced by Aristotle, and epitomized by Isaac Newton and René Descartes, and applied to biomechanics most notably by Borelli, the reductive path has led, in the physical medicine field, to books filled with goniometric angles, levers, and force vectors based on drawing each individual muscle's insertion closer to its origin (Fig. 1.5).[3]

While we have many researchers to thank for brilliant analysis and consequent therapies for specific muscles, individual joints, and particular impingements in the 20th century, the 21st is looking for a more integrated way of

Involvement of the Lines

SFL: Neck to Solar Plexus
Short and down
Rectus Abdominis
Long and down
Rectus Femoris
Short and down
Lower leg
Short and down

SBL: Occiput to C4
Short and down
Erectors C4 – T12
Long and wide
Erectors L1– Sacrum
Short and narrow
Hamstrings
Long and up
Calf and Plantar Fascia
Long and up

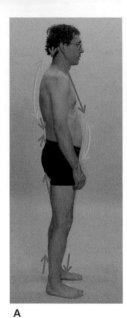

A

Strategies for the Lines

SFL: Neck to Solar Plexus
Lengthen and lift
Rectus Abdominis
Shorten
Rectus Femoris
Lengthen and lift
Lower leg
Lengthen and lift

SBL: Occiput to C4
Lengthen and lift
Erectors C4 – T12
Shorten and narrow
Erectors L1– Sacrum
Lengthen and widen
Hamstrings
Shorten and drop
Calf and Plantar Fascia
Shorten and drop

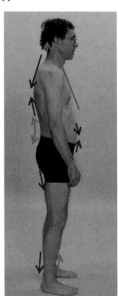

B

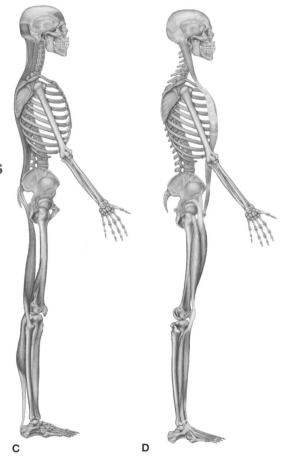

C **D**

• **Fig. 1.2** An analysis of shortness or weakness within any given myofascial meridian coupled with the relationship of that meridian to the others lead to whole-body strategies for improving posture and movement function. (**A**) A side view shows us the relationship between just the Superficial Back Line (pictured in **C**) and the Superficial Front Line (**D**). In **A**, a simple chart of the directionality in the fascial planes, and areas of likely hyper- and hypotonus in sagittal plane control. (**B**) A chart of the strategy to remedy the pattern via myofascial manipulation and movement education.

assessing movement.[4–7] If you kick a ball, about the most interesting way you can analyze the result is in terms of the mechanical laws of force and motion. The coefficients of inertia, gravity, and friction are sufficient to determine its reaction to your kick and the ball's final resting place. But if you should be so cruel as to kick a large dog, such a mechanical analysis of vectors and resultant forces may not prove as salient as the reaction of the dog as a whole. Analyzing individual muscles biomechanically likewise yields an incomplete picture of human movement experience (Fig. 1.6).

In the early 20th century, physics by means of Einstein and Bohr moved into a relativistic universe, a language of relationship rather than linear cause and effect, which Jung in turn applied to psychology, and many others applied to diverse areas. However, it took that entire century for this point of view to spread out and reach physical medicine. This book is one modest step in this direction – general systems thinking applied to postural and movement analysis (Fig. 1.7).

It is not very useful merely to say 'everything is connected to everything else', and leave it at that. Even though

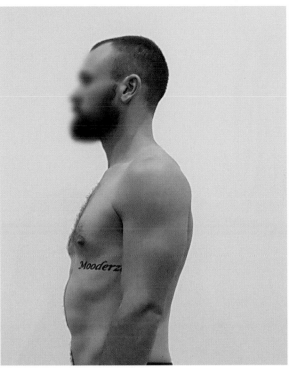
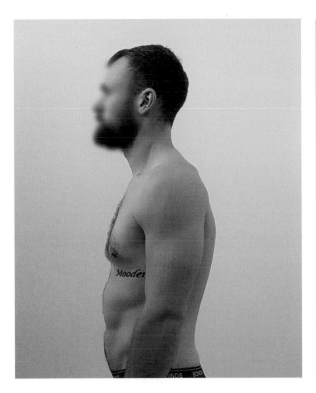

• **Fig. 1.3** Using the kind of strategies charted in Fig. 1.2, it is possible to effect significant changes in posture (and function, but a book limits us to photos). This recent student in our training classes shows significant changes in alignment. (www.anatomytrains.com – video ref: BodyReading, 101; see also Ch. 11.) (Photo courtesy of the author.)

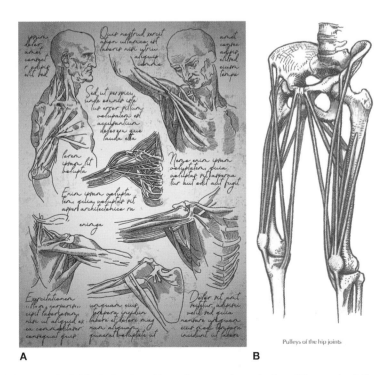

A   **B**

Pulleys of the hip joints

• **Fig. 1.4** (**A**) Leonardo da Vinci, drawing without the pervasive prejudice of the mechanistic muscle–bone viewpoint, drew some remarkably 'Anatomy Train'-like figures in his anatomical notebooks. (**B**) A few modern anatomists, like the delightful John Hull Grundy, have also applied systems thinking to musculo-skeletal anatomy. (A, Leonardo da Vinci/Shutterstock. B, Reproduced with kind permission from Grundy 1982.)

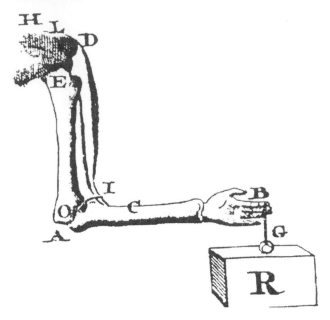

• **Fig. 1.5** The concepts of mechanics, applied to human anatomy, have given us much information about the actions of individual muscles in terms of levers, angles, and forces. But how much more insight will this isolating approach yield? (Historic Images/Alamy Stock Photo.[3])

these physicists assert that this is ultimately true, such a premise leaves the practitioner in a nebulous, even vacuous, world with nothing to guide him but lore or 'intuition'. Einstein's special theory of relativity did not negate Newton's laws of motion; rather it subsumed them in a larger scheme. Likewise, myofascial meridian theory does not eliminate the value of the many individual muscle-based techniques and analyses, but simply sets them in the context of the system as a whole.

Anatomy Trains is not a replacement for existing knowledge about muscles. Splenius capitis can still be seen to rotate the head and extend the neck, *and* it operates, as we shall see, as part of spiral and lateral myofascial chains to dampen any disruption to the teleceptors (eyes and ears and vestibular system) from the motion of the body below (Fig. 1.8).

These fascial lines within the musculoskeletal system only comprise one small pattern within our entire neuro-myofascial web, which is in turn one among the myriad rhythmic and harmonic patterns at play in the entire living body. As such, Anatomy Trains is a small part of a larger re-vision of ourselves, not as Descartes' 'soft machine' but

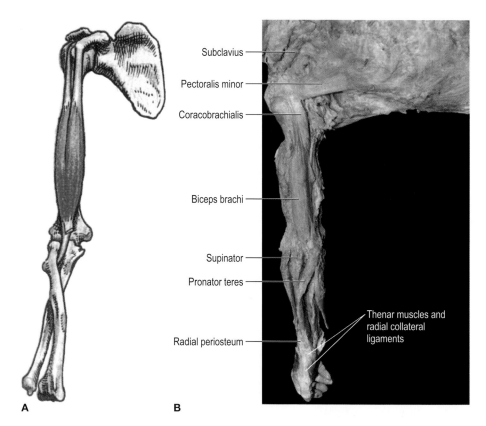

A   **B**

• **Fig. 1.6** **(A)** Individual muscles are universally described as the actuators of movement. Analyzing their action consists of isolating a single muscle on the skeleton, as in this depiction of the biceps, and determining what would happen if the two ends are approximated. This is a highly useful exercise, but hardly definitive, as it leaves out the effect the muscle could have on neighboring muscles and ligaments by tightening their fascia and pushing or pulling them. It also, by cutting the fascia at either end, discounts any effect of its pull on the proximal or distal structures beyond. These latter connections are the subject of this book. **(B)** The biceps can also be seen as part of a myofascial continuity from the axial skeleton to the thumb, termed here the Deep Front Arm Line (see also Fig. 7.1). (A, Reproduced with kind permission from Grundy 1982. B, Photo courtesy of the author.)

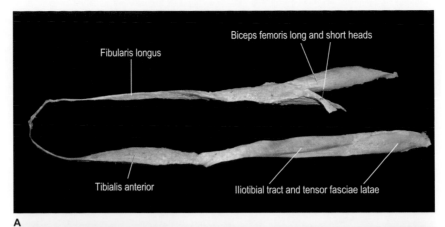

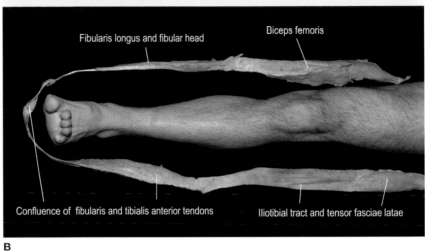

• **Fig. 1.7** New strategies occur when fascia-to-fascia linkages are considered. This dissection of the lower Spiral Line (see Ch. 6) shows how, by changing the angle of the scalpel, we can demonstrate the integrated action not of just one myofascial unit (muscle), but of several running. This specimen starts from the hip on the lower right, loops under the arch at the left, and carries on up to the ischial tuberosity with biceps femoris at the upper right. (www.anatomytrains.com – video ref: Anatomy Trains Revealed) (Photo courtesy of the author.)

as an integrated informational system, what non-linear dynamics mathematicians call autopoietic (self-forming) systems.[8–12] The fascial system is one of those complex fractals, hovering between order and chaos, but constantly remodeling and regulating itself to meet the challenge of forces within and around us.

The attempt to shift our conceptual framework in a relational direction may sound fuzzy at first, compared to the crisp 'if … then …' statements of the mechanists. Ultimately, however, this relativistic viewpoint produces powerful integrative therapeutic strategies – many of which we explore in these pages, while others are taught in our training courses and webinars. These new strategies include biomechanics but also go beyond to say something useful about synergy – emergent systemic properties of the body as a whole unpredicted by the sum of the behaviors of each individual muscle or joint.

The Discovery

Parallel to this modern application of systems theory to our body's design is the related discovery of the role of fascial webbing in body posture and movement (Fig. 1.9). While everyone learns something about bones and muscles, the origin and disposition of the fascinating fascial net that unites them is less widely understood (see Figs A1.10 & 1.10). The blunt statement is that, in 500 years of the Western tradition of anatomy, an entire bodily system has remained almost totally unseen, and certainly underappreciated. Termed by fascial researcher Dr Robert Schleip as 'the Cinderella of body systems', fascia has long been considered mere 'packing material', to be dissected and thrown away in order to see more interesting tissues. New research from a number of different angles confirms that fascia is a very interesting and communicative whole-body

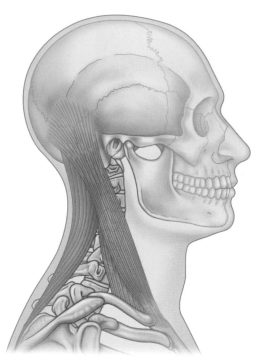

A

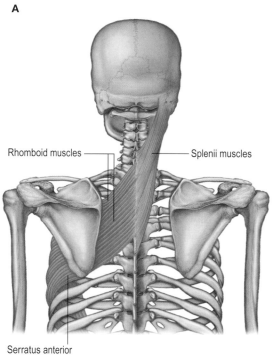

Rhomboid muscles — — Splenii muscles

Serratus anterior

B

• **Fig. 1.8** The splenius capitis muscle, when considered on its own, rotates and extends the head. In function it works as part of both the Lateral Line and the Spiral Line to keep the head and eyes steady while the body runs, hunts, or tends to children below.

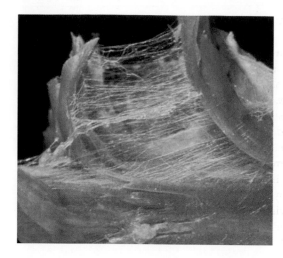

• **Fig. 1.9** This magnification of the myofascia – the 'cotton candy' (UK: candy floss) – is perimysial tissue enwrapping each fascicle (neuromotor unit). This fascia is thoroughly enmeshed with the fleshy (and teased up) muscle fibers. (Reproduced with kind permission from Ronald Thompson)

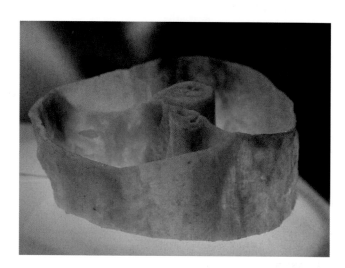

• **Fig. 1.10** A recent plastinated specimen from a part of the upper thigh showing the surrounding fascia lata and the two major fascial septa. The lateral wall to the left separates the quadriceps from the hamstrings, running from the surface to the periosteum at the linea aspera. The medial septum separates the quads from the adductors, likewise reaches to the linea aspera, and additionally provides protection for the neurovascular bundle, retained in this preparation. (© FasciaResearchSociety.org/Plastination)

system (see Appendix 1). Fascia is not inert, it performs as important a regulatory job as the nervous and circulatory systems, with profound implications for sport, rehabilitation, physical education, and – important to those of us with silver hair – aging gracefully.

The vast majority of the public – and even most therapists and trainers – still base their thinking on the limited idea that there are individual muscles that attach to bones that move us around via mechanical leverage. The very term 'musculoskeletal system' leaves out the complex of tissues through which muscles and bones are woven together – the fascial web.

When this book was first written, the accepted model was – and largely remains – that we move the skeletal frame via muscles that pull on tendons over joints whose movements are limited by bone shape and restricting ligaments. This leverage model falls apart as too simplistic when asked to explain the movements of embryological development or extreme athleticism, yet is far too complex to have easy explanatory power for common problems such as soft-tissue pain, gait anomalies, or faulty recruitment patterns.

Integrating the new findings about fascia into our strategic thinking about therapy and training is not quite as easy as simply adding a fascial overlay to what we already know. It requires a shift in our point of view.[13] Although increased research in the last twenty years has certainly broadened our knowledge, and while books, symposia, conferences and courses with 'Fascia' in the title abound,[14–17] the implications of fascia's 'discovery' are still unfolding, and even in its fourth edition this book is still an interim report. In any case, fascia has been investigated right along by a few outlying researchers, but without its full import being understood.[18–23]

The realization is dawning that all these trees might just amount to a forest, that all these individual sinews are functioning as part of a responsive whole, an extended mycelium-like 'root system' in the human body. This discovery has profound implications for our idea of the body – and for physical education, rehabilitation, and athletic training of all types.

Coupled with the work on cellular mechanotransduction at the microscopic end,[24] we are on the verge of an entirely new integrated understanding of how our biomechanical system seamlessly spans from within each cell to the bio-psychosocial organism.

Included in this edition is a compendium on contemporary understanding of fascial function as the first appendix of this book, where 'afascianados' (we are tired of being called 'fascists') can overview a more detailed understanding of fascial matrix's disposition, properties, abilities, and limitations. This appendix includes more recent research on remodeling after injury, the elastic response to new training challenges, new information on interoceptive sensing in fascia, as well as building the recently revealed story of the interstitial perfusion amongst the gels and cells of all other body systems.

Please note that this book presents a point of view, a particular set of arguments that build toward the Anatomy Trains concept. It is by no means the complete story on the roles or significance of fascia. Here, we go long on geometry, mechanics, and spatial arrangement, and drastically short on the relevant chemistry. We concern ourselves with the healthy supporting role of fascia in posture and movement, totally avoiding any discussion of pathology. Other diverse and excellent descriptions are referenced along the way for the interested reader.[25,26]

In simple terms, the fascia is the fabric of the body that holds our trillions of wet, greasy cells together. It is basically what used to be called 'sinews', and it forms a unitary, tough, and fibrous net that can be found everywhere in the body (Fig. 1.11; see Fig. A1.9B). If we were to render all tissues invisible in the human body except the fibrillar elements of the connective tissue – collagen, elastin and reticulin – we would see the entire body, inside and out, in a fashion similar to the more familiar neural and circulatory nets. (For a discussion of the holistic communicating

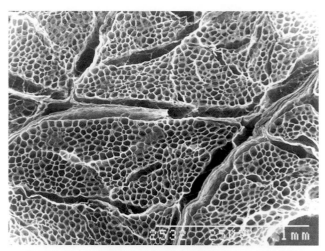

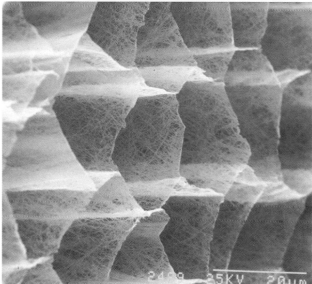

• **Fig. 1.11** These electron microscope images show that our fascial system nomenclature is an attempt to impose categories on a net that is continuous, seamless, and constantly self-repairing to meet the forces placed upon it. (Reprinted from Journal of Bodywork and Movement Therapies, Vol 14, Purslow PP, Muscle fascia and force transmission, pp. 411–417, Copyright 2010, with permission from Elsevier.)

networks, see Appendix 1, pp. 244–322.) Areas would differ in density – the bones, cartilage, tendons, and ligaments would be thick with leathery fiber, so that the area around each joint would be especially well represented. Each muscle would be sheathed with it, and infused with a cotton-candy net surrounding each muscle cell and bundle of cells (see Figs. A1.19 and A1.20). The face would be less dense, as would the more spongy organs like the thyroid or pancreas, though even these are encased by denser bags. Although it arranges itself in multiple folded planes, we emphasize once again that no part of this net is distinct or separated from the net as a whole, any more than there are isolated groups of nerves, or an island of capillaries separate unto itself. Each of these bags, strings, sheets, and leathery networks is meshed with each other into one net, birth to death and top to toe (Fig. 1.12).

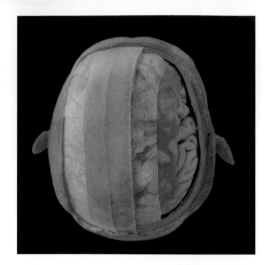

• **Fig. 1.12** The fascial system is widely depicted as being layered, as in this dissection of the layers in the head. From skin to a thin fatty layer to the galea aponeurotica to a loose layer that allows you to move the scalp on the bone, or actually on the pericranium, a tough fascial coating around each bone, before going into the other layers that surround and protect the brain. Although fascial layering is an obvious fact in the body, we should note that histologically there is always transition between layers, and only in the open spaces of synovial joints and lumens of fluid tubes are collagen fibers absent. In other words, all of these distinct layers are wedded to each other with force-transmitting collagen fibers. (Photo courtesy of Science Photo Library.)

The bald statement is that the fascial web so permeates the body as to be part of the immediate environment of every cell. Without its support, the brain would be runny custard, the liver would spread through the abdominal cavity, and we would end up as a puddle at our own feet. Only in the open lumens of the respiratory and digestive tracts is the binding, strengthening, connecting, and separating web of fascia absent.

In summary, including fascia and the new findings on how it works in movement requires that we see the body differently. The book you are holding is the author's attempt to make this shift of gears – between the 'isolated muscle' concept and the fascia system view – without too much grinding.

The Hypothesis

Whatever else they may be doing individually from origin to insertion, muscles also exert influence along functionally integrated body-wide continuities within the fascial webbing. These sheets and lines follow the grain of the body's connective tissue fabric, forming traceable 'meridians' of myofascia (Fig. 1.13). Muscles contract within these lines like fish in a net, transmitting myofascial force to create resilient stability or – less efficiently – to foster chronic tension and fixation. Most pertinent to this text, the resulting postural compensation patterns can be 'read' via these lines. (No claim is made, by the way, for the exclusivity of these lines. The functional myofascial lines noted by previous authors described later in this chapter, as well as

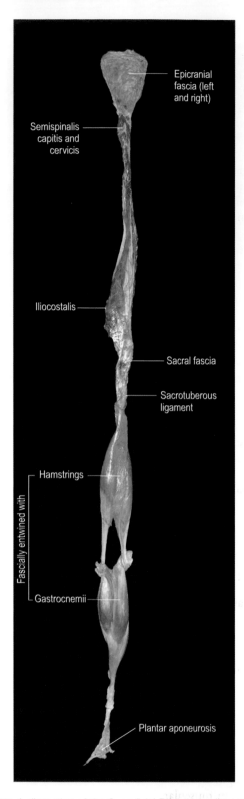

• **Fig. 1.13** A dissection of the Superficial Back Line, dissected intact from untreated tissue by Todd Garcia of the Laboratories of Anatomical Enlightenment (www.LofAE.com). (Photo courtesy of the author. Please note, this specimen is explained on video on the accompanying website.)

muscle attachments to the ligamentous bed described as the 'inner bag' in Appendix 1,[27] and the latitudinal shouldering of strain by neighboring muscles, as detailed in the work of Huijing et al.[28] in Appendix 1, are all valid alternative avenues for the efficient distribution of myofascial forces.)

Essentially, the Anatomy Trains map provides a 'longitudinal anatomy' – a sketch of the long tensile straps and slings within the musculature as a whole, offering a supplement to (and at times an alternative to) the standard analysis of muscular action.

Standard anatomical analysis could be termed the 'isolated muscle theory'. Almost every text presents muscle function by isolating an individual muscle on the skeleton, divided from its connections above and below, shorn of its neurological and vascular feeds, and divorced from regionally adjacent structures.[29–37] 'What would happen to the skeleton if this were the only muscle on the body?' – a muscle's function is defined solely by what happens in approximating the proximal and distal attachment points or to resist their being stretched apart (see Fig. 1.6). The overwhelmingly accepted view is that muscles attach solely from bone to bone, whereas in fact: (1) no muscle attaches to a bone anywhere in the body – muscle is hamburger without its attaching fascia – and (2) most muscles have a number of clinically relevant soft-tissue attachments beyond their origin and insertion (see Figs. 1.6 & 1.13).

Occasionally the role of myofascia relative to its neighbors is detailed, as in the role that the vastus lateralis takes as a 'hydraulic amplifier' in pushing out against and thus pre-tensing the iliotibial tract. In fact, such hydraulic amplification is occurring constantly all over the body (see the discussion of Tensegrity in Appendix 1). Almost never are the longitudinal connections between muscles and fasciae listed or their function discussed (as in, for instance, the consistent link between the iliotibial tract and the tibialis anterior muscle – see Fig. 1.7).

The absolute dominance of our current manner of defining muscles is largely an artifact of our method of dissection. With a knife in hand, the individual muscles are easy to separate from surrounding fascial planes. This does not mean, however, that this is how the body is biologically assembled or how it organizes movement. One may question whether a 'muscle' is even a useful division to the body's own kinesiology. No one has found a representation of the 'deltoid' in the brain. The brain 'thinks' in terms of individual neuromotor units, and thus divides the deltoid into at least seven different actuating units.[38]

Having the isolated muscle presentation as the first and last word in muscular anatomy (along with the reductionistic and ultimately naive conviction that the complex equation of human movement and stability can be derived by doing our sums on the action of all these individual muscles) leaves the current generation of therapists unlikely to conceive of movement in any other way.

The elimination of the muscle as a physiological unit may be too radical a notion for most of us to accept at this time, but we can at least assert that contemporary therapists need to think 'outside the box' of this isolated muscle concept (see Fig. A1.6). Research supporting this kind of systemic thinking is cited along the way as we attempt a move beyond a muscle's singular 'action' to reveal systemic function. Here we assemble linked myofascial structures into this image of the 'myofascial meridians'. We should be clear that 'Anatomy Trains' is not an established science – this book leaps ahead of the research – but at the same time, we have been pleased with how well the concepts play out in clinical practice and movement education.[39,40]

Once the pattern of these myofascial meridians is recognized and the connections grasped, they can be easily applied in assessment and treatment across a variety of therapeutic and educational approaches to movement facilitation (Fig. 1.14). The concepts can be presented at any of several depths. Thumb through the book to get the general idea, using the illustrations along with their captions to recapitulate the story. The text itself attempts to strike a balance that meets the needs of the informed therapist, while still staying within the reach of the interested athlete, client, or student (Video 6.25).

Aesthetically, a grasp of the Anatomy Trains scheme will lead to a more three-dimensional feel for musculoskeletal anatomy and an appreciation of whole-body patterns distributing compensation in both daily and performance functioning. The 'feel' of the Anatomy Trains is most easily accepted among dancers, fighters, and athletes because they live in their movement.

Clinically, facility with the myofascial meridians leads to a directly applicable understanding of how painful problems in one area of the body can be linked to a totally 'silent' area far removed from the presenting symptom. Unexpected new strategies for treatment, especially for chronic pain, arise from applying this 'connected anatomy' point of view to the practical daily challenges of manual and movement therapy.

Though some promising evidence from dissection is presented in this edition, it is too early in the research process to claim an objective reality for these lines. More examination of the mechanisms of communication across the myofascial net along these fascial meridians would be especially welcome, including immediate effects in terms of joint stability in athletics, and also to measure the result of sustained structural pulls on posture. So we present the Anatomy Trains merely as a potentially useful alternative map, a systems view of some longitudinal connections in the parietal myofascia.

Anatomy Trains and Myofascial Meridians: What's in a Name?

'Anatomy Trains' is a descriptive term for the whole schema. It is also a way of having a bit of fun with a fairly dense subject by providing a useful metaphor for the collection of continuities described in this book. The metaphor of tracks, stations, expresses and locals and so on is used throughout

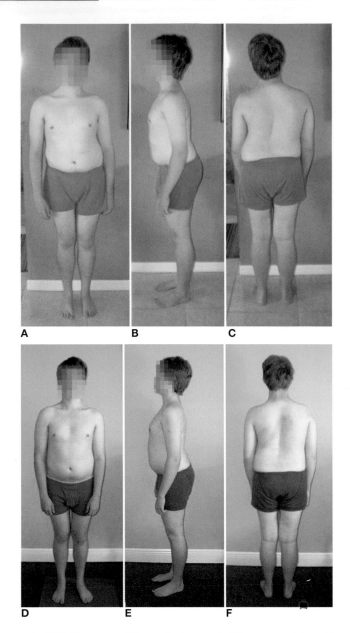

A B C

D E F

• **Fig. 1.14** Shortness within or displacement of the myofascial meridians can be observed in standing posture or in motion. These assessments lead to globally based treatment strategies. Can you look at (**A**)–(**C**) and see the shortnesses in the left Lateral Line and fascial plane shifts especially in the spine and neck after Structural Integration treatment in (**D**)–(**F**)? (www.anatomytrains.com – video ref: BodyReading, 101; for an explanation of the lines, see Ch. 11.) (Photos courtesy of the author.)

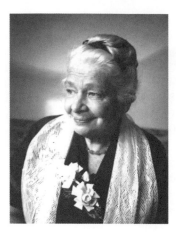

• **Fig. 1.15** Dr Ida P. Rolf (1896–1979), originator of the Structural Integration form of myofascial manipulation. (© Tom Myers, courtesy of Marvin Solit.)

the text. A single Anatomy Train is an equivalent term for a myofascial meridian.

The word 'myofascia' connotes the bundled together, inseparable nature of muscle tissue (myo-) and its accompanying web of connective tissue (fascia), which comes up for a fuller discussion in Appendix 1 (Video 6.20).

Manual therapy of the myofasciae has spread quite widely among massage therapists, osteopaths, and physiotherapists from several modern roots. These include the work of osteopaths, physiotherapists, and my own primary teacher, Dr Ida Rolf (Fig. 1.15),[41] and others, many of

whom make various claims to originality.[42] All of these, in fact, are part of an unbroken chain of hands-on healers running back to Asklepios (*Lat:* Aesculapius) and his first 'hospitals' in early Greece and back from there into the mists of pre-history.[43,44]

While the term 'myofascial' has steadily gained currency over the last couple of decades, replacing 'muscle' in some texts, minds, and brand names, it is still widely misunderstood. In many applications of myofascial therapies, the techniques taught are actually focused on individual muscles (or myofascial units, if we are to be precise), and fail to address specifically the communicating aspect of the myofasciae across extended lines and broad planes within the body.[45,46] The Anatomy Trains approach adds a dimension of connectivity to our visual, palpatory, and movement considerations in assessment and treatment that fills a current need for a global view of human structure and movement (Fig. 1.16).

In any case, the word 'myofascial' is a terminological innovation only, since it has always been impossible, under whatever name, to contact muscle tissue at any time or place without also contacting and affecting the accompanying connective or fascial tissues. Even that inclusion is incomplete, since almost all of our interventions will also necessarily contact and affect the function and perfusion in neural, vascular, and epithelial cells and tissues as well. Nevertheless, the approach detailed in this book largely ignores these other tissue effects to concentrate on one aspect of the patterns of arrangement – the design, if you will – of the 'fibrous body' in the upright adult human. This fibrous body consists of the entire collagenous net, which includes all the tissues investing and attaching the organs as well as the collagen in bones, cartilage, tendons, ligaments, skin, and the myofasciae.

'Myofasciae' specifically narrows our view to the muscle fibers embedded in their associated fasciae (as in Figs. 1. 9 & 1.11, A1.19). In order to simplify nomenclature and to emphasize a central tenet of this book – the unitary nature

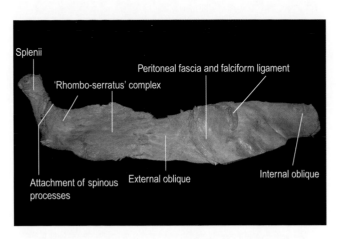

• **Fig. 1.16** The splenii in the neck (left) are connected across the spinous processes to the contralateral rhomboids, which are in turn strongly connected to the serratus, and on around through the abdominal fasciae to the ipsilateral hip. This set of myofascial connections, which are of course repeated in a mirror image on the opposite side, become a focus for the mammalian ability to rotate the trunk, and are detailed in Chapter 6 on the Spiral Line. (www.anatomytrains.com – video ref: Anatomy Trains Revealed) (Photo courtesy of the author.)

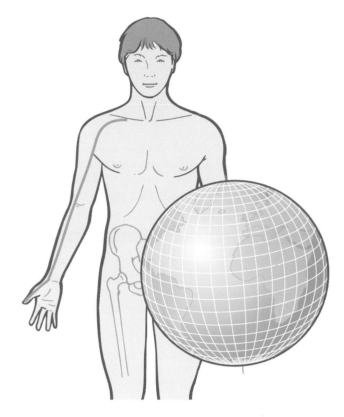

• **Fig. 1.17** Although the myofascial meridians have some overlap with Asian medicine's meridian lines, they are not equivalent. Think of these meridians as defining a 'geography' within the myofascial system. Compare the Lung meridian shown here to Fig. 7.1 – the Deep Front Arm Line. See also Appendix 4.

of the fascial web – this tissue will henceforth be referred to in its singular form: myofascia. There is really no need for a plural, because it arises from and remains all one structure. For the myofascia, only a knife creates the plural.

The term 'myofascial continuity' describes the connection between two longitudinally adjacent and aligned structures within the structural webbing. There is a 'myofascial continuity' between the serratus anterior muscle and the external oblique muscle (see Fig. 1.6). 'Myofascial meridian' describes an interlinked series of these connected tracts of sinew and muscle. A myofascial continuity, in other words, is a local part of a myofascial meridian. The serratus anterior and external oblique are both part of the larger overall sling of the upper Spiral Line that wraps around the torso (Fig. 1.16 and see Ch. 6).

The word 'meridian' is often used in the context of the energetic lines of transmission in the domain of acupuncture.[47–49] Let there be no confusion: the myofascial meridian lines are not acupuncture meridians, but lines of pull based on standard Western anatomy, lines which transmit strain and elastic recoil, facilitating movement and providing stability through the body's myofascia around the skeleton. They clearly have some overlap with the meridians of acupuncture, but the two are not equivalent (for a comparison, see Appendix 4, p. 339). The use of the word 'meridians' has more to do, in the author's mind, with the meridians of latitude and longitude that girdle the earth (Fig. 1.17). In the same way, these meridians girdle the body, defining geography and geometry within the myofascia, the geodesics of the body's mobile tensegrity.

This book considers how these lines of pull affect the structure and function of the body in question. While many lines of pull may be defined, and individuals may set up unique strains and connections through developmental

abnormality, injury, adhesion, or attitude (Video 1.4), this book outlines 12 myofascial continuities commonly employed around the human frame. The 'rules' for constructing a myofascial meridian are included so that the experienced reader can construct other lines that may prove useful in certain cases. The body's fascia is omnidirectionally versatile and can resist other lines of strain besides the ones listed herein as created by odd or unusual movements, readily seen in any roughhousing child. We are reasonably sure that a fairly complete therapeutic approach can be assembled from the 12 lines we have included, though we are open to new ideas that further exploration and more in-depth research will bring to light (see Appendix 3, p. 327).

Chapter 2 sets up these rules and the scope for constructing a myofascial meridian. Chapters 3–9 present the Anatomy Trains lines, and consider some of the therapeutic and movement-oriented implications of each line. Please note that in Chapter 3, the 'Superficial Back Line' is presented in excruciating detail in order to clarify the Anatomy Trains concepts. Subsequent chapters on the other myofascial meridians are laid out using the terminology and format developed in this chapter. Whichever line you are interested in exploring, it may help to read Chapter 3 first. Chapter 10 deals with applications to movement practice, and Chapter 11 addresses global assessment and strategy considerations, both attempts to be helpful in applying the Anatomy Trains concept, regardless of treatment method.

Following the 'lines' chapters, Appendix 1 includes more detail about various aspects of the fascial webbing, with updates on current research directions. This includes recent research on remodeling after injury and the elastic response to new training challenges, as well as building the recently revealed story of the 'interstitium' – how perfusion operates amongst the gels and cells of all other body systems. Also new to this edition is an initial attempt at mapping these lines in a quadruped, and an enhanced outline of the protocol taught in our Anatomy Trains Structural Integration certification.

History

The Anatomy Trains concept arose from the experience of teaching myofascial anatomy to diverse groups of 'alternative' therapists, including Structural Integration practitioners at Ida Rolf's school, massage therapists, osteopaths, physiatrists, midwives, dancers, yoga teachers, physiotherapists, rehabilitation specialists, and athletic trainers across the world. What began literally as a game, an aide-mémoire for my students, slowly during the 1990s coalesced into a system worthy of sharing. Urged to write by the late Dr Leon Chaitow, these ideas first saw light in the *Journal of Bodywork and Movement Therapies* in 1997.

Moving out from anatomical and osteopathic circles into the wider world of soft-tissue therapy, the concept that the fascia connects the whole body in an 'endless web'[50] has steadily gained ground. Given that generalization, however, the student can be justifiably confused as to whether one should set about fixing a stubborn frozen shoulder by working on the ribs or the hip or the neck. The next logical questions, 'how, exactly, are these things connected?', or 'are some parts more connected than others?', had no specific answers. This book is an attempt to answer these and other questions from my students.

In 1986, Dr James Oschman,[51,52] a Woods Hole biologist who has done a thorough literature search in fields related to healing, handed me an article by the South African anthropologist Raymond Dart on the double-spiral relationship of muscles in the trunk.[53] Dart had unearthed the concept not from the soil of the australopithecine plains of South Africa, but out of his experience as a student of the Alexander Technique.[54] The arrangement of interlinked muscles Dart described is included in this book as part of what I have termed the 'Spiral Line', and his article started a journey of discovery which extended into the myofascial continuities presented here (Fig. 1.18). Dissection studies, clinical application, endless hours of teaching, and poring through old books (including, courtesy of Dr Carla Stecco, the fascinating library of the University of Padua) have refined the original concept to its current state.

Over this decade, we have looked for effective ways to depict these continuities that would make them easier to understand and see (Video 2.2). For instance, the connection

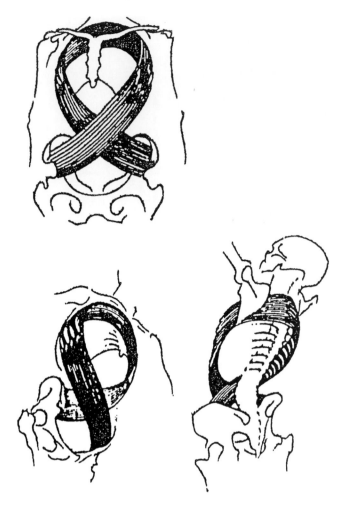

• **Fig. 1.18** Although Dart's original article contained no illustrations, this illustration from Manaka shows the same pattern Dart discussed, part of what we call the Spiral Line. (Reproduced with permission from Matsumoto K, Birch S, Hara Diagnosis: Reflections on the Sea. Paradigm Publications; 1988[33] with kind permission.)

between the biceps femoris and the sacrotuberous ligament is well documented, while the fascial interlocking between the hamstrings and gastrocnemii at the lower end of Fig. 1.19 is less often shown. These form part of a head-to-toe continuity termed the Superficial Back Line, which we have dissected out intact in both preserved and fresh-tissue cadavers (see Fig. 1.13).

The simplest way of depicting these connections is as a geometric line of pull passing from one 'station' (muscle attachment) to the next. This one-dimensional view is included with each chapter (Fig. 1.20). Another way to consider these lines is as part of a plane of fascia, especially in the superficial layers and the fascial 'unitard' of the profundis layer, so this two-dimensional 'area of influence' is also included for the surface lines (Fig. 1.21). Principally, of course, these chains of muscles and their accompanying fascia are a three-dimensional volume – and this volumetric view is featured in three views at the beginning of each chapter (Fig. 1.22).

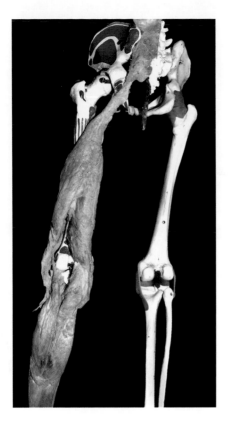

• **Fig. 1.19** The hamstrings have a clear fibrous fascial continuity with the sacrotuberous ligament fibers. There is also a fascial continuity between the distal hamstring tendons and the heads of the gastrocnemii, but this connection is often cut and seldom depicted. (Photo courtesy of the author; dissection by Laboratories of Anatomical Enlightenment.)

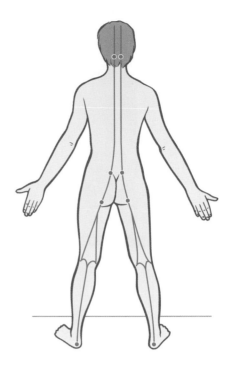

• **Fig. 1.20** The Superficial Back Line shown as a one-dimensional line – the strict line of pull.

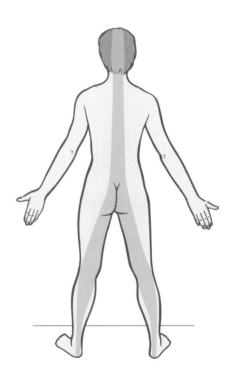

• **Fig. 1.21** The Superficial Back Line shown as a two-dimensional plane – the area of influence.

Additional views of the Anatomy Trains in motion have been and continue to be developed for our video series (Fig. 1.23). Stills from these sources have been used in this book when they shed additional light. As well, we have used still photos of action and standing posture with the lines superimposed to give some sense of the lines *in vivo* (Figs. 1.24 & 1.25; see Fig. 10.1; Video 6.25).

Although I have not seen the myofascial continuities completely described elsewhere, I was both chagrined (to find out that my ideas were not totally original) and relieved (to affirm that I was not totally off-track) to discover, after I had published an early version of these ideas,[55,56] that similar work had been done by some German anatomists, such as Hoepke and Benninghof-Guertler, in the 1930s, largely buried after the Third Reich (Fig. 1.26).[57] There are also similarities with the *chaînes musculaires* of Françoise Mézière[58,59] (further developed by Leopold Busquet), to which I was introduced prior to completing this book. These *chaînes musculaires* are based on *functional* connections – passing, for instance, from the quadriceps through the knee to the gastrocnemii and soleus, which are functionally connected in a leap – whereas the Anatomy Trains are based on direct *fascial* fabric connections. The more recent diagrams of the late German anatomist Tittel are likewise based on functional, rather than actual fabric linkages (Fig. 1.27).[60] All

of these 'maps' have some overlap with the Anatomy Trains, and their pioneering work is acknowledged with gratitude.

Since initial publication, I have also become aware of the work of Andry Vleeming and associates on 'myofascial slings' in relation to force closure of the sacroiliac joint,[61,62] especially as applied clinically by the incomparable Diane Lee[61,63] (Fig. 1.28). Vleeming's Anterior Oblique sling and

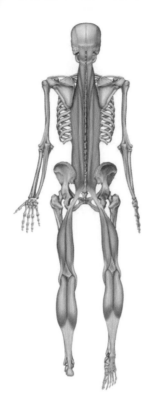

• **Fig. 1.22** The Superficial Back Line shown as a three-dimensional volume – the muscles and fasciae involved.

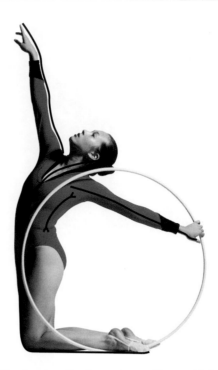

• **Fig. 1.24** The lines in action in sport – see Chapter 10. In this photo, the Superficial Front Line is lengthened, toned, and stretched by the backbend, flexed knee, and plantarflexed foot. The Superficial Back Arm Line on the right side sustains the arm in the air, and the Deep Front Arm Line on the left side is stretched from ribs to thumb. The Lateral Line on the left side is compressed in the trunk, and its complement is conversely open.

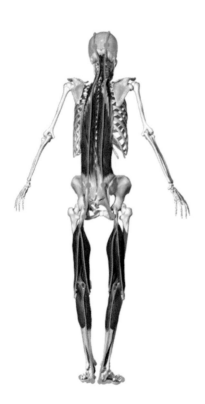

• **Fig. 1.23** A still from the Primal Pictures DVD-ROM program on the Anatomy Trains. (Image provided courtesy of Primal Pictures, www. primalpictures.com)

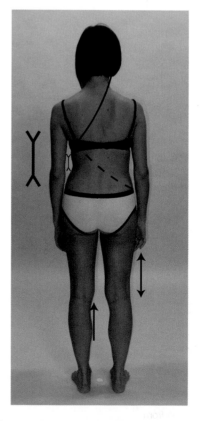

• **Fig. 1.25** Diagramming postural compensations – see Chapter 11. (Photo courtesy of the author.)

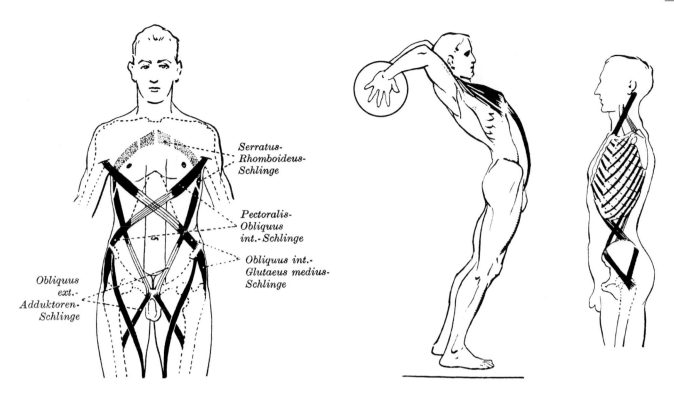

• **Fig. 1.26** The German anatomist Hoepke detailed some 'myofascial meridians' in his 1936 book, which translates into English as 'muscle-play'. Less exact but similar ideas can be found in Mollier's *Plastische Anatomie* (published by Bergmann, Munich; 1938). (Reproduced with kind permission from Benninghoff A, Lehrbuch der Anatomie des Menschen, 1939 Berlin: Lehmann's Verlag.)

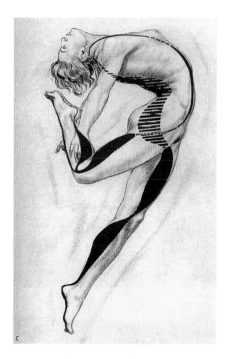

• **Fig. 1.27** The German anatomist Kurt Tittel also drew some marvelously athletic bodies overlaid with functional muscular connections. The difference is between these muscular functional connections, seen also in the work of Françoise Mézière, et al., which are movement-specific and momentary, and the Anatomy Trains fascial 'fabric' connections, which are more permanent and postural. (From Tittel 1956, with kind permission from Urban and Fischer.)

Posterior Oblique sling coincide generally with the Functional Lines to be found in Chapter 8 of this book, while his Posterior Longitudinal sling forms part of what is described in this book as the much longer Spiral Line (see Ch. 6). As stated previously, the presumptuous book you hold in your hand reaches ahead of the peer-reviewed research such as Vleeming's and Lee's, to present a point of view that seems to work well in practice but is yet to be validated in evidence-based publications.[38]

With the renewed confidence that comes from such confirmation accompanied by the caution that should pertain to anyone on such thin scientific ice, my colleagues and I have been testing and teaching a system of Structural Integration (www.anatomytrains.com, and see Appendix 3, p. 327) based on these Anatomy Trains myofascial meridians. Practitioners coming from these classes report significant improvement in their ability to tackle complex structural problems with increasing success rates. This book is designed to make the concept available to a wider audience. Since the publication of the first edition in 2001, this intent has been realized: the Anatomy Trains classes and materials are available to a broad variety of professions on the internet and in fifteen languages on every continent save Antarctica.

www.anatomytrains.com
www.anatomytrains.co.uk
www.anatomytrainsaustralia.com
www.anatomytrains.pl
www.anatomytrains.jp

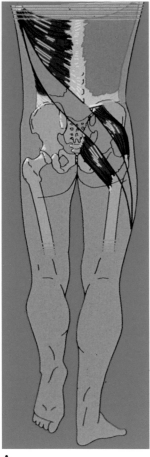

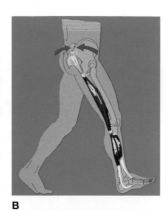

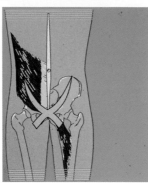

• **Fig. 1.28** Andry Vleeming and Diane Lee described the Anterior and Posterior oblique slings – very similar to the Front and Back Functional Lines described in this book (and very similar to the *ligne de fermeture* and *ligne d'ouverture* described by Mézière). Vleeming's Posterior longitudinal sling (**B**) is primarily contained within the Spiral Line in this text. (A, Modified from Vleeming et al.[61] with kind permission. B, Reproduced from Vleeming and Stoeckart[62] with kind permission. C, Reproduced from Lee[63] with kind permission.)

References

1. Pontzer H. Evolved to exercise. *Sci Am.* 2019;23–29.
2. Lieberman D. *The Story of the Human Body.* New York: Pantheon Books; 2013.
3. Borelli GA. *De motu animalium.* Lugduni in Batavis; 1685.
4. Kendall F, McCreary E. *Muscles, Testing and Function.* 3rd ed. Baltimore: Williams and Wilkins; 1983.
5. Fox E, Mathews D. *The Physiological Basis of Physical Education.* 3rd ed. New York: Saunders College Publications; 1981.
6. Alexander RM. *The Human Machine.* New York: Columbia University Press; 1992.
7. Hildebrand M. *Analysis of Vertebrate Structure.* New York: John Wiley; 1974.
8. Prigogine I. *Order Out of Chaos.* New York: Bantam Books; 1984.
9. Damasio A. *Descartes' Mistake.* New York: GP Putnam; 1994.
10. Gleick J. *Chaos.* New York: Penguin; 1987.
11. Briggs J. *Fractals.* New York: Simon and Schuster; 1992.
12. Sole R, Goodwin B. *Signs of Life: How Complexity Pervades Biology.* New York: Basic Books; 2002.
13. Schleip R, Findley TW, Chaitow L, et al., eds. *Fascia: The Tensional Network of the Human Body.* Edinburgh: Elsevier; 2012.
14. Lesondak D. *Fascia: What It Is and Why It Matters.* London: Handspring; 2017.
15. Avison J. *Yoga: Fascia, Anatomy and Movement.* Edinburgh: Handspring; 2015.
16. Schleip R. *Fascia in Sport and Movement.* Edinburgh: Handspring; 2015.
17. Larkam E. *Fascia in Motion.* Edinburgh: Handspring; 2017.
18. Scarpa A. *Commentarius De Penitiori Ossium Structura.* Lipsiae: Sumtibus J.F. Hartknoch; 1799.
19. Singer E. *Fascia of the Human Body and Their Relations to the Organs They Envelop.* Philadephia: Williams and Wilkins; 1935.
20. Ruffini A. *Di una particolare reticella nervosa e di alcuni corpuscoli del Pacini che si trovano in connessione cogli organi muscolo-tendinei del gatto.* Atti dell' Accademia nazionale dei Lincei; 1892.
21. Still AT. *The Philosophy and Mechanical Principles of Osteopathy.* Kansas City, MO: Hudson-Kimberly; 1902.
22. Sutherland WG. *Teachings in the Science of Osteopathy.* Cambridge, MA: Rudra Press; 1990.
23. Gallaudet BB. *A Description of the Planes of Fascia of the Human Body, With Special Reference to the Fascia of the Abdomen, Pelvis and Perineum.* New York: Columbia University Press; 1931.
24. Ingber D. Cellular mechanotransduction: putting all the pieces together again. *FASEB J.* 2006;20:811–827.
25. Stecco L. *Fascial Manipulation for Musculoskeletal Pain.* Padua: PICCIN; 2004.
26. Vaglio A, ed. *Systemic Fibroinflammatory Disorders.* Heidelberg: Springer Verlag; 2017.
27. Van der Waal JC. The architecture of connective tissues as parameter for proprioception – an often overlooked functional parameter as to proprioception in the locomotor apparatus. *Int J Ther Massage Bodywork.* 2009;2(4):9–23.
28. Huijing PA. Intra-, extra-, and intermuscular myofascial force transmission of synergists and antagonists: effects of muscle length as well as relative position. *Int J Mech Med Biol.* 2002;2: 1–15.
29. Biel A. *Trail Guide to the Body.* 3rd ed. Boulder, CO: Discovery Books; 2005.
30. Chaitow L, DeLany J. *Clinical Applications of Neuromuscular Techniques.* Vols 1, 2. Edinburgh: Churchill Livingstone; 2000.
31. Jarmey C, Myers TW. *The Concise Book of the Moving Body.* Berkely, CA: Lotus Publishing/North Atlantic Books; 2006.
32. Kapandji I. *Physiology of the Joints.* Vols 1–3. Edinburgh: Churchill Livingstone; 1982.
33. Muscolino J. *The Muscular System Manual.* Hartford, CT: JEM Publications; 2002.
34. Platzer W. *Locomotor System.* Stuttgart: Thieme Verlag; 1986.
35. Simons D, Travell J, Simons L. *Myofascial Pain and Dysfunction: The Trigger Point Manual.* Vol. 1. Baltimore: Williams and Wilkins; 1998.
36. Schuenke M, Schulte E, Schumaker U. *Thieme Atlas of Anatomy.* Stuttgart: Thieme Verlag; 2006.
37. Luttgens K, Deutsch H, Hamilton N. *Kinesiology.* 8th ed. Dubuque, IA: WC Brown; 1992.
38. Brown JMM, Wickham JB, McAndrew DJ, Huang XF. Muscles within muscles: coordination of 19 muscle segments within three shoulder muscles during isometric motor tasks. *J Electromyogr Kinesiol.* 2007;17(1):57–73.

39. Wilke J, Krause F, Vogt L, et al. What is evidence-based about myofascial chains: a systematic review? *Arch Phys Med Rehabil.* 2016;97:454–461.

40. Zügel M, Maganaris CN, Wilke J, et al. Fascial tissue research in sports medicine: from molecules to tissue adaptation, injury and diagnostics: consensus statement. *Br J Sports Med.* 2018;52(23):1497.

41. Rolf I. *Rolfing.* Rochester, VT: Healing Arts Press; 1977. *Further information and publications concerning Dr Rolf and her methods are available from the Rolf Institute, 295 Canyon Blvd, Boulder, CO 80302, USA.*

42. Chaitow L. *Soft-Tissue Manipulation.* Rochester, VT: Thorson; 1980.

43. Sutcliffe J, Duin N. *A History of Medicine.* New York: Barnes and Noble; 1992.

44. Singer C. *A Short History of Anatomy and Physiology From the Greeks to Harvey.* New York: Dover; 1957.

45. Barnes J. *Myofascial Release.* Paoli, PA: Myofascial Release Seminars; 1990.

46. Simons D, Travell J, Simons L. *Myofascial Pain and Dysfunction: The Trigger Point Manual.* Vol. 1. Baltimore: Williams and Wilkins; 1998.

47. Mann F. *Acupuncture.* New York: Random House; 1973.

48. Ellis A, Wiseman N, Boss K. *Fundamentals of Chinese Acupuncture.* Brookline, MA: Paradigm; 1991.

49. Hopkins Technology LLC. *Complete Acupuncture. CD-ROM.* Hopkins, MN: Johns Hopkins University; 1997. 2013.

50. Schultz L, Feitis R. *The Endless Web.* Berkeley: North Atlantic Books; 1996.

51. Oschman J. *Readings on the Scientific Basis of Bodywork.* Dover, NH: NORA; 1997.

52. Oschman J. *Energy Medicine.* Edinburgh: Churchill Livingstone; 2000.

53. Dart R. Voluntary musculature in the human body: the double-spiral arrangement. *Br J Phys Med.* 1950;13(12NS):265–268.

54. Barlow W. *The Alexander Technique.* New York: Alfred A Knopf; 1973.

55. Myers T. The anatomy trains. *J Bodyw Mov Ther.* 1997;1(2): 91–101.

56. Myers T. The anatomy trains. *J Bodyw Mov Ther.* 1997;1(3): 134–145.

57. Benninghoff A, Lehrbuch der Anatomie des Menschen, 1939 Berlin: Lehmann's Verlag.

58. Godelieve D-S. *Le Manuel Du Mezieriste.* Paris: Editions Frison-Roche; 1995.

59. Busquet L. *Les Chaînes Musculaires.* Vols 1–4. Frères, Mairlot: Maîtres et Cles de la Posture; 1992.

60. Tittel K. *Beschreibende Und Funktionelle Anatomie Des Menschen.* Munich: Urban & Fischer; 1956.

61. Vleeming A, Udzwaard AL, Stoeckart R, et al. The posterior layer of the thoracolumbar fascia: its function in load transfer from spine to legs. *Spine.* 1995;20:753.

62. Vleeming A, Stoeckart R. The role of the pelvic girdle in coupling the spine and the legs: a clinical-anatomical perspective on pelvic stability. In: Vleeming A, Mooney V, Stoeckart R, eds. *Movement, Stability & Lumbopelvic Pain, Integration of Research and Therapy.* Edinburgh: Elsevier; 2007.

63. Lee DG. *The Pelvic Girdle.* 3rd ed. Edinburgh: Elsevier; 2004.

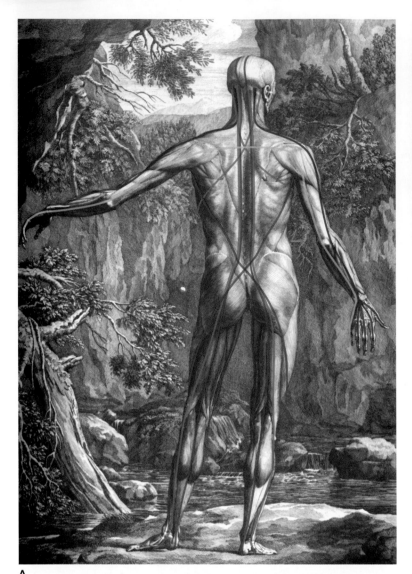

A

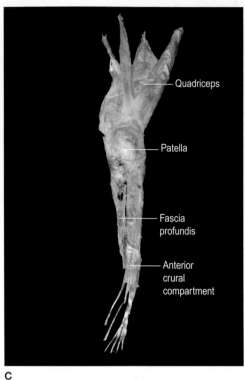

— Quadriceps

— Patella

— Fascia profundis

— Anterior crural compartment

C

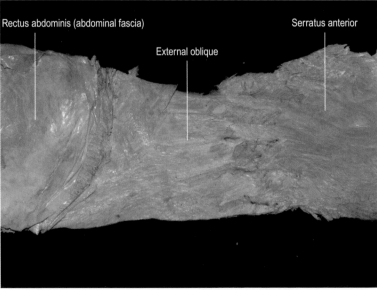

Rectus abdominis (abdominal fascia)

External oblique

Serratus anterior

B

• **Fig. 2.1** (**A**) A back view summary of the Anatomy Trains myofascial meridians described in this book, laid over a figure from Albinus (see also Fig. 1.1A). (**B**) A dissection of an Anatomy Trains 'station' between the serratus anterior and the lower slips of the external abdominal oblique, seen from the profound side, looking, as it were, out from the ribs. Notice how the zigzag attachments of both serratus and external oblique provide attachment to the periosteum of the ribs, but if those are detached, there is also a substantial fascial continuity between the two 'tracks'. (**C**) The lower section of the Superficial Front Line, showing a dissection of the continuous biological fabric which joins the anterior compartment of the lower leg – toe extensors and tibialis anterior – through the bridle around the patella and into the quadriceps, spread here for easy identification. Notice the inclusion of the fascia profundis (in this case, the crural fascial layer) over the tibia. This is explained more fully in Chapter 4, but serves here to demonstrate the concept of the complete myofascial 'track'. (www.anatomytrains.com – video ref: Anatomy Trains Revealed) (A, Reproduced with kind permission from Dover Publications, NY.)

2

The Rules of the Road

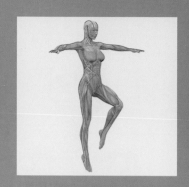

Although intended as a practical aid to working clinicians, 'Anatomy Trains' is most easily outlined as a game within this railway metaphor. There are a few simple rules, designed to direct our attention, among the galaxy of possible myofascial connections, toward those with common clinical significance (Fig. 2.1). Since the myofascial continuities described here are not exhaustive, the reader can use the rules given below to construct additional trains not explored in the body of this book. Those with serious structural anomalies – e.g. stroke victims, scoliotics or amputees – will create unique lines of myofascial transmission independent of the body's common design.

Simply stated, active myofascial meridians must proceed in a consistent direction and depth via direct fibrous connections capable of force transmission. It is also clinically useful to note where the fascial trains attach, combine, divide, or display alternative routes.

From time to time, we will find places where we have to bend or break these rules (Video 1.4). These breaks in the rules are given the name 'derailments' and a rationale is offered for persisting in spite of the break.

1. 'Tracks' Proceed in a Consistent Direction Without Interruption

To look for an Anatomy Train, we look for 'tracks' made from myofascial or connective tissue units (i.e. muscles and ligaments – which are human distinctions, not divine, evolutionary, or even anatomically discrete entities). These structures must show a continuity of fascial fibers creating lines of force transmission through the myofascia. Like a real train track, the lines must run fairly straight or change direction only gradually. Some myofascial connections are only pulled straight in certain positions or load conditions.

Likewise, since the body's fascia is largely arranged in planes, jumping from one depth to another among the planes amounts to jumping the tracks. Radical changes of direction or depth are thus not allowed (unless it can be demonstrated that the fascia itself actually acts across levels); nor are 'jumps' across joints or through sheets of fibers that run counter to the tracks. Any of these would nullify the ability of the tensile fascia to transmit force from one link of the chain to the next.

A. Direction

As an example, the pectoralis minor and the coracobrachialis are clearly connected fascially at the coracoid process (Fig. 2.2A, and see Ch. 7). This, however, cannot function as a myofascial continuity when the arm is relaxed by one's side, because there is a radical change of direction between these two myofascial structures. (We will abandon this awkward term in favor of the less awkward 'muscles' if the reader will kindly remember that muscles are mere ground beef without their surrounding, investing, and attaching fasciae.) When the arm is aloft, flexed as in a tennis serve or when hanging from a chinning bar or a branch like the simian in Fig. 2.2B, then these two line up with each other and *do* act in a chain that connects the ribs to the elbow (and beyond in both directions – the Deep Front Arm Line connecting to the Superficial Front Line – from thumb to pelvis).

The usefulness of the theory comes with the realization that the presenting problem with the tennis serve or the chin-up may show up in the function of either of these two muscles or at their connecting point, and yet have their source in structures farther up or down the tracks. Knowing the trains allows the practitioner to make reasoned holistic decisions in treatment strategy, regardless of the method employed.

On the other hand, fascial structures themselves can in certain cases carry a pulling force around corners. The fibularis brevis takes a sharp curve around the lateral malleolus, but no one would doubt that the myofascial continuity of action is maintained (Fig. 2.3). Such pulleys, when the fascia makes use of them, are certainly permitted by our rules.

B. Depth

Although we live in one single fascial net, it is folded in embryological development again and again to form fascial planes (Fig. 2.4). Each myofascial meridian stays on its given fascial plane, without jumping from one to another.

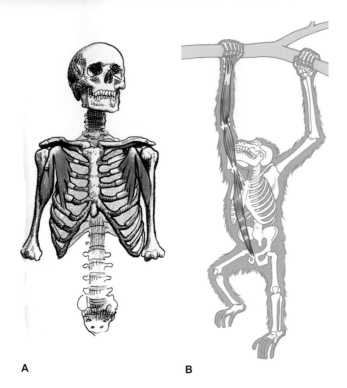

A   **B**

• **Fig. 2.2** While the fascia connecting the muscles that attach to the coracoid process is always present (**A**), the connection only functions in our game of mechanical tensile linkage when the arm is above the horizontal (**B**). (A, Reproduced with kind permission from Grundy 1982.)

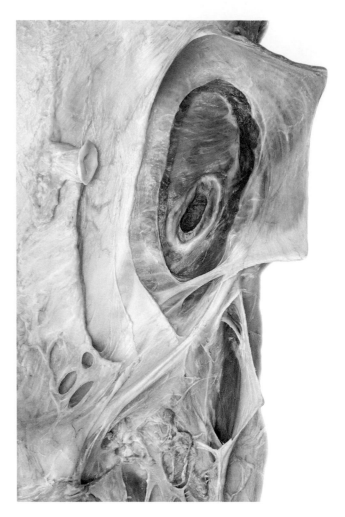

• **Fig. 2.4** The unitary fascial net is folded into layers during embryological development in the most complicated feat of origami imaginable. Here, progressive layers in the trunk are revealed. Depending on the speed of the motion and condition of the tissues, both movement and force transmission can occur among layers. Each Anatomy Train, however stays on one given layer. (Photo courtesy of Dr Hanno Steinke and Anna Rowedder.)

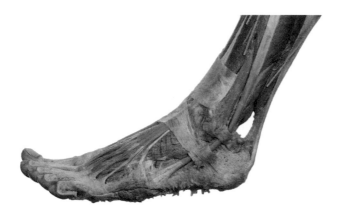

• **Fig. 2.3** Tendons acting around corners like pulleys around bones or under retinaculae are an acceptable exception to the 'no sharp turns' rule. (© Ralph T. Hutchings. Reproduced from Abrahams, et al. 1998.)

Like abrupt changes of direction, abrupt changes of depth – shifting from a superficial fascial plane to a deeper one, e.g., – are also frowned upon. For example, when we look at the torso from the front, the logical connection in terms of direction from the rectus abdominis and the sternal fascia up the front of the ribs would clearly be the infrahyoid muscles running up the front of the throat (Fig. 2.5A). The error of making this 'train' becomes clear when we realize that the infrahyoid muscles attach to the posterior of the sternum, thus connecting them to a deeper ventral fascial plane within the rib cage (part of the Deep Front Line). The superficial plane actually continues to the skull via the sternocleidomastoid (Fig. 2.5B).

C. Intervening Planes

Resist the temptation to carry an Anatomy Train through an intervening plane of fascia that goes in another direction, for how could the tensile pull be communicated through such a wall? As an example, the adductor longus comes down to the linea aspera of the femur, and the short head of the biceps goes on from the linea aspera in the same direction. Surely that constitutes a myofascial continuity? In fact it does not, for there is the intervening plane of the adductor magnus, which would cut off any direct tensile communication between longus and biceps (Fig. 2.6). There may be some mechanical connection between these two

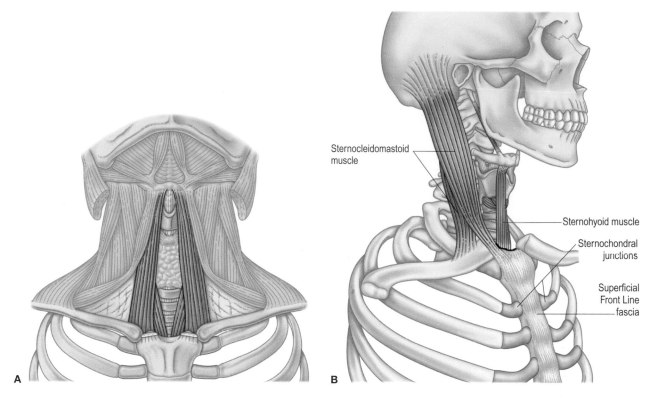

Sternocleidomastoid muscle

Sternohyoid muscle

Sternochondral junctions

Superficial Front Line fascia

A   B

• **Fig. 2.5** Although a mechanical connection can be felt from chest to throat when the entire upper spine is hyperextended, there is no direct connection between the superficial chest fascia and the infrahyoid muscles because of the difference in depth of their respective fascial planes. The infrahyoids pass deep to the sternum, connecting them to the inner lining of the ribs and the endothoracic fascia and transversus thoracis (**A**). The more superficial fascial planes connect the sternocleidomastoid to the fascia on the superficial side of the sternum and sternochondral junctions (**B**).

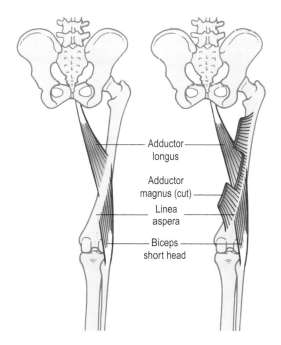

Adductor longus

Adductor magnus (cut)

Linea aspera

Biceps short head

• **Fig. 2.6** If we just look at adductor longus and the short head of the biceps femoris (as on left), they appear to fulfill the requirements for a myofascial continuity. But when we see that the plane of adductor magnus intercedes between the two (as on the right) to attach to the linea aspera, we realize that such a connection cannot transmit force.

through the bone, but myofascial force transmission is negated by the fascial wall between.

2. These Tracks Are Tacked Down at Bony 'Stations' or Attachments

In the Anatomy Trains concept, muscle attachments ('stations') are seen as places where some underlying fibers of the muscle's epimysium or tendon are enmeshed or continuous with the periosteum of the accompanying bone, or, less often, with the collagen matrix of the bone itself. In other words, a station is where the outer myofascial bag attaches itself onto the inner 'osteoarticular' wrapping.

The more superficial fibers of the myofascial unit, however, can demonstrably be seen to run on, and thus communicate, to the next piece of the myofascial track. For instance, in Fig. 2.7 we can see that some of the fibers at the end of the myofascia on the right are clearly tied to the periosteal wrap around the scapula, while some fibers continue on into the next 'track' of myofascia. There remains a strong and substantial sheet of biological fabric connecting splenius to rhomboids to serratus anterior. In fact, one can argue that dividing them into separate muscles is a convenient fiction.

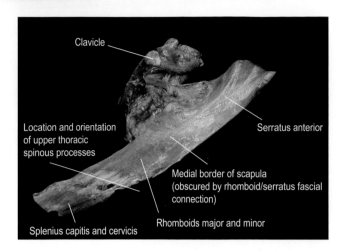

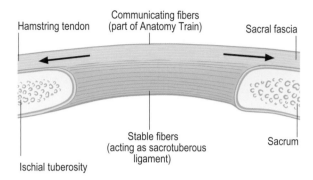

• **Fig. 2.9** The deeper fibers of a station 'communicate' less along the tracks, while the superficial fibers – the ones we can more easily reach manually – communicate more.

• **Fig. 2.7** In this photo of a recent dissection, a series of muscles were detached from their periosteal attachments to show the continuity of fascial fabric from the splenius attachment to the skull on the left to the serratus anterior attachment to the lateral ribs on the right. Please note that we are looking at the anterior (deep) surface of the muscles, such that the scapula is, in this view, under the 'rhombo-serratus' muscle (see Ch. 6).

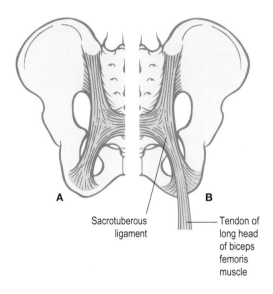

• **Fig. 2.8** A traditional view of the sacrotuberous ligament (**A**) shows it linking the ischial tuberosity to the sacrum. A more inclusive view (**B**) shows the hamstring tendons – especially that of the biceps femoris – being continuous with the surface of the sacrotuberous ligament and then on up into the sacral fascia.

Thus, for example, the hamstrings clearly attach on the posterior side of the ischial tuberosities. Just as clearly, some fibers of the hamstring myofascia continue on over and into the sacrotuberous ligament and up onto the sacrum (Fig. 2.8). These ongoing connections have been de-emphasized in most contemporary texts that tend to treat muscles or fascial structures singularly in terms of their actions from origin to insertion. Contemporary musculoskeletal illustrations tend to reinforce this impression.

Most stations have more communication with the next myofascial linkage in the superficial rather than the deeper

fibers, and the sacrotuberous ligament is a convenient example. The deeper layers clearly join bone to bone and have very limited movement or communication beyond that connection. The more superficial we go, the more communication through to the other myofascial tracks there is (Fig. 2.9). Too much movement in the deeper layers approximates a 'lax' ligament. Too little 'give' in the tissue courts injury through rigidity or immobility reducing the body's ability to adjust resiliently in movement.

3. Tracks Join and Diverge in 'Switches' and the Occasional 'Roundhouse'

Fascial planes frequently interweave, joining with each other and splitting from each other, which we will call 'switches' (UK: points) in keeping with our train metaphor. The fascial laminae of the abdominal muscles, for example, arise together from the lumbar transverse processes, divide into the three differently grained layers of the obliques and transversus muscles at the lateral raphe, only to split uniquely around the rectus abdominis, join into one at the linea alba, and repeat the whole process in reverse on the opposite side (Fig. 2.10) to complete the 'belt'. As another example, many laminae of fascia intermingle in the thoracolumbar and sacral area, where they blend into stronger sheets, often inseparable in dissection.

Switches require the body – and sometimes the therapist – to make choices. The rhomboids span from the spinous processes to the medial scapular border. At the scapula, there is a clear fascial connection to both the serratus anterior (especially from the fascia on the profound side of the rhomboids), which carries on around under the scapula to the rib cage, but also (from the fascial layer on the superficial side of the rhomboids) to the infraspinatus, which carries on out the arm (Fig. 2.11). We will often see fascial and myofascial planes divide or blend, and the force transmission will emphasize one track or another depending on body position and outside forces. Which Anatomy Train to use in any given posture or activity is not a matter for

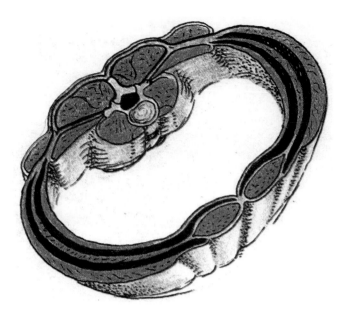

• **Fig. 2.10** The layers of abdominal fasciae converge and diverge in a complex functional pattern. (Reproduced with kind permission from Grundy 1982.)

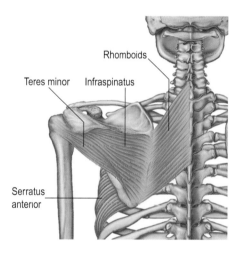

• **Fig. 2.11** An example of a 'switch': from the rhomboid major we could transmit force either into the serratus anterior with one track around the trunk (red muscle under scapula – part of the Spiral Line, see Fig. 2.7 and Ch. 6), or over into the infraspinatus with another track out the arm (part of the Deep Back Arm Line, see Ch. 7).

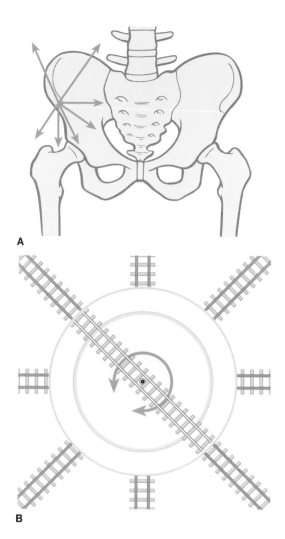

A

B

• **Fig. 2.12** Many competing vectors of myofascial force proceed out in all directions from the 'roundhouse' (**B**) of the anterior superior iliac spine (**A**)

landmarks, noting their position is crucial to an Anatomy Trains analysis of structure.

4. 'Expresses' and 'Locals'

Polyarticular muscles (crossing more than one joint) abound on the body's surface. These muscles often overlie a series of monarticular (single-joint) muscles, each of which duplicates some single part of the overall function of the polyarticular muscle. When this situation occurs within an Anatomy Train, we will call the multi-joint muscles 'expresses' and the underlying single-joint muscles 'locals'.

As an example, the long head of biceps femoris runs from 'above' the hip joint to below the knee, hence it is an express affecting both joints. Deep to it lie two locals: the adductor magnus – a one-joint local crossing the hip and extending as well as adducting it – and the short head of the biceps – a one-joint muscle crossing only the knee to flex and rotate it (Fig. 2.13).

It is our contention that general postural 'set' is determined less by the superficial expresses and more by the

voluntary choice, though individual patterns of muscle contraction will be a factor, and adjustments – as one makes in a yoga pose or loaded lifting – will change the exact route of force transmission. By and large, however, the amount of force transmission down any given track is determined by the physics of the situation.

A 'roundhouse' is where many myofascial force vectors meet and/or cross, the pubic bone or the anterior superior iliac spine being prime examples (Fig. 2.12). Because of the competing tugs on these roundhouses, which are often bony

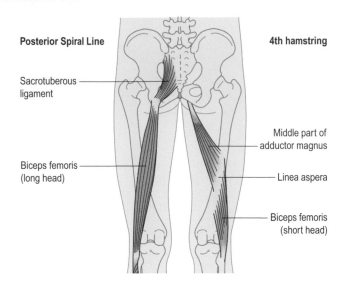

• **Fig. 2.13** The long head of the biceps femoris is a two-joint 'express', part of the Spiral Line (left). Beneath it lie the one-joint 'locals' of the short head of the biceps connecting across the linea aspera to the middle of the adductor magnus muscle (right), with considerable fascial fabric overlap between the two. The two locals closely mirror individually the collective action of the single express.

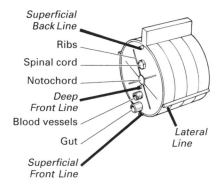

• **Fig. 2.14** The five more or less straight longitudinal lines (counting the left and right Lateral Lines as two) identified on a cross-section of the basic vertebrate body plan (as if you are looking at a section cut from a fish). Note the relationship among the lines themselves, as well as to major organic structures.

deeper locals, which are too often ignored because they are 'out of sight, out of mind'. This would suggest, for instance, that an anterior tilt of the pelvis (postural hip flexion) would yield more to release in the pectineus and iliacus (single-joint hip flexors) than to release in the rectus femoris or sartorius, or that chronic flexion of the elbow would best be treated by release of the brachialis rather than concentrating all our attention in the more obvious and available biceps brachii.

Summary of Rules and Guidelines

While we have attempted to be fairly thorough in presenting the principal large myofascial meridians at work in the human body (Fig. 2.14), readers can find and construct

their own by following these rules. (Some students and colleagues have attempted, for instance, to lay out a convincing 'Deep Back Line' myofascial meridian according to these rules, but the author remains sceptical.)

• Follow the grain of the connective tissue, maintaining a fairly steady direction without jumping levels or crossing through intervening planes of fascia.
• Note the stations where these myofascial tracks tie down to the underlying tissues.
• Note any other tracks that diverge or converge with the line.
• Look for underlying single-joint muscles that may affect the working of the line.

What the Anatomy Trains Is Not

A Comprehensive Theory of Manipulative Therapy

This book and the Anatomy Trains theory deals only with the 'outer bag' of parietal myofascia as described in Appendix 1. The whole area of joint manipulation is left to the osteopathic and chiropractic texts, and is beyond the scope of the myofascial meridians concept. Certainly, we have found that balancing the lines eases joint strain and thus perhaps extends joint life. Attention to the 'inner bag' of peri-articular tissues, however, as well as dorsal and ventral cavity connective tissue complexes (cranial and visceral manipulation), is essential, advisable, and simply not covered by this book.

A Comprehensive Theory of Muscle Action

Anatomy Trains theory is not designed to replace other findings of muscle function, but to add to them. The infraspinatus is still seen to be active in laterally rotating the humerus and in preventing excessive medial rotation, and in stabilizing the shoulder joint. Here we simply add the idea that it *also* operates as part of the Deep Back Arm Line, a functionally connected meridian of myofascia that runs from the little finger to the thoracic and cervical spine.

Also, while this book includes most of the body's named muscles within the lines, certain muscles are not easily placed within this metaphor. The deep lateral rotators of the hip, for example, are construed fascially to be part of the Deep Front Line. They do not really lend themselves, however, to being part of any long line of fascial transmission. These muscles are most easily seen as combining with others around the hip to present a series of three interlinked fans.[1]

Those muscles not named as part of the Anatomy Trains map are obviously still active in a coordinated fashion with others in the body, but may not be operating along these articulated chains of myofascia.

A Comprehensive Theory of Movement

While some movements definitely take place along the meridian lines, anything more complex than the simplest reflex or gesture defies description in terms of the action of a single line. Splitting wood with an axe involves shortening the Superficial Front Line with elongation of the Superficial Back Line, but shifting the axe head around back on your dominant side for another blow involves a shifting complex of lines – Spiral, Functional, Lateral. Global actions involved in joint fixation or trunk stabilization, or whole-body stretches are more amenable to Anatomy Trains analysis and readily conform to the meridians. Thus the system lends itself to postural analysis, which depends primarily upon fixation.

Each meridian describes one very precise line of pull through the body, and most complex movements, of course, sweep across the body, changing their angles of pull second by second (for example, the footballer kicking or the discus thrower). Although an Anatomy Trains analysis could probably be made of complex movements, it is not clear that this would add a great deal to contemporary kinesiological discussion. On the other hand, an analysis of which lines restrict the response of the body to the primary movement or stabilize to enable the primary movement – in other words, which lines of stabilization are overly tight, unnecessarily held, not engaging, or dangerously lax – is very useful and leads to new strategies for structural unfolding toward balance.

The Only Way to Parse Body Structure

Many forms of structural analysis are abroad in the world.[2–4] The method described in Chapter 11 has shown itself to be useful in practice, and has the advantage of being psychologically neutral. Some approaches overlay a grid, plumb line, or some form of platonic 'normal' or neutral on the varieties of human physique. We prefer to keep the frame of reference to relationships within the individual only.

A Complete Anatomy Text

Although the subject of this book is musculoskeletal relationships, it is not designed as a comprehensive anatomy text. Anatomy Trains could be described as a 'longitudinal anatomy'. The use of any good regionally organized anatomy atlas as a supplement to the text and illustrations included here is recommended[5–9] (www.anatomytrains.com – video ref: Myofascial Meridians).

A Scientifically Supported Theory

The concepts in this book are backed by the anecdotal evidence of years in practice, and are successfully being applied by therapists in a number of different disciplines. The evidence from dissection included is an early indication that supports the ideas, which have not yet been confirmed by detailed dissection or other scientifically reliable evaluation. Caveat emptor – Anatomy Trains is a work in progress.

How We Present the Lines

Presentation of three-dimensional, living and moving anatomy on the quiet two-dimensional page has plagued anatomy teachers since Renaissance times when Jan Stefan van Kalkar started drawing for Andreas Vesalius. The myofascial meridians can be described in a variety of ways: as a strict one-dimensional line, as an articular chain of myofascia, as part of a broader fascial plane, or as a volumetric space (see Figs. 1.20–1.22). We have attempted to blend all four of these in this book, in hopes of catching the reader's imagination with one or more of them. The medium of the map is, as always, inadequate to the territory, but nevertheless can be helpful.

The precise lines with their tracks and stations, with summaries of postural and movement function, are laid out at the beginning of each chapter, with the articulated chains of myofascia described in the chapter body. Larger issues around the lines are discussed at the end of each chapter; smaller issues are noted in the text via the icons. The first line described (Ch. 3, the Superficial Back Line) lays out the terminology and concepts used throughout the rest of the chapters, and is thus worth reviewing first.

Each chapter also contains a guide to palpation and movement of the line, designed as a guide for both consumer and practitioner. While some clinical approaches are discussed, individual techniques, many of which come from the library of Structural Integration,[2] are presented sparsely for several reasons.

For one, the Anatomy Trains can be successfully applied across a variety of manual and movement techniques; presentation of any one set of techniques would be unnecessarily exclusive of others. It is the author's intention for this theory to contribute to the dialogue and cross-pollination across technical and professional boundaries.

Given the limitations in presenting a living technique in a book, the author prefers teaching from hand to hand with a feeling unattainable in book form. If the reader acquires an appetite for techniques to deal with the patterns revealed by the meridians analysis, so much the better. Seek out a class or a mentor – though despite the limitations, many of the techniques referred to are covered in a parallel book.[10] Online education concerning our fascial release techniques are available from www.anatomytrains.com.

Chapters 10 and 11 present specific applications of the system in terms of structural and movement analysis of some applications with which the author has some familiarity. It is fervently hoped that practitioners in other disciplines will carry this type of analysis into their own field of expertise.

References

1. Myers T. Fans of the hip joint. Massage Magazine No. 75, 1998.
2. Rolf I. *Rolfing*. Rochester, VT: Healing Arts Press; 1977.
3. Aston J. *Aston Postural Assessment Workbook*. San Antonio, TX: Therapy Skill Builders; 1998.
4. Keleman S. *Emotional Anatomy*. Berkeley, CA: Center Press; 1985.
5. Netter F. *Atlas of Human Anatomy*. 2nd ed. East Hanover, NJ: Novartis; 1997.
6. Clemente C. *Anatomy: A Regional Atlas*. 4th ed. Philadelphia: Lea and Febiger; 1995.
7. Biel A. *Trail Guide to the Body*. Boulder, CO: Discovery Books; 1997.
8. Ross L, Lamperti E. *Atlas of Anatomy*. New York: Thieme; 2006.
9. Gorman D. *The Body Moveable*. Guelph, Ontario: Ampersand Press; 1978.
10. Earls J, Myers T. *Fascial Release for Structural Balance*. 2nd ed. Berkeley: North Atlantic; 2017.

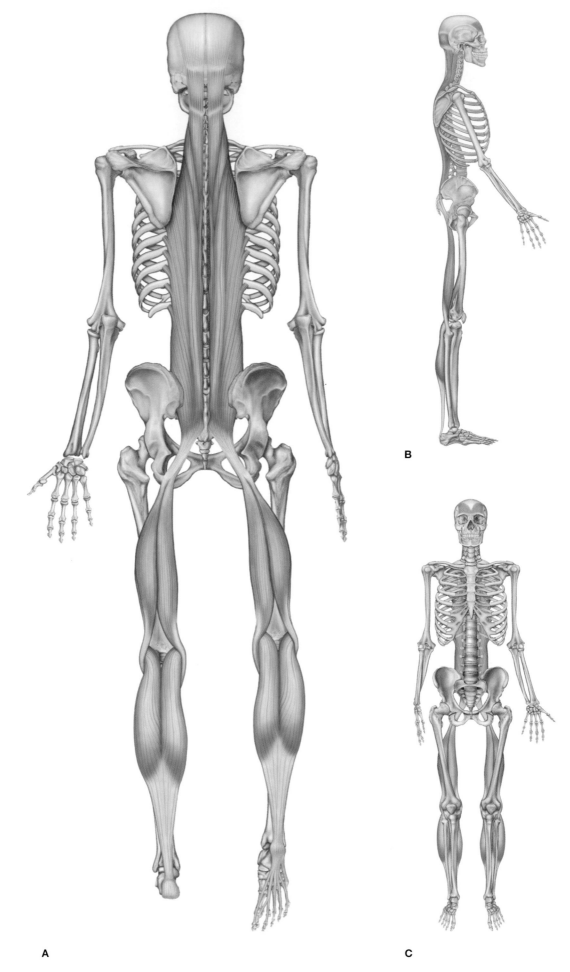

A

B

C

• **Fig. 3.1** The Superficial Back Line.

3

The Superficial Back Line

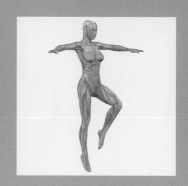

This first line, the Superficial Back Line (SBL) (Fig. 3.1), is presented in considerable detail, in order to clarify some of the general and specific Anatomy Trains concepts. Subsequent chapters employ the terminology and format developed in this chapter. Whichever line interests you, it may help to read this chapter first.

OVERVIEW

The Superficial Back Line (SBL) connects and protects the entire posterior surface of the body like a carapace from the bottom of the foot to the top of the head in two pieces – toes to knees, and knees to brow (Fig. 3.2/Table 3.1; Videos 2.2, 6.15). When the knees are extended, as in standing, the SBL functions as one continuous line of integrated myofascia. The SBL can be dissected as a unity, seen here both on its own and laid over a plastic skeleton (Figs. 3.3 and 3.4, see also Fig. 1.13; Video 4.3).

Postural Function

The overall postural function of the SBL is to support the body in full upright extension, to prevent the tendency to curl over into flexion exemplified by the fetal position. This all-day postural function requires a higher proportion of slow-twitch, endurance muscle fibers in the muscular portions of this myofascial band. The constant postural demand also requires extra-heavy sheets and bands in the fascial portion, as in the plantar aponeurosis, Achilles tendon, within the hamstrings, the sacrotuberous ligament, thoracolumbar fascia, the 'cables' of the erector spinae, and the sweeping nuchal ligament at the occipital ridge.

The exception to the extension function comes at the knees, which, unlike other joints, are flexed to the rear by the muscles of the SBL. In standing, the interlocked tendons of the SBL assist the cruciate ligaments in maintaining the postural alignment between the tibia and the femur.

Movement Function

With the exception of flexion from the knees on down, the overall movement function of the SBL is to create extension and hyperextension. In human development, the muscles of the SBL lift the baby's head from embryological flexion, with progressive engagement and 'reaching out' through the eyes, supported by the SBL down through the rest of the body to the ground – belly, seat, knees, feet – as the child achieves stability in each of the developmental stages leading to upright standing about one year after birth (Fig. 3.5, see also Figs. 10.38–10.44).

Because we are born in a flexed position, with our focus very much inward, the development of strength, competence, and balance in the SBL is intimately linked with the slow wave of maturity, as we move from this primary flexion into a full and easily maintained extension. The author of Psalm 121, who wrote 'I will lift up mine eyes unto the hills, from whence cometh my help', is enabled to do so by the Superficial Back Line.

The Superficial Back Line in Detail

NOTE: We begin most of the major 'cardinal' lines (those lines on the front, back, and sides) at their distal or caudal end. This is merely a convention; we could have as easily worked our way down from the head. The body will frequently create and distribute tension either way, or a bind in the middle will work its way out toward both ends. No causation is implied in our choice of where to start.

General Considerations

The most general statement that can be made about any of these Anatomy Trains lines is that strain, tension (good and bad), trauma, and the force that movement creates tend to be passed through the structure along these fascial lines of transmission.

The SBL is a cardinal line primarily mediating posture and movement in the sagittal plane, either limiting forward movement (flexion) or exaggerating or maintaining excessive backward movement (extension).

Although we speak of the SBL in the singular, there are, of course, two SBLs, one on the right and one on the left, and imbalances between the two SBLs should be observed

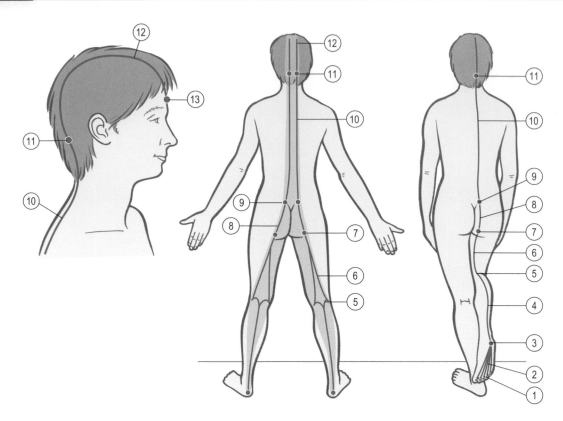

• **Fig. 3.2** Superficial Back Line tracks and stations. The shaded area shows where it affects and is affected by the more superficial fasciae (dermis, adipose, and the deeper fascia profundis). (Video 6.15)

TABLE 3.1	Superficial Back Line: Myofascial 'Tracks' and Bony 'Stations' (Fig. 3.2)	
Bony Stations		**Myofascial Tracks**
Frontal bone, supraorbital ridge	13	
	12	Galea aponeurotica/epicranial fascia
Occipital ridge	11	
	10	Sacrolumbar fascia/erector spinae
Sacrum	9	
	8	Sacrotuberous ligament
Ischial tuberosity	7	
	6	Hamstrings
Condyles of femur	5	
	4	Gastrocnemius/Achilles tendon
Calcaneus	3	
	2	Plantar fascia and short toe flexors
Plantar surface of toe phalanges	1	

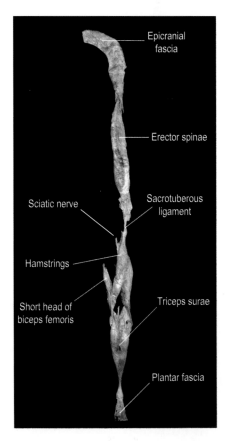

• **Fig. 3.3** The Superficial Back Line dissected away from the body and laid out as a whole. The different sections are labeled, but the dissection indicates the limitation of thinking solely in anatomical 'parts' in favor of seeing these meridians as functional 'wholes'.

and corrected along with addressing bilateral patterns of restriction in this line.

Common postural compensation patterns associated with the SBL include: ankle dorsiflexion limitation, knee hyperextension, hamstring shortness (often as a substitution for inadequate deep lateral rotators), anterior pelvic shift, sacral nutation, lordosis, extensor widening in thoracic flexion, suboccipital limitation leading to upper cervical hyperextension, anterior shift or rotation of the occiput on the atlas, and eye–spine movement (oculo-motor reflex) disconnection.

From Toes to Heel

Our originating 'station' on this long line of myofascia is the underside of the distal phalanges of the toes. The first 'track' runs along the under surface of the foot. It includes the plantar fascia and the tendons and muscles of the short toe flexors originating in the foot.

These five bands blend into one aponeurosis that runs into the front of the heel bone (the antero-inferior aspect of the calcaneus). The plantar fascia picks up an additional and important 6th strand from the 5th metatarsal base, the lateral band, which blends into the SBL on the outside edge of the heel bone (Figs. 3.6 and 3.7).

These fasciae, and their associated muscles that pull across the bottom of the foot, form an adjustable 'bowstring' to the longitudinal foot arches. This bowstring helps to approximate the two ends, thus maintaining the heel and the 1st and 5th metatarsal heads in a proper relationship (Fig. 3.8). The plantar aponeurosis constitutes only one of

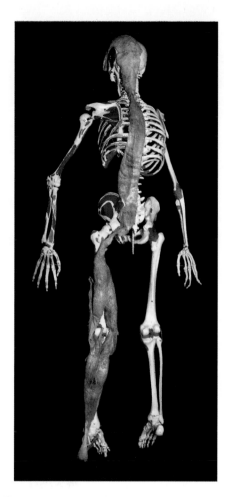

• **Fig. 3.4** The same specimen laid out on a classroom skeleton to show how the whole is arrayed. The cadaver was a good deal taller than the skeleton. (Video 4.3)

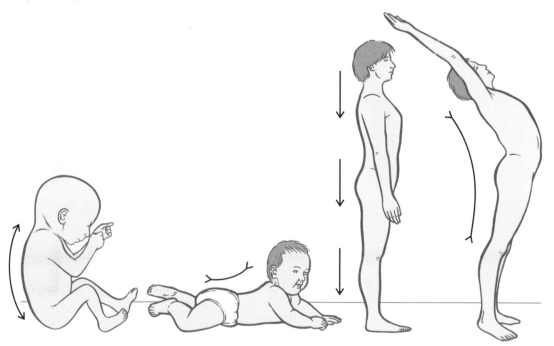

• **Fig. 3.5** In development, the SBL shortens to move us from a fetal curve of primary flexion toward the counterbalancing curves of upright posture. Further shortening of the muscles of the SBL produces hyperextension.

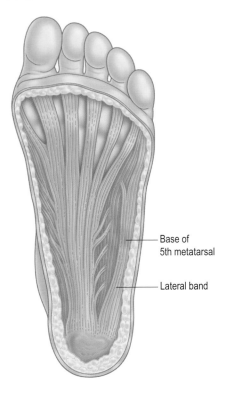

• **Fig. 3.6** The plantar fascia, the first track of the SBL, including the lateral band.

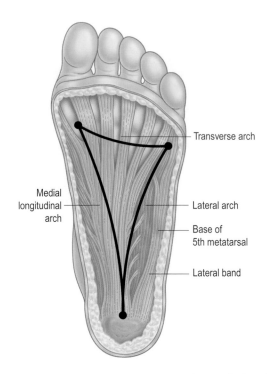

• **Fig. 3.8** The plantar aponeurosis forms a 'trampoline' under the arches – one springy arch between each point of contact: the 5th metatarsal head, the 1st metatarsal head, and the heel. (Video 3.4)

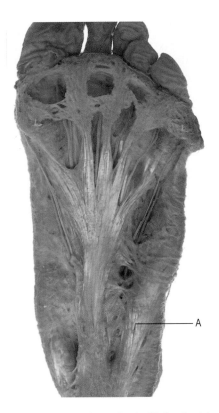

• **Fig. 3.7** A dissection of the plantar fascia. Notice the lateral band (A) comprising a somewhat separate but related track. (© Ralph T. Hutchings. Reproduced from McMinn, et al. 1993.)

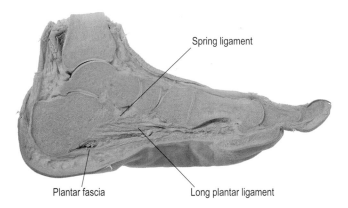

• **Fig. 3.9** A sagittal section of the medial longitudinal arch, showing how the plantar fascia and other tissues deep to it form a series of 'bowstrings' which help to hold up and act as springs for the medial arch. (© Ralph T. Hutchings. Reproduced from Abrahams, et al. 1993.)

these bowstrings – the long plantar ligament and spring ligament also provide shorter and stronger bowstrings deeper (more cephalad) into the tarsum of the foot (visible below the subtalar joint in Fig. 3.9, see also Fig. 3.34).

❧ ❖ The Plantar Fascia

The plantar aponeurosis of the foot is often a source of trouble that communicates up through the rest of the line. Limitation here often correlates with tight hamstrings, lumbar lordosis, and resistant hyperextension in the upper cervicals. Although structural work with the plantar surface often involves a lot of knuckles and fairly hefty stretching of this dense fascia, any method that aids in releasing it will communicate to the tissues above (www.anatomytrains.com – video ref: Superficial Back Line, 10:57–16:34). If your hands are not up to the task, consider using the 'ball under the foot' technique described below in 'A simple test'.

Compare the inner and outer aspect of your client's foot. While the outer part of the foot (base of little toe to heel) is always shorter than the inner aspect (from base of big toe to heel), there is a common balanced proportion. If the inner aspect of the foot is proportionally short, the foot will often be slightly lifted off the medial surface (as if supinated or inverted) and seemingly curved toward the big toe in a 'cupped hand' pattern, as if a slightly cupped hand were placed palm down on the table. In these cases, it is the medial edge of the plantar fascia that needs opening.

The plantar surface of the foot is often a source of trouble that communicates up through the leg. If the outer aspect of the foot is short – if the little toe is retracted or the 5th metatarsal base is pulled toward the heel, or if the outer aspect of the heel seems pulled forward – then the outer edge of the plantar fascia, especially its lateral band, needs to be lengthened (www.anatomytrains.com – video ref: Superficial Back Line, 20:29–22:25). This pattern often accompanies a weak inner arch and the dumping of the weight onto the inner part of the foot, but can occur without the fallen arch.

Even in the relatively balanced foot, the plantar surface can usually benefit from enlivening work to make it more supple and communicative, especially in our urbanized culture where the feet stay locked up in leather coffins all day (Video 3.5). A default approach to the plantar tissues is to lengthen between each of the points that support the arches: the heel, the 1st metatarsal head, and the 5th meta-tarsal head (see Fig. 3.8; Video 3.4).

❖ ❖ *A Simple Test*

For a sometimes dramatic and easily administered test of the relatedness of the entire SBL, have your client do a forward bend, as if to touch the toes with the knees straight (Fig. 3.10). Note the bilateral contour of the back and the resting position of the hands. Draw your client's attention to how it feels along the back of the body on each side.

Have your client return to standing and roll a tennis ball (or a golf ball for the hardy) deeply into the plantar fascia on one foot only (usually the side with more limited move-ment), being slow and thorough with the pressure rather than fast and vigorous. Keep it up for at least a couple of minutes, making sure the whole territory is covered from the ball of all five toes back to the front edge of the heel, the whole triangle shown in Fig. 3.8.

Now have the client do the forward bend again and note the bilateral differences in back contour and the distance of each hand from the floor (and draw the client's attention to the difference in feeling). In most people this will produce a dramatic demonstration of how working in one small part can affect the functioning of the whole. This will work for many people, but not all: for the most easily assessable

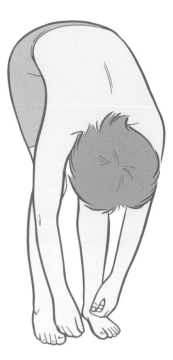

• **Fig. 3.10** A forward bend with the knees straight links and challenges all the tracks and stations of the Superficial Back Line. Work in one area, e.g. the plantar fascia, can affect motion and length anywhere and everywhere along the line. After work on the right plantar surface, the right arm hangs lower.

results, avoid those with a strong scoliosis or other blatant bilateral asymmetries.

Since this also functions as a treatment, do not forget to carry out the same procedure on the other side after you both assess any difference.

It is difficult in this test to determine how much of the effect is neurological and how much is due to a physiologi-cal change in the fascia. For our purposes, the cause is less important than the sense of how regions of the body are connected longitudinally by these continuities.

❖ ❖ *Heel Spurs*

It is 'common knowledge' that the muscles attach to bones – but this commonsense view is simply not the case for most myofasciae. The plantar fascia is a good case in point. People who run on the balls of their feet, for instance, or others who, for some reason, put repetitive strain on the plantar fascia, tug constantly on the calcaneal attachment of the plantar fascia. Since this fascia is not really attached to the calcaneus but rather blends into its periosteal 'plastic wrap' covering, it is possible in some cases for the periosteum to be progressively tugged away from the calcaneus, creating a space, a kind of 'tent', between this fabric and the bone (Fig. 3.11).

Between most periostea and their associated bones lie many osteoblasts – bone-building cells. These cells are con-stantly cleaning and rebuilding the outer surface of the bone. In both the original creation and the continuing maintenance of their associated bone, the osteoblasts are programed with a simple commandment: Thou shalt fill in

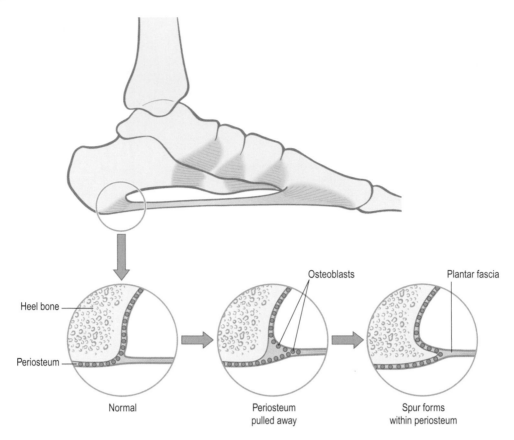

• **Fig. 3.11** The formation of a heel spur by the osteoblasts, which fill in bony matrix under the pulled-away periosteum, illustrates both the adaptability of the connective tissue system and one limitation of the simplistic 'muscles attach to bones' concept.

the bag of the periosteum. Clients who create repetitive strain in the plantar fascia are likely to create plantar fasciitis anywhere along the plantar surface where it tears and inflames. If instead the periosteum of the calcaneus gives way and comes away from the bone, then the osteoblasts will fill in the 'tent' under the periosteum, creating a bone spur. The spur itself and the spurring process are natural and not inherently painful; the pain comes if the spur interferes with a sensory nerve, as a heel spur often does with the fibular nerve.

🌸 From Heel to Knee

As discussed in Chapter 2, the fasciae do not just attach to the heel bone and stop (as implied in Fig. 3.11). They actually attach to the collagenous covering of the calcaneus, the periosteum, which surrounds the bone like a tough plastic wrapping. If we begin to think in this way, we can see that the plantar fascia is thus continuous with anything else that attaches to that periosteum. If we follow the periosteum around the calcaneus, especially underneath it around the heel to the posterior surface (following a thick and continuous band of fascia – see Figs. 3.12 and 3.15B), we find ourselves at the beginning of the next long stretch of track that starts with the Achilles tendon (Figs. 3.12 and 3.13).

Because the Achilles tendon must withstand so much tension, it is attached not only to the periosteum but also into the collagenous network of the heel bone itself, just as a tree is rooted into the ground. Leaving the calcaneus and its periosteum, our train passes up the Achilles, getting wider and flatter as it goes (see Fig. 3.12). Three myofascial structures feed into the Achilles tendon: the soleus from the profound side, the gastrocnemius from the superficial side, and the little plantaris in the middle.

Let us take this first connection we have made – from the plantar fascia around the heel to the Achilles tendon – as an example of the unique clinical implications that come out of the myofascial continuities point-of-view.

🌸 ❖ 🌸 *Heel as Arrow*

In simple terms, the heel is the patella of the ankle, as we can see in the X-ray of a foot (Fig. 3.14). From a 'tensegrity' point of view, the calcaneus is a compression strut that pushes the tensile tissues of the SBL out away from the ankle to create proper tone around the back of the tibio-talar fulcrum, with the soft tissue spanning from knee to toes. (Contrast this leverage with the proximity of the joint-stabilizing muscles: the fibularii (peroneals) of the Lateral Line that snake right around the lateral malleolus. Similarly, the long toe flexors of the Deep Front Line pass close behind

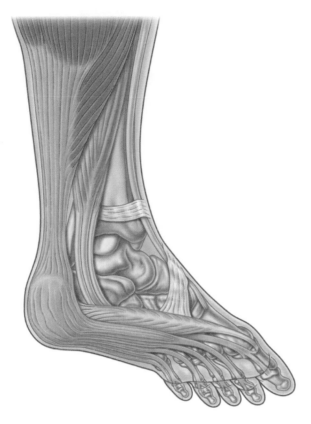

• **Fig. 3.12** Around the heel, there is a strong and dissectable fascial continuity between the plantar fascia and the Achilles tendon and its associated muscles.

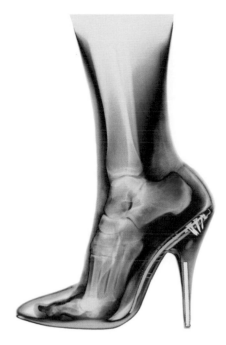

• **Fig. 3.14** This X-ray of a dancer's foot shows how the calcaneus functions in a way parallel to the patella – what the patella does on the front of the knee, the calcaneus does on the back of the ankle – namely, pushing the soft tissue away from the fulcrum of the joint to give it more leverage. (© Bryan Whitney, reproduced with permission.)

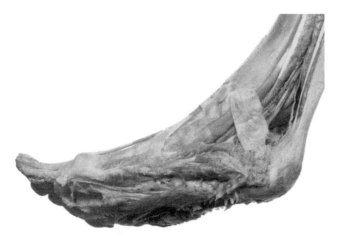

• **Fig. 3.13** A dissection of the heel area demonstrates the continuity from plantar tissues to the muscles in the superficial posterior compartment of the leg. (© Ralph T. Hutchings. Reproduced from Abrahams, et al. 1998.)

the medial malleolus, lending them more ankle stabilization advantage, but less leverage for jumping.)

To see the clinical problem this patterning can create, imagine this lower section of the Superficial Back fascial line – the plantar fascia and Achilles-associated fascia – as a bowstring, with the heel notched into it like an arrow (Fig. 3.15; Video 6.7). As the SBL chronically over-tightens (common in those with the ubiquitous urban postural fault

of a forward lean of the legs and an anterior shift of the pelvis), it is capable of pushing the heel forward into the subtalar joint; or, in another common pattern, such extra tension can bring the tibia–fibula complex posteriorly on the talus, which amounts to the same thing.

To assess this, look at your client's foot from the lateral aspect as they stand, and drop an imaginary vertical line down from the lower edge of the lateral malleolus (or, if you prefer, place your index finger vertically down from the tip of the malleolus to the floor). See how much of the foot lies in front of this line and how much behind. Anatomy dictates that there will be more foot in front of the line, but, with a little practice, you will be able to recognize a normal proportion (Fig. 3.16A) versus comparatively little heel behind this line (Fig. 3.16B).

Measure forward from the spot below the lateral malleolus to the 5th metatarsal head (toes are quite variable, so do not include them). Measure back from the spot to the place where the heel leaves the floor (the limit of its support). On a purely empirical clinical basis, this author finds that a proportion of 1 : 3 or 1 : 4 between the hindfoot and the forefoot offers effective support. A ratio of 1 : 5 or more indicates minimal support for the back of the body. This pattern can not only *result* in tightness in the SBL but can also *cause* more tightness as well, as it is often accompanied by a forward shift at the knees or pelvis to place more weight on the forefoot, which only tightens the SBL further. As long as this compensation pattern remains, it will prevent the client from feeling secure as you attempt to rebalance the hips over the feet.

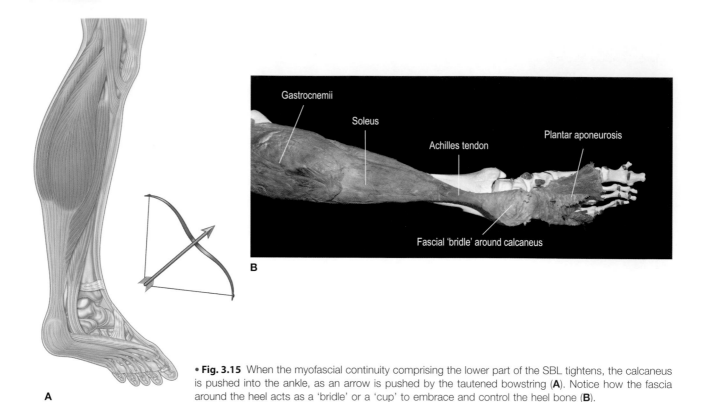

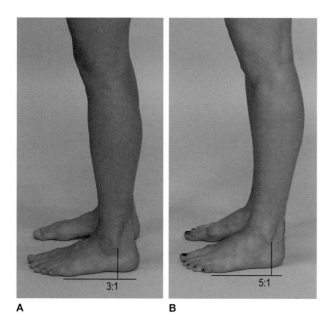

A

B

• Fig. 3.15 When the myofascial continuity comprising the lower part of the SBL tightens, the calcaneus is pushed into the ankle, as an arrow is pushed by the tautened bowstring (**A**). Notice how the fascia around the heel acts as a 'bridle' or a 'cup' to embrace and control the heel bone (**B**).

A   **B**

• Fig. 3.16 The amount of the foot in front of the ankle joint should be balanced by about ⅓ to ¼ behind the ankle joint, as in (**A**). Without this support for the back body, as in (**B**), the upper body will lean forward to place the weight on the front of the foot.

To those who say that this proportion is determined by heredity, or that it is impossible for the calcaneus to move significantly forward or backward in the joint, we suggest trying the following:

- release the plantar fascia, including the lateral band, in the direction of the heel (www.anatomytrains.com – video ref: Superficial Back Line, 10:57–16:34, 20:29–22:25);

- release the superficial posterior compartment of the leg (soleus and gastrocnemius) down toward the heel (www.anatomytrains.com – video ref: Superficial Back Line, 22:27–24:30);
- mobilize the heel by stabilizing the front of the tarsum with one hand while working the heel through its inversion and eversion movements in your cupped hand.

In more recalcitrant cases, it may be necessary to further release the ligaments of the ankle by working deeply but slowly from the corner of each malleolus (avoiding the nerves) diagonally to the postero-inferior corner of the heel bone. The result will be a small but visible change in the amount of foot behind the malleolar line, and a very palpable change in support for the back of the body in the client. Therefore, strategically, this work should precede any work designed to help with an anterior pelvic shift.

Please note that the mark of success is a visibly increased amount of heel when you reassess using the malleolus as your guide. Repetition may be called for until the forward lean in the client's posture is resolved by your other efforts (e.g. freeing the distal ends of the hamstrings, lifting the rectus femoris of the Superficial Front Line, etc.).

❖ ❖ ❧ 'Expresses' And 'Locals'

Two large muscles attach to the Achilles band: the soleus from the deep side, and the gastrocnemius from the superficial side (see Fig. 3.15A). The connection of the SBL is with the superficial muscle, the gastrocnemius. First, however, we have an early opportunity to demonstrate another Anatomy Trains concept, namely 'locals' and 'expresses'.

The importance of differentiating expresses and locals lies in this: postural position is most often held in the underlying locals, not in the more superficial expresses. Express trains of myofascia cross more than one joint; locals cross, and therefore act on, only one joint. With some exceptions in the forearms and lower leg, the locals are usually deeper in the body – more profound – than the expresses. (See Ch. 2 for a full definition and examples.)

This superficial posterior compartment of the lower leg is not, however, one of these exceptions: the two heads of the gastrocnemius cross both ankle and knee joints, and can act on both. The deeper soleus crosses only the ankle joint – passing from the heel to the posterior aspects of the tibia, interosseous membrane, and fibula – and acts only on this joint. (The so-called ankle joint is really two joints, consisting of the tibio-talar joint, which acts in plantar- and dorsiflexion, and the subtalar joint, which acts in what we will call inversion and eversion. Though the triceps surae – plantaris, gastrocnemius and soleus together – does have some effect on the subtalar joint, we will ignore that effect for now, designating the soleus a one-joint muscle for the purposes of this example.)

If we took the soleus local, we could keep going on the same fascial plane and come onto the fascia on the back of the popliteus, which crosses the knee and flexes it (and also rotates the tibia medially on the femur when the knee is flexed, though that is outside our current discussion). The gastrocnemius express can thus participate in both plantarflexion and knee flexion, while each of the two locals provides one action only. We will see this phenomenon repeated throughout the myofascial meridians.

❖ ✿ Derailment

Following the SBL via the gastrocnemius, we come to the first of many bends in the Anatomy Trains rules, which we will term 'derailments'. Derailments are exceptions to the Anatomy Trains rules, which can be explained in useful terms for soft-tissue and movement work. In a derailment, the Anatomy Trains still communicate, but only under particular conditions.

In order to understand this first important exception, we need to look more closely at the interface between the two heads of the gastrocnemius and the tendons of the three hamstrings (Fig. 3.17).

It is easy to see from comparing Fig. 1.1A with Fig. 3.17 that the gastrocnemius and hamstrings are both separate and connected. In dissection, strong areolar fascia clearly links from near the distal ends of the hamstrings to near the proximal ends of the gastrocnemii heads. In Fig. 3.17 this tissue has been dissected away; in Fig. 3.3 it has been retained. Such areolar tissue, long thought to be simply a passive 'filler', has now been shown to be an effective force transmitter when tightened.[1]

In practice, then, flexion of the knees delinks the upper leg from the lower in the back. While by strict Anatomy Trains rules they are not a myofascial continuity, they do function as one primarily when the knee is extended. The

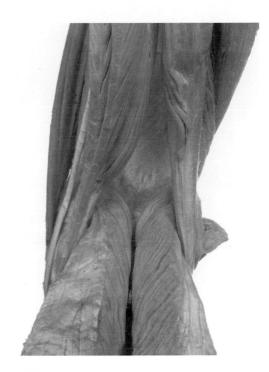

• **Fig. 3.17** The relationship between the heads of the gastrocnemii and the tendons of the hamstrings in the popliteal space behind the knee provide the key to the 'derailment' of the SBL. See also Fig. 3.3. (© Ralph T. Hutchings. Reproduced from Abrahams, et al. 1998.)

gastrocnemii heads reach up and around the hamstring tendons to insert onto the upper portions of the femoral condyles. The hamstrings reach down and around the gastrocnemii to attach to the tibia and fibula. As long as the knee is bent, these two myofascial units go their own ways, neighboring but loosely connected (Fig. 3.18A). As the knee joint comes into extension, however, the femoral condyles come back into this tendon complex, engaging these elements with each other, and making them function together almost as if they were two pairs of hands gripped at the wrists (Fig. 3.18B–C). This configuration also bears a strong resemblance to a square knot, loosened when the knee is bent, drawn taut as the knee straightens.

This provides a long-winded but accurate explanation of why it is less of a stretch to pick up your dropped keys from the floor by flexing your knees rather than keeping them extended (Fig. 3.19). A very slight flexion of the knees is sufficient to allow significantly more forward bend in the spine and hips. The traditional explanation is that the hamstrings are eased by the knee flexion, thus freeing the hips to flex more. In fact, bending the knees only a tiny amount, e.g. moving the knees forward a mere inch or a few centimeters, does not shorten the distance from the ischial tuberosity to the lower leg appreciably (apply Pythagoras' theorem), and yet it frees the hip flexion considerably. Our explanation would be that even a slight flexion loosens the square knot, unlinking the lower part of the SBL from the upper. The linked SBL is harder to stretch into a forward fold; the unlinked SBL is easier.

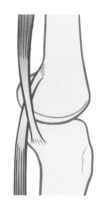
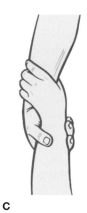
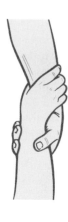

Femur

Hamstring

Tibia

Gastrocnemius

A B C

• **Fig. 3.18** When the knee is flexed, the myofascia of the thigh and the myofascia of the lower leg function separately (**A**). When the knee is extended, these myofasciae link into one connected functioning unit (**B**), like the interlocked hands of a pair of trapeze artists (**C** – compare to Fig. 3.17). The configuration is reminiscent of a reef or square knot; able to form a tight knot, yet readily loosened as well.

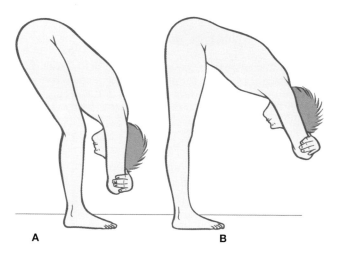

A B

• **Fig. 3.19** When the knees are bent (**A**), the upper and lower parts of the SBL are relatively separate, and it is easier to fold at the hips. With the knees extended (**B**), the SBL from toes to sacrum is linked into one unit, and a forward bend may not be as easy.

The entire SBL is a continuity in a regular standing posture. In yoga, for instance, postures (asanas) which utilize a forward bend with straightened legs (as in the Downward-Facing Dog, Plow, Forward Bend, or any simple hamstring stretch) will engage the SBL as a whole, whereas forward bends with the knees bent (e.g. Child's pose) will engage only the upper myofascia of the line, except in those with very short SBLs, for whom even flexing the knees is not enough to allow a full forward bend.

❖ ✿ *The Distal Hamstrings*

The interface between the heads of the gastrocnemii and the 'feet' of the hamstrings can get tied up; the result is usually not a flexed knee but a tibia that seems to sit posteriorly to the femur when viewed from the side.

This technique requires some finger strength, but tenacity will be rewarded. It also requires precise finger placement

to avoid pain for the client. Have your client lie prone, with one knee bent to near 90°. Support this foot with your sternum or shoulder, so that the hamstring can temporarily relax. Hook your fingers, palms facing laterally, inside the hamstrings at the back of the knee, 'swimming' in between these tendons (two on the inside and one on the lateral side) to rest on the heads of the gastrocnemii (see Fig. 3.17). Be sure to take a little skin with you and keep your fingers moving out against the hamstring tendons to avoid pressuring the endangerment site in the middle of the popliteal space. This technique should not produce any nerve pain, parasthesia, or radiating sensations. Have your client retake control over her leg, then remove your support. The hamstring tendons will pop out as they tense, so keep your fingers in position against the posterior surface of the distal femur.

Have your client slowly lower her foot to the table (extending the knee) as you move slowly up the inside of the hamstring tendons (but mostly simply maintaining your position, while the client does the work). The client will be lengthening both the hamstrings and gastrocnemii in eccentric contraction, freeing their distal ends from each other. When effectively done, this 'pin & stretch' will result in the tibia moving forward under the femur (www.anatomytrains.com – video ref: Superficial Back Line 25:56–28:45).

✿ From Knee to Hip

Assuming, then, that the legs are straight and the knees extended, we continue up the myofascial continuity provided by the hamstrings, which takes us to the posterior side of the ischial tuberosities (Fig. 3.20). The dual medial hamstrings, the semimembranosus and semitendinosus, are complemented by the single lateral hamstring, the biceps femoris (although the outer leg can also be seen as having two 'hamstrings' – see Ch. 6, p. 104). All three of our hamstrings are expresses, affecting both knee and hip.

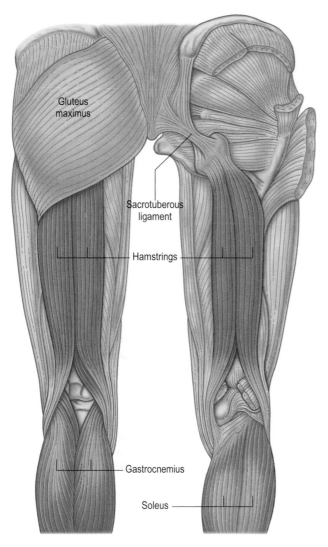

• **Fig. 3.20** A superficial view (left) shows the hamstrings disappearing under the gluteus maximus, but despite the gluteus being a superficial muscle on the back, it is not part of the SBL. It is disqualified by involving both a change in direction, and a change of level. Remove the gluteus (which will show up later as part of other lines) to see the clear connection from the hamstrings to the sacrotuberous ligament.

❖ ❖ Separating the Hamstrings

Much has been written about the hamstrings, but very little about the separate functions of the hamstrings. The medial hamstrings (semitendinosus and semimembranosus) create medial tibial rotation when the knee is flexed. The lateral hamstring (biceps femoris) creates lateral rotation of the lower leg on the femur in the same situation. To perform these separate functions, the two sets of muscles must be able to work separately. This differential movement between inner and outer hamstrings is especially important in sports or activities where the hips move side-to-side while there is pressure on the knee, as in jazz dance, slalom skiing, or dodging in football or rugby. In straightforward running – pure flexion and extension – this separation is not required as the inner and outer hamstrings always work in tandem.

To feel how far the inner and outer hamstring function is separated, have your client lie prone with the knee flexed for easier access. Begin to feel your way up the space between the two sets of hamstrings, just above the endangerment area in the popliteal space (see Figs. 3.17 and 3.20). Here it will be easy to feel the medial to lateral separation, for all three are quite tendinous, and at least an inch or two (3–5 cm) apart. Now move up toward the ischial tuberosity, being careful to stay in the 'valley' between the two sets of muscles. How far up can you feel a palpable valley? For some people, the entire group of three muscles will be bound together a few inches superior to the popliteal space; for others a division will be palpable halfway or more to the ischial tuberosity. In dissection the muscles can be separated up to within a few inches, around 10 cm, of the ischial tuberosity.

To test this functionally, have your prone client bend the knee you are assessing to a right angle, and then twist that foot to the limits of medial and lateral rotation – "Turn your shin in; turn your shin out" – while you rest a hand across the hamstring muscles and palpate to feel if they are working separately.

To treat bound hamstrings, insert (or wiggle or swim) your fingers in between the muscles at the lowest level of binding as your client continues to slowly rotate the lower leg medially and laterally with the knee bent. The binding fascia will gradually release, allowing your fingers to sink toward the femur. Continue working upward a few inches at a time until you reach the limit of that technique (www.anatomytrains.com – video ref: Superficial Back Line, 31:08–33:57).

❖ ❖ ❖ Rotation at the Knee

Although functional rotation of the knee is only possible when the knee is flexed, postural rotation of the tibia on the femur, medial or lateral, is quite common. Although several factors, including strain in peri-articular tissues and strains coming up from the foot, can contribute to this pattern, working differentially on the two sets of hamstrings can be very helpful in releasing the leg back into alignment.

If the tibia is medially rotated (as measured by the direction in which the tibial tuberosity faces relative to the patella – the outside edges of the patella and tibial tuberosity should form an isosceles triangle), then manual or stretching work on the medial set of hamstrings (semitendinosus and semi-membranosus) is required. If the tibia is turned laterally, work on the biceps femoris (both heads, but especially the short head) is necessary. The tissues should be worked toward the knee. Begin with whatever general stretching or work with the hamstrings you had planned, then do additional work on the relevant hamstring to reduce the rotation, using the client's slow eccentric lengthening of the tissues occasioned by bringing the knee from flexion to extension. The tissues that maintain these rotations are located deep within the hamstring myofascia. If this is not effective, delve further into possible strains deriving from foot position, pelvic torsions, or the Spiral Line (see Ch. 6).

Hip to Sacrum

If we are still thinking in terms of muscles, it is difficult to see how we can continue from here using the Anatomy Trains rules, for no muscle attaches to the ischial tuberosity in a direction continuous with the hamstrings. The gluteus maximus goes over the hamstring attachment, but it clearly runs in a more superficial fascial plane. Going onto the quadratus femoris, the adductor magnus, or the inferior gemellus, which are on a similar plane, would all involve a rule-breaking radical change of direction. If we think fascially, however, we are not stymied at all: the sacrotuberous ligament arises from the back of the tuberosity, demonstrably as a continuation of the hamstrings, and passes across to the lateral border of the sacrum, just above the sacrococcygeal junction (see Fig. 3.20).

The inferior end of the ligament is continuous with the hamstrings. In fact the tendon of the lateral hamstring, the biceps femoris, can actually be separated in dissection and traced up to the sacrum. (This part of the ligament is probably a degenerated muscle; we have only to look at our close mammalian friend, the horse, to see a biceps femoris muscle that runs all the way up to the sacrum. A horse sacrum, of course, bears less proportionate weight than our own and is allowed a good deal more freedom of movement than a human sacrum could possibly enjoy.)

Stations

Let us be clear about fascial communication at the stations, or attachments. Here we pause again for a fuller explanation, as this is a good example of the general functioning of an Anatomy Trains station. We are not saying that the entire sacrotuberous ligament is an extension of the hamstrings. The very strong, almost bone-like tensile connection between the sacrum and the ischial tuberosity is absolutely necessary for upright human posture and pelvic integrity. Without it, our 'tail' would pop up into the air, painfully and irretrievably, the very first time we bent over. The ligament is absolutely tacked down to the bones (at least to the periosteal wrapping) and cannot slide significantly as a whole either toward the hamstrings or the sacral fascia.

What we *are* saying is that the more superficial layers of fascia are continuous with the myofascia on either side, and are, or should be, able to communicate both movement and strain across the fascial fibers adjacent to the surface of the ligament (see Figs. 2.8 and 2.9). How many layers are able to communicate and how many are stuck down varies from person to person and depends on the person-specific mechanical needs of the area. In extremely stuck cases, the dermis of the skin will be tied down to other layers (sometimes creating a dimple in the skin), a sure indication of a station that is not communicating. In extremely loose cases, usually after some trauma, but sometimes due to overstretching or overmanipulating or simple 'ligamentous laxity' in their overall tissue tone, layers which should be intrinsic to the local stations become too communicative,

requiring extra myofascial tightening elsewhere to maintain some form of integrity at the sacroiliac joint.

The superior end of the deep ligament is likewise firmly joined to the sacrum, but more superficial connections spread to the other fasciae in the area, specifically down to the coccyx and up onto the posterior spine of the ilium. In dissection, it is possible to lift the superficial communicating fibers of the sacrotuberous ligament off the body maintaining their strong connection with the hamstrings and erector spinae fascia (as in Fig. 3.3).

The Sacrotuberous Ligament

The following, then, does not address the sacrotuberous ligament per se, but rather the tissue of the SBL that passes over the sacrotuberous ligament on its way from the hamstrings to the sacral fascia. Because the medial edge of the gluteus maximus attaches over the tissue we want to access, enter from the medial side of the heavy ligamentous line from the lower lateral aspect of the sacrum down, drawing the tissue down and laterally to the ischial tuberosity, or vice versa, depending on the pattern.

This tissue should generally be carried in a downward direction for those with an anterior tilt to the pelvis, and carried upward in those with a flat lumbar spine or a posterior tilt to the sacrum (www.anatomytrains.com – video ref: Superficial Back Line 35:03–36:35). Use a deep, firm, and consistent pressure, without chopping or digging, feeling for the slight but deep feeling of release.

From Sacrum to Occiput

From the superior end of the sacrotuberous ligament, our rules require that we keep going in roughly the same direction, and we have no trouble doing that: the erector spinae arise from the layers of sacral fascia continuous with the sacrotuberous ligament (Fig. 3.21; Video 3.7) (www.anatomytrains.com – video ref: Superficial Back Line, 1:04:24–1:06:52). The erector spinae span the spine from sacrum to occiput, with the expresses of the longissimus and iliocostalis complex overlying the ever deeper and shorter locals of the spinalis, semispinalis, and multifidus (Fig. 3.22). The deepest layer, the transversospinalis group, provides the shortest one-joint locals, which reveal the three basic patterns followed by all the erector muscles (Fig. 3.23). The functional anatomical details of all these muscle complexes have been ably covered elsewhere.[2–4]

The most superficial express layers of fascia in this complex tie sacrum to occiput. We should note that even though the erectors are part of what is termed the Superficial Back Line, several layers of even more superficial myofascia overlie the line here in the form of the serratus posterior muscles, the splenii, the rhomboids, the levator scapulae, and the superficial shoulder musculature of the trapezius and latissimus dorsi. These muscles form parts of the Spiral, Arm, and Functional Lines, and are addressed in Chapters 6, 7, and 8, respectively.

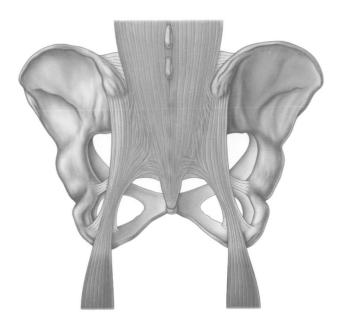

• **Fig. 3.21** With a knife, it is possible to isolate the sacrotuberous liga-ment as a separate structure. In life, though, it (at least superficially) connects both up to the sacral fascia and the erector spinae and down to the biceps femoris and the medial hamstrings as well. (Video 3.7)

❖ ❖ ❖ *Erector Spinae Fascia*

The methods for treating the back muscles are myriad and so diverse that many books would be required to detail all of them. We include a few global considerations and techniques.

Since the erector spinae cover the posterior side of the spinal curves, they co-create the depth of these curves, along with the muscles and ligaments that attach to the front of the spine in the neck and the lumbars (see Ch. 9 on the Deep Front Line). With that in mind, our first consideration is the depth of the curves in the spine: is there a lumbar or cervical lordosis, or a thoracic kyphosis? Observe: do the spinous processes protrude like bumps or a ridge beyond the surrounding tissue (are they 'mountains'?); or do they sink below the surrounding myofascial tissue in a groove (do they form 'valleys'?).

The general rule is counter-intuitive: pile up on the mountains, and dig out the valleys. Myofascial tissue has spread away from the spinous processes that protrude (as in a hyperkyphosis), first widening and subsequently adher-ing to surrounding layers. These tissues ask to be moved medially, toward the spinous processes, not only to free the tissues for movement, but also to give some forward impetus to those vertebrae that are too far back. Conversely, when the vertebrae are buried deep (as in a hyperlordosis), contiguous myofascial tissues migrate medially and tighten, forming the bowstring to the bow in that part of the spine. These tissues must be lengthened but also moved laterally, progressively from superficial to deep. This will allow the buried vertebrae some room and slack into which they can move back.

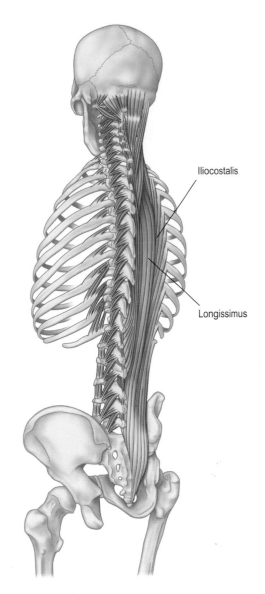

• **Fig. 3.22** The erector spinae form the next track of the SBL. The muscles run from the sacrum to the occiput; the fascia runs from the sacrotuberous ligament to the scalp fascia. On the left are some of the underlying 'locals' of the transversospinalis – intertransversarii, rotatores, and levatores costarum.

To assess the ability to lengthen at various levels of the spine, seat your client on a stool (or on the edge of a treat-ment table, provided it is low enough for the client's feet to be comfortably on the floor). Help your client assume an upright posture, with the weight on the ischial tuberosities and the head lengthened away from the floor but still hori-zontal (looking straight ahead). Instruct your client to drop his chin toward his chest until he feels a comfortable stretch in the back of the neck. Let the weight of his forehead begin to carry him forward, 'one vertebra at a time', while you stand beside him and watch. Look for places where the individual spinous processes do not move away from each other like a train pulling out of the station one car at a time. In all but the healthiest of spines, you will find places where a couple or even a whole clump of vertebrae move together,

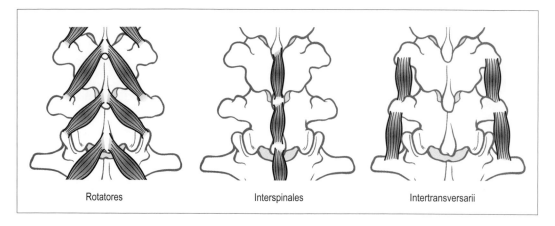

Rotatores   Interspinales   Intertransversarii

• **Fig. 3.23** The deepest level of the spinal musculature demonstrates three primary patterns: spinous process to transverse process, spinous process to spinous process, and transverse process to transverse process. The more superficial muscles can be seen as ever-longer express versions of these primary local functions.

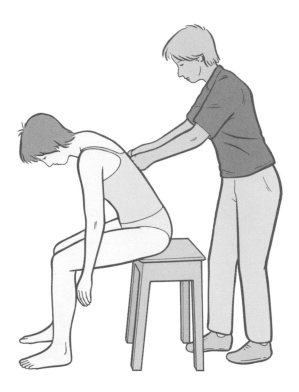

• **Fig. 3.24** Working the erector spinae and associated fascia in eccentric contraction from a bench is a very effective way of creating change in the myofascial function around the spine.

without any differentiation. Really bound clients may move the spine as a whole, getting most of their forward motion through flexion at the hips, rather than by curling or flexing the spine itself (Fig. 3.24).

The assessment can turn into treatment very easily by putting your hand gently on a stiff area and encouraging your client to find the bend or movement in that part of the spine. More assertive manual treatment can follow for defiantly stiff areas. Stand behind the bench, and as the client begins to roll forward with the chin slightly tucked,

place the dorsal surface of all the proximal phalanges (in English: an open, soft fist) on both sides of the spine at the level of the cervicothoracic junction. Move down as the client curls forward, keeping pace with him, moving tissue down and out or down and in (depending on the 'mountains' and 'valleys') as you go. You should reach the sacral fascia at about the same time he is fully forward, chest to thigh (www.anatomytrains.com – video ref: Superficial Back Line, 36:44–57:04).

It is very important that the client stay grounded, pushing back against your pressure from his feet, but not from the back or neck. For best results, it is important that the client's feet not be hanging, but rather firmly planted. This technique should be totally comfortable for the client; desist immediately if it is painful in the low back (but because of the eccentric load on the muscles and fascial sheets, those with low back problems are often fine with this technique). Your pressure should be more down the back than forward into it.

For more specific work, a knuckle may be used as an applicator, and a 'seeing' elbow is also good for opening heavier fascial sheets and ropes.

There is a variation that can be good in the case of a kyphotic spine, but may only be applied to those with a strong lower back. Lower back pain during this technique contraindicates the treatment. Have your client begin the spinal flexion movement as detailed above. When your applicator (fist, elbow, knuckle) is at the most posterior part of the thoracic curve (which is likely to be the tightest, most frozen area as well), instruct your client to 'curve in the opposite direction; bring your sternum to the wall in front of you' like the Sphinx or a Cobra in yoga. Maintain your position in the back as he opens into hyperextension with flexed hips (somewhat like a figurehead on the old ships). This can produce dramatic opening in the chest and thoracic spine.

These techniques can be repeated a number of times, within a session or in successive sessions, without negative effect – as long as it remains pleasurable, not painful, for the client.

❖ ❧ ❖ ❧ The Suboccipitals

Many techniques for general traction and stretching of neck tissues, as well as muscle-specific techniques for cervical musculature, have been well documented elsewhere, and these can be effectively used in terms of the SBL (www.anatomytrains.com – video ref: Superficial Back Line, 1:00:00–1:02:20). The deepest layers of posterior cervical muscles (the suboccipital 'star') are crucial to opening up the entire SBL; indeed, the rectus capitis posterior and obliquus capitis muscles can be considered the functional centerpieces of the SBL (Fig. 3.25). The high number of stretch receptors in these tissues, and their essential link from the eye movements to coordination of the rest of the back musculature, ensure their central role. These muscles have been shown to have 36 muscle spindles per gram of muscle tissue; the gluteus maximus, by contrast, has 0.7 spindles per gram.[5] Thus the suboccipitals might be said to be around 50 times 'smarter' than the gluteus – but look in vain to find a machine for exercising these essential muscles in any modern gym.

To feel this linkage for yourself, put your hands up on either side of your head with your thumbs just under the back of your skull. Work your thumbs gently in past the superficial muscles so that you can feel the deeper tissues under the occipital ridge. Close your eyes. Now, move your eyes right and left, while your palms, essentially over your ears, ensure that your head is still. Can you feel the small changes of muscle tonus under your thumbs? Even though your head is not moving, these ancient and primary muscles are responding to your eye movements. Look up and down and you will feel other muscles within this set engage in a similar way. Try to move your eyes without these muscles moving; you will find that it is nearly impossible. They are so fundamentally connected – and have been for nearly our entire vertebral history – that any eye movement will produce a change in tonus in these suboccipitals. Altering this deep neural 'programming' is difficult, but is sometimes necessary for vision or reading disorders, and certain

problems of the neck.* The rest of the spinal muscles 'listen' to these suboccipitals and tend to organize by following their lead.

The adage 'A cat always lands on its feet' is also an illustration of this concept. When a cat finds itself in the air, it uses its eyes and inner ear to orient its head horizontally. This puts certain tensions into these suboccipital muscles, which the brain reads from the myriad stretch receptors, and then reflexively orders the rest of the spinal muscles to re-organize the entire spinal orientation from the neck down, so that the cat's feet are under it before it ever hits the carpet. Though our spines are upright, our head–neck–upper back relationship functions in much the same way. Thus, how you use your eyes, and more particularly, how you use your neck, determines the tonus pattern for the rest of your spinal musculature. This plays into a number of postural patterns we see every day in our practice: loosening, lengthening, and organizing the neck is often key to intransigent problems between the shoulder blades, in the lower back, and even in the hips.

Retracting the neck and head is also a fundamental part of the fear response. Most animals respond to fear with a retraction of the head, and humans are no exception (Video 3.6). Since most of us do not get out of childhood without some unresolved fear, this retraction, either as a habit before we begin a movement or as a permanent postural state, becomes built into our movement as a socially acceptable, unobserved, but ever-so-damaging state of being. Being so deep and of such long standing, such a habit is not easy to root out – teachers of the Alexander Technique spend years at it – but the effort is worthwhile for the psychological and physical feeling of freedom it gives.

The four suboccipital muscles which are a part of the SBL are the rectus capitis posterior minor (RCPM), the rectus capitis posterior major (RCPMaj), the obliquus capitis superior (OCS), and the obliquus capitis inferior (OCI). They run among the occiput, the atlas (C1), and the axis (C2). The transverse processes (TPs) of C1 are quite large, while the spinous process (SP) is quite small. To feel the relative position of the C1 TPs, have your client lie supine, and sit at the head end of the table with your hands around the skull such that the *intermediate* phalanx of both your index fingers lies against the mastoid processes, leaving the distal bone free. Your wrists should be close to or on the table, so that your index finger follows roughly the direction of the sternocleidomastoid (SCM). Now gently flex the distal part of your index fingers into the flesh just inferior to the mastoid. If your wrists are too far off the table and your fingers are pointing down at it, you will miss the atlas. If your wrists are too low or your index finger is in front of the mastoid, you will go into the space between the jaw and the mastoid, which is definitely not recommended. Sometimes you can feel the TPs directly, just inferior and anterior

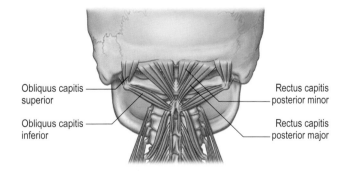

Obliquus capitis superior

Obliquus capitis inferior

Rectus capitis posterior minor

Rectus capitis posterior major

• **Fig. 3.25** The small but central suboccipital set of muscles is the functional centerpiece of the SBL – thus requiring more detailed views than this one directly from the back.

*Moshe Feldenkrais developed a series of elegant 'lessons' for disengaging these habits, to be found in his book *Awareness Through Movement*.

to the mastoid; sometimes, because so many muscles are competing for attachment space on the TP, you can only feel them by implication. If, however, you keep the middle phalanx in contact with the mastoid process, with a little practice you will be able to feel accurately whether one TP is more prominent than the other (indicating a lateral translation or shift to the prominent side); or forward of the other (indicating a rotation at the atlanto-occipital (O-A) joint), or closer to the skull than the other (indicating a lateral flexion or tilt between the two).

The OCI is badly named, since it does not attach directly to the head, but runs from the large SP of the axis to the large TPs of the atlas, somewhat like the reins on a horse (Fig. 3.26). This muscle parallels the splenius capitis and provides the deepest and smallest muscle of ipsilateral rotation, creating that 'no' motion, the rotation of the atlas and occiput together on the axis. You can find this muscle by locating the TPs of the atlas and the SP of the axis, positioning your index fingertips right between the two (in most clients there is an indicative 'divot' there between the trapezius and SCM), fixing the skull with your thumbs, and calling for head rotation against the resistance – the deep muscle will 'pop' into your fingertips, and the difference in tone between the two sides is assessed.

The other three suboccipital muscles run down from deep underneath the occipital shelf. Going from medial to lateral, the RCPM runs from the occiput to the spinous process of the atlas, crossing only the O-A joint. But we have already said that the atlas does not have much of a spinous process, so what is unclear in most anatomy atlases is that this muscle runs inferiorly *and very much forward* to do this (Fig. 3.27).

The next muscle laterally, the RCPMaj, runs down to the SP of the axis, but since that bone has such a huge spinous process, this muscle runs pretty much straight up and down. This points to a difference in function between these two muscles: the RCPM, among its other functions, tends to pull the occiput *forward* on the atlas (occipital protraction, or an anterior shift of the occiput on the atlas), while the

RCPMaj creates pure hyperextension in both the A-A (atlanto-axial) and the O-A joints. (The RCPM cannot pull the atlas posteriorly because the dens of C2 prevents this motion.)

The most lateral of these three, the obliquus capitis superior (OCS), runs down and forward again from the posterolateral part of the occiput, this time to the large TPs of the atlas. This muscle, which runs on a parallel course to the RCPM, will have the same effect – pulling the occiput forward on the atlas (as well as helping to create a postural rotation in the O-A joint if it is shorter on one side than the other).

Though treatment of these muscles can be a complex process of unwinding, given the connection 'upward' to the eyes, and downward to the entire spine, we can facilitate palpation. Once again, your supine client's head rests in your hands, but this time the occiput is cradled in your palms, so your fingers are fully free. Curl your fingers fully up under the occiput (so that they point toward you, not toward the ceiling), swimming in past the trapezius and semispinalis to these deep little muscles. Leave the little fingers on the table, and let your ring fingers touch at the client's nuchal midline, so that six fingertips are arrayed along the bottom of the occiput (Fig. 3.28). With adjustments for differently sized hands and heads, your ring fingers will be in contact with the RCPM, your middle fingers on the RCPMaj, and your index fingers on the OCS. Strumming back and forth with the middle finger will often (but not always) reveal the more prominent band of the RCPMaj, and the two other fingers can be placed evenly on either side of it (www.anatomytrains.com – video ref: Superficial Back Line, 1:02:20–1:04:22).

To reverse the common postural problem of the occiput being held forward on the atlas you need to create length and release in the muscles under your index and ring fingers. To combat postural hyperextension of the neck, you need to release the slightly more prominent RCPMaj under your middle fingers (while getting your client to engage the longus muscles in the front of the neck by sliding the back

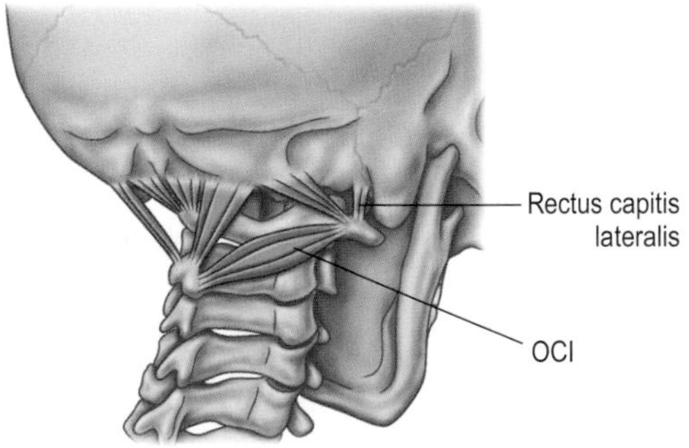

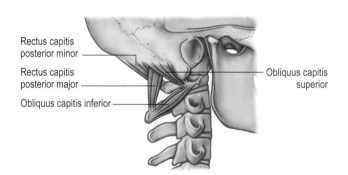

• **Fig. 3.26** An oblique view of the suboccipitals gives a much better sense of how the muscles relate to each other and to head movement. The OCI, running between the SP of C2 and TPs of C1, is a fundamental modulator of rotation in the spine.

Rectus capitis lateralis
OCI

Rectus capitis posterior minor
Rectus capitis posterior major
Obliquus capitis inferior
Obliquus capitis superior

• **Fig. 3.27** A lateral view of the suboccipitals shows us how the RCPM and OCS pull the skull down and forward, whereas the RCPMaj tends to pull the skull down and just a little back. In extreme cases, they all work together, but in 'fine tuning' a head–neck relationship, differentiating among them is essential to integrating the myofascial work on the large spinal muscles into proper functional movement.

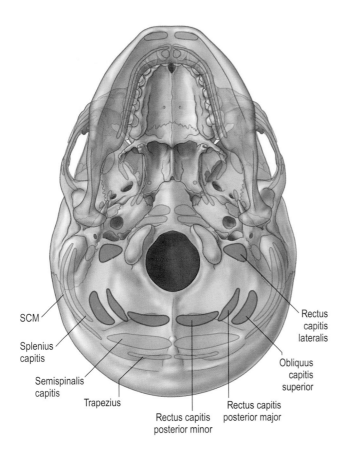

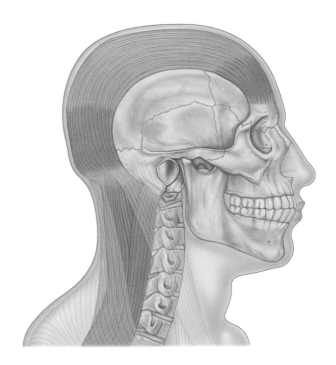

• **Fig. 3.29** From the erector fascia the SBL travels over the top of the skull on the galea aponeurotica, or scalp fascia, to attach firmly onto the frontal brow ridge.

• **Fig. 3.28** A view looking up at the skull from below. The three middle fingers of each hand usually correspond 'handily' to the origins of the three suboccipital muscles at the deepest level of the upper spine.

of their head toward you and flattening the neck against the table). While these two patterns often accompany each other in determined head forward posture, they also occur separately, so that this distinction becomes useful.

From Occiput to Supraorbital Ridge

From the occipital ridge the SBL continues up and over the occiput as these layers blend into the galea aponeurotica, or scalp fascia, which includes the small slips of the occipitalis and frontalis muscles, all clearly oriented in the same direction as the SBL. It finally comes to rest in a strong attachment at the brow or supraorbital ridge, on the frontal bone just above the eye socket (Fig. 3.29).

The Scalp

Though the scalp may seem plastered down to the skull and largely amuscular, it is still an active area within the SBL and other lines, where much relief can be obtained. The scalp is the terminus of several of the longitudinal lines, so tugging and releasing here can be like playing with the strings of a marionette for the skilled manual therapist. Larger areas of tension can be 'scraped' caudally with the fingertips working in extension. In those with a head forward posture, the fascial attachments of the erectors

'creep' up the back of the occiput, seeking higher leverage on the skull, just as a quadruped's erectors do – one reason your cat or dog loves to be scratched behind the ears. Part of the solution, besides easing pulls from the Superficial and Deep Front Lines and correcting faulty breathing, is to release these extra fascial attachments at the back of the scalp to allow the head to rise.

A detailed examination of the scalp from the occipital ridge to the brow ridge will also reveal little spindle-shaped fascicles that, though sometimes difficult to find because they are so small, are often extraordinarily tight and painful to the touch (Video 6.8). They can be released through steady finger (or even fingernail) pressure, applied to the very center of the knot (use client feedback to locate yourself) for around a minute or until the knot or trigger point is entirely melted. Effectively applied, this can often occasion blessed relaxation through the entire affected line.

Care must be taken to notice the orientation of the spindles, since several lines melt into the scalp fascia, and the spindle will line up like a compass needle along the direction of pull. Pulls from any of the cardinal lines – Front, Back, or Lateral – plus the Spiral Line, Deep Front Line, or the Superficial Back Arm Line, can all show up here.

A generally over-tight scalp can be released more gently by applying the fingerpads slowly in a circular motion, moving the skin on the bone until you feel the scalp melt itself free from the skull beneath. This method can be particularly effective if you stay with the pads, not the fingertips, and stay with melting, not forcing (www.anatomytrains.com – video ref: Superficial Back Line, 57:05–59:59).

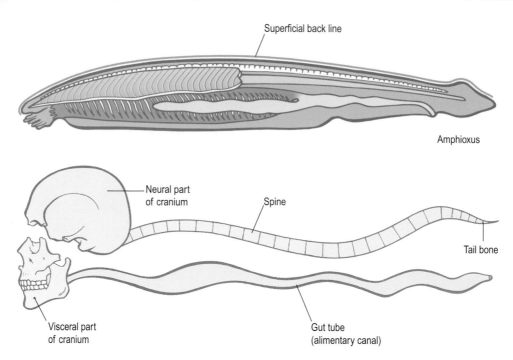

Superficial back line

Amphioxus

Neural part
of cranium

Spine

Tail bone

Visceral part
of cranium

Gut tube
(alimentary canal)

• **Fig. 3.30** Our seemingly solid, one-piece skull is actually formed from two different embryological sources. Looking at the skull of primitive chordates and early fish, we see that these animals had a cranium but no facial bones. The neurocranial part of our skull is an extension of the spine, while the viscerocranial facial structures develop from our branchial apparatus. The SBL stops near the forward end of the neurocranium.

The Neurocranium and the SBL

Although there are further fascial connections from the brow down onto the face, they are very superficial and loose, and do not constitute a line of structural pull. The facial muscles are loosely set into the superficial fascia, readily palpable as you move the tissue of the face around (compare to the minimal movement available in the fascia under the skin in the forehead). The brow ridge is the effective end of the SBL.

It also makes sense for the SBL to end above the eye socket when we consider its evolutionary origins. In the earliest vertebrates, the agnathous (jawless) fishes, the skull ended just above the eyes. The underside of the eyes and the mouth were all defined by soft tissue alone. It was some millions of years later that the bony structure of the gill arches 'migrated' up into the face to form the zygomatic, maxillary, and mandibular arches that now join with the more ancient neurocranium to form our familiar skull (Fig. 3.30).

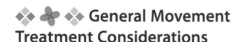 General Movement Treatment Considerations

A generally mobile and motile SBL allows trunk and hip flexion with the knees extended, and creates trunk hyperextension, knee flexion, and plantar flexion. Thus, the various types of forward bends are all good ways to stretch the line as a whole or to isolate parts, while postural hyperextension is a mark of hypertonus or shortening of the SBL

myofascia. Extension exercises would engage the SBL and tonify it where necessary.

Overall Stretches

NOTE: These stretches, mostly drawn from yoga asanas, are included for clarity and inspiration. Attempting them yourself or putting clients into the stretches without proper preparation and training can cause an injury or negative result. Use caution, get trained, or refer.

Overall stretches (in an ascending scale of difficulty) include a Seated Forward Bend (Fig. 3.31A), Standing Forward Bend (Fig. 3.31B), the Downward-Facing Dog (Fig. 3.31C), and the Plow position (Fig. 3.31D).

The Child's pose (see Fig. 10.46C, p. 202) can be used to stretch the thoracolumbar fascia and the erectors. A Shoulder Stand is specific to the upper back and cervical part of the SBL. A forward bend leaning onto a table will isolate the leg portion of the SBL.

For those with access, rolling prone over a large physioball provides a good way to foster relaxation in the SBL as a whole.

Specific Areas

• *Plantar*: Taking the SBL from the bottom, overly dense plantar fascia will limit foot and toe mobility as well as limit movement in the SBL as a whole. A simple but effective technique calls for having your client stand barefoot and do a forward bend with straight knees, just

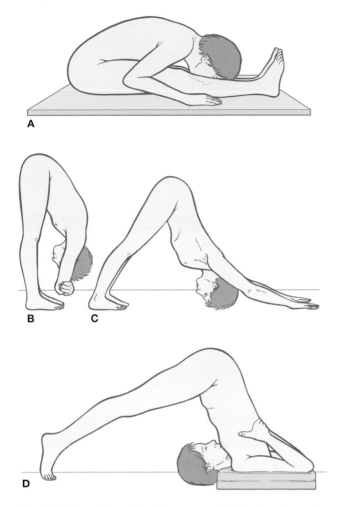

• **Fig. 3.31** Many different stretches, easy and difficult, reach parts or the whole of the SBL.

to see how it feels. Then have the client (standing again) place a tennis or small therapy ball under her foot. Now have her give weight into various parts of the plantar surface from the front of the heel out to the ball of the foot, looking for places that hurt or feel tight. She should give enough weight to reach that point between pleasure and pain, and should sustain the pressure on each point for at least 20 seconds. The whole exercise should take a few minutes.

• Remove the ball and have her lean forward again, and call her attention to the difference in feeling between the two sides of the SBL. Often the comparison is quite dramatic. Have her do the other foot, of course, and check if the forward bend is once again even, though more mobile. A more advanced, limber, or masochistic client can use a harder ball.

• Any movement that requires dorsiflexion and toe hyperextension will stretch the plantar-calf section of the SBL around the heel. A simple but effective stretch for the plantar fascia and its connection around to the Achilles is to kneel with the feet dorsiflexed and the toes hyperextended under you, and then sit on (or toward, for the stiffer among us) your heels. For the more limber, 'walk'

the knees back toward your fixed toes to feel the stretch increase along the plantar surface.

• *Calf*: Leaning forward and resting your forearms on a wall, the lower leg section of the SBL can be stretched by putting one foot back and resting into the heel. If the heel reaches the floor easily, flex the knee forward toward the wall to increase the stretch on the soleus. Dropping the heel off the back of a stair step is a time-tested and effective way of stretching the calf.

• *Hamstrings*: Any of the forward bends described above will help lengthen the hamstring group. Swing the upper body left and right during these bends to ensure that the entire muscle group, not just one line through it, gets activated and stretched.

• *Spine*: Inducing wave motions throughout the SBL, especially in the erector spinae and surrounding tissues, is very good for loosening and waking up neurology of the SBL. Have your client lie prone, or in any comfortable lying position. Ask the client to tighten the belly muscles, so a wave of flexion goes through the low back and pelvis. Encourage this wave of motion to spread progressively out across the entire back or even down the legs. Watch the motion, and observe where there are 'dead' spots – places where the motion is stifled and does not pass through. Place your hand on the dead spot and encourage the client to bring motion to that area. Clients will frequently try ever-larger efforts to force the motion through the dead spot, but smaller motions, with pauses for absorption, are often more effective. While restrictions most often occur in the flexion–extension pattern, waves involving lateral flexion or rotation can be helpful also.*

• *Neck*: The suboccipital area at the top of the neck is an area that often holds excess tension and immobility. The importance of the rectus and obliquus capitis muscles, which mediate between eye movements and spinal movements, to the general mobility of the SBL can hardly be overstated. These muscles create the beginnings of hyperextension and rotation, and occipital protraction (an anterior shift of the head on the neck). They are stretched by upper cervical flexion, rotation, and sliding the occiput posterior on the condyles of the atlas.

To induce movement in this area requires some concentration to focus the movement at the top of the neck, since similar movements can be produced in the lower cervicals by the expresses that overlie these essential, ancient, and tiny locals. Lying supine, and keeping attention at the top of the cervicals under the skull, slide the back of your head up away from the body, but without lifting it off the surface you are lying on. Maintaining this position of upper cervical flexion and length, move slowly into rotation, again focusing on the upper cervicals.

---

*This simple movement has been beautifully elaborated by Continuum, which can be explored via www.continuummovement.com, or www.continuummontage.com, or in Anita Boser's books on Undulation.

Again, the 'Awareness Through Movement' lessons of Moshe Feldenkrais, which separate eye movements from neck and body movements, are unequaled in their ability to clarify and differentiate these muscles and this area.[6]

❦ ❖ Palpation Guide for the SBL

Beginning again from the distal end of the SBL, the first station is at the underside of the tips of the toes, which we cannot feel very well through the pads, but we can find the tendons of the short toe flexors under the thinner-skinned proximal part of the toes. The plantar fascia really begins at the ball of the foot station, narrowing as it passes back toward the front of the heel, where it is less than an inch (2 cm) wide. Pulling the toes up into extension brings the plantar fascia into sharp relief, where its edges can be easily felt. The lateral band is hard to feel directly through the thick overlying padding, but can be inferred by putting your finger or knuckle into the line that runs between the outer edge of the heel to the 5th metatarsal base, a clearly palpable knob of bone halfway between the heel and the little toe (see Figs. 3.6 and 3.7, p. 32). The lateral band, an extension of the accompanying abductor digiti minimi can be found between the base of the 5th metatarsal and the outer edge of the calcaneus.

The track runs around and through the heel, which is hard to feel through the tough padding on the bottom, but can be felt on the back of the heel bone. Put your fingers on the heel bone while you flex and extend the toes to feel the effect on the fascia around the heel (see Fig. 3.12, p. 34).

The Achilles tendon is easily felt and familiar to most, but follow it up the calf as it widens and thins. If your model is standing on the balls of her feet, the lower edges of the gastrocnemii heads are easily palpable where they attach to this aponeurosis. Relax the ankle, and the large soleus is easily felt deep to this fascial sheet.

The next station, the heads of the gastrocnemii, lies between the strong tendons of the hamstrings behind and above the knee at the back of the femoral condyles (see Fig. 3.17, p. 37). The hamstrings reach down with their tendons below the knee: the two semis (semimembranosus and semitendinosus) to the medial part of the tibia, the singular biceps femoris to the fibular head on the lateral part of the lower leg. Follow the hamstrings up to the posterior aspect of the ischial tuberosity (see Fig. 3.20, p. 39). Having your model flex the knee or extend the hip against resistance will convince you how far posterior on the tuberosities the hamstring fascia lies.

If you reach under the medial edge of the gluteus maximus just above the tuberosity, you can find the almost bone-like sacrotuberous ligament – the shortest, most dense track of this line. Reach in along its medial side, following it up to the lower, outer edge of the sacrum (see Fig. 3.21, p. 41).

From this station of the sacrum, between the two posterior superior iliac spines, the erector spinae and the underlying transversospinalis traverse the entire spinal column in a long track up to the occipital ridge. The innermost of the erector spinae, the spinalis muscle, less than a half-inch wide in most cases, can be felt right up against the spinous processes, most easily at the mid-thoracic, 'bra line', level (see Fig. 3.22, p. 41).

The middle of the erector spinae group, the longissimus, is easily felt as a series of strong cables just lateral to the spinalis. The most lateral of the muscles, the iliocostalis, can be felt between the cables of the longissimus and the angle of the ribs. The slips of this muscle often feel like the raised ridges of corduroy as you strum them horizontally at this level. Any of these muscles can then be traced up or down from where you locate them.

At the top of the neck, the semispinalis muscle is easily palpable under the trapezius (especially when your model pushes their head back against resistance) as two vertical cables narrowing down from the occiput. The palpation of the underlying suboccipitals has already been laid out in the section on this important group on pages 43–45.

From the station at the occipital ridge, the epicranial fascia, or galea aponeurotica, runs up over the occipital bone (containing, in most people, slips of the occipitalis muscle), over the top of the head and down the forehead (enveloping the frontalis muscle) to attach to its final station, the brow ridge (see Fig. 3.29, p. 45).

DISCUSSION 3.1

❖ ❦ ❦ The SBL and the Waves of the Spine

The SBL provides a functional link across the waves that constitute the primary and secondary curves of the spine and legs. In the plantigrade human posture, the body arranges itself in an alternating series of counterbalancing curves. Traditional anatomical thinking recognizes the thoracic and sacrococcygeal curves of the spine, which are concave to the front of the body, as primary curves, that is, curves that still reflect the flexed position of fetal development.

During late pregnancy and in the first year of life, the secondary curves form in sections within the baby's primary flexion curve. Activating the neck muscles (to lift the head) and later the lower back muscles (to sit and crawl) changes the shape of the intervertebral discs to reverse the convexity of the cervical and lumbar curves respectively (see Figs. 10.38–10.44, pp. 198–200). In the standing posture, however, we can expand our view of the spinal undulation to the whole body, seeing the cranial curve as a primary curve, the cervical as secondary, the thoracic as primary, the lumbar as secondary, and the sacrococcygeal as primary.

Extending this point of view down the legs, the slight flex of the knees can be seen as secondary, the curve of the heel as primary, and the arch of the foot as secondary, and the ball of the foot as primary. The knee 'curve' forms in the process of learning to stand, and the final secondary curve, to form the foot arches, takes final shape as the child strengthens the deep calf muscles in walking.

While these curves are not all developmentally equivalent, this concept is quite practical, and admits wide application in the field of manual and movement therapy. All the primary curves are more or less maintained by the shape of the surrounding bones. The cranium is interlocked to itself, the thoracic curve is maintained by the ribs and sternum complex, the sacrococcygeal curve by the hip bones and pelvic ligaments, and the heel by the shape of the foot bones (Fig. 3.32).

All the secondary curves, however, are more dependent on the balance of myofascia, first to create and then to maintain their position. Thus the cervicals and lumbars, being the free-standing sections of the spine, depend more heavily on the guy-wires of the surrounding myofascia for their stability and positioning. The bones and ligaments leave the knee free to run from full flexion to hyperextension; muscle balance determines where the knees habitually rest. The arches of the foot are likewise pulled into final position as the child stands and pushes off in walking, and their maintenance depends as much on the successful

balance of soft tissues in the leg and foot as on any actual arch in the bones. (The muscles that reach down from the calf to pull up on the various arches will turn up later as the lower ends of other major train lines – see Chs 5, 6, and 9 on the Lateral, Spiral, and Deep Front Lines.)

In functional posture and movement, all of these secondary curves are also related to each other. Lack of balance in one often asserts a compensatory pattern into other nearby secondary curves. The illustrated relation between the knees and lower back is readily seen in day-to-day observation (Fig. 3.33).

Proper balance among all the primary and secondary curves, accompanied by an evenness of tone in the SBL tissues, can be seen as a balanced unfolding into 'maturity' from the embryonic fetal curve. Postural flexion or hyperextension patterns can be related to areas where full maturation was not complete. Chronic flexion of the hips is often occasioned by the failure of the hips to fully extend as the child grows; this lack of extension will require indicative, 'readable' compensation in the SBL. A person who is completely 'evolved' (in its literal sense of 'unfolded') displays a 'tensegrity' balance of the body's alternating sagittal waves.

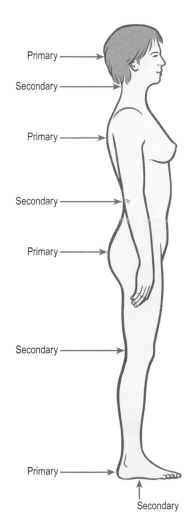

Primary
Secondary
Primary
Secondary
Primary
Secondary
Primary
Secondary

• **Fig. 3.32** The alternation of primary and secondary curves in the spine can be seen as extending across the whole back of the body. The SBL extends behind all these curves, and the tone of its tissues is instrumental in maintaining an easy balance among them.

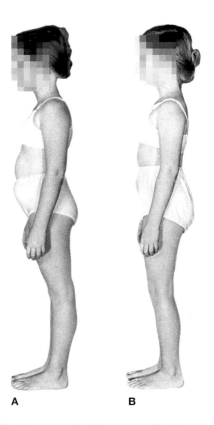

A   B

• **Fig. 3.33** The hyperextended knees can be viewed, in Anatomy Trains terms, as a secondary curve problem. (**A**) Before treatment, the secondary curve of the knee has been reversed to a primary curve, exporting extra strain to the other secondary curves – in this case the lumbar and cervical areas. (**B**) After Structural Integration processing, the knee curve has normalized, and so have the rest of the secondary curves. (From Toporek (1981), reproduced by kind permission of Robert Toporek (www.newbabymassage.com).)[7]

The SBL links the posterior aspect of all these curves together, from top to bottom. The general tenet of the myofascial meridians approach is that force and ultimately strain travel up or down along these lines. Thus, problems in any of these curves may create undue stress anywhere along that line. The converse also works: stubborn pain problems may best be served by extending our assessment and treatment to other parts of the line, often quite distant from the site of pain. This book is an extended plea to create time and space in which to consider such an overall systemic view of the interaction along an entire myofascial meridian, or, as we proceed, among the meridians, instead of focusing solely on single muscles or individual fascial structures as culprits. Do not punish the victims for what the criminals are doing.

DISCUSSION 3.2

 Is There a Deep Back Line?

According to standard anatomical nomenclature, if there is a Superficial Back Line, there should be a Deep Back Line. Besides, if there is clearly a Deep Front Line as well as a Superficial Front Line, does symmetry not require that there be a Deep Back Line? In fact, whether symmetry requires it or not, anatomically, there is no Deep Back Line. Though there are isolated areas along the SBL where there are distinct deeper layers of myofascia, there is no consistent and connected layer deeper than the one already discussed (see, however, the discussion of the Deep Dorsal Line in horses in Appendix 5, p. 349).

Taking a brief look at these areas is instructive. In the plantar surface of the foot, for instance, many layers lie superior (profound) to the plantar fascia. These layers contain the short flexors and the ab- and adductors of the toes and their associated fascia, as well as the long plantar and spring ligaments that underlie the tarsal arches. The plantar fascia was described above as the bowstring of the arches' bow, but of course the bow is not static, given the many possible motions of the foot in daily and sporting life. In motion, all of these successively deeper layers of myofascia and ligament are active in sustaining the arches (Fig. 3.34 and see Fig. 3.9).

These constitute layers that are deeper than the SBL, but when we come to their proximal or distal ends, we cannot point to specific fascial continuity with any other sections of the body, beyond the 'everything-is-connected-to-everything-else-in-the-fascial-net' generalization.

In the lower leg, there is the deeper set of locals (soleus and popliteus) that underlie the gastrocnemii, but they are still part of the SBL, being attached simply to the underside of the Achilles fascia (and we include little plantaris in this group also).

There is a group of muscles deep to the soleus, between it and the back surface of the interosseous membrane – the deep posterior compartment – consisting of the long toe flexors and the tibialis posterior (Fig. 3.35). These muscles, despite their position posterior to the bones in this segment of the body, will be very clearly shown to be part of the Deep Front Line (see Ch. 9), and thus do not qualify as a Deep Back Line. The fibularii muscles, in the lateral compartment, will be clearly shown to be part of the Lateral Line (see Ch. 5).

In the thigh, the hamstrings overlie the short head of the biceps and the adductor magnus, which constitute a local under the express of the long head of the biceps (see the section on the 4th hamstring in Ch. 6). So all of the hamstring group, right down to the bone, can be thought of as part of the SBL, and not a Deep Back Line.

There is another story in the back of the hip. Although they do not directly underlie the structures of the SBL, the deep lateral rotators nevertheless act like a Deep Back Line in this area, limiting hip flexion along with the hamstrings, as well as helping to keep the spine aloft and in balance. In this light, this group might better have been named *extensor coxae brevis*, the short extensors of the hip.[8] These muscles, from piriformis down through the obturators and the gemelli to the quadratus femoris, have a continuity of function with each other, but no directional fiber continuity with other local myofascial structures. These deep lateral

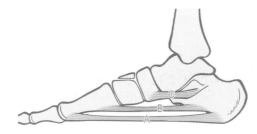

• **Fig. 3.34** The plantar fascia (**A**) is, in fact, only the most superficial of several layers of myofascia, including the long plantar ligament (**B**) and the spring ligament (**C**), that act to support the arches (compare to Fig. 3.9).

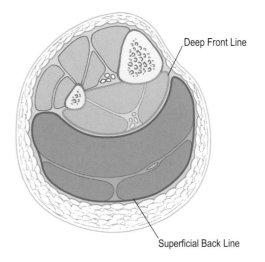

• **Fig. 3.35** The SBL occupies the entire superficial posterior compartment of the lower leg. The deep posterior compartment belongs not to a Deep Back Line but, paradoxically, to the Deep Front Line.

rotators are best thought of as a branch of the Deep Front Line in the myofascial meridians theory (see Ch. 9), though their lack of linear connections makes them difficult to place in the Anatomy Trains metaphor. They are best considered in light of another concept, a series of fans of the hip joint.[9]

In the spinal area, it could be argued that the muscles we have included as part of the SBL fall into two major fascial planes, the more superficial erector spinae (spinalis, longissimus, and iliocostalis) and the deeper transversospinalis (semispinalis, multifidus, rotatores, interspinous, and intertransversarii). While it is true that there is a fascial plane dividing these two groups, it is argued here quite firmly that this is simply a massively complicated set of locals and expresses, with the tiny monarticular locals forming three distinct patterns over the 26 bones from sacrum to occiput (see Figs. 3.22 and 3.23, pp. 41–42). These patterns – spinous process to spinous process, transverse process to transverse process, and spinous process to transverse process – are repeated with ever-greater polyarticular intervals by the overlying semispinalis and erectors.

In the last part of the SBL, the scalp fascia, there is clearly only one thick layer of fascia between the periosteum of the skull and the dermal layer of the skin, and several lines and levels of myofascia, as we mentioned earlier, blend into this layer.

The answer to our question, therefore, is that there is no myofascial Deep Back Line, whether symmetry requires it or not. The argument for symmetry falls away in any case as we examine our evolutionary history and realize that the Deep Front Line began as the original soft-tissue 'carapace' of our tunicate 'gut body' self (Fig. 3.36). (See also the general discussion of the Deep Front Line in Ch. 9.)

An argument can be made for a 'Deep Back Line' that would consist of the connective tissue that surrounds the central nervous system, the dura, and its extension into the neural and neurovascular bundles that snake through the limbs. This has an attraction in that the Deep Front Line surrounds the ventral organs, and its projections into the arms (via the Deep Front Arm Line) and legs can be seen as the extension of these organs into the arms and legs. Likewise, the dura surrounds the organs of the dorsal cavity, and thus its extensions into the limbs could be termed the Deep Back Line, especially the sciatic nerve. As more work is done with the connections of dural and nerve sheath anatomy, we may find this argument has merit, but given that (1) this fascial configuration would be associated with no muscles except perhaps the piriformis, and (2) the fascial extensions of the dura follow the nerves everywhere in the body (front, back and sides, not just the inner back of the leg), we choose to stay with the idea that there is simply no coherent myofascial continuity that could be termed the Deep Back Line.

There are, as we have seen, several places on the SBL where important locals underlie the multi-joint expresses. Because the skeleton underlying the SBL undulates with primary and secondary curves, we can note that these locals tend to congregate around the secondary, posteriorly convex curves – under the foot arches, around the knee, and in the lumbars and cervicals. The exception here is of course the thoracic area, where just as many locals underlie the expresses around a primary curve. This provides the opportunity for local strain, and thus for many tenacious trigger points which, paradoxically, are often best addressed posturally from the front (see the section on the interaction between the SBL and the Superficial Front Line in Ch. 4, pp. 68–70).

References

1. Huijing PA, Baan GC, Rebel GT. Non-myotendinous force transmission in rat extensor digitorum longus muscle. *J Exp Biol.* 1998;201:682–691.
2. Bogduk N. *Clinical Anatomy of the Lumbar Spine and Sacrum.* 3rd ed. Edinburgh: Churchill Livingstone; 1997.
3. Gorman D. *The Body Moveable.* Guelph, Ontario: Ampersand; 1978.
4. Kapandji I. *The Physiology of the Joints.* Vol. 3. Edinburgh: Churchill Livingstone; 1974.
5. Peck D, Buxton D, Nitz A. A comparison of spindle concentrations of large and small muscles. *J Morphol.* 1984;180:245–252.
6. Feldenkrais M. *Awareness Through Movement.* New York: Penguin; 1977.
7. Toporek R. The promise of Rolfing children. *Transformation News Network.* 1981.
8. Myers T. Extensor coxae brevis. *J Bodyw Mov Ther.* 2009;12(3): 62–68.
9. Myers T. Fans of the hip joint. *Massage Magazine.* 1998;No. 75.

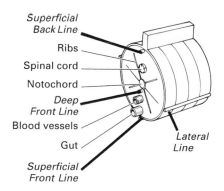

Superficial Back Line
Ribs
Spinal cord
Notochord
Deep Front Line
Blood vessels
Gut
Superficial Front Line
Lateral Line

• **Fig. 3.36** The location of the cardinal lines on a generalized vertebrate body plan. Notice that the SBL lies behind the spine, while the Deep Front Line lies just in front of the spine, and the Superficial Front Line in front of the organs. From the beginning of vertebrate evolution, the left–right symmetry of the musculoskeletal system has not been matched by a front–back symmetry.

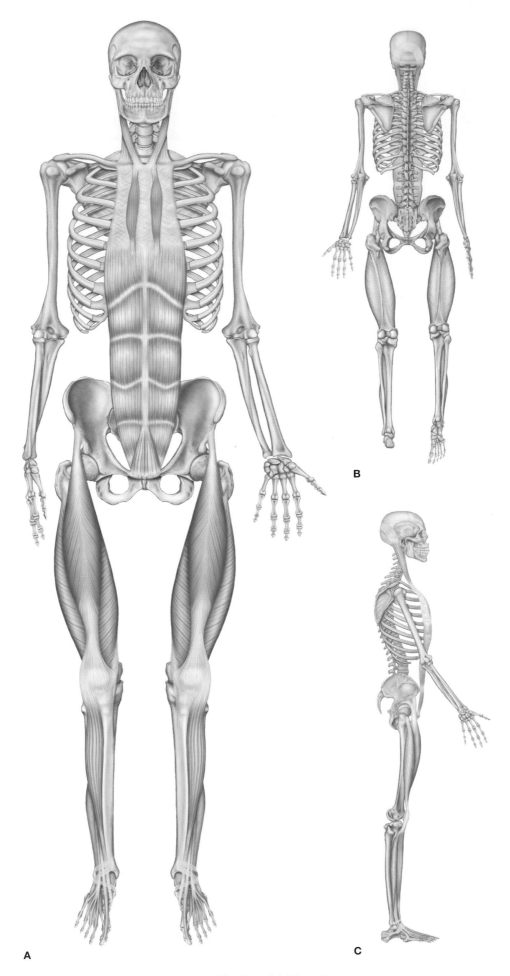

A

B

C

• **Fig. 4.1** The Superficial Front Line.

4

The Superficial Front Line

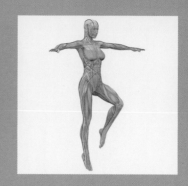

OVERVIEW

 The Superficial Front Line (SFL) (Fig. 4.1; Video 2.1) connects the entire anterior surface of the body from the top of the feet to the side of the skull in two pieces – toes to pelvis and pelvis to head (Fig. 4.2/Table 4.1) – which, when the hip is extended as in standing, function as one continuous line of integrated myofascia.

Postural Function

The overall postural function of the SFL is to balance the Superficial Back Line (SBL), and to provide tensile support from the top to lift those parts of the skeleton which extend forward of the gravity line – the pubis, rib cage, and face. Myofascia of the SFL also maintain the postural extension of the knee. The muscles of the SFL also stand ready to protect the viscera of the ventral cavity and defend the soft and sensitive parts that adorn the front surface of the human body (Fig. 4.3).

The SFL begins on the tops of the toes. By the 'everything-connects-to-everything-else' fascial principle, the SFL technically joins with the SBL through the periostea around the tip of the toe phalanges, but there is no discernible 'play' across this connection. Functionally these two Anatomy Trains lines oppose each other, the SBL being responsible for flexing the toes, and the SFL taking on the job of extending them, and so on up the body. More practically, in postural terms, the dorsiflexors act to restrain the tibia–fibula complex from moving too far back into plantarflexion, and the plantarflexors prevent it from leaning too far forward into dorsiflexion.

Sagittal postural balance (A–P balance) is primarily maintained throughout the body by either an easy or a tense relationship between these two lines (Fig. 4.4). In the trunk and neck, however, the Deep Front Line must be included to complete and complicate the equation (see Fig. 3.36 and Ch. 9).

When the lines are considered as parts of fascial planes, rather than as chains of contractile muscles, it is worth noting that in by far the majority of cases, the SFL tends to shift caudally down, and the SBL tends to shift up rostrally in response (Fig. 4.5).

Movement Function

The overall movement function of the SFL is to create flexion of the trunk and hips, extension at the knee, and dorsiflexion of the foot (Fig. 4.6), or to resist their opposite. The SFL performs a complex set of actions at the neck level, which comes up for discussion below. The need to create sudden and strong flexion movements at the various joints requires that the muscular portion of the SFL contain a higher proportion of fast-twitch muscle fibers. The interplay between the predominantly endurance-oriented SBL and the quickly reactive SFL can be seen in the need for contraction in one line when the other is stretched (Fig. 4.7).

❖ ❖ ❖ General Manual Therapy Considerations

As with the SBL, there are actually two SFLs, one just to the right and one just to the left of the midline. Viewing the client from the front will help assess differences between the right and left sides of this line, though a good first course of action in the majority of cases is to resolve any general shortness in the SFL. Viewing the client from the side reveals the state of balance between the SFL and SBL, and gives a good indication of where to open and lengthen the line in general (see Fig. 1.2).

The SFL, along with the SBL, mediates movement in the sagittal plane. When it malfunctions it acts to create forward movement (flexion) or to restrict backward movement (extension). Trouble abounds when the SFL myofascia starts to pull inferiorly on the skeleton from a lower stable station, rather than pulling superiorly from an upper stable station, i.e. the belly muscles start acting to pull the ribs toward the pubic bone, instead of bringing the pubic bone up toward the ribs.

Common postural compensation patterns associated with the SFL include: ankle plantarflexion limitation, knee hyperextension, anterior pelvic tilt, anterior pelvic shift, breathing restrictions in the anterior ribs, and forward head posture.

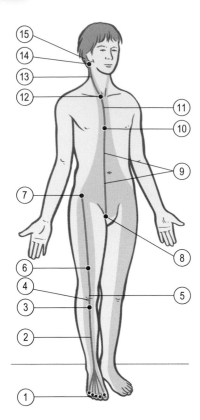

• **Fig. 4.2** Superficial Front Line tracks and stations. The shaded area shows the area of superficial fascial influence.

TABLE 4.1	Superficial Front Line: Myofascial 'Tracks' and Bony 'Stations' (Fig. 4.2)	
Bony Stations		**Myofascial Tracks**
	15	Scalp fascia
Mastoid process	14	
	13	Sternocleidomastoid
Sternal manubrium	12	
	11	Sternalis/sternochondral fascia
5th rib	10	
	9	Rectus abdominis
Pubic tubercle	8	
Anterior inferior iliac spine	7	
	6	Rectus femoris/quadriceps
Patella	5	
	4	Patellar tendon
Tibial tuberosity	3	
	2	Short and long toe extensors, tibialis anterior, anterior crural compartment
Dorsal surface of toe phalanges	1	

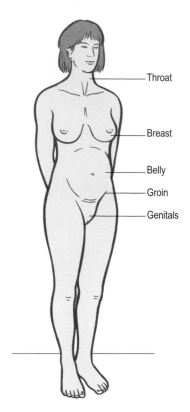

• **Fig. 4.3** Human beings' unique plantigrade way of standing presents all their most sensitive and vulnerable areas to the oncoming world, all arrayed along the SFL. Compare this to quadrupeds, who protect most or all of these vulnerable areas (see Fig. 4.31).

The Superficial Front Line in Detail

The five tendons that originate on the top of the toes form the beginning of the SFL. Moving up the foot, the SFL picks up two additional tendons (Fig. 4.8). On the lateral side, we get the fibularis (peroneus) tertius (if there is one) originating from the 5th metatarsal shaft. From the medial side, we find the tendon of the tibialis anterior from the 1st metatarsal on the medial side of the foot. The SFL includes both the short extensor muscles on the dorsum of the foot and the long tendons from the lower leg.

The Shin

The fascial plane of the SFL passes up into the anterior compartment of the lower leg, but on its way it passes under the extensor retinaculum. The retinaculum is essentially a thicker extension of an even more superficial fascial plane, the deep investing crural fascia that surrounds the lower leg. This retinacular thickening is necessary to hold the tendons down (otherwise your skin between the foot and the middle of the shin would pop out every time the muscles contracted – Fig. 4.9). Because the tendons run around a corner (allowed by our rules in this case because of the clear fascial and mechanical continuity), lubricating tissues wrap around the tendons to ease their movement under the retinacular strap. Far from a simple

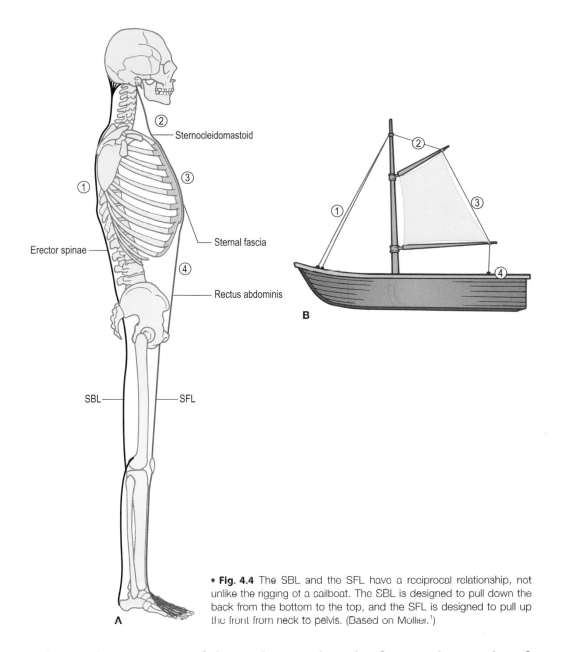

Sternocleidomastoid

Sternal fascia

Erector spinae

Rectus abdominis

SBL ———   ——— SFL

A

B

• **Fig. 4.4** The SBL and the SFL have a reciprocal relationship, not unlike the rigging of a sailboat. The SBL is designed to pull down the back from the bottom to the top, and the SFL is designed to pull up the front from neck to pelvis. (Based on Mollier.[1])

'strap', however, the complex intertwining of the crural fascia, tendons, and retinacular layers, as well as the higher number of proprioceptive sensors within this tissue make it a potent area for creating functional change through manual or movement intervention.

Above the retinaculum, the SFL passes up the front of the lower leg. On the lateral side, it contains the muscles of the anterior compartment – the tibialis anterior and the extensor digitorum and hallucis longus – in the scooped-out shape anterior to the interosseous membrane. On the medial side, we have found that, for best effect, the crural fascia must also be included where it overlies the tibia and its periosteum (compare Fig. 4.10 to Fig. 2.1C, p. 18).

🍀 ❖ The Anterior Crural Compartment

The tibialis anterior is generally the strongest muscle of the anterior compartment, but the compartment as a whole produces dorsiflexion and resists plantarflexion. Here we deal with the two most common pattern problems in this compartment.

When the series of tendons from this compartment pass under the restraining strap of the retinaculum, they can get restricted in terms of free movement. Presumably the lubricating continuities of the peritendinous sheaths adhere locally to the investing crural fascia above and below the retinacular layers. This is usually due to lack of full-range movement use and thus being 'set' at a constant tension. Whatever the cause, the solution is fairly simple and straightforward, and often produces surprised pleasure on the part of the client due to increased ease of movement after just a few passes.

Have your client supine, with the heels just off the end of the table. Have her dorsiflex and plantarflex, checking to see that she is 'tracking' straight with the ankle, so that the foot is headed directly toward the knee, not up and in or

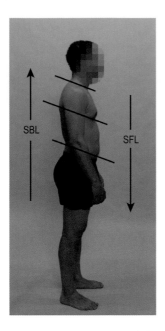

• **Fig. 4.5** It is a very common pattern for the SFL to be pulled down in the front while the SBL hikes up in back (vertical lines). This creates a disparity between the corresponding fascial planes in the front and back of the body represented by the horizontal lines. This fascial plane shift is a relatively new concept in training and bodywork, and is not the same as string and weak muscles or short or long myofascia. Those issues will accompany this pattern, but if nothing is done to 'level the playing field' in terms of a plane shift back towards balance, muscle imbalances will keep reasserting themselves.

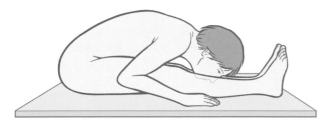

• **Fig. 4.6** Contraction of the SFL extends the toes, dorsiflexes the ankles, extends the knees, and flexes the hips and trunk, like a regular forward fold – excepting that the SFL, as here, hyperextends the upper neck.

up and out. You can add more muscular differentiation by adding toe flexion and extension to the ankle movement.

Apply a broad surface of a loose fist to the dorsum of your client's foot distal to the retinacula. While the other hand guides the client's dorsi- and plantarflexion, have your client move slowly through the sequence of motion as you pass slowly up the front of the foot and ankle, working gently to open the retinaculum and up onto the crural layer beyond (Video 3.2). If the retinacula are too tight, or if the tendons are stuck, you will feel 'slowed' in your progress up the shin. Using the client's movement, repeat the pass (perhaps using a bit more pressure) until the feeling of restriction is gone, both from your sensing hand and from the client's feeling within the movement (www.anatomytrains.com – video ref: Superficial Front Line, 11.16–19:24).

Where you stop above the retinacula varies from client to client. In some people you run out of 'juice' just above

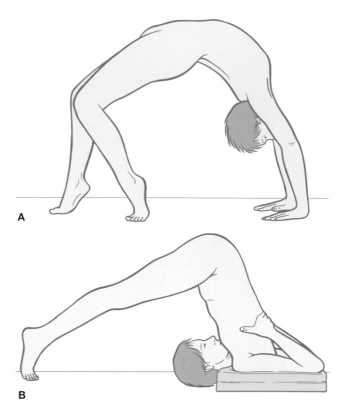

• **Fig. 4.7** The reciprocal relationship between the SBL and SFL can be seen in these two poses. In (**A**), the SBL is contracted and the SFL stretched, vice versa in (**B**).

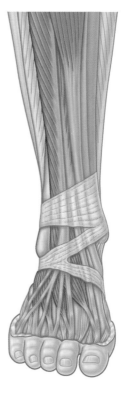

• **Fig. 4.8** The initial track of the SFL consists of seven tendons running under the even more superficial retinacula to combine into the anterior compartment of the leg.

the ankle; in others you feel as if you are 'skating' over the surface of the shin. If so, stop at this point. For some, the feeling of engagement and freeing extends well up the shin toward the knee, and you may continue on up as far as you still feel work is being done.

When your work does extend above the ankle, pay attention to which side of the shin is more restricted – the medial

or the lateral. Since you began on the tendons, the natural progression is up onto the muscles of the anterior compartment, on the lateral side of the anterior shin. The SFL, however, also includes the crural and superficial fascial layers that pass over the tibia on the anteromedial side (see Figs. 2.1C, 4.10 and 4.11).

We have arrived at the second common pattern problem in this area, so let us define the problem before we finish with the technique. In any kind of forward lean of the legs, where the knee rests posturally on a line anterior to the ankle, the posterior calf muscles tighten (eccentrically loaded in the muscle and locked long in the fascia), and the anterior muscles and tissue move down (and tighten concentrically, locking the fascia short). One of the best remedies for this is to move the tissue of the anterior surface up again (while easing the corresponding tissues of the SBL down).

So, above the ankle, superior to the retinacula, you can work both the muscle surface and the shinbone surface. Since they are at angles with each other, they can be worked sequentially, or both at once with two hands (Video 6.10). The two-handed technique involves putting both hands into a loose fist, with the proximal phalanges against the surface, one hand conforming to the front of the anterior compartment of muscles, the other to the anterior surface of the tibia above (www.anatomytrains.com – video ref: Superficial Front Line, 19:24–25:53). In this position, your right and left sets of knuckles (PIPs) rest near or against each other. Sink into the tissue enough to engage, and move along parallel to the bone, not with digging pressure that would cause pain to the tibial periosteum.

Let your hands work upward in time to the client's movement, pausing as she stretches out from under you in plantarflexion, carrying the tissue cephalad as she dorsiflexes,

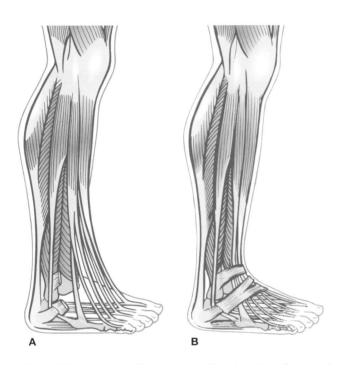

• **Fig. 4.9** The retinacula, thickenings in the deep investing crural fascia, provide a pulley to hold in the tendons of the SFL and direct their force from the shin muscle to the toes. It is also a rich area for proprioception.

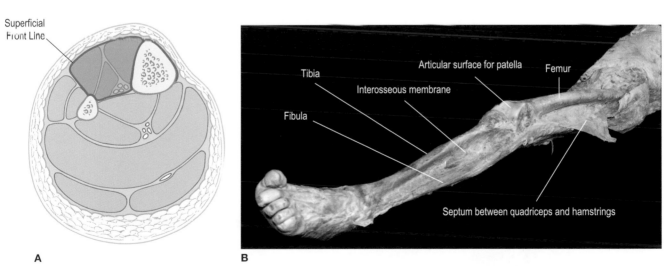

• **Fig. 4.10** The SFL occupies the anterior compartment of the leg, and the tissues on the front of the tibia (shinbone) as well. In (**B**), we see how little of the leg is left when the SFL is removed. We can see the interosseous membrane under where the anterior compartment has been removed, and the femur is almost fully exposed without the quadriceps in place. See also Fig. 2.1C, where both these parts of the crural fascia have been dissected as one piece – the anterior compartment and the surface fascia profundis coating the tibia. Where holes appear in this fascia are likely places where the person suffered trauma to the shin (as in playing football or falling upstairs), resulting in the crural fascia adhering to the periosteum underneath. (www.anatomytrains.com – video ref: Anatomy Trains Revealed)

until you run out of effectiveness or reach the top of the muscle compartment, whichever comes first.

Do not fail to have your client dorsi- and plantarflex after you have finished the treatment, since you will often be rewarded by the exclamation of increased freedom.

✿ The Thigh

Although the muscles themselves have attachments within the anterior compartment to the tibia, fibula, and interosseous membrane, the next station for the SFL is at the top of both the medial and lateral side of this track, the tibial tuberosity and condyles (Fig. 4.11).

Continuing in a straight line upward is no problem: the quadriceps begin their upward sweep here with the patellar tendon. The SFL includes the patella, the large sesamoid bone designed to hold the SFL away from the knee joint fulcrum so that the tissues of the quadriceps have more leverage for extending the knee. The patella rests in a channel (trochlea) in the femur, which also assures that the quadriceps, with its several different directions of pull, still tracks directly in front of the hinge of the knee joint.

The three vastii of the quadriceps all grab onto various parts of the femoral shaft, but the fourth head, the rectus femoris, continues bravely upward, carrying the SFL to the pelvis (Fig. 4.12). Although the rectus occupies the anterior surface of the thigh, its proximal attachment is not so superficial. Its upper end dives beneath the tensor fasciae latae and the sartorius to attach to the anterior inferior iliac spine (AIIS), a little bit below and medial to the anterior superior iliac spine (ASIS). There is a small but important head of the rectus that wraps around the top of the hip joint. Palpation and experience with dissection reveals that in some undetermined percentage of the population there is an additional significant fascial attachment of this muscle to the ASIS.

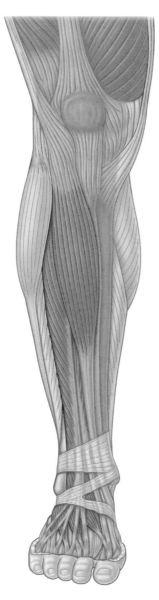

• **Fig. 4.11** The top of the anterior compartment leads past the tibial tuberosity onto the patellar tendon, a 'bridle' of retinacular tissue around the knee, and the quadriceps complex.

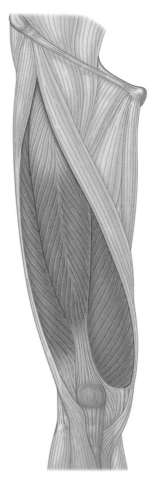

• **Fig. 4.12** The penumbra of the SFL could be said to include the entire quadriceps group, but a stricter interpretation sticks with the rectus femoris part of this group, passing up onto the anterior inferior iliac spine.

▶ ❁ ◆ The Quadriceps (Video 6.21)

The strictest interpretation of the SFL would include only the rectus femoris, not the entire quadriceps. For the freedom of this line, we must ensure that the rectus, being a two-joint muscle, is free to do its job at both hip and knee. Repetitive motion patterns, especially in athletics, can result in the rectus being stuck down to the underlying vasti, limiting glide, or restriction with the suprapatellar bursa.

The following technique requires a careful set-up of client movement. What we are after here is the client's use of his ankle movement to flex the knee and the hip. Your client lies supine with his heels on the table. Place a finger or hand against the bottom of the client's heel, to keep the heel from moving downward. Have your client dorsiflex; the heel will press down against your restraining hand, and the client's femur will be pressed into his hip. Have him dorsiflex again, adding just a minimal lifting/flexing of the knee. This time, your hand acts as an anchor (you can add the suggestion, 'Imagine the back of your heel is glued to the table while you flex your ankle'), and the knee and the hip will flex as the ankle 'pumps' or levers the knee up.

Watch the hip. If the client's ASIS moves toward the knee (producing lumbar hyperextension) as the knee rises, have him be as passive as possible in the hip. The hip should remain neutral or even fall back (into posterior pelvic tilt or hip extension) as the foot is dorsiflexed and the knee flexes. If the hip is actively flexing, work with the client's movement until it is minimally disturbing to the knee and hip, and most of the work is taking place at the ankle.

Place whatever applicator you wish to use just above the patella (feel free to use everything from fingertips to elbows depending on the body type and muscular development of the client). Work slowly cephalad up the rectus femoris, while the client repeats the dorsiflexing movement, keeping the heel 'glued' to the table. Pay particular attention to the receptor-rich area between the patella and the belly of the muscle. You can follow it, especially in those with an anterior pelvis, all the way to the AIIS (remember to track the muscle into its attachment, deeper and lower than the ASIS). Your goal is to free the two-joint rectus from its monarticular knee extensors below; the client's movement is essential help (www.anatomytrains.com – video ref: 🌐 Superficial Front Line, 25:44–33:12).

❁ Branch Lines

Returning to the upper part of the shin, there are alternative routes or switches here (Fig. 4.13). Instead of going straight up with rectus femoris, we could choose to follow the anterior edge of the iliotibial tract (ITT) from the tibialis anterior muscle (as we will in Ch. 6 with the Spiral Line), which would carry us laterally up the thigh to the ASIS. This could be seen to link to the internal oblique.

On the medial side of the knee, we could follow the sartorius from its distal attachment on the periosteum of the tibia around the medial thigh, again arriving at the

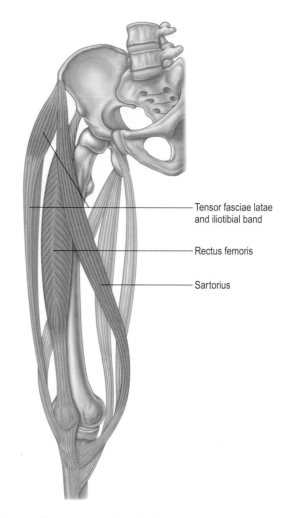

• **Fig. 4.13** There are two branch lines or alternative routes to the rectus femoris from the knee to the hip. The sartorius curves up from the inside to the anterior superior iliac spine, and the anterior edge of the iliotibial tract does the same on the outside of the leg.

Tensor fasciae latae and iliotibial band

Rectus femoris

Sartorius

ASIS, though this time the 'follow through' north of the ASIS would be the external oblique (see the Ipsilateral Functional Line in Ch. 8). These various branch lines of pull coming off the 'roundhouse' of the ASIS would allow us to travel in various ways up the abdomen to the ribs (Fig. 4.14). While these trains are obviously in use in daily rotations in gait and the activities of daily life, we are choosing to emphasize, in this chapter, the direct and vertical link up the front of the body.

◆ ❁ Derailment

At the upper station of the rectus femoris, our Anatomy Train seems to come to a halt. No muscle or fascial structure takes off from the AIIS or even the ASIS in a generally superior direction. The abdominal obliques take off at angles (see Fig. 4.14A). The muscle contiguous to the rectus femoris on the medial side is the iliacus, so an argument could be made for some kind of linkage between the two structures, but the iliacus is part of a deeper plane, the Deep

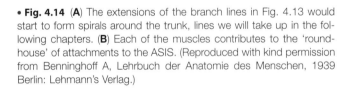

A

B

• **Fig. 4.14** (**A**) The extensions of the branch lines in Fig. 4.13 would start to form spirals around the trunk, lines we will take up in the following chapters. (**B**) Each of the muscles contributes to the 'roundhouse' of attachments to the ASIS. (Reproduced with kind permission from Benninghoff A, Lehrbuch der Anatomie des Menschen, 1939 Berlin: Lehmann's Verlag.)

Front Line (Fig. 4.15). For the SFL, we are looking for the surface continuity up the front. The rectus–iliacus connection is a special case that we will consider when we consider the interactions between the SFL and the Deep Front Line in Chapter 9.

The myofascia that clearly continues the run up the front line of the body is the rectus abdominis, so we will simply have to break the Anatomy Trains rules to make a logical jump over to the pubis. The rationale for this jump is as follows: the AIIS and the pubis are part of the same bone (at least in anyone over one year in age) (Fig. 4.16A). So, for every millimeter the pubis is pulled up by the rectus abdominis, the rectus femoris must lengthen by a millimeter to allow it to happen. If both contract, the front of the

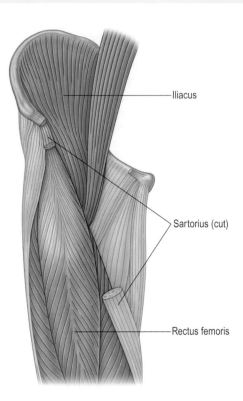

• **Fig. 4.15** Once you travel up the rectus femoris, what train can you take from there? No muscle goes directly in a cranial direction (see also Fig. 4.14B). The iliacus continues this direction, but there are two problems with this track: (1) the rectus femoris and the iliacus, though nearly contiguous, do not connect fascially, and (2) this portion of the iliacus is only a temporary surfacing of a deeper track, the Deep Front Line (see Ch. 9).

rib cage and the knee will approximate (Fig. 4.16B). If the body is arched into hyperextension, both must stretch reciprocally. If one cannot elongate, the other must make up for it or pass the strain up or down the train (Fig. 4.16C,D).

Thus, even though there is not a myofascial continuity, there is a mechanical continuity through the hip bone. This Anatomy Train works as a single track as long as we limit our discussion to movement in or near the sagittal plane. The SFL will not work as a continuous band in movements that involve strong hip or trunk rotations, but does act as a continuity in posture, running, and in sagittal stretches and movements (Fig. 4.17).

The Abdomen

Having now reseated ourselves on the top of the pubis, we can ride up on the abdominal fascia, including the muscular elements of the pyramidalis and rectus abdominis, and the fascial layers that surround the rectus from the obliques and transversus (Fig. 4.18; Video 6.16).

The Rectus Abdominis

The poor rectus abdominis: over-exercised by the 'go for the burn' crowd, and under-treated by the manual therapist. It

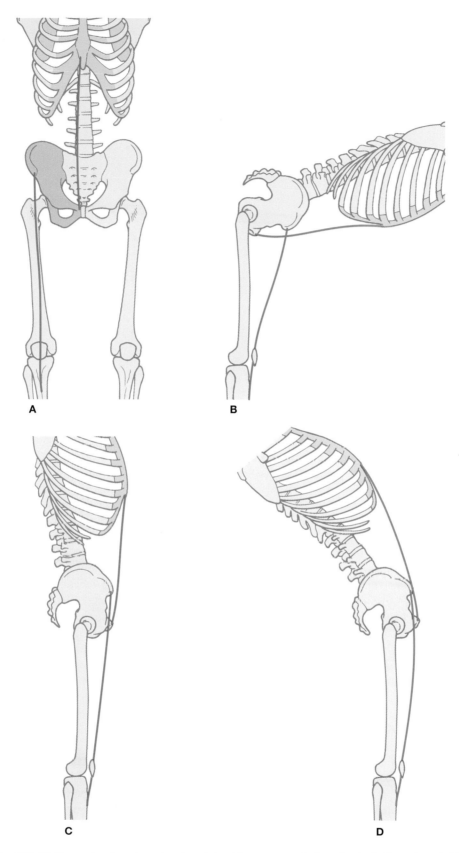

• **Fig. 4.16** (**A**) The rectus femoris and rectus abdominis are connected mechanically through each hip bone. (**B**) If both contract, the hip and trunk flex to approximate the rib cage and the knee. (**C**) In standing, relative tonus will help determine pelvic tilt. (**D**) In hyperextension, both are stretched away from each other – if one part is inelastic, the other must make up for it or pass the strain up or down the SFL. While this separation breaks the SFL into two slings, they are mechanically connected for all flexion and extension movements in the hip and trunk.

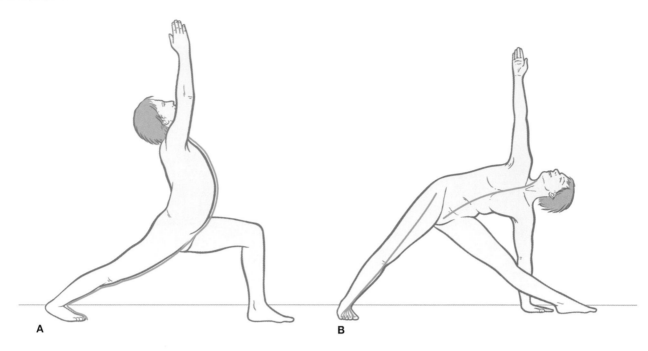

• **Fig. 4.17** (**A**) Purely sagittal (flexion–extension) movements will engage the SFL as a whole. (**B**) Rotational movements through the hips or trunk disengage the upper portion of the SFL from the lower.

is important to understand that the SFL involves at least three layers at this level: the fascial aponeurosis that runs in front of the rectus, the muscle itself, and the fascial sheet that runs behind it (see Fig. 4.18). These aponeuroses are shared with the other abdominal muscles, and will come up for consideration with other lines (see Chs 5, 6, 8, and 9). For now, we will concern ourselves with the span of the rectus itself between the pubis and the costal margin of the rib cage.

As we view the rectus, then, we must assess three separate parts: the tonus of the muscle itself, and the tonus of the two enveloping sheaths, in front and behind the muscle. If the rectus is flat – a set of 'six-pack' abs – then we can suspect high tonus in the superficial sheet and in the muscle itself. If the rectus bulges out, we must assess the tonus of the muscle, but we can be fairly sure that the deeper sheet behind the muscle, the transversalis fascia, is shortened (www.anatomytrains.com – video ref: Superficial Front Line, 33:15–35:05).

To free the front sheet and the muscle, have your client lie supine with his knees up, feet on the table. Facing cephalad, hook the tips of flexed fingers into the lower part of the muscle and move tissue upward, toward the ribs, taking a new purchase each time you reach one of the tendinous inscriptions in the rectus. You can repeat this move as necessary to continue the process of freeing the superficial aspect of the rectus up to the 5th rib.

To reach the posterior lamina of the rectus requires a more invasive but very effective technique. First, we must assess the nature of the shortness. If the lumbars are hyperextended into a lordosis, or the pelvis is held into an anterior tilt, the lumbars may simply be pushing the abdominal contents forward into the restraining rectus. In that case, it is necessary to free the SBL in the lumbars to give the abdomen more room to drop back (see Ch. 3).

If this is not the case, the bulging abdomen can also be due to enlargement of the abdominal contents caused by overeating or bloating, which must be solved by dietary means. Or, of course, there can be excess fat, either subcutaneously or, especially in men, in the visceral omental adipose layer underlying the peritoneum.

In any case, even if the belly sticks out and the muscle tonus seems low, it is possible that the tonus of the wall behind the rectus is quite high, tight, and responsible for restricting breathing or pulling on the back. With no bones near to work against, how can we isolate the sheath that runs behind the rectus but in front of the peritoneum? Since the back of the rectus sheath is part of the Deep Front Line, see Chapter 9 for the answer (or www.anatomytrains.com – video ref: Deep Front Line, Part 2).

The various tracks which crisscross the abdomen will be discussed in Chapters 6 and 8 (Video 6.9); for the moment we are moving due north on the rectus and its accompanying fascia. Of course, these abdominal lines all interact, but the SFL runs on a straight (though widening) track up to its next station at the 5th rib. The rectus must reach as high as the 'true' 5th rib to achieve sufficient stability for all the strong actions it must perform. The lower 'abdominal' ribs, with their long cartilaginous attachments to the sternum, would be too mobile to provide a stable attachment for the SFL, especially considering their large excursion during breathing, and the strong forces generated by the rectus abdominis in a tennis smash.

Mobilization and freeing extra adhesions where the rectus abdominis attaches and the abdominal fascia blends into the pectoral fascia is frequently rewarded with expanded

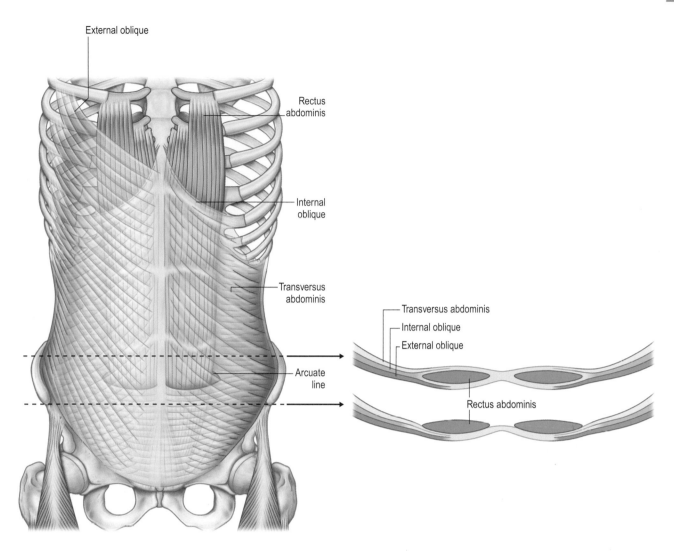

• Fig. 4.18 The rectus abdominis is the most superficial muscle of the abdomen all the way from the chest to the pubic bone. In terms of fascial layering, however, the rectus begins as superficial at the 5th rib, but shortly dives under the external oblique fascia within a few inches. Two inches (5 cm) lower than that, the internal oblique fascia splits to surround the rectus. Below the navel at the arcuate line pocket, the rectus passes through the transversalis fascia behind the transversus abdominis to become, at the pubic bone, the deepest muscle of the abdomen. Such an understanding of fascial, as opposed to simply muscular, anatomy leads to different strategies for 'Spatial Medicine'.

 breathing movement (www.anatomytrains.com – video ref: Superficial Front Line, 40:38–45:26).

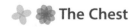 **The Chest**

From the 5th rib we can continue in the same direction via the sternalis muscle (if present) or its associated fascia (which almost always is), including the sternal fascia passing up the surface of the sternum, along with the fascia underlying pectoralis major out as wide as the sternochondral joints at the lateral edge of the sternum (Fig. 4.19). (The rectus attachment at the 5th rib will make another appearance when we consider, in Chapter 7, the anterior Arm Lines, which both start from the 5th rib attachment of the pectoralis minor and major. The rectus fascia thus shows a 'switch' here, a choice point, where strain or tension could follow either line, depending on the circumstances of movement, posture, and the necessities of physics.)

The sternalis, however, is an anomalous, capricious and surface muscle, though it is often expressed fascially even when it is not expressed muscularly. Whether or not the sternalis muscle or fascia can be detected, the SFL continues up from the rectus by means of fascial layers, which are readily palpable, over the sternum, the sternochondral joints, and the costal cartilages, up to the origin of the sternocleidomastoid. We suspect that stronger forces are transmitted mechanically through the sternum, as well as fascially via these layers and the pectoral fasciae as well.

It is interesting to note that Vesalius shows the rectus fascia proceeding under the pectoralis major almost all the way to the clavicle (Fig. 4.20). Modern anatomists think he may have been making a deliberate reference to canine

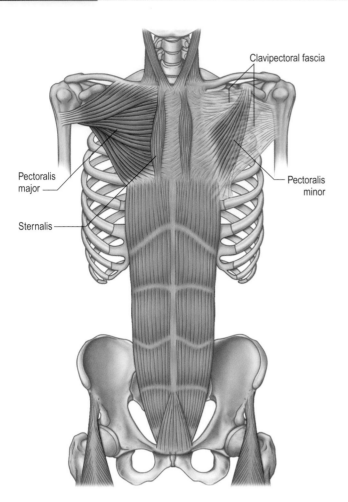

Clavipectoral fascia

Pectoralis major

Pectoralis minor

Sternalis

• **Fig. 4.19** The rectus abdominis attaches strongly to the 5th rib, but the fascia is continuous up the sternalis myofascia and with the fascia running along the sternochondral joints. The rectus also links fascially into the pectoralis major and minor, connecting the SFL to both the Front Arm Lines (see Ch. 7).

anatomy, but perhaps he was reflecting the fascial reality of his time. Could it be that the predominant activities at that period – chopping and agricultural work in general; in other words, active flexion movements – resulted in the laying down of increased sagittally oriented fascia traversing the front of the trunk (Video 6.14)?

Our initial attempts to make a similar dissection have fallen short of Vesalius's picture (Fig. 4.21). On the basis of a few attempts at dissection, we were able to follow the fascia up the sternum, but not any wider on the cartilaginous 'breastplate' to either side of the sternum, where our results could best be described as 'lacy'. More recently, we have found vertical fibers in the fascia on the profound side of the epimysium of pectoralis major, which do indeed connect from the rectus attachment to the lower part of the fascia colli superficialis (and sternocleidomastoid). By previously removing the pectoralis major from the cadaver prior to searching for the SFL, we had inadvertently eliminated these fibers, and thus a major part of the soft-tissue track along the front of the chest. In examining fascia as a system, our old muscular habits die hard.

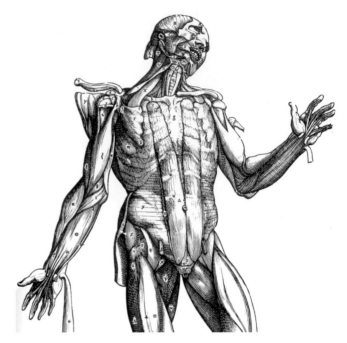

• **Fig. 4.20** Vesalius, in an early precursor of the myofascial meridians theory, shows the rectus abdominis fascia going up the rib cage nearly to the collarbone. Why? (Reproduced with permission from Saunders JB, O'Malley C. Dover Publications; 1973.)

❖ The Sternal Area

Above the costal arch, the rectus may be lifted headward from the front with extending fingertips or the heel of the hand. Although the rectus formally stops at the 5th rib, the SFL does not, and you can continue up the sternal area (Video 3.3), including the tissues superficial to the sternum itself, especially the tissue overlying the sternochondral joints between the sternum and the medial edge of the pectoralis major. Generally, this tissue wants to be moved cephalad, but sometimes, as in the case of a pinched or narrow chest, it also requires a lateral vector (www.anatomytrains.com – video ref: Superficial Front Line, 33:05–40:38).

The SFL in the Neck

Following the SFL upward on these tissues between and beneath the two medial edges of the pectoralis major muscles, we come to the top of the front of the sternum. A superficial glance at standard anatomy plates seems to indicate that the logical direction from here is to keep going straight, right up the front of the throat to the lower part of the jaw using the infrahyoid muscles (see Fig. 2.5A). These muscles would connect through the hyoid to the mandible, and from the mandible via the jaw muscles onto the lower part of the cranium, temptingly close to the upper end of the SBL on the brow ridge.

But this beautiful theory is about to be destroyed by an ugly fact: the lower attachments of these hyoid muscles do not attach to the front of the sternum, but tuck behind it into the posterior aspect of the sternal manubrium. Thus

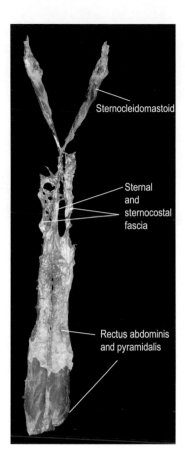

Sternocleidomastoid

Sternal and sternocostal fascia

Rectus abdominis and pyramidalis

• **Fig. 4.21** Our attempt to reproduce, in a fresh tissue cadaver, what Vesalius indicates as a connection from the rectus on up the chest yielded a disappointing lacework, at least on the part lateral to the sternum over the chondral portion of the ribs. Given the palpable layer of tissue that can be felt in this area, subsequent dissections have included investigation of the posterior pectoral major fascia as part of this line.

they are not on the same fascial plane as the SFL myofasciae (see Fig. 2.5B, p. 21). In fact the hyoid grouping is part of the visceral cylinder of the neck, joined to the thoracic viscera through the thoracic inlet, and will be seen again as one route in the Deep Front Line (see Ch. 9).

The mechanical connection from the chest to these muscles can be felt by hyperextending the neck and pointing the chin up into the air. The discerning will notice, however, that most of that pull extends down the inside of the rib cage with the Deep Front Line, not down the superficial surface with the SFL.

To continue up the SFL, we must look at what attaches to the outside of the top of the sternum. What does attach here, of course, is our familiar friend and member of the superficial cylinder of the neck (fascia colli superficialis), the sternocleidomastoid (SCM). The sternal head, in particular, of the SCM myofascia attaches firmly to the top and front of the sternum, interfacing with the sternal layer that comes up under the pectoralis fascia. This important track leads up laterally and posteriorly to the mastoid process of the temporal bone, and onto the postero-lateral galea aponeurotica (Fig. 4.22).

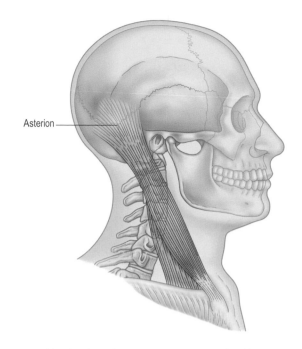

Asterion

• **Fig. 4.22** The fourth and uppermost portion of the SFL is the sternocleidomastoid (SCM) muscle, which tracks back along the neck onto the posterior portion of the temporal bone and the asterion – the sutural junction among the temporal, parietal, and occipital bones, and a major attachment of the tentorium cerebelli on its profound side.

The fact that the myofascial pull running up the sensitive front of the body makes a sudden jump to the back of the skull via the SCM produces a very interesting counterintuitive situation. Tightening the SFL causes flexion of the hips and trunk, either in motion or in posture, but produces hyperextension at the top of the neck (Fig. 4.23).

The SCM can participate in pure neck flexion in the supine position, as in a sit-up, when it is lifting the head against the force of gravity. Even in standing, put your hand against your forehead and push forward and down with your head, and you will feel the SCM contract. In standing posture, however, because it attaches to the mastoid process, it runs posterior to the hinge of the atlanto-occipital and atlanto-axial joints. Thus it works with gravity to help produce lower neck flexion and (a bit unexpectedly) upper neck hyperextension.

❖ The Sternocleidomastoid

The sternocleidomastoid (SCM) is a difficult muscle to stretch, the more so because often the underlying scalenes and suboccipitals are so short that they may reach their limitation long before the superficial SCM is brought into a stretch (see Ch. 9 for a discussion of these underlying muscles).

To stretch and open the superficial fascial cylinder in general, and the SCM in particular, stand beside your supine client and place your open fist along the SCM on one side of her neck, with your fingers pointing posteriorly. The direction of your pressure is crucial here: *do not push*

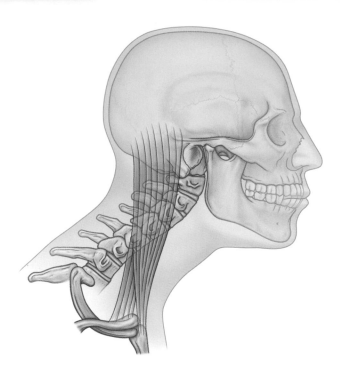

• **Fig. 4.23** The SCM is uniquely positioned, in standing posture, to create lower cervical flexion at the same time that it creates upper cervical hyperextension. The exact cervical level where this switch is made varies with posture, but is usually between C2-C3, or C3-C4.

into the neck (Video 3.1). The idea is to peel the superficial layer off the underlying layers, not to mash the SCM into submission. The direction of your stretch is to follow your fingers back, around the neck along its 'equator', without significant pressure into the viscera. The design is to pull the superficial fascia (and the SCM) toward the back, not to occlude the carotid artery or jugular vein. Any significant change of color in the client's face or report of intracranial pressure should cue you to desist.

As you begin your move, have your client assist by rotating her head away from you, taking the tissue out from under your hand as you move along the neck toward the back. Make sure your client is rotating around the axis of the neck, not simply rolling her head away from you on the table. You can use your other hand to guide her head, and you can also cue her: if she is really rotating her head, she will be able to hear her hair on the table. Just rolling the head on the table will not create the same noise to the client's ear (www.anatomytrains.com – video ref: Superficial Front Line, 46:58–52:45). Have her go to the limit of her easy range of motion, or to a full 90 degree side turn if that range is available.

❖ ♣ The Scalp

The line of pull from the SFL up onto the skull overlies and particularly affects strains at the asterion, the juncture among the occiput, parietal, and temporal bones (which, on the inside of the skull, is a major attachment point of

the tentorium cerebelli). Consider the line of pull of both SFLs, especially if they are tight (as in extreme forward head posture) – they can form a functional loop up and over the occiput at or about the lambdoidal suture (Fig. 4.24; Video 6.8). This loop can be palpated and released (www.anatomytrains.com – video ref: Superficial Back Line, 57:03–59:55). Otherwise, the fascia of the SFL blends with that of the SBL through the posterior part of the scalp fascia.

Where the fascia of the SCM and the superficial cylinder of the neck join the galea aponeurotica of the scalp, the same considerations and techniques as were already discussed in terms of the SBL (Ch. 3, p. 45) apply equally to the SFL: look for spindles of extra-tight fascia aligned along the direction of the SCM above and behind the mastoid process, right over or near the asterion.

❖ ♣ General Movement Treatment Considerations

The muscles of the SFL create dorsiflexion at the ankle, extension at the knee, and flexion of the hip and trunk. In the neck, the action of the SFL depends on one's position relative to gravity: while lying, it flexes the head on the neck; while in standing, the SCM creates lower cervical flexion and upper cervical hyperextension (see Discussion 4.2 below). At the same time, the SFL elongates to allow for full extension and hyperextension of the trunk and flexion at the knee. Various degrees of backbends and front of the leg stretches like lunges can thus be used to mobilize the SFL. Postural flexion of the trunk, forward head posture, or locked knees are all signs of excessive contraction in the SFL.

NOTE: Once again, as with the stretches offered in Chapter 3, caution is urged in assigning or attempting these stretches (see note on p. 46).

- Kneeling on the toes in plantarflexion and sitting into the heels is an easy way to test the ability of the lowest part of the SFL to stretch, from the back of the toes across the retinaculum to the knee.
- The 'cobra' stretch is an easy way to extend the stretch into the belly from the toes (Fig. 4.25A). Be aware of the head: if there is too much hyperextension in the neck, the stretch in the belly will be counteracted by the shortening of the SCM. Keep the chin tucked in a little, and the head high.
- Arching back into hip extension (fully supported for most beginners; meaning enough support to completely avoid lumbar strain or pain) extends the stretch of the SFL above the knee to the hip (Fig. 4.25B).
- The 'bridge' provides another intermediate stretch for the upper part of the SFL (Fig. 4.25C). Keep the neck flat to extend the mastoid process away from the sternal notch. Keep the toes pointed in plantarflexion to include the legs.

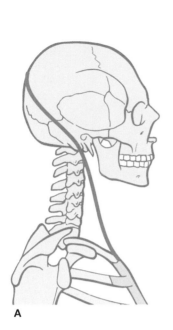

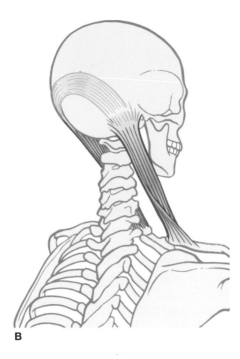

A

B

• **Fig. 4.24** The SCM muscle stops on the mastoid process, but the line of pull continues over the head, roughly along the line of the lambdoidal suture, connecting with the other SCM to form a scarf-like loop. (Video 6.8.)

• The backbend is the most complete stretch for the SFL, for those with the strength and flexibility to sustain it. It is not recommended for the beginner, though a physioball is a great support to give the beginner a feeling for what a full opening of the SFL would involve (see Fig. 4.7A). Pinching in the lower back is a sign to go more slowly into the stretch, that more preparatory work is needed in the core muscles.

❖ ❖ ❖ Palpating the Superficial Front Line

The departing station of the SFL is clearly palpable on the tops of the five toes, with the first track running back with the tendons onto the dorsum of the foot. The short extensor muscles of the toes can be felt on the lateral side of the upper foot, while the long tendons stay the course under the retinaculum and on up into the leg. The tibialis anterior tendon can be clearly seen and felt when the foot is dorsiflexed and inverted. If you dorsiflex and evert the foot, you may find the peroneus tertius tendon (if you or your model has one), just lateral to the little toe tendon, going down to the middle of the 5th metatarsal (see Fig. 4.11).

All of these tendons run under the retinacula to gather into the anterior compartment of the leg. The thickened areas of the retinacula can sometimes be felt when the foot is strongly dorsiflexed, just to either side of these tendons, running to both malleoli. The sharp edges of the retinacula seen in anatomy atlases are not often palpable, as it fades off into the crural fascia – the sharp edges are created with a scalpel.

In the leg, the individual toe extensor muscles disappear under the tibialis anterior, which can be followed right up

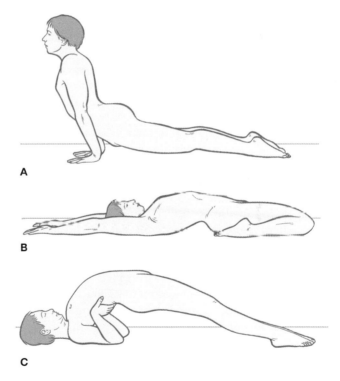

A

B

C

• **Fig. 4.25** Common stretches for parts or all of the SFL.

to the bump of the tibial tuberosity below the knee. The lateral edge of the anterior compartment is marked by the anterior intermuscular septum, which can be traced by walking your finger up from the lateral malleolus while dorsiflexing and plantarflexing the foot. The tibialis – anterior to the malleolus – will be active on dorsiflexion, while the neighboring fibularii, in the compartment posterior and superior to the malleolus, will be active on plantarflexion. The septum is the wall between the two. If you follow it accurately, you will reach the top of the septum just in front of the fibular head.

The sub patellar (quadriceps) tendon can be easily palpated between the tibial tuberosity and the patella. With an extended knee, the tendon of the rectus femoris is also easily palpable above the knee, as is the muscle, which can usually be 'strummed' horizontally most of the way up to the AIIS. As you approach the top of the thigh, the sartorius and tensor fasciae latae can be felt converging toward the ASIS, while the rectus, in most cases, dives down between these two, creating a small but palpable 'pocket' on its way to the AIIS (see Fig. 4.12). (Can you feel a strong tendon-like fascia going to the ASIS? Though never listed in the books, we have found such alternative attachments fairly often in cadaver dissection.)

The rectus abdominis is easily felt between the pubis and the ribs by having the client lift his head and chest as in a sit-up. It begins as two round tendons palpable on the superior aspect of the pubic bone. It widens as it passes up the body to the 5th rib (see Fig. 4.19). The outside edge of the rectus tracks a fascial structure called the semilunar line. Tendinous inscriptions within the muscle of the rectus abdominis create the 'six-pack' (which is actually an 'eight-pack').

Reach around the rectus at the level of the umbilicus and pick it up (toward the ceiling with a supine model). The umbilicus joins all the layers from the skin to the peritoneum as a type of fascial grommet, so that when you lift it, you affect the falciform and round ligament going to the liver, and lift the entire peritoneal contents, all the way around to the retroperitoneal kidneys.

The sternalis and its fascia can sometimes be 'strummed' horizontally above the 5th rib and medial to the pectoralis, but the fascia over the sternochondral joints can be readily felt at the bumpy outer edges of the sternum.

The SCM can also be easily distinguished by having the supine client rotate the head to one side and lift it against resistance, such as a hand resting on the forehead (see Fig. 4.22). Both the sternal head and the clavicular head can be felt, the more if you have them turn their head from side to side, and the muscle followed up to its attachment to the mastoid process, with a thin fascial layer going beyond the muscle attachment onto the skull.

DISCUSSION 4.1

❧ ❖ ❧ Balance Between the Superficial Front and the Superficial Back Lines

The first aspect of the SFL to note is its disjointed, disparate nature compared to the long conjoined flow of the SBL. In contrast, the SFL shows more discrete functioning of its constituent parts: the anterior crural compartment, the quadriceps, the rectus abdominis, and the SCM. Though they often work together to create consistent pulls along the

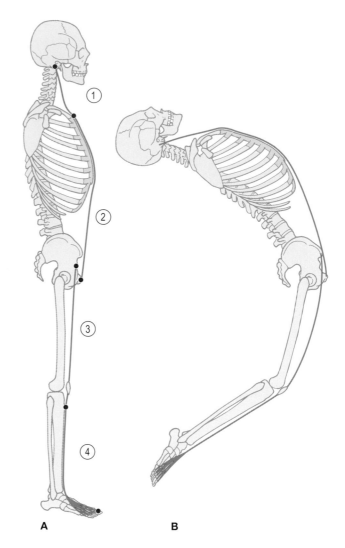

• **Fig. 4.26** With the Superficial Back Line 'turned on' in its postural role of holding us up, the four tracks of the SFL are able to work individually while standing, but will conjoin in trunk hyperextension.

SFL, they tend to conjoin truly into a single band only in relatively extreme hyperextended postures such as a backbend (Fig. 4.26 or Fig. 4.7A), or in extreme contraction (see Fig. 4.30).

This brings us to the obvious, but complex, relationship between the SFL and the SBL, the two lines that traverse the front and back aspects of the body. In the example of the 'military' or 'compensated oral' postural preference, the SBL (or some portion of it) is 'locked short' like a bowstring (Fig. 4.27). In the same example, the SFL (or some portion of it) will be 'locked long' – i.e. strained or eccentrically loaded, with the visceral contents of the ventral cavity pushed forward against its restraining tension. If the SBL is acting like a bowstring, the SFL starts to act like the wood on the front of the drawn bow.

Imagine a strip of balsa wood with an elastic stretched along both sides (Fig. 4.28A). As the elastic on one side was shortened, the wood would bend, stretching, perforce, the elastic on the other side (Fig. 4.28B).

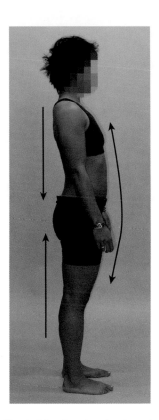

• **Fig. 4.27** The 'military' style of posture involves shortening and tightening the SBL, especially the middle part, while the SFL must lengthen in some other part to accommodate it.

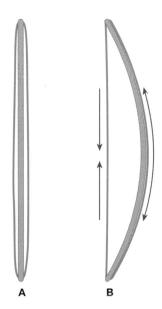

• **Fig. 4.28** (**A**) Myofascial units are often arranged in antagonistic pairs on either side of the skeletal armature. (**B**) When one side is chronically shortened, either muscularly concentrically loaded or fascially locked short, the other side is stretched tight (eccentrically loaded on the muscle and locked long in the fascial elements).

A commonly observed pattern shows the hamstrings and the muscles surrounding the sacrum becoming shortened and bunched, pushing the pelvis and hip forward. The muscles on the front of the hip then become tight as they are stretched and strain to contain the forward push from

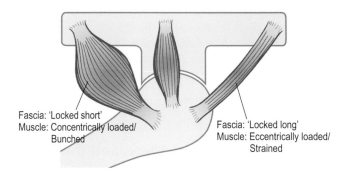

Fascia: 'Locked short'
Muscle: Concentrically loaded/ Bunched

Fascia: 'Locked long'
Muscle: Eccentrically loaded/ Strained

• **Fig. 4.29** The eccentrically loaded muscles are often the noisy ones in terms of pain and active trigger points, but the locked short muscles, often silent, are the ones that need to be opened and stretched for permanent resolution of the pattern.

the back. It is very important clinically to distinguish between the muscle that is tense because it is concentrically loaded, and the muscle that is tense because it is eccentrically loaded, as treatment of the two conditions will differ (Fig. 4.29).

Just as often, however, we see the opposite pattern between the SFL and the SBL: the front is locked short, rounding the thoracic spine or flattening the lumbar curve, creating a collapsed or 'overburdened' posture (see Fig. 11.12, p. 234).

In considering a fully lengthened, easily maintained posture, it is hard to escape the idea that the muscles of the SFL are designed to pull 'up'. Now muscles, as far as is known, show no propensity or even possibility for determining their direction of pull. They simply pull on the surrounding fascial net, and physics determines whether the result pulls origin toward insertion, insertion toward origin, or neither, as in an isometric or eccentric contraction.

Nevertheless, if we consider the SFL from the top down, we could see that the SCM portion originating from the mastoid process would ideally be the origin of postural stability, helping to pull up on the top of the rib cage via the sternum (see Fig. 4.4). In turn, the rectus abdominis could pull up on the pubic bone, helping to prevent a slump into an anterior tilt of the pelvis. Too often, however, the very opposite occurs, and the rectus pulls down on the rib cage, depressing the ribs and restricting breathing. This pull is conveyed through the sternalis and sternum to the SCM, which pulls down, in its turn, on the head, bringing it forward (see Fig. 4.5; Video 6.25).

When this occurs, an extra burden is shifted onto the SBL: in addition to supporting the back of the body in extension, it must now counteract the downward pull of the SFL. This often leads to super-tight muscles and to extra fibrotic and stuck-down fascia along the back line of the body, tissue that aches and cries out to be worked on. The practitioner viewing this pattern, however, is well advised to work up the front of the body, freeing the SFL so that the SBL can return to its proper job. Working only the SBL and back in cases like these will result in only temporary relief and, over time, an even worse posture. How many bodywork clients say, 'Just work my back and shoulders today, please, that's what's really aching'? The knowledgeable practitioner turns his or her attention to other places along the front line, or to postural re-education.

DISCUSSION 4.2

❖ ♣ ♣ The SFL, the Neck, and the Startle Response

'All negative emotion', says Feldenkrais, 'is expressed as flexion'.[2] The general truth of this simple statement is brought home to any observer of human behavior every day. We see the hunch of anger, the slump of depression, or the cringe of fear many times and in many different forms. They all involve flexion.

Among the quadrupeds, as we have noted, only humans put all their most vulnerable parts literally 'up front' for all to see (or cut or bite) (see Fig. 4.3). Subtly or obviously, people protect those sensitive parts: a retraction in the groin, a tight belly, a pulled-in chest. It is natural enough that when they feel threatened, humans should return toward a younger (primary fetal curve) or more protected (quadrupedal) posture.

There is, however, one notable exception to Feldenkrais's observation: negative emotion regularly produces hyperextension of the upper neck, not flexion (Fig. 4.30). We can see this very clearly in the reaction called the startle response (what Thomas Hanna referred to as the 'red light' reflex[3]).

What we can see very clearly is that the startle response is not, strictly speaking, a total flexion response, but is more accurately seen as a shortening and tightening along the SFL. The clear indication of this general response is that the mastoid process is brought closer to the pubic bone. This not only protects the organs along the front, but also retracts the neck into hyperextension, bringing the head forward and down. There have been several theories put forward as to why this pattern of contraction may have been evolutionarily advantageous. The most tellingly obvious is that in the quadruped, where the SFL shows up more or less in its current form from head to pubis, contracting the SFL would bring the head closer to the ground without sacrificing the ability to see and hear the threat (Fig. 4.31). A hedgehog, obviously, has adopted the full flexion strategy.

The muscles of the Superficial Front Arm Line also frequently join in this response, bringing elbow flexion and shoulder protraction into this picture. The total posture, then, of the startled person involves rigidity in the legs, plus trunk and arm flexion, coupled with upper neck hyperextension.

The problem comes when the startled posture is maintained, which humans are perfectly and repeatedly capable of doing over an extended period (Fig. 4.32). This posture and its variants can affect nearly every human function negatively, though breathing in particular is restricted by

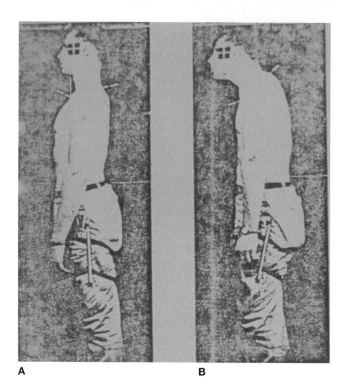

A   **B**

• **Fig. 4.30** A famous photo, from the world of the Alexander Technique, of a subject (**A**) just before and (**B**) just after a blank gun was fired behind him. The startle response is cross-cultural, and can be viewed as a sudden contraction of the SFL, which serves to protect the spine as well as all the sensitive parts on the front of the body shown in Fig. 4.3. (Reproduced with kind permission from Frank Jones.[4])

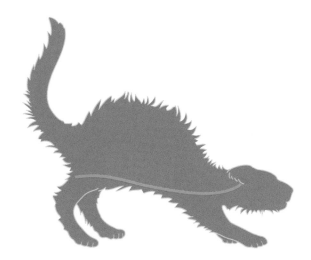

• **Fig. 4.31** In a quadruped, the SFL runs along the underside of the body, but passes up behind the head. When it contracts, the back arches in flexion, but the neck extends so the face and eyes stay in contact with the outside world.

shortening of the SFL. Easy breathing depends on upward and outward movement of the ribs, as well as a reciprocal relationship between the pelvic and respiratory diaphragms. The shortened SFL pulls the head forward and down, requiring compensatory tightening in both the back and the front that restricts rib movement. Shortening in the groin,

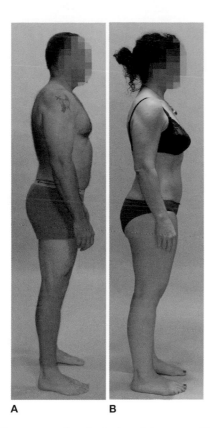

A   **B**

• **Fig. 4.32** Can you see the shortening of the upper SFL underlying (**A**)'s posture? (**B**)'s SFL is open in the chest, but short in the lower leg. Humans can manage to maintain a postural version of the startle response, along with its underlying psycho-emotional state, for many years, until structural or psychological intervention (**A**). In some cases, a shortened portion of the SFL is compensated by a shortening in the SBL (see Fig. 4.27). We are looking for balanced tone between the tissues of the SFL and SBL as is approximated in (**B**), without regard, for the time being, to whether that tone is high or low. Get balance first, then go for proper tone. (www.anatomytrains.com – video ref. Body Reading, 101)

if the protective tightness proceeds beyond the rectus abdominis into the legs, throws off the balance between the respiratory and pelvic diaphragms, resulting in over-reliance on the front of the diaphragm for breathing.

The real, original startle response is marked by an explosive exhale; the maintained startle response shows a decided postural tendency to be stuck on the exhale side of the breath cycle, which in turn can accompany a trip through depression. A slow and thorough journey up the SFL, freeing these tissues and learning to lift each element of the SFL from the top can relieve the somatic element of burden from such clients, often to very positive effect.

References

1. Mollier S. *Plastische Anatomie*. 2nd ed. Munich: Bergman Verlag; 1938.
2. Feldenkrais M. *Body and Mature Behavior*. New York: International Universities Press; 1949.
3. Hanna T. *Somatics*. Novato, CA: Somatics Press; 1968.
4. Jones FP. *Freedom to Change*. 3rd ed. London: Mouritz; 1997.

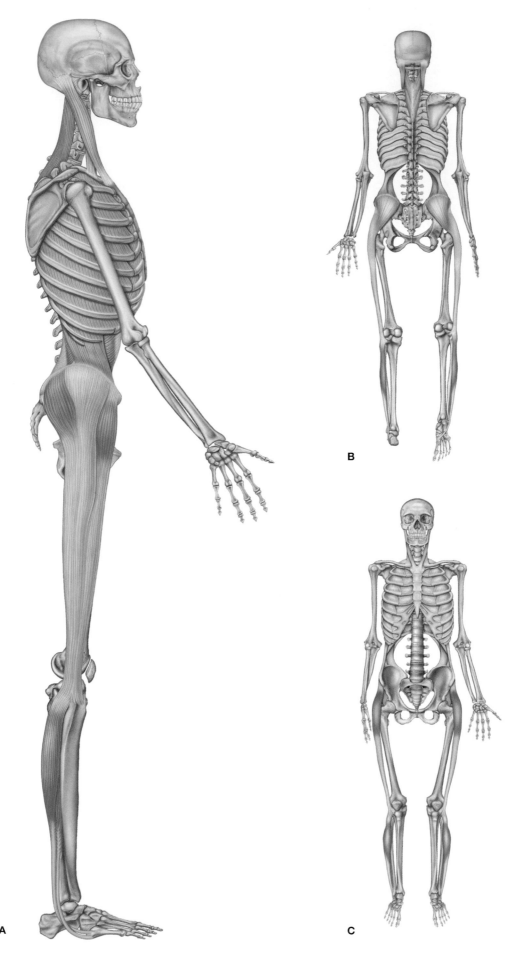

A

B

C

• **Fig. 5.1** The Lateral Line.

5

The Lateral Line

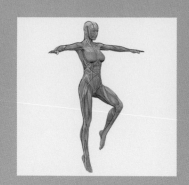

OVERVIEW

The Lateral Line (LL) (Fig. 5.1) brackets each side of the body from the medial and lateral mid-point of the foot around the outside of the ankle and up the lateral aspect of the leg and thigh, passing along the trunk in a 'basket weave' (crossed-shoelace) pattern under the shoulder to the skull in the region of the ear (Fig. 5.2/Table 5.1; Video 2.3).

Postural Function

The LL functions posturally to balance front and back, and bilaterally to balance left and right (Fig. 5.3). The LL also mediates forces among the other superficial lines – the Superficial Front Line, the Superficial Back Line, all the Arm Lines, and the Spiral Line. The LL often acts in a coordinated manner as an outer stabilizing system for the trunk and legs to prevent buckling of the structure during activity. (The inner stabilizing system is found in the Deep Front Line – see Ch. 9.)

Movement Function

The LL participates in creating a lateral bend in the body – lateral flexion of the trunk, abduction at the hip, and eversion at the foot – but also functions as an adjustable 'brake' for lateral and a 'watch spring' for rotational movements of the trunk (Fig. 5.4).

General Manual Therapy Considerations

Although both of the other 'cardinal' lines have both a right and a left side, the two Lateral Line myofascial meridians are sufficiently far from each other and from the midline to exert substantially more side-to-side leverage on the skeleton than either the SFL or the SBL, into both of which the Lateral Line blends at its edges (Fig. 5.2A). The LL is usually essential in mediating left side–right side imbalances, and these should be assessed and addressed early in a global treatment plan.

Common postural compensation patterns associated with the LL include: ankle pronation or supination, ankle dorsiflexion limitation, genu varus or valgus, adduction restriction/chronic abductor contraction, lumbar side-bend or lumbar compression (in bilateral LL contraction), side shifts or tilts of the rib cage on the pelvis, shortening of depth between sternum and sacrum, and shoulder restriction due to over-involvement with head stability, especially in head forward posture.

The Lateral Line in Detail

The LL manages to connect both the medial and the lateral side of the foot to the lateral side of the body. We begin – at the lowest point again, simply as a convenience – with the joint between the 1st metatarsal and 1st cuneiform, about halfway down the foot on its medial side, with the insertion of the tendon of fibularis longus (Fig. 5.5). Following it, we travel laterally under the foot, and, via a channel in the cuboid bone, turn up toward the lateral aspect of the ankle.

The LL picks up another connection, the fibularis brevis, about halfway down the lateral side of the foot. (The peroneal muscles were renamed as the 'fibularis' muscles; despite a lifetime of habit, we will follow the new convention.) From its insertion at the base of the 5th metatarsal, the fibularis brevis tendon passes up and back to the posterior side of the fibular malleolus, where the two fibularis muscles comprise the sole muscular components of the lateral compartment of the lower leg (see Fig. 2.3, p. 20). Thus both sides of the metatarsal complex are strongly tied to the fibula, providing support for the lateral longitudinal arch along the way (Fig. 5.6).

❖ The Lateral Arch

The lateral band of the plantar fascia was included in the Superficial Back Line (Ch. 3, p. 33). Although it is technically not part of the LL per se, it merits a mention as a factor in lateral balance. If the lateral muscles are so short as to evert the foot, or the foot is pronated in any case, the lateral band of the plantar fascia, running from the outer

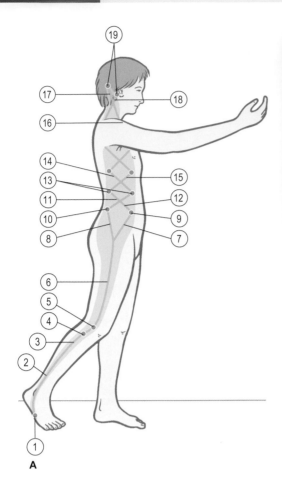

A

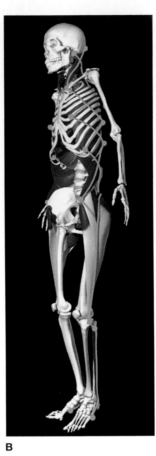

B

• **Fig. 5.2 (A)** Lateral Line tracks and stations. The shaded area shows the area of superficial fascial influence. **(B)** Lateral Line tracks and stations using the Primal Pictures Anatomy Trains program. (B, Image provided courtesy of Primal Pictures, www.primalpictures.com.)

lower edge of the calcaneus straight forward to the 5th metatarsal base, will commend itself to work in the side-lying position, spreading the tissue between the two attachments (www.anatomytrains.com – video ref: Lateral Line, 10:27–13:00).

❖ ❖ The Fibularii (Peroneals)

The depth of the fibularis longus tendon on the underside of the foot and the brevity of the fibularis brevis make it impossible to accomplish anything useful with the LL below the malleolus, so we begin with the lateral crural compartment (Fig. 5.7; Video 6.24). Fibularis longus and brevis blend together in this compartment, which is bounded by septa (fascial walls) on either side. The anterior septum can be found on a line that runs roughly between the lateral malleolus and the front of the head of the fibula. The posterior septum, between the fibularii and the soleus, can be traced from the open space just in front of the Achilles tendon up to just behind the fibular head. (See the palpation section below for more detail.) These septa and the overlying crural fascia are primary places to ease and open first in addressing all forms of compartment syndrome.

As well as direct work to open these septa, the fibular myofascial units themselves can be lengthened and softened by work at right angles to the muscle fiber direction:

spreading the tissue of this compartment both to the anterior and the posterior of the lateral line with fingertips or knuckles, while the client moves through the dorsiflexion–plantarflexion range (www.anatomytrains.com – video ref: Lateral Line, 12:51–19:12).

The fibularii are often used posturally to prevent dorsiflexion, as in standing. They can create excessive eversion when they are too loaded or short.

❀ ❀ The Thigh

Although the fibularis brevis originates on the lower half of the fibula, the longus (and thus the fascial compartment) and this train of the LL continue on up to the fibular head. The obvious, straight-ahead connection from this point is to continue on to the biceps femoris, and this myofascial meridian connection will be explored in the next chapter on the Spiral Line. The continuation of the LL, however, involves a different switch, going slightly forward onto the anterior ligament of the head of the fibula onto the tibial condyle and blending into the broad sweep of the inferior fibers of the iliotibial tract (ITT) (Fig. 5.8).

The ITT begins its upward journey here, starting from the lateral tibial condyle as a narrow, thick, and strong band that can be clearly felt on the lateral aspect of the lower thigh. Like the Achilles tendon, the ITT widens and thins

TABLE 5.1	Lateral Line: Myofascial 'Tracks' and Bony 'Stations' (Fig. 5.2)	
Bony Stations	**Myofascial Tracks**	
Occipital ridge/ mastoid process	19	
	17,18	Splenius capitis/ sternocleidomastoid
1st and 2nd ribs	16	
	14,15	External and internal intercostals
Ribs	13	
	11,12	Lateral abdominal obliques
Iliac crest, ASIS, PSIS	9,10	
	8	Gluteus maximus
	7	Tensor fasciae latae
	6	Iliotibial tract/abductor muscles
Lateral tibial condyle	5	
	4	Anterior ligament of head of fibula
Fibular head	3	
	2	Fibularii muscles, lateral crural compartment
1st and 5th metatarsal bases	1	

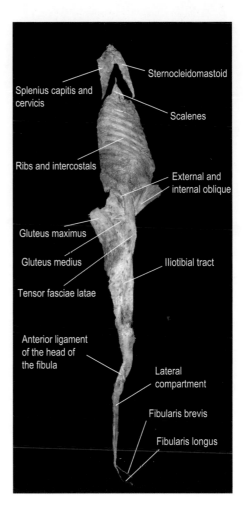

• **Fig. 5.3** Here we see a dissection from an embalmed cadaver of the Lateral Line, including the two fibularii (peroneals), connecting through tissues at the lateral knee to the iliotibial tract and abductors, which are fascially continuous with the lateral abdominal obliques. The ribs from the sternochondral junction in the front to the angle of the ribs posteriorly are included with their corresponding intercostal layers. The scalenes, attached to the upper two ribs, are included here, but the quadratus lumborum is not. The upper two muscles, the sternocleidomastoid and splenii looking like a chevron, do not attach to the rest of the specimen because they both attach inferiorly near or at the midline, whereas the specimen includes only about 30° each side from the coronal midline. (www.anatomytrains.com – video ref: Anatomy Trains Revealed)

as it passes superiorly. By the time it reaches the hip, it is an aponeurosis wide enough to hold the greater trochanter of the femur in a fascial cup or sling (Fig. 5.9). The tension on the ITT sheet, which is maintained and augmented by the abductors from above and the vastus lateralis hydraulically amplifying from beneath, helps keep the ball of the hip in its socket when weight is placed on one leg. This arrangement also acts as a simple tensegrity structure. By acting as a 'backstay', some of the direct compressive stress of our body weight is taken off the femoral neck by the ITT, whose leverage can be augmented by the stiffening created by a contraction of the underlying vastus lateralis.

The LL continues to widen above the trochanter, to include three muscular components: the tensor fasciae latae along the anterior edge, the superior fibers of the gluteus maximus along the posterior edge, and the gluteus medius, which attaches to the underside, the profound side, of the ITT's fascial sheet (see Figs. 5.3 and 5.4).

All these myofasciae tack down onto the outer rim of the iliac crest, stretching from the ASIS to the PSIS. This entire complex is used in the weighted leg in every step to keep the trunk from leaning toward the unweighted leg. In other words, the abductors are used less often to create abduction, but are used in every step to prevent hip adduction. This

requires a stabilizing tension along the whole lower LL to the next stable area: where the foot meets the floor.

❖ The Iliotibial Tract

In terms of its role in the LL, the ITT can be considered to begin at a point at the bottom (the tibial condyle, but really the whole outside of the knee), spreading upward to three points at the top (the ASIS, PSIS, and the strong fascial attachment at the heavy middle portion of the iliac crest). Depending on the postural angle of the pelvis, it may be advisable to work the leading or following edge of the ITT more strongly (Video 3.9). Left–right imbalances in ITT

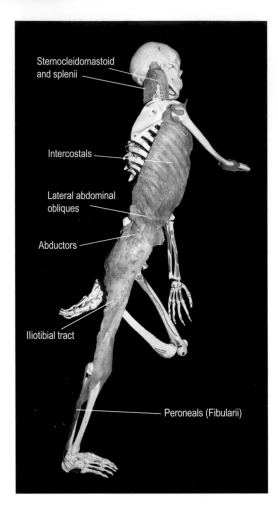

Sternocleidomastoid and splenii

Intercostals

Lateral abdominal obliques

Abductors

Iliotibial tract

Peroneals (Fibularii)

• **Fig. 5.4** Here we see the same specimen laid into a classroom skeleton. The position is not quite accurate because the scapula was fixed and could not be moved or removed, but this photo nevertheless gives a sense of how the Lateral Line is used to stabilize coronal and rotational movements of the body during our predominantly sagittal motivation.

tone will be present in lateral tilts of the pelvis. Imbalance between the ITT and adductor muscles will be present in *genu varum* and *valgum* (laterally or medially shifted knees).

The ITT can be worked in a manner similar to the fibularii: with the client side-lying and the knee supported, the practitioner can work either up or down the ITT and associated abductors, spreading laterally from the lateral midline with knuckles or loose fists. Since fibers of the ITT are

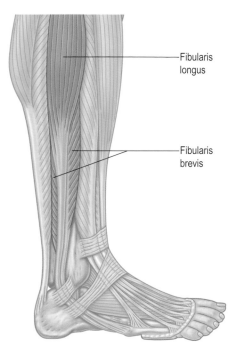

Fibularis longus

Fibularis brevis

• **Fig. 5.6** The first track of the Lateral Line joins the metatarsal complex to the lateral side of the fibula, supporting the lateral longitudinal arch along the way.

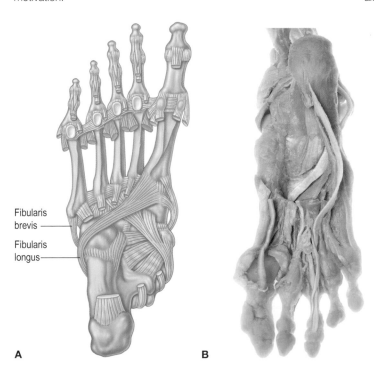

Fibularis brevis

Fibularis longus

A   B

• **Fig. 5.5** (**A**) The Lateral Line begins in the middle of the medial and lateral arches of the foot, at the bases of the 1st and 5th metatarsals. (**B**) The foot from below, with superficial structures resected to reveal the fibularis longus tendon, strapping in the lateral and proximal transverse arches with a strong (white) band snugged up to the 1st metatarsal base, cuneiforms, and the cuboid bones. This is the starting point for the journey up the Lateral Line. (B, Photo courtesy of Anna Rowedder)

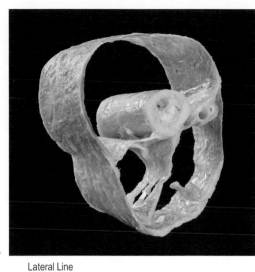

Lateral Line
(fibularii and fascial septa)

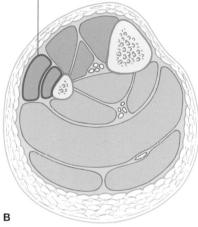

B

• **Fig. 5.7** (**A**) The thigh dissected and plastinated to show the lateral intermuscular septum diving from the fascia lata and iliotibial tract for the linea aspera on the femur. (**B**) The lateral compartment consists of the deeper fibularis brevis and the overlying fibularis longus. This compartment is bound by septa on both anterior and posterior aspects, separating it from the anterior compartment (SFL) and the superficial posterior compartment (SBL) respectively. (Video 6.24)

meshed with the circumferential fibers of the fascia lata, it can also be useful to work the side of the leg vertically. Use the flat of the ulna, placing one just under the iliac crest, the other just above the greater trochanter. Slowly but deliberately bring the lower forearm toward the knee, stimulating the ITT. The client can help by bringing the knee forward and back (www.anatomytrains.com – video ref: Lateral Line, 19:13–25:51).

The ITT is far too tough to get longer, even with strong pressure, so 'stretching' the ITT is likely stretching the truth. We can possibly help hydrate the dense fascia of the ITT, certainly improve its proprio- and interoception, or likely ease its glide on the underlying vastus lateralis muscle, but lengthening the ITT through either manual therapy, yoga-type sustained stretch, or via foam rolling or self-myofascial release tools is physically unlikely.[1]

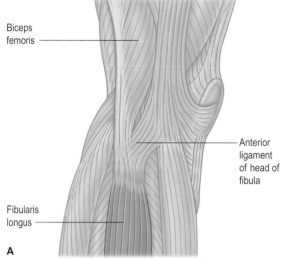

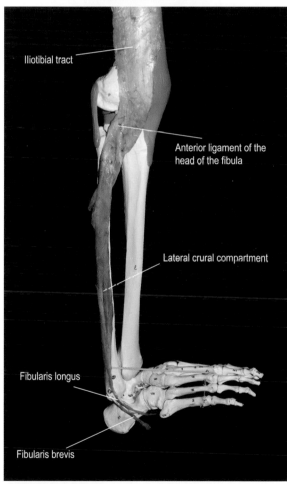

• **Fig. 5.8** (**A**) The Lateral Line goes from the lateral compartment via the anterior ligament of the head of the fibula to the bottom of the iliotibial tract. (**B**) Tissues of the lower end of the iliotibial tract in fact have attachments to the tibia, the fibula, and the fascia of the lateral as well as the anterior crural compartment.

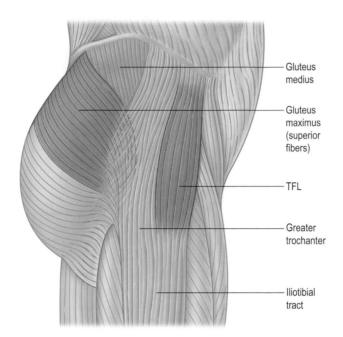

• **Fig. 5.9** The second major track of the Lateral Line consists of the iliotibial tract and the associated abductor muscles, the tensor fasciae latae (TFL), the gluteus medius, and the superior fibers of the gluteus maximus.

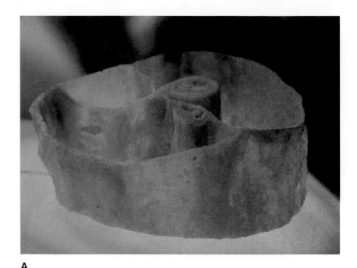

A

THE LOWER LIMB

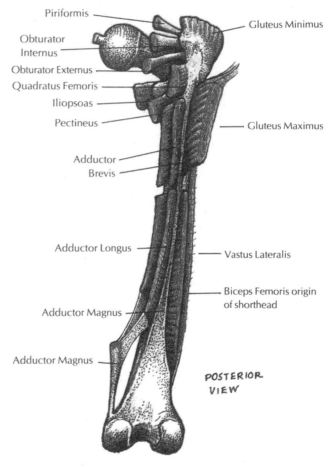

Posterior view of muscle insertions of the Femur

B

Work here is nevertheless helpful. Searching fingers can assess: Is the anterior edge of the ITT proportionally thicker, more fixed, or tighter than the posterior edge? If so, then the angle of the forearm on the leg can be adjusted, as in changing the angle of a violin bow to sound another string, to emphasize either the anterior, middle, or the posterior portion.

The posterior portion of the ITT blends with the fascia lata into a strong wall, the lateral intermuscular septum, which dives in to divide the vastus lateralis from the biceps femoris (Fig. 5.10A). This septum runs from the posterior surface of the inferior part of the greater trochanter where the gluteus maximus ends, and attaches onto the linea aspera all along its length to the lateral epicondyle above the knee (Fig. 5.10B). Much attention has been given to the ITT by the foam rollers, but we need to attend (often with your elbow) to the posterior ITT, working your way down between the muscle groups, seeking the edge of the linea aspera.

This work is especially called for in those whose pelvis is anteriorly shifted relative to their feet. Working the tissue toward the knee, while the supine client slowly flexes and extends the knee can help the duck-footed or the 'uptight' regain an adaptable balance. This heavy septum, which participates with the SFL and SBL, also needs to be opened, hydrated, and revivified if the client is 'leaning into the tissues' of the leg to stand up, rather than letting the weight fall through the bones. When the Lateral Line is straight from trochanter to malleolus, the SBL and SFL in the leg are likely to be balanced as well.

• **Fig. 5.10** (**A**) The lateral intermuscular septum is continuous with the iliotibial tract, the fascia lata, and the epimysial coverings of the biceps femoris and vastus lateralis. (**B**) This septum reaches into the linea aspera on the posterior edge of the femur right between the short head of the biceps femoris and the vastus lateralis. (B, Image from John Hull Grundy)

❖ The Abductor Muscles and the Greater Trochanter

The abductor muscles themselves, tensor fasciae latae and the three gluteal muscles, can be worked generally with the point of the elbow or well-placed knuckles to move the tissue in a radiating pattern away from the greater trochanter toward and up to the iliac crest. You may wish to work these tissues differentially in the case of anteriorly tilted pelvis, say, where the anterior tissues, acting as flexors, will be very much shorter and denser. Do not neglect the 'facets' of the greater trochanter itself, which, when freed in detail, can be very productive of new movement (www.anatomytrains.com – video ref: Deep Front Line, Part 1: 25:52–30:57).

✿ Derailment

As we move from the appendicular portion to the axial portion of the LL, we face another derailment – a break with the general Anatomy Trains rules. The ITT – in fact, the whole lower LL – looks a bit like the letter 'Y' (see Fig. 5.9). To follow the rules we would have to keep going up and out on the upper prongs of the 'Y' (as in Fig. 5.11A) with sheets or lines of myofascia that continued to fan outward and upward from the ASIS and PSIS. We will find these continuations in the Spiral and Functional Lines (Chs 6 and 8). If, however, we look at how the myofascia arranges itself along the lateral aspect of the trunk from here on up, we find that the fascial planes cross back and forth in a basket weave arrangement (Figs. 5.2 and 5.11B).

Although these sharp changes in direction break the letter of the Anatomy Trains rules, the overall effect of these series of 'X's (or diamonds, if you prefer) is to create a mesh or net which contains each side of the body as a whole – a bit like the old Chinese finger traps. The resultant structure is a wide net of a line that contains the lateral trunk from hip to ear (see Fig. 5.2).

❖ The Iliac Crest and Waist

The upper edge of the iliac crest provides attachments for the latissimus dorsi and the three layers of the abdominal muscles. The outer two of these, the obliques, form part of the LL, and are fascially continuous with the ITT over the edge of the iliac crest (see Fig. 5.3). The external oblique attaches to the outside edge of the iliac crest, the internal oblique to the top of the iliac crest, and the transversus abdominis (which is part of the Deep Front Line) to the inside edge. Practitioners can affect different layers by adjusting their pressure, angle, and intent accordingly.

In terms of the LL, the iliac crest is a frequent site of connective tissue accumulation, especially posteriorly, and 'cleaning' these layers off the bone can be helpful in coaxing length from the LL (www.anatomytrains.com – video ref: Lateral Line, 30:50–35:38). Direction matters here: in cases where the pelvis is in anterior tilt, the tissue needs to be moved posteriorly; in cases of posterior tilt, the inverse is true. In cases with neutral pelvic tilt, tissue can be spread in either direction from the midline (www.anatomytrains.com – video ref: Lateral Line, 35:39–37:23).

When the rib cage is shifted posteriorly relative to the pelvis, the lower lateral ribs move closer to the posterior

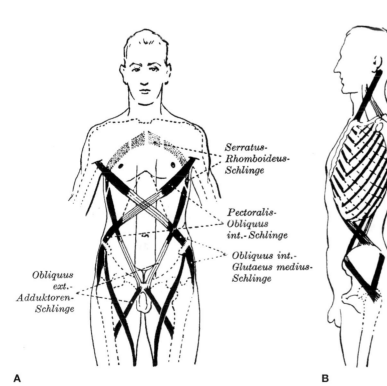

Serratus-
Rhomboideus-
Schlinge

Pectoralis-
Obliquus
int.-Schlinge

Obliquus int.-
Glutaeus medius-
Schlinge

Obliquus
ext.-
Adduktoren-
Schlinge

A

B

• **Fig. 5.11** Anatomy Trains rules would require that the 'Y' of the iliotibial tract continue out and around the body in spirals as in (**A**), but the actuality of the Lateral Line is that it starts a series of crisscrossing 'X's up the lateral aspect of the trunk, essentially like shoelaces weaving the front and back together via the sides (**B**). (Reproduced with kind permission from Benninghoff and Goerttler 1975.)

aspect of the iliac crest. In these cases, it is necessary to focus more on the internal oblique part of this local 'X', to get it to relent and allow these ribs to lift superior and anterior. In the far rarer case where these lower ribs move down and forward toward the pelvis, the external oblique would need to be lengthened.

So we turn a sharp switchback from the PSIS on the most posterior fibers of the internal oblique, which head upward and forward to the lower ribs. Laid over this is the more superficial track from the ASIS, consisting of the anterolateral fibers of the external oblique, which go upward and backward (Video 3.8). The fibers of both these muscles are nearly vertical along the lateral aspect of the trunk, but still take an oblique direction so that they form an 'X' (Fig. 5.12). If you pinch your waist at the side, the fibers of the external oblique, running up and back from the ASIS, will be more superficial. Deep to this will be the internal oblique, palpably running up and forward. Turn your rib cage toward and away from your hand to feel the difference in these thin but strong layers. This myofascia can be worked individually by layer in rotational patterns, or collectively just to lift the ribs off the pelvis (www.anatomytrains.com – video ref: Lateral Line: 37:24–41:00).

The Lateral Ribs

These abdominal obliques attach to the lower floating and abdominal ribs. We can move up from here using both the ribs themselves and the muscles between them. The lateral aspect (around 60° worth) of the rib cage is likewise crisscrossed with a similar pattern of myofasciae (Video 3.10): the external intercostals running backward and up, the internal intercostals running forward and up. These muscles continue the same pattern all the way up the rib cage, under the overlying shoulder girdle and its associated muscles, up to the first ribs at the bottom of the neck (see Fig. 5.10B).

Although the intercostals follow the same design as the obliques, they are much shorter, being interspersed with ribs, so they do not respond in the same manner. The fascia over the ribs can be stretched or moved with broad sweeps. The intercostals can be affected somewhat by a fingertip inserted between the ribs from the outside, but the amount of change is limited (www.anatomytrains.com – video ref: Lateral Line, 41:00–43:42).

A hand from the outside can be a cue for clients to help themselves by breathing the ribs open from the inside. Do not neglect the lateral aspect of the upper ribs, which can be reached by putting the flat of the hand on the ribs with the fingertips into the armpit between the pectoralis and latissimus muscles. By sliding the hand gently into the armpit, you can reach the side of ribs 3-5, either for direct manual work or to bring awareness there for increased movement in breathing (www.anatomytrains.com – video ref: Deep Front Line, 42:45–44:27).

✿ ◆ The Neck

In the neck, from the ribs to the skull, the 'X' pattern repeats itself, and once again the forward and up portion lies deep to the backward and up portion (Fig. 5.13).

We have already addressed the 'backward and up' portion, the sternocleidomastoid (see Ch. 4 or www.anatomytrains.com – video ref: Superficial Front Line, 46:58–52:45 – the SCM can be worked in side-lying as well as supine). Since this myofascial unit participates in both the SFL and LL, if the SFL is pulled downward, the LL will be adversely affected.

The counterpart to the SCM in the LL is the splenius capitis, the 'forward and up' leg of this topmost cervical 'X'. The splenius capitis originates on the spinous processes of the lower cervicals and upper thoracics and ends on the lateral border of the occiput and posterior portion of the temporal bone. To lengthen the splenius, have your client supine. Support the occiput in one hand, and reach under the occiput with the other hand to the side you wish to affect. Grip your fingers against the bone just where the mastoid process joins the occipital ridge, so that one fingertip is just above the ridge, one just below. Slowly but firmly bring the tissue at this line in toward the midline, as the client turns his head in time with you toward the side you are working (www.anatomytrains.com – video ref: Lateral Line, 57:55–59:06). Splenius cervicis, going to the transverse processes of the atlas and axis, also can be included in this technique.

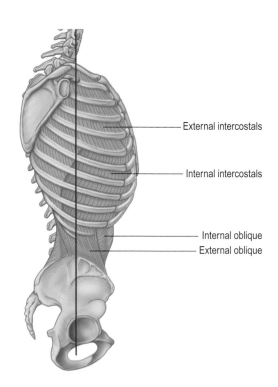

External intercostals

Internal intercostals

Internal oblique
External oblique

• **Fig. 5.12** The abdominals form a large 'X' on the side of the abdomen, and the intercostals continue with smaller Xs. Taken altogether they describe a line up the side.

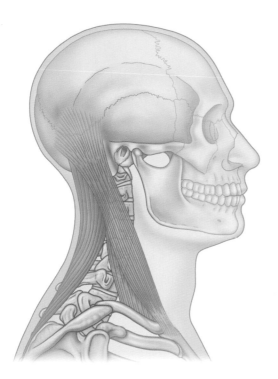

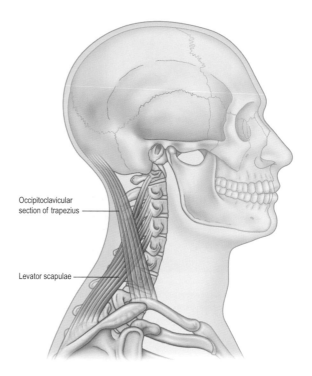

Occipitoclavicular
section of trapezius

Levator scapulae

• **Fig. 5.13** In the neck, the final 'X' of the Lateral Line consists of the sternocleidomastoid muscle (especially the clavicular head) on the outside with the splenius capitis muscle forming the other leg underneath.

• **Fig. 5.14** The levator scapulae would seem to fulfill the same requirements as the splenius as part of the Lateral Line, but this is a common 'mistake' that the body sometimes makes, involving the shoulder in the stability of the trunk. A similar 'mistake' is made in substituting the anterior edge of the trapezius for the sternocleidomastoid. (Video 6.25)

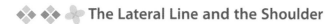 ## The Lateral Line and the Shoulder

Clearly, the LL and the arms are related: the arms hang off the side of the body, covering the lateral ribs and the myofascia of the LL. Please note, though, that the LL itself does not involve the shoulder girdle directly; in the trunk it is a line of the axial skeleton. This is a conceptual separation only – the tissues of the arm lines of course blend right in to the tissues of the Lateral Line.

This conceptual separation has an important practical aspect, however, because it is our contention that support of the head is best accomplished as an entirely axial event, so that the shoulders are absolutely free of any postural role in supporting the head. The tensional balance between the SCM and splenii is sufficient to accomplish outer lateral support of the head, if the underlying structure of the rib cage is in place.

While evident in posture, this four-muscle complex – both splenii and both SCMs – is in constant action during walking and running. All four of these muscles are rotators of the head on the torso, the splenii as ipsilateral rotators and the SCMs as contralateral rotators. As the torso rotates in gait, these four tense and relax in turn to keep the teleceptors (eyes, ears and vestibular system) steady and focused while the body moves underneath. The right SCM and the left splenius resist the tendency of the head to rotate to the right, while the converse muscles resist rotation to the left – with the result that the head stays 'still' relative to the object in focus – a ball, prey, or another dangerous human.

There are a couple of Arm Line myofasciae, however, that can get inadvertently caught up in this Lateral Line job, and involve the shoulder in this core steadying function. One of these muscles is the levator scapulae, which connects the transverse processes of the cervicals with the apex of the scapula. (Notice that Hoepke, in Fig. 5.10B, makes the same error by including levator scapulae in his 'lateral line'.) This muscle parallels the splenius and is well situated to counterbalance any anterior pull on the cervicals or head (Fig. 5.14; Video 6.25). The problem is that the scapula is not a firm base of support, and the result of reversing the origin and insertion to use levator scapulae as 'cervicus-preventus-going-forwardus' is often that the scapula begins to be pulled up toward the back of the neck. Clients will often report pain and trigger points at the lower attachment of the levator, ascribing it to 'stress', when the actual cause is their reaction to the ubiquitous 'head forward' posture (Fig. 5.15), which is itself a common reaction to stress. To relieve this common pattern, pat the poor victimized levator scapulae on the back and proceed to lift the head back onto the body from the all-too-common forward head posture.

The leading edge of the trapezius, attached to the outer edge of the clavicle, can similarly substitute for the more stable and axial sternocleidomastoid, again drawing the shoulder assembly into the support of the head. This pattern can now be understood as a misuse of the LL, which should underlie and be relatively independent of the shoulder

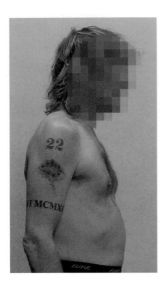

• **Fig. 5.15** The 'head forward' posture necessitates the involvement of the shoulder girdle with the stability of the head on the trunk, a common but inefficient compensatory pattern.

assembly. It is when the dynamic balance of the 'X's of the LL get disturbed that the levator and/or trapezius try to take over the job. (See also the discussion of the levator and trapezius in their proper role, as part of the Arm Lines, in Ch. 7.)

◆ General Movement Treatment Considerations

Almost any kind of lateral flexion of the trunk and abduction of the leg will involve the LL, stretching it on one side until it engages as a stabilizer and contracting or relaxing the tissues on the shortening side, depending on the body's relationship to gravity.

Since the muscles of the LL create lateral flexion, restrictions in the myofascia or excess muscle tensions will show up in postures involving lateral flexion or in restrictions to free movement on the opposite side, i.e. restriction of lateral flexion to the right usually resides in the left Lateral Line.

Since the LL from trochanter to ear is a series of short arcs or switchbacks, the involvement of this line with spiral and rotational movement is worth noting, as we have in the section below on walking. Rotational movement will be taken up more fully in Chapters 6 and 10.

Assessment and Stretches

• Assessing the LL from the front or back in standing posture is the quickest and easiest way to catalogue differences between the right and left LLs. Tilts in the shoulder or hip girdles can be traced to skeletal anomalies, twists, or soft-tissue shortening in the LL north or south of the girdles themselves. Because most everyone reflexively tunes their body so that their eyes and inner ears are level in gravity, shortness in the trunk on one

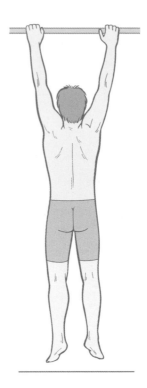

• **Fig. 5.16** Aside from simply viewing the body from the front or back, having your client hanging from a chinning bar allows you another avenue to see underlying patterns of imbalance in the two Lateral Lines.

side is often counterbalanced by shortness in the neck on its opposite.

• Another way to assess the LL is to stand in a doorway (or anywhere where you or the client can get a firm grip on a bar or something steady overhead) and hang from the hands (Fig. 5.16). For self-observation, you can feel where the tissues of the LL resist the call of gravity. When observing a client, look for asymmetries in the two sides as the person hangs from the arms.

• In terms of overall stretches, the half-moon stretch, a simple lean to one side with the arms overhead, is the most obvious overall stretch for the LL (see also Fig. 10.32, p. 195). The LL links into the Arm Lines seamlessly, but for now it is not important to our purposes that the arm be stretched overhead. It is, however, very necessary to be aware during the side-bend whether the upper body leans forward or backward from the hip (in other words, does their side bend include a rotation of the trunk?). The best assessment depends on achieving pure lateral flexion, without sagittal flexion or extension. The head moves away from the neck, the neck from the rib cage, and the ribs should fan away from each other. As the waist opens, the ribs move away from the hip, the iliac crest moves away from the trochanter.

• The Triangle pose and its variants (see Fig. 4.17B and Ch. 10) are a good stretch for the lower part of the LL; the inversion at the ankle ensures a stretch in the fibular (peroneal) compartment as the subtalar joint is passively inverted. In other words, the distance between the outside of the foot and the iliac crest is maximized. In general, inversion and dorsiflexion of the foot done at the same time will stretch the fibularii, while eversion and plantarflexion is created by their contraction.

- An interesting stretch for the ITT–abductor portion of the line is to stand with one foot placed in front of and outside the other. Do a forward bend, and the ITT of the posterior leg will be engaged.
- The lateral portion of the trunk and neck may be stretched through a variety of common stretches, such as *Parighasana* or the Gate pose in yoga.

In movement terms, the lateral flexion movement through the spine is a primary foundation stone for walking. Lying prone on the floor and developing a slow and even eel-like undulation contributes to integration through this line. In a therapeutic setting, the practitioner can observe this side-to-side movement and either use it as an assessment for where to work, or use a hand to bring the client's attention to where lateral flexion movement is not happening.

❖ Palpating the Lateral Line

You can find the originating points of the LL on both the medial and lateral sides of the foot (see Fig. 5.5). On the medial side, we are looking for the distal insertion of fibularis longus. Although it is hard to touch directly, we can locate it by starting with the big toe and walking our fingers up its 1st metatarsal extension until we come to a bump on the top inside of the foot about two inches (5 cm) in front of the ankle. From here, walk your fingers down the inside of the foot toward the underside, keeping in contact with the little valley that represents the joint between the 1st metatarsal and 1st cuneiform. As you pass to the underside of the foot, you will encounter the overlying tissues which make the deep fibularis tendon hard to palpate, but the end point of this muscle, and thus the beginning of the LL, lies just on the inferior and lateral part of this joint.

The other origination of the LL is easily felt when you run your fingers up along the lateral edge of the foot from the little toe. You will encounter the clearly palpable knob of the 5th metatarsal base, and it is from here that the fibularis brevis makes its way up toward the back of the fibular malleolus.

By everting and plantarflexing the foot, you can feel these two tendons just below the lateral malleolus, passing behind it to fill the lateral compartment of the leg (see Fig. 5.6). Of the two tendons, the brevis is the more prominent, the longus disappears rapidly into the flesh below the malleolus.

It is an easy and worthwhile job to find and assess the septa (fascial walls) that border this compartment: for the anterior septum, start with the fibular malleolus, and walk your fingers upward along the bone (see Figs. 5.6 and 5.7). As the bone begins disappearing into the flesh, look for a valley between the anterior and lateral compartments. It may feel like a valley, or alternatively, in the very tight or very toxic, like a string of small beads or pearls. These 'pearls' (principally calcium lactate and other metabolites) have no value, and can be worked out with vigorous manual therapy or very specific foam roller work, resulting in increased freedom of movement for the recipient (with the occasional post-session feeling of slight nausea for the client as these metabolites are processed by the liver). Movement can be very helpful to your search if the valley (the compartmental division) is difficult to feel. Plantarflexion will engage the fibularii, while stretching the anterior compartment muscles; dorsiflexion and toe extension will engage the muscles of the anterior compartment and stretch those in the lateral compartment. By placing your fingerpads on the outside of the leg where you think the valley is, you will be able clearly to distinguish the area where these two opposing movements meet. That place is the septum between the two compartments.

Obviously, this anterior crural septum will end just in front of the fibular head. If you draw a mental line between the lateral malleolus and just in front of the fibular head, the septum will lie close to this line.

Many people confuse the soleus with the fibularii, because in plantarflexion the squeezed soleus often bulges out on the lateral side of the leg, looking for all the world like the fibularii. To avoid this error, start in the clear division between the fibular malleolus and the Achilles tendon. Work upward, staying in the valley between them. The lateral compartment is very small at the inferior end, so use eversion to pop those tendons so that you can stay clearly behind the lateral compartment. This septum should end just behind the fibular head. Here, the lateral compartment (and thus the fibularii) attaches to the lateral aspect of the head of the fibula, whereas the soleus attaches to the posterior aspect of the fibula (see Figs. 5.7, 5.8).

By alternately pressing the toes into the floor and lifting them while your hands explore the area of the head of the fibula, you will be able clearly to distinguish the tibialis anterior (anterior compartment, SFL) and the soleus (superficial posterior compartment, SBL), and by default, the top of the fibularis longus in between (lateral compartment, LL).

While the tendon of the lateral hamstring is the most prominent structure attaching to the head of the fibula, the LL continues by way of the anterior ligament of the head of the fibula (see Fig. 5.8A). This fascial link can be felt coming into tension just anterior and superior to the head of the fibula when the leg is actively abducted while side lying, or supine when the leg is medially rotated and the foot is lifted from the ground (see Fig. 5.8B). It forms a clearly palpable connection between the head of the fibula running slightly anterior toward the lateral tibial condyle and into the ITT.

The ITT, the next fascial element of the LL, is clearly palpable on the lateral aspect of the thigh at or just above the femoral condyle, as a strong superficial band. Follow it upward to feel it widen and thin out along the thigh superficial to the muscular feel of the vastus lateralis, which can be contracted by extending the knee fully.

Above the level of the greater trochanter, the LL includes more muscular elements: the tensor fasciae latae can be easily felt by placing your fingers just under the lateral lip of the ASIS, and then medially rotating the hip (turning the knee in) (see Fig. 5.9). The upper fibers of the gluteus can be similarly felt by placing your fingers under the lateral aspect of the PSIS and then laterally rotating and abducting the hip.

Between these two, the strong central part of the ITT can usually be felt passing up to the middle of the iliac crest, with the gluteus medius muscle lining it on the inside. This muscle can be clearly felt in abduction.

To feel the parts of the abdominal obliques involved in the LL, pinch the waist along the lateral aspect (see Fig. 5.12). Providing that muscle can be felt, the more superficial external oblique will have a 'grain' that runs down and forward toward the hip. A deeper pinch contacts the internal oblique whose grain runs the other way: down and back from the ribs to the hip. Having your client perform small trunk rotations is helpful in differentiating these two layers. Both muscles are closer to vertical out here on the side than they are in the anterior abdominal region, but the distinction in direction can still be clearly felt.

The external intercostals can be felt between the ribs, especially just superior to the attachments of these abdominals, before the ribs are covered over by various layers of shoulder musculature. The internal intercostals are difficult to feel through the externals, but can be felt by implication in forced expiration or in rotation of the rib cage to the same side as the palpation.

The three layers of myofascia in the neck are all accessible to palpation. The SCM, clearly palpable on the surface, has already been covered in our discussion of the SFL (see Fig. 5.13). The splenius capitis is most easily palpated by putting your hands on your supine client's head so that the palpating fingers are just under and slightly posterior to the mastoid processes, but with your hand arranged so that your thumbs on the parietals can offer some resistance to head rotation (www.anatomytrains.com – video ref: Lateral Line, 58:00–59:05). Have your client rotate his head into your resistance and you will feel the splenius contract on the same side he is turning toward, just under the superficial (and usually quite thin) trapezius muscle.

The deepest layers of neck myofascia involved with the LL (see Discussion 5.1 below) require precision and confidence to palpate. To find the anterior scalene, have your client lie supine, and gently lift the SCM forward with the fingernail side of your fingers, hands palm down, and press in gently with your fingertips to feel the solidity of the motor cylinder (the scalenes and the other muscles surrounding the cervical vertebrae) (see Fig. 5.17). The most lateral of these muscles is the middle scalene (www.anatomytrains.com – video ref: Lateral Line, 1:00:25–1:01:47).   Slide the pads of your fingers along the front of the motor cylinder, not pressing into it, nor shying away from it, with your ring finger just above the collar bone. (The client will feel pain or tingling in his fingers or a drawing pain in the scapula if you are pressing on the brachial plexus; if so, move or back off your

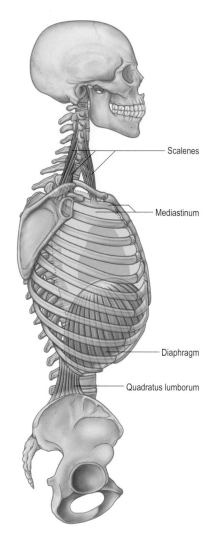

• **Fig. 5.17** Two deeper concomitants of the LL, although both structures are technically part of the Deep Front Line, are the scalenes and the quadratus lumborum, which suspend the rib cage between them.

pressure.) The half-inch band under your fingertips is the anterior scalene. Have the client breathe deeply; the anterior scalene should engage during, and for many especially at the top of, the inhalation (www.anatomytrains.com – video ref: Lateral Line, 59:05–1:00:25).

The other end of this line, the obliquus capitis superior, can be felt by bringing your hands around to cup the occiput in your palms, so that your fingers are free and under the back of the neck. Curl your fingers under the occiput and insinuate your fingertips under the occipital shelf, mindful that you must feel through the trapezius and the underlying semispinalis muscles. Come to rest with fingertips under the occiput, with three fingertips in a row, preferably the ring, middle, and index fingers, with the ring fingers almost touching at the midline, and the index fingers medial to where the occiput begins to curve around toward the mastoid process. Sizes of hands and skulls vary, but for most the six fingertips will be comfortably together on either side of the midline. The occipital attachment of the obliquus capitis superior is just under your index finger, and can be tractioned by pinning the index finger to the inferior surface of the occiput and pulling posteriorly and superiorly with a gentle hand.

The other end of the 'Deep Lateral Line', the quadratus lumborum (QL), can be palpated in the side-lying client by hooking one's fingertips over the superior edge of the iliac crest near the ASIS and walking the fingers back toward the PSIS. At or just behind the midline, tracking the inside edge of the iliac crest, you will encounter the leading edge of the QL fascia, often very tough and termed by some the 'lateral raphe', which leads the fingers away from the crest toward the lateral end of the 12th rib – a clear indication that you have accurately found the QL. This will not work if your fingers are walking back on the top or outside of the iliac crest; because of the depth of the QL, your fingertips must be on the inner rim of the iliac crest to reach this fascial layer.

To work the QL toward greater length and responsiveness, work along this outer edge, freeing it from the iliac crest toward the 12th rib (www.anatomytrains.com – video ref: Lateral Line, 52:58–57:09).

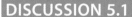

DISCUSSION 5.1

The Deep Lateral Line

There are two sets of myofascia that need to be considered for a complete view of our lateral line, even though they clearly belong to (and will be further discussed with) the Deep Front Line (Ch. 9). Together, these lateral elements of the Deep Front Line comprise a 'Deep Lateral Line', which is included here because working with these structures will frequently improve your results with LL issues, especially with breathing but also with bilateral asymmetries (www .anatomytrains.com – video ref: Lateral Line 52:57–58.10).

The quadratus lumborum (QL) is part of a layer deep to the transversus abdominis and thus not fascially connected to the superficial abdominal muscles of the LL. We cannot, however, ignore its congenial relationship with the LL. Running essentially from the iliac crest up to the 12th rib, it is the real paraspinal muscle in the lumbars. Though the erectors of the SBL (iliocostalis especially) can be involved in lateral flexion, they are more often employed to create extension and hyperextension. The rectus abdominis (SFL) creates primarily trunk flexion. The psoas (the medial portion of the Deep Front Line in this area, see Ch. 9) can create a complex of moves, including flexion, hyperextension, lateral flexion, and rotation in the lumbars. The QL, however, is uniquely placed to mediate a fairly pure lateral flexion. Therefore any work with the LL should also include some attention to the tone and fascia of the QL, even though it is not, by Anatomy Trains' rules, directly part of the LL.

At the other end of the rib cage, we have a similar deep layer in the neck, the scalenes and associated fascia. The scalenes form a kind of skirt around the cervical vertebrae, acting to create or stabilize lateral flexion of the head and neck, in a similar fashion to the QL. We can imagine the

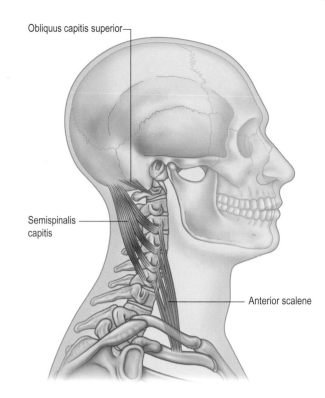

• **Fig. 5.18** Another inner leg of lateral stability consists of the anterior scalene linked to deeper structures of the back of the neck, such as the upper part of semispinalis and obliquus capitis superior. Together, they form two locals that echo the express of the sternocleidomastoid.

rib cage (and indeed the lungs) as being suspended between the QL pulling from one end and the scalenes pulling from the other (Fig. 5.17).

We can also see another leg of an 'X', parallel to but deeper than the SCM. This innermost layer consists of the anterior scalene muscle, running up and back from the 1st rib to the transverse processes of the middle cervicals. The pull of this muscle forms a functional connection, if not a fascial continuity, with the suboccipital muscles, most particularly the obliquus capitis superior or upper semispinalis capitis (Fig. 5.18). These muscles take the occiput into protraction or anterior translation, and the upper cervical joints into hyperextension, while the anterior scalene pulls the lower cervicals into flexion. The combination helps to contribute to a familiar form of the 'head forward' posture.

DISCUSSION 5.2

The Lateral Line and Fish: Vibration, Swimming, and the Development of Walking

Sensing Vibration

The top of the LL terminates at the ear, located in the temporal bone on the side of the head; indeed, the ideal of

Lateral Line posture is always described as passing through the ear. The entire ear, of course, contains structures sensitive to vibratory frequencies from about 20 Hz to 20 000 Hz, to gravitational pull, and to accelerating motion. The ear is a sophisticated rendering of vibratory sensors that are set along the entire lateral line of many ancient and some modern fish, such as sharks, who 'hear' the thrashing of their prey from their sides (Fig. 5.19). Later vertebrates such as ourselves seem to have concentrated most of their vibratory sensitivity at the leading end of the organism. Some connection seems to remain, however, in the way that left/right differences can reflect coordination balance problems more than front/back differences.

Swimming

Almost all fish swim with a side-to-side motion. This obviously involves the contraction of the two lateral 'contractile fields' in succession.[3] Perhaps the original creator for

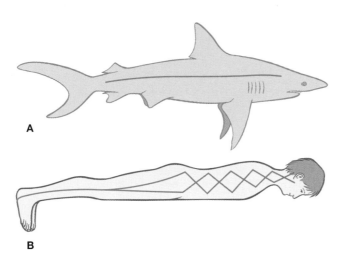

• **Fig. 5.19** Some fish such as sharks have a line of vibratory sensors running down their lateral line. Humans seem to have concentrated most of that vibratory sensitivity in the ear at the top of the line. Can you hear with your 'inner fish'?[2]

this movement (and thus the deepest expression of the Lateral Line) is found in the tiny intertransversarii muscles that run from transverse process to transverse process in the spine. When one side contracts, it stretches the corresponding muscle on the other side (Fig. 5.20). The spinal stretch reflex, an ancient spinal cord movement mediator, causes the stretched muscle to contract, thus stretching the first muscle on the opposite side, which contracts in its turn, and so on. In this way, a coordinated swimming movement (in other words, coordinated waves running down the lateral musculature) can occur with minimal involvement by the brain. A lamprey eel, a modern equivalent to ancient fish, can be decerebrated, and when it is placed in flowing water, it will still swim upstream in a blind, slow, but coordinated fashion, working only through spinal mechanisms – the stimulation from the vibratory sensors on the lateral skin linking to its stretch reflex.

Of course, corresponding movements remain in humans. There are many movements such as walking that work through reciprocal stretch reflexes. The side-to-side motion itself is less visible in regular adult walking, but its underlying primacy is indicated in the infant at about 3–6 months, when the side-to-side movement of creeping begins. This movement will later be replaced by the more sophisticated crawling movement, which combines flexion/extension and rotation along with the lateral flexion.[4]

Walking

When we assess adult walking, excessive side-to-side motion is seen as an aberration. We expect to see the head and even the thorax moving along fairly straight ahead, with most of the side-to-side accommodation handled at the waist and below. From the point of view of myofascial meridians, the entire LL is involved in such adjustments, and should be considered in correcting deviations of too much or too little lateral flexion in the underlying pattern of walking.

For our primary forward motivating force we humans use flexion/extension, sagittal motion (as the dolphins and

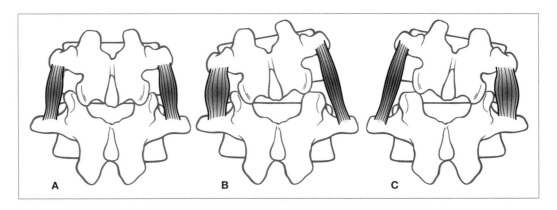

• **Fig. 5.20** Lateral movement, the kind involved in the swimming motions of a fish or forward motion of an eel or snake, consists of reciprocal reflexes flowing down the musculature in waves. When one side is contracted, the other side is stretched, inducing a contraction in it, which stretches the first side, so it contracts, and so on and on upstream.

whales do as well), not side-to-side motion as the fish do. Our walking involves a little side-to-side accommodation, as we have noted, but the contralateral motion of human walking involves a lot of rotation, especially through the waist and lower rib cage, which mediate between opposed oscillations of the pelvic girdle and the shoulder girdle.

The series of 'X's or the basket weave that characterizes the LL in the trunk and neck are perfectly situated to modulate and brake these rotatory movements. Therefore, the woven structure of the LL in the trunk can be seen as partial arcs of spirals that are used like springs and shock absorbers to smooth out the complexities of walking. In this way, we can see the slanted direction of the intercostals as acting almost like a watch spring, storing up potential energy when the rib cage is twisted one way, releasing it into kinetic energy as the rib cage rotates in the other direction (Fig. 5.21). We have found interesting results treating the intercostals primarily as muscles of walking rather than as muscles of breathing (an idea first proposed to us by Jon Zahourek of Zoologik Systems).

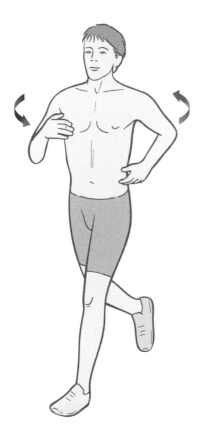

• **Fig. 5.21** The intercostals can be seen as operating like a watch spring, winding and unwinding the rib cage reciprocally with each step. As you take a step forward with the left foot and the rib cage rotates to the left, the external intercostals on the right are being contracted, while the internal intercostals on the left are contracting to create the movement. Their complements are being stretched, storing an elastic recoil to take the rib cage back the other way. If this watch spring mechanism is not working – if the ribs are rigidly held in gait, a common pattern for large men among others – the acceleration of the thighs will have to be counteracted solely by the arms. (www.anatomytrains. com – video ref: Body Reading 101)

Lateral vs Sagittal Movement

In the early 1980s, in a suburb near London, I was just beginning a Saturday seminar to a group of aerobic instructors when the cheerful cacophony of a school band drowned me out. I went over to the window to see, and called my students over to witness a simple but telling phenomenon. We were looking down from the 6th floor at a Remembrance Day parade. From above, we could see the parade starting out, with the heads of the World War II veterans clearly moving from side to side, while the heads of the teenage band members were just as clearly bobbing up and down (Fig. 5.22).

The message was clear: the older veterans had diminished accommodation in the lateral lines around the waist (and perhaps some degenerative arthritis in their hips as well). They were thus compelled, as they 'marched', to shift their weight from one foot entirely onto the other, causing their heads to move from side to side. The teenagers carrying the instruments were doing just fine on the side-to-side accommodation, but (we surmise) the collision between increased hormone levels and Britain's general reticence about sex had possibly caused a spot of tension in the hip flexors at the front of the pelvis, so that all the up and down motion in dorsiflexion was being transferred right through the hip up to the spine and head.

Whatever the cause, the veterans were exhibiting LL problems as a group, and the teenagers were showing SBL and SFL restrictions.

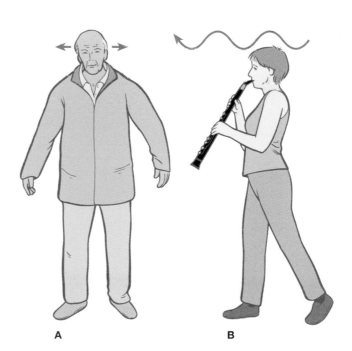

A   B

• **Fig. 5.22** Older people tend to walk with a greater side-to-side movement of the head due to the decreasing ability of the hips and waist to accommodate shifting weight. Teenagers tend to walk with the head steady in the right–left dimension, but not infrequently their heads will shift up and down as they walk, due to chronic shortness in the flexors of the hips.

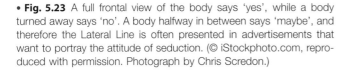

• **Fig. 5.23** A full frontal view of the body says 'yes', while a body turned away says 'no'. A body halfway in between says 'maybe', and therefore the Lateral Line is often presented in advertisements that want to portray the attitude of seduction. (© iStockphoto.com, reproduced with permission. Photograph by Chris Scredon.)

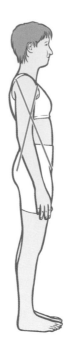

• **Fig. 5.24** An imaginary 'X', one leg drawn from the spinous process of C7 to the pubic bone and the other drawn from the sternal notch to the top of the sacrum, is a simple way to assess the summary of 'X's across the trunk.

DISCUSSION 5.3

The Lateral Line and Seduction

If presenting the SFL to the world, in all its sensitivity and erogenous zones (see Ch. 4, Discussion 4.2, p. 70) is essentially a statement of trust, or a 'Yes', and presenting the SBL, the carapace ('turning your back') is essentially an expression of protection, or 'No', what is the meaning of the presentation of the side, or Lateral Line? The answer is 'Maybe'. Therefore, presentation of the Lateral Line can be associated with the complex reeling in known as seduction. This ties into issues that link safety to sensuality and sexuality. Any perusal of the ads or fashion shoots in *Vogue* or the Sunday Fashion Supplements will reveal how often presentation of the body's side is used to sell clothes, perfume, jewelry, make-up, or the other accoutrements of the play of seduction (Fig. 5.23). (This psychobiological idea comes courtesy of *Born to Walk* author James Earls.)[5]

DISCUSSION 5.4

The Summary Lateral 'X'

Since we are more or less bilaterally symmetrical (at least in the musculoskeletal system), it is a fairly simple matter to examine our clients from the front or back to detect any differences in how the Lateral Lines are handled from left to right, and correct any imbalance by lengthening the shortened tissues. Looking at the basket weave of the LL from the side is a bit more complex, but just as useful. We can assess the individual 'X's as they run along the trunk, or we can take an overview and assess the trunk as a whole.

To do this: look at your client from the side (or yourself in a mirror or photo). Imagine that one leg of the 'X' runs from the spinous process of the 7th cervical vertebra to the pubic bone, while the other runs from the sternal notch to the apex of the sacrum (Figs. 5.24 and 5.25, compare with Fig. 5.11). Is one of these legs significantly longer than the other? Nearly all of those with a depressed or 'burdened' body type will display a sternum-to-sacrum line that is visibly shorter than the 7th cervical-to-pubis line (see Fig. 5.25B). The 'military' type of posture usually throws the sternum well up and forward, but often at the expense of bringing the sacrum up and forward also, so that this leg of the 'X' is not lengthened, merely moved (see Fig. 5.25C; Video 6.5). Infrequently (at least in Western cultures) the rib cage will be shifted down and forward compared to the pelvis, and the sternum–sacrum line will be the longer of the two.

Even though the more common pattern in regard to this 'X' is that the line from the sternal notch to the sacrum is too short, it is difficult to reach the tissues responsible. The internal oblique is one possible avenue, but often this pattern is buried in the crural section of the diaphragm, quadratus lumborum, or mediastinal structures (Fig. 5.26 and see Ch. 9). An approach through breathing awareness is often more effective and less invasive.

With your client standing sideways in front of you, place your hands on the manubrium of the sternum and on the

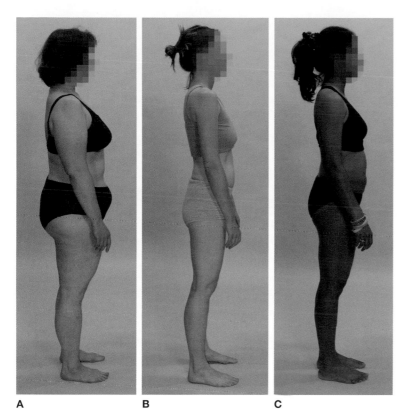

A   **B**   **C**

• **Fig. 5.25** A balanced structure shows an even balance of all the 'X's in the trunk (**A**). Having the sternum fall close to the sacrum is a very common Western pattern (**B**). Pulling the sacrum forward with an anterior pelvic tilt and sticking the chest out, as in a military posture, simply changes the compensatory pattern, but not the underlying structure (**C**). Much rarer is the pattern where the rib cage collapses forward on the pelvis, bringing C7 closer to the pubic bone (not pictured – www.anatomytrains.com – video ref: Body Reading, 101).

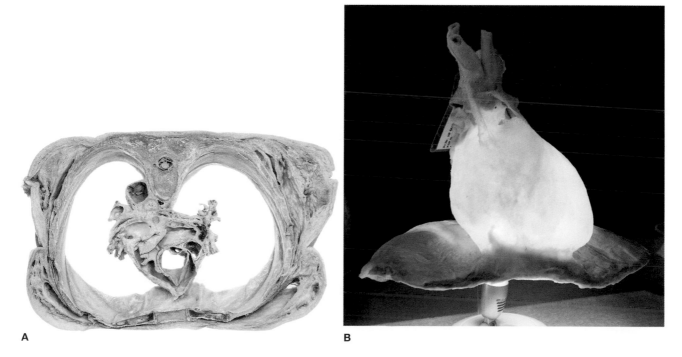

A   **B**

• **Fig. 5.26** Lengthening the line between the sternal notch and sacral promontory involves the inward and difficult-to-change tissues of the central tendon of the diaphragm and mediastinum. (**A**) The mediastinal tissues from the back of the sternum to the front of the thoracic spine. (**B**) The diaphragm showing the connection from the fascial central tendon to the fascial pericardium – lit from below. (A, photo courtesy of Anna Rowedder. B, © FasciaResearchSociety.org/Plastination).

low back at the sacrolumbar junction. Follow your client's breathing for a few cycles, noticing whether and how your hands are moved during inhalation. Then encourage your client to move your two hands apart from each other as they inhale, and allow them to fall together on the exhale. Some clients, by increasing the inhale, will increase the excursion between your hands; others will work hard but only succeed in bringing the upper hand forward at the cost of bringing the lower hand forward and up as well, resulting in no net gain in the length of this line. By encouraging movement with your hands and words, you can help the client induce an actual change in the length of the line, the sternum going up and forward while the sacrum drops in counternutation. Ask your client to repeat the move a number of times between sessions to reinforce length along this line.

References

1. Chaudhry H, Schleip R, Ji Z, et al. Three-dimensional mathematical model for deformation of human fasciae in manual therapy. *J Am Osteopath Assoc.* 2008;108(8):379–390.
2. Shubin N. *Your Inner Fish.* NY: Pantheon Books; 2008.
3. Beach P. *Muscles and Meridians.* Edinburgh: Churchill Livingstone; 2010.
4. Bainbridge-Cohen B. *Basic Neurocellular Patterns.* El Sobrante CA: Burchfield Rose Pub; 2018.
5. Earls J. *Born to Walk.* London: Lotus; 2016.

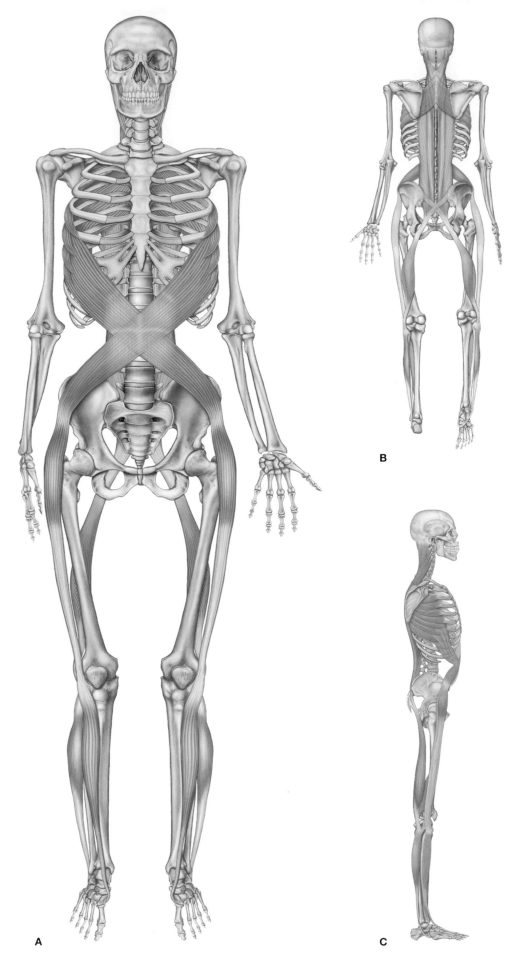

• **Fig. 6.1** The Spiral Line.

6

The Spiral Line

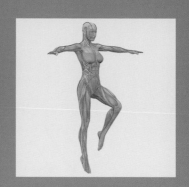

OVERVIEW

The Spiral Line (SPL) (Fig. 6.1; Video 2.4) loops around the body in two opposing helices, right and left, forming a double lattice joining each side of the skull across the upper back to the opposite shoulder, and then around the ribs to the front to cross again at the level of the navel to the hip. From the hip, the Spiral Line passes like a 'jump rope' along the anterolateral thigh and across the shin to the medial longitudinal arch, passing under the foot and running up the posterolateral side of the leg to the ischium and into the erector spinae myofascia (of either side, depending on posture or activity) to end very close to where it started on the skull.

Postural Function

The SPL functions posturally to wrap the body in a double spiral that helps to maintain balance across all planes (Fig. 6.2A–C/Table 6.1). The SPL connects the foot arches with the pelvic angle, and helps to determine efficient knee-tracking in walking. In imbalance, the SPL participates in creating, compensating for, and maintaining twists, rotations, and lateral shifts in the body. Depending on the posture and movement pattern, especially which leg is characteristically or momentarily more weighted, forces from the legs can travel up the same side or cross to the opposite side of the body at the sacrum, especially in the contralateral motion of walking (see Ch. 10).

Much of the myofascia in the SPL also participates in the other cardinal meridians (SBL, SFL, LL) as well as the Deep Back Arm Line (see Ch. 7). The SPL is involved in a multiplicity of functions, so that dysfunction in the Spiral Line can affect the easy functioning of these other lines. Because most people worldwide have a dominant and recessive hand, leg, and eye, the Spiral Line is rarely perfectly balanced side-to-side, but is functionally adaptable within fairly wide tolerances.

Movement Function

The overall movement function of the SPL is to create and mediate oblique spirals and transverse plane rotations in the body, and, in eccentric and isometric contraction, to steady the trunk and leg to keep it from folding into rotational collapse.

❖ ❖ ✿ General Manual Therapy Considerations

The SPL cuts across many of the other lines as a 'parasite', meaning that most of the structures involved in the SPL also take part in other lines as well. Techniques for the splenius capitis, tensor fasciae latae, and fibularii (peroneals) can be found in Chapter 5 (or the Lateral Line video at www.anatomytrains.com). There is more on the rhomboids with the Deep Back Arm Line in Chapter 7, on the biceps femoris and erector spinae in Chapter 3 (or the Superficial Back Line video at www.anatomytrains.com), and on the tibialis anterior and abdominal muscles in Chapter 4 (or the Superficial Front Line video at www.anatomytrains.com). Here in this chapter we focus on additional techniques aimed at areas exclusive to the Spiral Line.

Common postural compensation patterns associated with the SPL include: ankle pronation/supination, knee rotation and medial shift, pelvic rotation on feet, rib rotation on pelvis, one shoulder lifted or anteriorly shifted, and head tilt, shift, or rotation.

The Spiral Line in Detail

For convenience, we will change tactics and begin detailing the SPL from the top, keeping in mind that *in vivo* any of these lines can and do create myofascial force transmission from either end or out from nearly any 'station' along the 'tracks' in either direction.

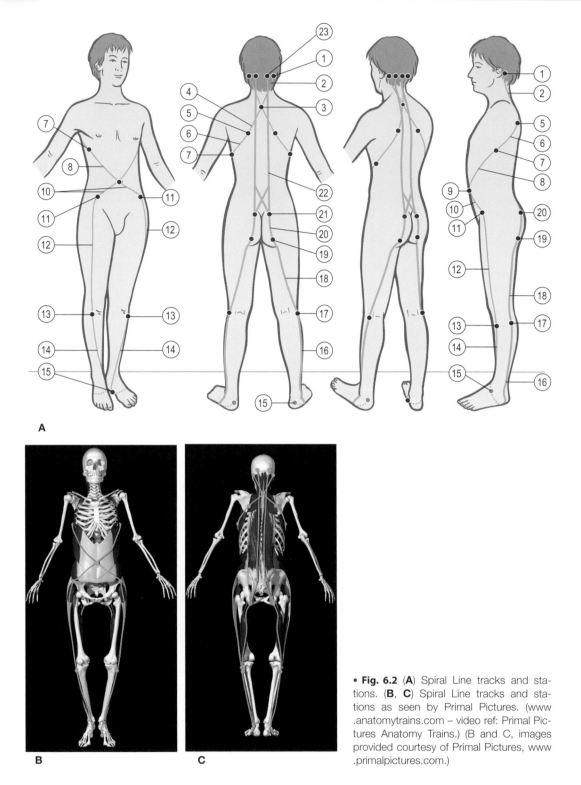

• **Fig. 6.2** (**A**) Spiral Line tracks and stations. (**B**, **C**) Spiral Line tracks and stations as seen by Primal Pictures. (www.anatomytrains.com – video ref: Primal Pictures Anatomy Trains.) (B and C, images provided courtesy of Primal Pictures, www.primalpictures.com.)

The SPL begins on the side of the skull, at or above the lateral portion of the nuchal line, at the junction between the occiput and temporal bone, sweeping down and in via the splenius capitis muscle. On its way, it picks up the splenius cervicis from the atlas and axis, spanning down to the spinous processes from C6 to T5 (Fig. 6.3A).

Crossing over the tips of the spinous processes with a continuous fascial sheet, we pick up the rhomboids major

and minor on the other side as part of the same fabric (see Figs. 1.16 and 2.7, pp. 11 and 22). (A smaller mechanical link runs from the splenius to the thinner serratus posterior superior which underlies the rhomboids and attaches to the ribs just lateral to the erectors – Fig. 6.3B; Video 4.5). The rhomboids carry us along the same line of pull over to the medial border of the scapula, thus connecting the left side of the skull to the right scapula and vice versa (Fig. 6.4; Video 4.4).

TABLE 6.1	Spiral Line: Myofascial 'Tracks' and Bony 'Stations' (Fig. 6.2)	
Bony Stations		**Myofascial Tracks**
Occipital ridge/mastoid process atlas/axis TPs	1	
	2	Splenius capitis and cervicis
Lower cervical/upper thoracic SPs	3	
	4	Rhomboids major and minor
Medial border of scapula	5	
	6	Serratus anterior
Lateral ribs	7	
	8	External oblique
	9	Abdominal aponeurosis, linea alba
	10	Internal oblique
Iliac crest/ASIS	11	
	12	Tensor fasciae latae, iliotibial tract
Lateral tibial condyle	13	
	14	Tibialis anterior
1st metatarsal base	15	
	16	Fibularis longus
Fibular head	17	
	18	Biceps femoris
Ischial tuberosity	19	
	20	Sacrotuberous ligament
Sacrum	21	
	22	Sacrolumbar fascia, erector spinae
Occipital ridge	23	

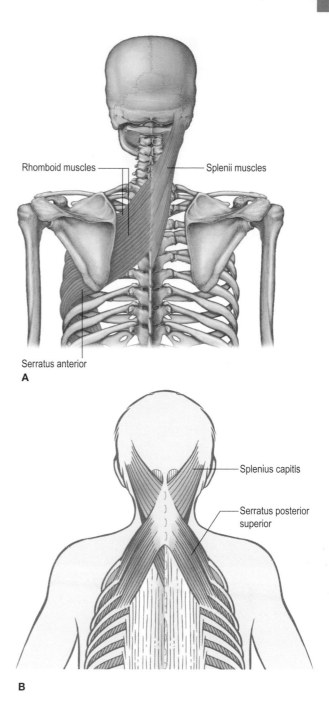

Rhomboid muscles — Splenii muscles

Serratus anterior

A

Splenius capitis

Serratus posterior superior

B

• **Fig. 6.3** The opening myofascial continuity of the Spiral Line is a fascial connection from the splenii over the spinous processes (**A**) to the rhomboids that pass to the contralateral scapula. A 'branch line' connection could also be made (**B**) to the serratus posterior superior muscle, which goes underneath the rhomboids but over the erector fascia to attach to the ribs.

From the medial border of the scapula, there is a direct fascial connection to the infraspinatus and subscapularis of the rotator cuff, which we will explore with the Arm Lines in the next chapter. The SPL, however, continues on a less obvious but nevertheless very strong fascial connection with the serratus anterior, deep to the scapula (Fig. 6.5). In dissection, the connection of the rhomboids to the serratus anterior is stronger and more 'meaty' than the connection of either muscle to the scapula itself.

The rhomboids connect to a goodly portion of the serratus, which is a complex muscle with many internal fiber directions. The SPL track as described above passes primarily through the lower part of the serratus anterior muscle. The serratus originates on the profound side of the medial border of the scapula and passes to attachments on the first nine ribs, but the part that attaches to ribs 5 through 9 provides the spiral continuity we are following (see Discussion 6.2, the SPL and Forward Head Posture, p. 106, to follow another of the directions within the serratus). In dissection, the fascial continuity with the rhomboids is very clear. If we could fold the glenoid section of the scapula back to expose the serratus, we would see clearly that there

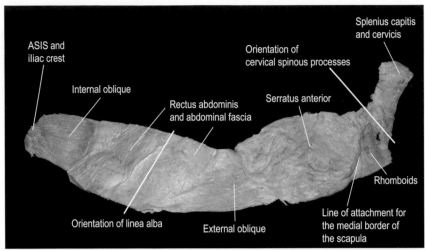

ASIS and
iliac crest

Splenius capitis
and cervicis

Internal oblique

Orientation of
cervical spinous processes

Rectus abdominis
and abdominal fascia

Serratus anterior

Rhomboids

Orientation of linea alba

External oblique

Line of attachment for
the medial border of
the scapula

A

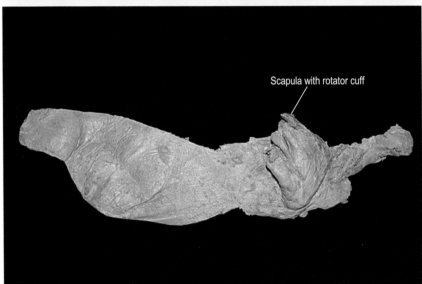

Scapula with rotator cuff

B

• **Fig. 6.4** (**A**) A dissection of the upper Spiral Line, showing the clear fascial continuities wrapped from the skull to the hip, by way of the splenii, rhomboids, serratus anterior, and abdominal fasciae containing the oblique muscles. The scapula has been removed from this specimen, leaving a visible line, but no break in the rhombo-serratus part of the sheet. The longer and heavier indicator lines indicate the median sagittal midline, front (left) and back (right). (**B**) The same dissection with the scapula (and rotator cuff muscles) still attached to the 'rhombo-serratus' sling (see also Figs. 2.1 & 2.7). (www.anatomytrains .com – video ref: Anatomy Trains Revealed; Video 4.4)

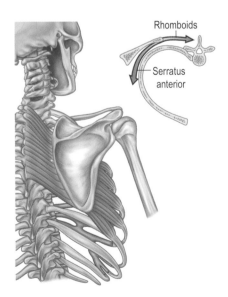

Rhomboids

Serratus
anterior

• **Fig. 6.5** Taken together, the rhomboids and serratus anterior, the next continuity in the Spiral Line, form a myofascial sling for the scapula. Thus the scapula is suspended between them, and its position will depend on the relative myofascial tone of these two.

is one muscle – the rhombo-serratus muscle, so to speak – with the medial border of the scapula glued into its fascia about halfway in its journey from the upper thoracic spinous processes to the lateral ribs (Fig. 6.6). If the scapula is cut away from the underlying tissues, the connection between the rhomboids and serratus remains very strong (see Fig. 6.4 and Fig. 6.7).

❖ The Rhombo-Serratus Muscle

The rhombo-serratus muscle (the rhomboid–serratus anterior sling) often shows medial to lateral or side-to-side imbalance that can be corrected manually. Taking the medial to lateral differences first: a common pattern is that the rhomboids are locked long (overstretched, eccentrically loaded) with the serrati locked short (concentrically loaded), pulling the scapula away from the spine. This pattern will show up commonly in body-builders, and those with a tendency to the kyphotic spine (anterior thoracic bend). In these cases, the therapist wants to lengthen the serrati while the client engages the rhomboids.

Seat your client on a low table or a bench with his feet on the floor and the knees lower than the hips. Have him bend slightly forward at the mid-chest. Move in behind him so that your chest is close to his back. (Use a pillow between you if this is uncomfortable, but you must be close for this technique to be supportable for the practitioner and to work for the client.) Put your open fists out on the lateral rib cage, just outside of or just on the lateral border of the scapula and the lateral edge of the latissimus dorsi, with your proximal phalanges rolling in to rest on the client's ribs, and your elbows as wide and forward as you can

comfortably position them. Peel the tissue around the rib cage toward your chest and his back, bringing the latissimus and scapula with you toward the posterior midline. Do not dig into the rib cage, but rather bring the entire shoulder structure around the ribs. At the same time have the client lift his chest in front with a big, proud inhale. With a little practice this will stretch the myofasciae of the serratus anterior, and encourage the rhomboids to assume proper tone (www.anatomytrains.com – video ref: Spiral Line, 16:00–20:28).

If there is a right–left difference between the two scapulae, use the same positioning, but merely emphasize the pressure to create change on the one side while stabilizing both the client and yourself with the other.

The converse pattern is less common, but still encountered frequently, where the rhomboids are locked short and the serrati locked long. In these patterns, the scapulae tend to be held high and close to the spinous processes, a pattern which often accompanies a flat (extended) thoracic spine.

To address this pattern in the SPL, have your seated client bend forward a little (not so far that he can rest his elbows on his knees) to expose the area between the thoracic spine and the vertebral border of the scapula. Standing behind, work out from the center line toward the scapula using your knuckles or elbows, lengthening in both directions away from the spine. The client can help in two ways: by pushing up from the feet into your pressure, the client will help keep the back sturdy and create more of a roundness (flexion). To get extra stretch out of the rhomboids, have the client reach out in front and bring the arms across each other as if giving someone a big slow hug (www.anatomytrains.com – video ref: Spiral Line, 20:28–25:53).

To emphasize one side more than the other, merely increase the pressure on the shorter side. Alternatively, cross your hands over each other, with one against several thoracic spinous processes, and the other against the vertebral border, and by pushing your hands apart, induce a stretch in the rhomboids (as well as, perforce, the middle trapezius) (Video 3.12).

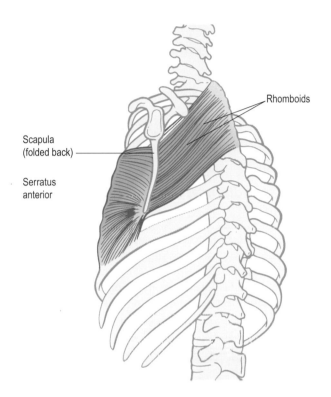

Scapula (folded back)

Serratus anterior

Rhomboids

• **Fig. 6.6** If we fold the scapula back, we can see how there is really a 'rhombo-serratus' muscle with the medial border of the scapula essentially 'glued' into the middle of this myofascial sheet.

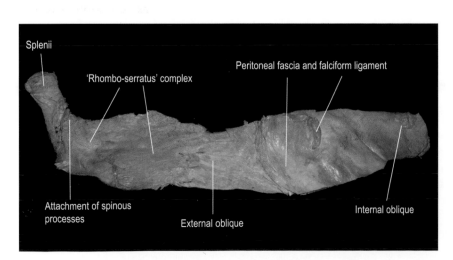

Splenii

'Rhombo-serratus' complex

Peritoneal fascia and falciform ligament

Attachment of spinous processes

External oblique

Internal oblique

• **Fig. 6.7** The same specimen as Fig. 6.4, viewed from the profound side. The peritoneum and transversalis fascia, as well as the remnants of the falciform ligament, can be seen in the lower (right) part of the specimen. The saw-tooth attachments of the serratus and external obliques to the ribs can be seen, as well as the stark fact of the stronger attachment that both muscles have for each other than either has for the ribs.

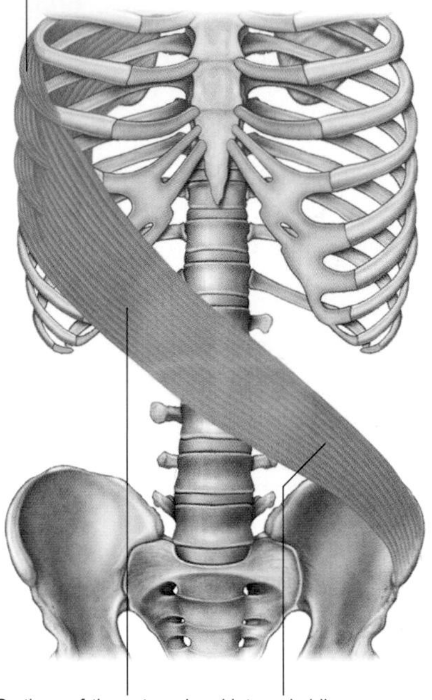

Serratus anterior

Portions of the external and internal oblique

• **Fig. 6.8** The next set of continuities in the Spiral Line carries it from the serratus anterior onto the external oblique, on through the linea alba, and over to the anterior superior iliac spine via the contralateral internal oblique.

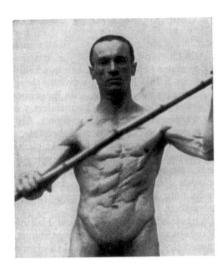

• **Fig. 6.9** The Spiral Line connections in the abdomen in action. Note that it is the left Spiral Line (running from the fellow's right ribs to left pelvis) that is being contracted, while the other side is being stretched. Consistent postural positioning of one set of ribs closer to the opposite hip is a red flag for Spiral Line treatment. (Reproduced with kind permission from Hoepke 1936.)

The Internal and External Oblique Complex

From the lower attachments of the serratus, our way forward is clear: the serratus anterior has strong fascial continuity across the serrated attachments on the lateral ribs with the external oblique (Figs. 6.7 and 6.8). The fibers of the external oblique blend into the lamina of the superficial abdominal aponeurosis, which carries over to the linea alba, where they mesh with the opposing fibers of the internal oblique on the opposite side (see Fig. 6.7). This carries us to our next 'station', the ASIS (anterior superior iliac spine) and an opportunity for a brief sidetrack, or, in this case, a roundhouse (see 'Roundhouse: the anterior superior iliac spine' below; Video 6.1).

In the abdomen, one set of external/internal oblique (abdominal ribs to opposite pelvis) complex may be visibly shorter than the other (Fig. 6.9). To assess imbalance, measure from where the outside edge of the rectus abdominis crosses the costal cartilage to the contralateral ASIS, and compare it with its complement on the other side. If the difference is significant, position the fingertips into the superficial layers of abdominal fascia and lift them diagonally and superiorly toward the opposite ribs (www.anatomytrains.com – video ref: Spiral Line, 12:28–16:00). This will usually serve to correct this imbalance, although more complex counterbalancing patterns often involve the psoas and its rotational moment as well (see Ch. 9).

Roundhouse: the Anterior Superior Iliac Spine

The SPL passes over the anterior superior iliac spine (ASIS), touching there as a station before passing down the leg. The ASIS is of such central importance to structural analysis in general, and myofascial continuity theory in particular, that we must pause here to note the various mechanical pulls from this point. It could be compared to a clock or a compass, but since we are mired in train images for this book, we will call it a roundhouse (Fig. 2.12B, p. 23).

The internal oblique pulls the ASIS in a superior and medial direction (see Fig. 2.12A). Other internal oblique fibers, as well as fibers from the transversus abdominis, pull directly medially. Still other fibers of the internal oblique fan, plus the restraining cord of the inguinal ligament, pull medial and inferior. The sartorius, attaching to the ASIS on its way to the inner knee, pulls mostly down and slightly in. The iliacus, clinging to the inside edge of the ASIS, pulls straight down toward the inner part of the femur.

The rectus femoris, as we noted in discussing the Superficial Front Line, does not attach to the ASIS in most people; nevertheless it exerts a downward pull on the front of the hip from its attachment a bit lower on the AIIS. The tensor fasciae latae pulls down and out on its way to the outer aspect of the knee. The gluteus medius pulls down and back toward the greater trochanter, the transversus abdominis pulls back nearly horizontally along the iliac crest, and the external oblique pulls up and back toward the lower edge of the rib cage.

Getting all these forces to balance around the front of the hip in both standing and gait involves an attentive eye, progressive work, and more than a little patience. This balance involves at least three of the Anatomy Trains lines –

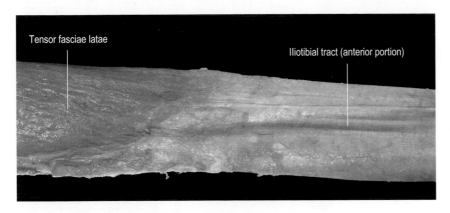

Tensor fasciae latae

Iliotibial tract (anterior portion)

• **Fig. 6.10** The myofascial blend we call the tensor fasciae latae muscle becomes the iliotibial tract as the muscle attenuates to nothing – but it is all one fascial sheet from iliac crest to tibial condyle. (www .anatomytrains.com – video ref: Anatomy Trains Revealed; Video 3.9)

this Spiral Line, the Lateral Line, the Deep Front Line, and, by mechanical connection, the Superficial Front Line. Proper assessment involves weighing an ever-shifting dance of pulls created by a host of myofascial units across each semi-independent side of the pelvis.

Because of the many pulls and tracks competing to set the position of the ASIS, the SPL does not always win out in communicating between its upper track (the skull to ribs to hip portion we have just covered) and its lower track (the 'jump rope' around the arches we are about to cover). Therefore, we often assess and consider these two halves of the line separately.

✿ The Lower Spiral Line

The lower SPL is a complex sling from hip to arch and back to the hip again.

Continuing on from the ASIS, we must keep going in the same direction to obey our rules. Rather than sharply switching our course onto any of these other lines of pull, we pass directly across, connecting from the internal oblique fibers to the tensor fasciae latae (TFL) from the underside of the ASIS and lip of the iliac crest. Fig. 6.10 shows how the TFL blends with the anterior edge of the iliotibial tract (ITT) (Video 3.9), which passes down to attach strongly to the lateral condyle of the tibia (Fig. 6.11).

This time, however, instead of jogging over to the peroneals, as we did with the Lateral Line, we will keep going straight, with a more obvious fascial connection, especially for the anterior edge of the ITT, onto the tibialis anterior (Fig. 6.12). This connection is easily dissected (Fig. 6.13).

❖ *The 'Violin' of the Iliotibial Tract*

In the legs, lengthening this section of the SPL from the ASIS to the outer knee can be accomplished through a stroke, either up or down, designed to free the anterior edge only of the ITT. Usually the flat of the ulna is used, with the client side-lying. In this position, the ITT curves over the surface of the thigh like the strings of a violin. Your ulna then acts like a bow: by altering the angle of your arm, you can emphasize the connection from the gluteus maximus to the posterior part of the ITT (more a part of the Lateral or Back Functional Line), or (as suggested here for the SPL)

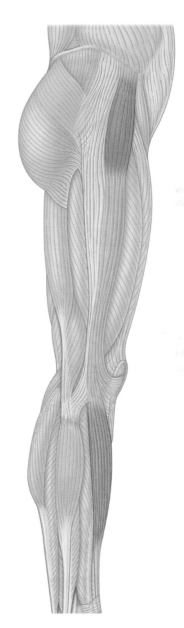

• **Fig. 6.11** From the ASIS, the Spiral Line passes down the anterior edge of the iliotibial tract and directly onto the tibialis anterior.

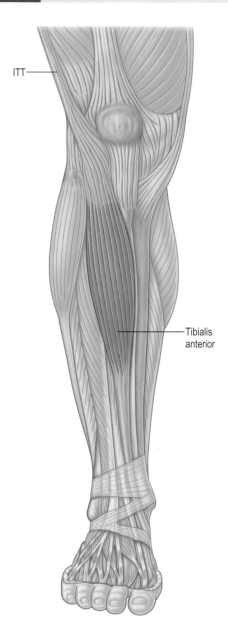

ITT

Tibialis anterior

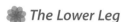

• **Fig. 6.12** The tibialis anterior continues the spiral from the outside of the knee across the shinbone to the inside of the ankle.

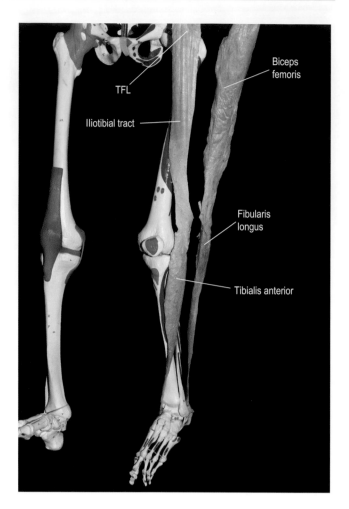

Biceps femoris

TFL

Iliotibial tract

Fibularis longus

Tibialis anterior

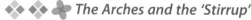

• **Fig. 6.13** The fascial continuity between the ITT and tibialis anterior is very strong and easily dissected. The lower Spiral Line resembles a jump rope from the anterior pelvis to the posterior pelvis by way of the arch of the foot.

concentrate on the anterior portion from the TFL to the tibialis anterior just below the knee. Near the knee, the anterior edge of the ITT is easy to feel; nearer the hip, stay on a line from the ASIS to the middle of the lateral part of the knee (www.anatomytrains.com – video ref: Spiral Line, 25:53–29:32).

Since this area can be quite painful when first approached, several repetitions in a more gentle fashion will often answer well.

🌸 The Lower Leg

The tibialis anterior passes down and in, crossing the lower shinbone to attach to the joint capsule between the 1st cuneiform and 1st metatarsal. In standard anatomy, this would seem to be the end point of the SPL until we look around to the other side of that joint capsule to find a direct

fascial connection with the peroneus longus, likewise with a bifurcated tendon into those same bones and joint capsule (Fig. 6.14). In other words, there is both a fascial and mechanical continuity between the tibialis anterior and the fibularis longus. Again, this can be easily dissected to maintain the fascial continuity of this 'sling' (Fig. 6.15; Video 3.11). This connection has been noted before, but can now be understood as part of a larger picture (see Fig. 6.16 and Discussion 6.3 on the SPL and foot arches at the end of this chapter).

❖ ❖ 🍀 The Arches and the 'Stirrup'

The stirrup under the arch is fairly inaccessible in the foot itself, and can best be worked from the lower leg. Oddly, the two ends of this sling, the tibialis anterior and the fibularis (peroneus) longus, lie next to each other on the anterolateral aspect of the lower leg (see Fig. 6.12). As we noted in looking at the Lateral Line (Ch. 5), there is a fascial septum between the two muscles (see Fig. 5.7). Thus, the two muscles could be seen as a sling or stirrup under the foot, with both muscles originating, at least in part, from this intermuscular septum.

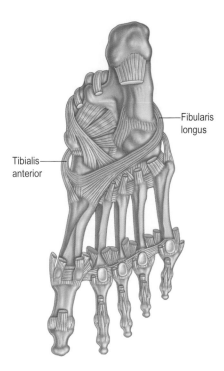

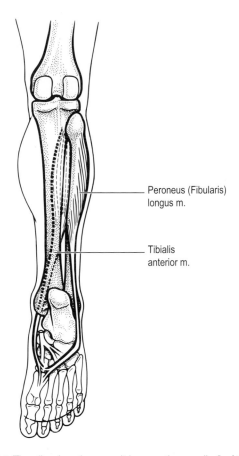

• **Fig. 6.14** The sole of the foot, showing the traditional view of the biomechanical connection between tibialis anterior and the fibularis longus at the 1st cuneiform/1st metatarsal joint.

• **Fig. 6.16** The sling (or stirrup, as it is sometimes called) of the tibialis anterior and the fibularis longus connects the medial longitudinal arch to the upper calf. (Adapted from Clemente.[1])

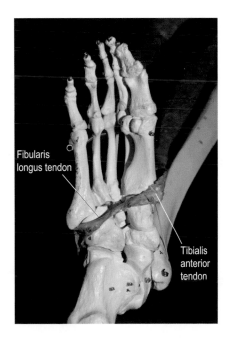

• **Fig. 6.15** The connection between the tibialis anterior and fibularis longus tendons can be dissected intact. They each attach to the periostea of the 1st metatarsal and 1st cuneiform, but they also attach to each other (Video 3.11). This connection is seldom displayed in contemporary anatomy books or dissections. Here the same specimen as in Fig. 6.19 is set in place on a plastic skeleton.

In the case of a pronated foot, you will often find that the tibialis anterior is locked long or eccentrically loaded, and the fibularis longus locked short (Video 6.24). Therefore, in these cases, the fascia of the tibialis anterior needs to be lifted and that of the fibularis lengthened inferiorly, and the tibialis often needs additional strengthening work. In a supinated foot, the reverse treatment applies: drop and lengthen the tibialis anterior, while lifting, freeing, and finally strengthening the fibularis longus (www.anatomytrains.com – video ref: Spiral Line, 33:50–46:44).

The Back of the Leg

Once onto the fibularis, we pass easily along it to the head of the fibula, as we did with the LL, but this time we take the more obvious route from the head of the fibula onto the biceps femoris, the lateral hamstring (Fig. 6.17). The long head of the biceps carries us up to the ischial tuberosity. This whole complex – TFL to ITT to anterior tibialis to fibularis longus to biceps femoris long head – can be seen as a conjoined 'jump rope' that travels from hip to arch down the anterolateral portion of the leg, and then arch to hip up the posterolateral aspect of the leg (Figs. 6.13, 6.18 and 6.19).

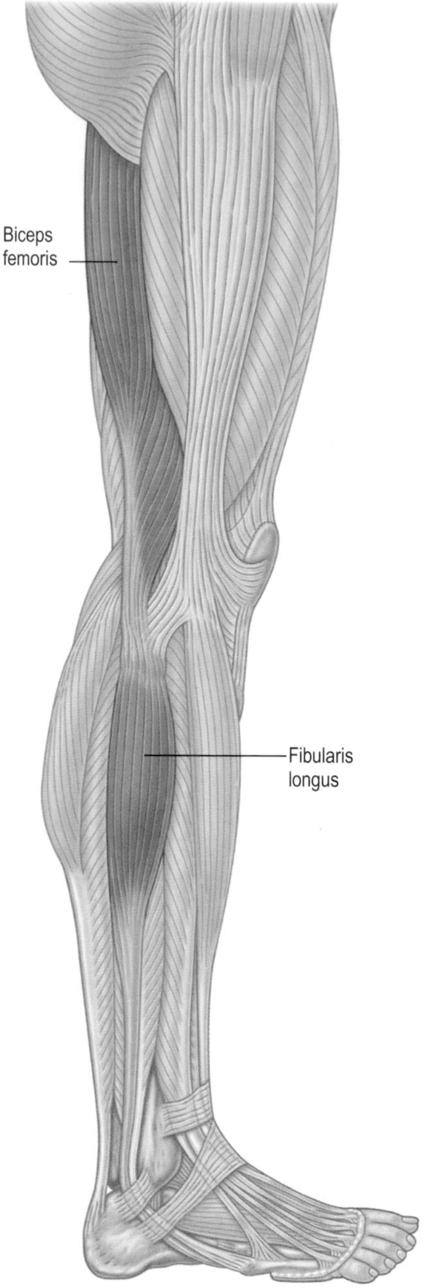

Biceps femoris

Fibularis longus

• **Fig. 6.17** There is a clear and direct fascial connection at the head of the fibula between the fibularis longus and the biceps femoris muscle.

❖ ❀ ❖ *The 4th Hamstring*

Deep to the biceps femoris long head, which is an express crossing both hip and knee, lies an important and not so obvious set of locals. This underlying connection can sometimes provide the answer to recalcitrant hamstring shortness and limitations to hip flexion and hip–knee integration. The first of these two locals is the short head of the biceps, which starts from the same tendinous attachment at the head of the fibula as the long head and passes to the linea aspera about one-third of the way up the femur (Figs. 6.19 and 6.20). Here there is a fascial continuity with the

middle section of the adductor magnus, which passes up beneath the rest of the biceps femoris to attach to the inferior aspect of the ischial ramus, just anterior to the hamstring attachments.

The short head of the biceps component may be overactive in chronically flexed knees or with a lateral postural rotation of the lower leg on the femur, while the adductor magnus component may contribute to a posteriorly tilted pelvis, or the inability of the hip joints to flex or 'sashay' properly.

Reaching this '4th hamstring' requires precision in getting under the superficial hamstrings. Find the singular biceps femoris tendon on the posterolateral side of the knee, coming up from the fibular head. The short head of the biceps can be found by reaching around this tendon on both its medial and lateral sides. It may be easier to reach the belly of the short head from one or the other side due to individual variation in the anatomy. With your client lying prone with the knee flexed, pin the muscle (but not the tendon) against the back of the femur, which will be stretched and lengthened as your client slowly lowers the leg and foot to full knee extension. The short head can also be reached side-lying, with the knee on the edge of the treatment table, still using moving from flexion to knee extension to stretch it (www.anatomytrains.com – video ref: Spiral Line, 29:33–33:49).

The adductor magnus (which makes another appearance as part of the Deep Front Line in Ch. 9) can most easily be reached by having your client side-lying with the upper knee and hip flexed (and the thigh resting on a pillow so that the pelvis is not rotated – one hip joint directly above the other is what you want) with the medial aspect of the underlying leg open for work (www.anatomytrains.com – video ref: Deep Front Line – Part 1, 37.32–41:59).

Find the hamstring attachments on the posterior aspect of the ischial tuberosity, and palpate along the bottom edge of the ischial tuberosity anterior about an inch (3 cm) to find the strong adductor magnus attachment. Instructing the client to lift the knee toward the ceiling will isolate this tendon from the hamstrings. Once found, work the adductor magnus down from its attachment toward the middle of the femur, remembering that this is a substantial piece of myofascia and several passes may be necessary to achieve the necessary depth.

Movement teachers can isolate this part of the adductor magnus by having their students stretch into hip flexion while keeping the knees slightly flexed. The stretch will be felt to run a bit deeper in the back of the thigh than the usual straight-legged forward bend.

❀ ❀ The Posterior Spiral Line

From the lateral hamstring, we can follow the SPL onto the sacrotuberous ligament, across the sacral fascia onto the contralateral dorsal sacroiliac ligament (which is really part of a whole 'bed' of ligaments), and on up the erector spinae on that contralateral side. Depending on the postural

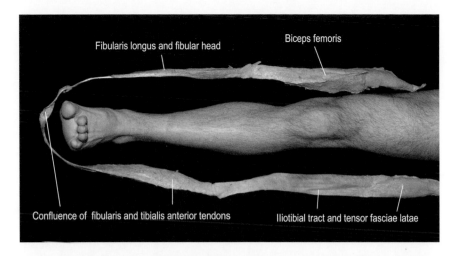

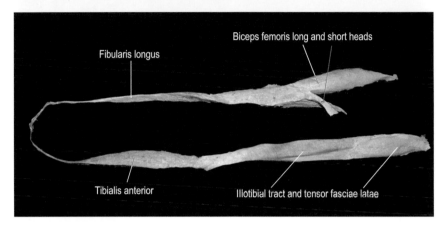

• **Fig. 6.18** In this dissection laid around a living leg, we see how the arch stirrup has connection right up the leg to the pelvis. (www.anatomytrains.com – video ref: Anatomy Trains Revealed.)

• **Fig. 6.19** The 'jump rope' of the lower Spiral Line, on its own, with the short head of the biceps femoris reflected away.

pattern and the dominant leg, however, the forces coming up the leg could track the SBL – transferring tension up the same side of the sacral fascia from the sacrotuberous ligament to the ipsilateral dorsal sacroiliac ligament to the spinal muscles (see Fig. 6.2A). These patterns have to do with differential leg length, lateral pelvic tilt, which leg is more heavily weighted, and can change from moment to moment in dynamic patterns like a football game.

This final track of the erectors thus passes close to the very beginning of this Spiral Line, passing under the rhomboids, splenius capitis and cervicis, to attach to the occiput (Fig. 6.21). Thus the SPL comes to rest on the back of the occiput, quite close to where we began many pages and several meters of fascia ago.

This line – which is of course expressed on both sides – joins each side of the skull across the back of the neck to its opposite shoulder, continuing around the belly in front to the hip on the same side as it started. From here the line drops down the outside of the thigh and knee, but crosses over the front of the shin to form a sling under the inner arch, which rises up the back of the body to rejoin the skull just medial to where it started.

The helical routes around the body are not by any means limited to the Spiral Line described here. See the discussion at the end of Chapter 8 (Functional Lines) and in Chapter 10 for a more expanded view.

❖ ❖ General Movement Considerations: Reciprocity

Obviously, the SPL will be both stretched and engaged by rotational and twisting movements. The currently popular 'crunch' (upper body sit up) with a twist, where one elbow heads for the opposite knee, engages the upper part of the SPL. Yoga 'twists' will stretch the upper SPL, and the Triangle pose and its variations in particular are designed to engage the entire line (Fig. 6.22). There is a clear reciprocal relationship between the two sides of the line; sitting (to fix the pelvis) and twisting the entire upper body to look over the right shoulder will stretch the upper left SPL while it employs the upper right SPL in concentric contraction. It is worth observing whether such movement is coordinated – using all parts of the line in an even way on the contracting side, and stretching all parts of the line evenly on the lengthening side. As we add in the core rotational pattern in Ch 9, the complexity of human rotational movement will be abundantly apparent.

❖ ❖ Palpating the Spiral Line

Though the SPL begins in the adherent fascia on the posterolateral aspect of the skull, its first real station is at the

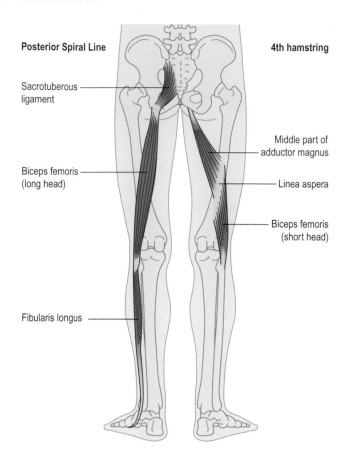

Posterior Spiral Line

4th hamstring

Sacrotuberous ligament

Biceps femoris (long head)

Fibularis longus

Middle part of adductor magnus

Linea aspera

Biceps femoris (short head)

• **Fig. 6.20** Beneath the express of the long head of the biceps femoris (left) lies a set of two locals termed the '4th hamstring' (right). It consists of the short head of the biceps running from the fibula up the linea aspera of the femur, and the middle section of the adductor magnus running from the same place on the femur up to the ischial ramus just in front of the hamstrings.

occipital ridge extending laterally onto the mastoid process, and the first track is the splenius capitis and cervicis, which we first encountered as part of the Lateral Line (see Fig. 6.3A). It can be clearly felt below the occipital ridge, slanting in from the side toward the cervical spinous processes below the superficial trapezius. It will pop into your fingers when the head is turned to the same side against resistance. To feel the splenii, have your client lie supine, with their head resting in your hands. Sink your fingers gently into the soft tissue below the occiput, a bit away from the midline. Have your thumbs alongside the client's head. As the client turns into the resistance of your thumbs, the splenii, with their fibers slanting down and in toward the upper thoracic spine, will be clearly felt on the same side just deep to the thin trapezius.

The rhomboids, the next track on this line, can be more easily seen and felt on someone else, since they occupy that space on your back that is so difficult to scratch when it itches. Have your model bring their shoulder blades up and together, and on most people you will see the shape of the rhomboids pushing out against the overlying trapezius.

If you can insinuate your fingers under the vertebral border of your model's scapula, you can feel where the

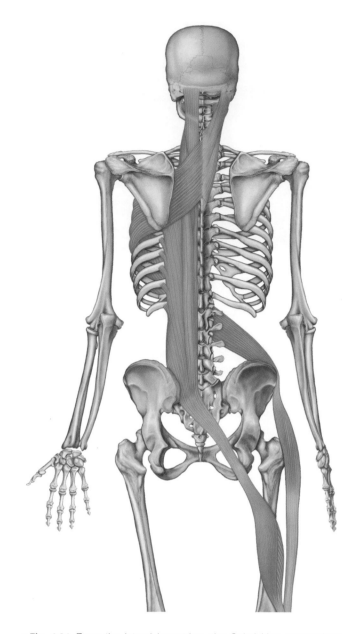

• **Fig. 6.21** From the lateral hamstring, the Spiral Line connections parallel the Superficial Back Line connections onto the sacrotuberous ligament, but cross to the other side and on up the erector spinae to the back of the skull, just next to where it began.

rhomboids continue on into the serratus anterior. Most of that large sheet of muscle, however, is invisible under the scapula. In thin individuals, the lower four or five slips (which are the part under discussion here) can be seen outside the edge of the latissimus when the model contracts the muscle (e.g. in a push-up or plank).

The link from the anterior part of the lower serratus onto the external oblique, across the linea alba into the internal oblique on the opposite side, is well known and can be easily palpated or observed, as in Fig. 6.9. This brings us to the connection of the internal oblique onto the anterior iliac crest and ASIS.

To continue down from here, place your fingers under the edge of the anterior iliac crest, then abduct and medially

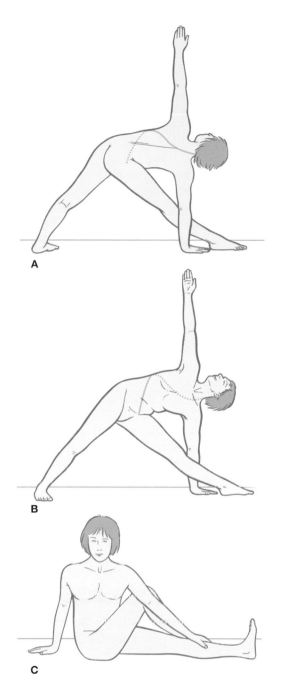

• **Fig. 6.22** Spinal twist poses, such as the Triangle pose or Seated Twist, are custom-made to stretch the upper portion of the Spiral Line on one side, while engaging it on the other.

rotate the hip joint (see Fig. 6.11). The tensor fasciae latae (TFL) muscle will pop your fingers out. From here, the iliotibial tract (ITT) can be felt, dimly at the top of the thigh but more distinctly as you pass down toward the knee. With the hip abducted and the foot off the ground and dorsiflexed, the connection from the ITT across the knee joint to the tibialis anterior can be clearly felt (see Figs. 6.12 and 6.13).

Follow the tibialis anterior down the front of the shin next to the tibia and find its strong tendon emerging from under the retinacula on the medial side of the front of the ankle. Strongly dorsiflex and invert the foot to feel the

tendon as far down as you can toward its station between the 1st metatarsal and 1st cuneiform (see Fig. 6.14).

The fibularis longus starts just on the other side of this attachment, with a fascial continuity through the fascia of the joint capsule, but this is very difficult to feel, except by implication, owing to the overlying myofascia and fascial padding on the bottom of the foot (see Fig. 6.15). The fibularis longus tendon passes under the foot deep to almost everything else, running through a canal in the cuboid (again very difficult to feel) and emerging to our fingers just under the lateral malleolus of the ankle (see Fig. 6.17). Two tendons will be palpable here, but the fibularis brevis tendon (which is part of the LL but not the SPL) will be superior to our fibularis longus tendon and clearly heading for, and attached to, the 5th metatarsal base.

The fibularis longus myofascia passes up the outside of the leg to the fibular head, where there is a clear, palpable, and easily dissected connection to the lateral hamstring, the biceps femoris. Follow the hamstring tendon up the outside back of the leg to arrive at the ischial tuberosity. From here the SPL connection passes onto the sacrotuberous ligament, the sacral fascia, and the erector spinae. (Palpation of these structures is discussed in connection with the Superficial Back Line in Ch. 3, p. 48, so we will not repeat it here.)

DISCUSSION 6.1

❖ ❖ ❀ The Upper Spiral Line and Postural Rotations of the Trunk

Because of the mechanical rather than direct connection across the pelvis at the ASIS, and the roundhouse of vectors that affect the ASIS position, the upper and lower portions of the SPL frequently, although not always, work separately; in any case they are most easily discussed separately. The two parts remain linked, of course, and can work in concert, but are also capable of singing counterpoint.

The upper portion of the SPL, from the occiput around the contralateral shoulder girdle to the ASIS (see Fig. 6.7), is in a perfect position to mediate rotations in the upper body (Fig. 6.23; Video 6.26). 'Mediate' because clinical experience suggests that the Spiral Line is only sometimes the *cause* of such postural rotations or twists, but is at least as often involved in compensating for deeper spinal twists which may come from any of a number of structural or functional sources (see also Ch. 9 on the Deep Front Line).

Thus the SPL complex of myofascia can be used to create twists in daily movements or specific exercises, or it can be used as a superficial postural bandage over a deeper scoliosis or other axial rotation. Any core rotation will affect the superficial lines, and none more than the SPL, which is often locked in a compensatory pattern. If the core pattern in the spine is a right rotation, the sleeve pattern in the SPL usually involves a counterbalancing shortness in the left SPL. This has the effect of making the body look straight

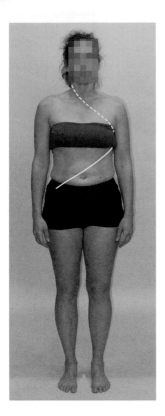

• **Fig. 6.23** A common postural pattern involving a shortening of one side of the upper Spiral Line – in this case, the right SPL is consistently short from the right side of the head to the right hip by way of the left shoulder and ribs. A head shifted and/or tilted to one side, differences in the scapular positions, and a shift or twist in the rib cage – all of which are present in this model – any of these should alert the practitioner to a possibility of Spiral Line imbalance in the pattern.

in the end, but in fact the body will be both restricted and short. (Take a towel and twist it, and notice it shorten in length – any fabric that is twisted will become shorter and fascial fabric is no exception.)

Once this pattern is recognized, it is important to release the sleeve first, before attempting to release the core muscles on the front and back of the spine. This is the intent of the work on the SPL in these patterns. Please note well: when one releases such a compensatory pattern in the sleeve-like SPL, the core rotation will usually become more apparent, so that the client may report feeling or looking more twisted at this juncture in their work with you. It is important to educate them as to what is unfolding – because only when the sleeve rotation in the SPL is removed can one effectively step in to work with the core rotation in the Deep Front Line or deep spinal muscles. The inverse statement is worth repeating: attempting to unravel core rotational patterns before the superficial sleeve rotational pattern is slackened is an exercise in frustration for both the practitioner and the subject.

Because of the interplay between deeper and superficial patterns, the number of specific modifications and individual ways of using the SPL in rotation are legion. Postural shortening directly up the line from the ASIS to the skull produces a characteristic posture, which any practitioner will recognize from Fig. 6.23.

As the line pulls through the abdominal fascia via the internal and external obliques from the hip onto the opposite serratus, it protracts the rib cage on that side, with the shoulder usually coming along for the ride. This usually pulls the upper back and/or lower neck toward that shoulder, so that the head shifts toward the shoulder, sometimes tilting to the opposite side – all of this visible in Fig. 6.23. The pattern is discernible in the absence of, or sometimes in competition with, other forces. An individually tight muscle (e.g. infraspinatus) or a competing pull from another line (e.g. a short Lateral Line on the same side as the SPL in question) will modify and perhaps obscure, but not obliterate, the pattern created by shortness in the upper SPL.

Owing to the weight and competing forces in the pelvis, the SPL rarely pulls the ASIS out of place from above, from the shoulder or ribs. It is, however, quite common to have parts of this line tighten without transferring the tension throughout the line. Thus, one section of the SPL may shorten without the shortness being passed to succeeding sections. In some cases, the section from the skull to the serratus tightens without the involvement of the belly, or the belly can pull through to the neck without the shoulder being protracted in the process. For this reason, we often assess the SPL from the ASIS toward the head, rather than the other way around.

Practice is necessary to discern the specific modifications in the pattern, but there are four 'red flags' that should alert the practitioner to possible or probable imbalance in the SPL: (1) shifts or tilts in the head position relative to the rib cage, (2) one shoulder more forward than the other, (3) lateral rib cage shifts relative to the pelvis, or (4) differences in the direction of the sternum and pubis, which usually can also be read as marked differences in the measurement from one costal arch (where the outside edge of the rectus abdominis crosses the costal cartilages at the 7th rib) to the opposite ASIS. In Fig. 6.9, for example, the measurement from his left ribs to right hip is clearly longer than the corresponding measurement from the right ribs to the left hip. In Fig. 6.23, it is shorter from the left ribs to right hip than its converse, but this is not so easily detected in a small photo. Exacting measurement is not necessary; if you need a micrometer to tell which of these lines is shorter, then there is probably not a significant SPL issue at this level.

Fig. 6.24 shows examples of other patterns of imbalance, mostly in the right Spiral Line that sweeps around the left shoulder and ribs.

DISCUSSION 6.2

❖ ❖ 🍀 The SPL and Forward Head Posture

The serratus anterior, as we noted above, is a complex muscle, a broad combination of a quadrate and triangular muscle that both stabilizes and controls scapular positioning.

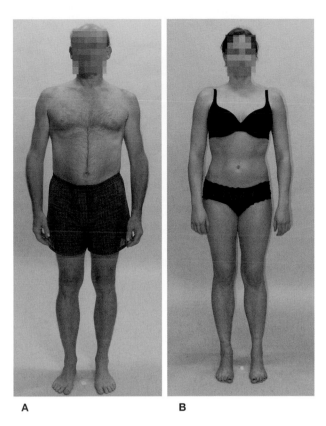

A **B**

• **Fig. 6.24** More common Spiral Line patterns, as seen in standing posture. In (**A**) the right SPL is pulled all the way to the right ankle. In (**B**) the left SPL is pulling the upper body onto the left leg.

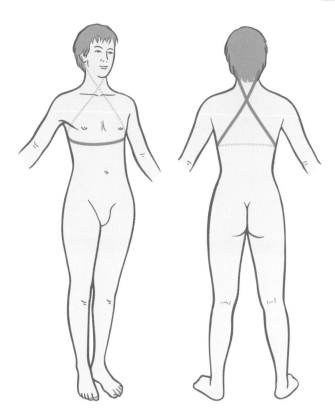

• **Fig. 6.25** The connection between the two serrati across the bottom of the sternum just below the pectoral muscles can be seen to continue up the SPL to connect forward head posture and restricted breathing.

Earlier in our phylogenetic history, the serratus was primarily responsible for creating a sling to support the rib cage within the uprights of the scapulae (see Ch. 7 or www .anatomytrains.com – video ref: Shoulder and Arm Lines, 3:22–5:07).

The lower slips of serratus definitely belong to the SPL, but the middle slips form a connection with each other across the center line at the bottom of the sternum, under the pectoralis major, at the level of the 'bra line'. (See also Appendix 2 – this corresponds to Schultz's chest band.) This creates a 'branch line' for the SPL of interest where you see the ubiquitous forward head posture.

If we follow this line from the midline just above the xiphoid process, around the middle slips of the serratus to the middle of the rhomboid and across to the splenius capitis, we end up on the skull on the opposite side (Fig. 6.25). To see or feel this for yourself – and it is worthwhile to understand this pattern – take a six- to eight-feet strip of fabric like a yoga belt or a length of gauze, stand behind your model, place the middle of the strip above the xiphoid at the bra line and bring the two ends behind the model, crossing them up between the shoulder blades to 'attach' them to the skull by holding them there with your hands. (It is possible to do this on yourself, but difficult to avoid getting tangled up.)

Now have the model jut their head forward of the rest of the body. Feel the strip tighten and pull back on the sternum. So many of those with forward head posture also have the tight chest band, and this is a major avenue for the force transmission of the compensation. If you wish to see the chest band loosen its hold on your model's breathing, progressively get the head back up on top of the body as you progressively loosen the fascial band connecting the two serrati. That will ease this line and help restore the full excursion of the chest in breathing.

DISCUSSION 6.3

❖ ❖ 🌸 The Foot Arches and Pelvic Tilt

Understanding patterns leads to highly specific, logical, and effective soft-tissue interventions. It has long been recognized that the tibialis anterior and the fibularis (peroneus) longus together form a 'stirrup' under the arch system of the foot. The tibialis pulls up on a weak section of the medial longitudinal arch, the fibularis tendon supports the cuboid, the keystone of the lateral arch, and together they help to prevent the proximal part of the transverse arch from dropping (see Fig. 6.15).

Furthermore, there is a reciprocal relationship between the two: a lax (or 'locked long') tibialis coupled with a contracted (or 'locked short') fibularis will contribute to an everted (pronated) foot, with the tendency toward a drop

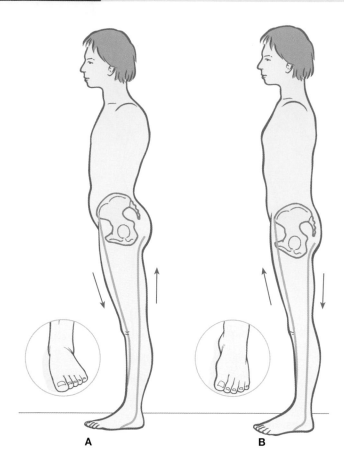

• **Fig. 6.26** The pattern of the sling under the foot can be extended, via the Spiral Line, to connect with the angle of pelvic tilt.

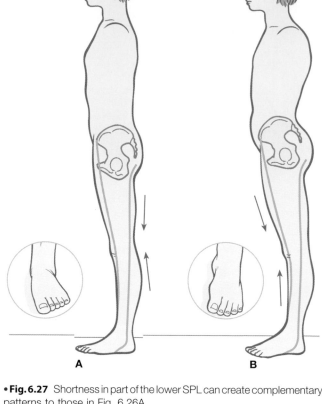

• **Fig. 6.27** Shortness in part of the lower SPL can create complementary patterns to those in Fig. 6.26A.

in the medial arch (see Fig. 6.16). The opposite pattern, a shortened tibialis and a strained fibularis, tends to create an inverted (supinated) foot with an apparently high arch and the weight shifted laterally on the foot.

With the entire SPL in mind, we can expand this concept to include the entire leg: the tibialis connects to the rectus femoris (SFL), the sartorius (SFL alternate route) and the ITT and TFL (SPL). All of these connections go to the very front of the hip bone: the ASIS or AIIS. The fibularis connects through the long head of the biceps femoris to the ischial tuberosity, or in other words to the very back of the hip bone (see Fig. 6.19).

Thus, the stirrup or 'sling' created by the tibialis and fibularis extends up the leg to the pelvis and relates to pelvic position (Fig. 6.26): an anterior pelvic tilt would bring the ASIS closer to the foot, and thus remove upper tensional support from the tibialis, creating a tendency (but not a certainty) toward a fallen medial arch (Fig. 6.26A). Conversely, a posterior pelvic tilt would tend to pull up on the tibialis and slacken the fibularis, creating the tendency toward an inverted foot (Fig. 6.26B).

Take note of the further implication: a shortened SPL in the back of the leg could overcome the front of the SPL and produce both a posterior pelvis *and* an everted foot (Fig. 6.27A). When we view this pattern, we know that the back of the lower SPL must have some significant shortening

somewhere along these tracks. In the reverse pattern (Fig. 6.27B), an inverted foot with an anterior tilt pelvis points to shortness along the front of the lower SPL (tibialis anterior – anterior ITT), though this pattern can also be linked to a shortened Deep Front Line (see Ch. 9).

DISCUSSION 6.4

❖ ✿ The Lower Spiral Line and Knee Tracking

The SPL can affect knee tracking (the ability of the knee to track straight forward and back in walking, keeping more or less the same directional vector as the hip and ankle).

To assess knee tracking, you can watch your client walk straight at you or straight away and see how the knees travel during the different phases of gait. An alternative assessment is to have your client stand in front of you with her feet parallel (meaning the 2nd metatarsals are parallel). Have her bring both knees forward, with her feet on the floor and while maintaining the upper body erect – neither sticking her bum back behind her nor seriously tucking it under to cause a backward lean in the rib cage – and see how the two knees track (Fig. 6.28). If one or both knees are heading

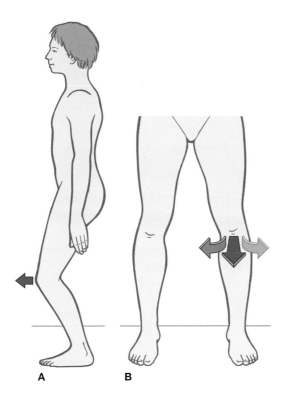

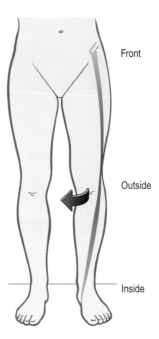

• Fig. 6.29 Because the Spiral Line passes from the front of the hip to the outside of the knee to the inside of the ankle, tightening this line can tend to induce medial rotation at the knee.

• Fig. 6.28 In assessing knee tracking, let both knees come straight forward with the pelvis tucked under and the heels on the ground, and watch the 'headlight' of the patella to see whether it tracks at all to the inside or outside as it comes forward or back.

inward, toward the other, as she brings them forward, the entire lower SPL sling may be tight on that side.

When we note how the SPL runs from the ASIS in the front of the pelvis to the outside of the knee and then down to the inside of the ankle, we can clearly see how tightening it can affect knee direction, by pulling the outside of the knee toward a line running straight from the ASIS to the medial ankle (Fig. 6.29). Loosening this line from above or below prior to local soft-tissue work, or prior to assigning remedial exercise to restore proper knee tracking, will greatly increase the efficacy of the treatment (www.anatomytrains .com – video ref: Spiral Line, 46:45–51:37). If the knee runs laterally during standing flexion, increasing standing tone in the lower anterior SPL can help steady this tendency.

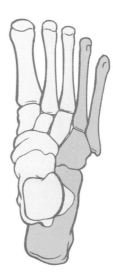

• Fig. 6.30 The foot parses fairly neatly into the bones of the medial arch and those of the lateral arch. Some dancers call this the 'toe foot' and the 'heel foot', respectively.

DISCUSSION 6.5

✿ The 'Heel Foot' and the Sacroiliac Joint

It has long been noted that the bones of the foot divide fairly neatly down a longitudinal axis into the bones that comprise the medial arch and those that comprise the lateral arch (Fig. 6.30).

Borrowing terms from dance, these could be referred to as the 'heel foot' and the 'toe foot'. The toe foot is clearly designed to take the primary weight: if you stand and let your weight swing onto your toes, you will feel the pressure

in the first three metatarsal heads on up to the talus. Seeing how the talus lines up with the main weight-bearing bone of the shin, the tibia, only reinforces our conviction. Swinging forward off your heel and keeping your weight on the two outside toes, unless you are quite accustomed to it, is quite difficult to do, and nearly impossible to maintain.

The heel, of course, does take weight in standing and walking, but the outer two toes and the associated bones (4th and 5th metatarsals and the cuboid) are really designed more as balancers, outriggers for the foot's canoe (Fig. 6.31).

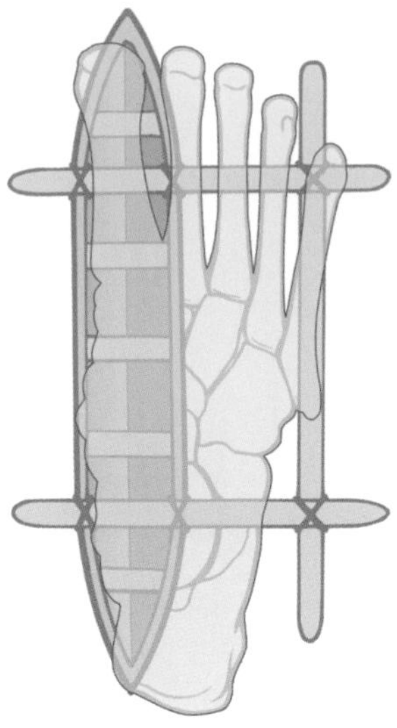

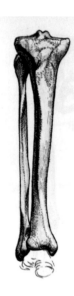

• **Fig. 6.31** In terms of function, the medial arch bones can be seen to be the major weight-bearing 'canoe', while the outer arch bones act like an 'outrigger', balancing and stabilizing but not bearing so much weight.

• **Fig. 6.32** Above the lateral arch bones is the fibula, which is clearly not positioned to transfer weight downward. On the contrary, its position, tucked under the condyle of the tibia, suggests that it is designed instead to resist upward pull. (Reproduced with kind permission from Grundy 1982.)

Looking above the heel foot, we find the fibula, uniquely placed in being tucked under the tibial condyle (Fig. 6.32). It is very badly positioned to bear weight, and in fact looks better placed to resist being pulled up, rather than pulled down. Although eight muscles pull down on the fibula from the foot, one very large one, the biceps femoris, pulls directly up and in on it.

If we trace this entire linkage, we can link the heel foot – in other words, the lateral arch – to the sacroiliac joint via the fibulari, the biceps femoris, and the sacrotuberous ligament (see Fig. 6.20). The success and holding power of the sacroiliac joint manipulations of our chiropractic and osteopathic colleagues can be markedly increased, in our clinical experience, through creating more soft-tissue balance of the heel foot, fibularii, head of the fibula, and lateral hamstring. In other words, heel position and the lateral arch relate to sacroiliac joint stability via the lower posterior SPL.

DISCUSSION 6.6

❖ ❖ 🍀 The Spiral Line Midline Crossing at the Sacrum in Walking

The third crossing of the Spiral Line at the midline rests on the observation of pelvic stability requirements. The complex movements of the sacrum and the two innominates in gait have been well documented elsewhere.[2] Here we focus on the role of the Spiral Line in modulating these movements, keeping the sacrum mobile within stable bounds.

In the push-off phase from the left foot, with the right foot forward between heel strike and weight acceptance, the sacrotuberous ligament on the right side, linked by stretched and tensed fascia to the right heel, prevents excess nutation of the sacrum, while the long dorsal sacroiliac ligament on the left side prevents excessive sacral counternutation as the front of the left pelvis is pulled into flexion.

These two coordinated ligamentous limitations are linked across the sacrum by the fascial tissues of the Spiral Line. There is thus a fascial continuity from the right ischial tuberosity across the midline and superiorly to the left posterior superior iliac spine (Fig. 6.33). As the gait proceeds through the swing phase, both sets of ligaments relent to allow the SI joint movement from nutation to counternutation or vice versa on the opposite side (Video 6.6). As we get to the push-off phase on the right foot, with the right SI joint closed in counternutation and left in nutation, the left sacrotuberous ligament and the right long dorsal sacroiliac ligament link across the sacrum from the left IT to the right PSIS during heel strike and weight acceptance onto the left foot.

This complex, whose tension is dynamically modulated by the hamstrings from below and the sacral multifidus and iliocostalis lumborum from above (see Fig. 6.21), thus links the entire posterior Spiral Line into pelvic stability in gait. If this system is not working properly – and significantly asymmetrical movements here are more common than not, often accompanied by pain patterns – requires a global view.

Attention to the internal mechanics of the pelvis (osteopathic or chiropractic manipulation) will be enhanced by soft-tissue balance of these ligamentous structures and by muscular stretching or toning to even out the forces crossing the sacrum from step to step. This points out the need for multidisciplinary clinics or multi-talented practitioners who can address all the elements of this situation: the joint kinematics, the ligamentous bed, myofascial tone, and recruitment coordination.

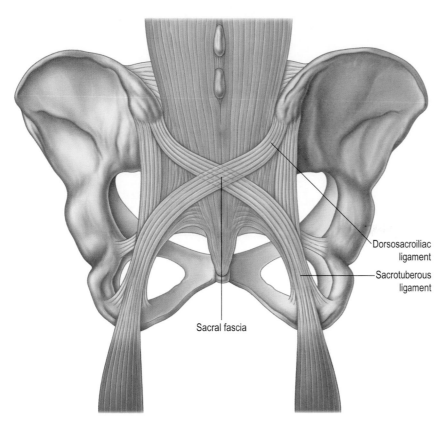

Dorsosacroiliac ligament

Sacrotuberous ligament

Sacral fascia

• **Fig. 6.33** In a step forward with the right foot, the right sacrotuberous and the diagonal portion of the left long dorsal sacroiliac ligaments combine to limit intrapelvic movement at the sacroiliac joints while their complements are eased. The opposite occurs when the left leg goes forward and the right comes back.

References

1. Clemente C. *Anatomy, a Regional Atlas of the Human Body*. 3rd ed. Philadelphia: Lea and Febiger; 1987. Fig. 506.

2. Vleeming A, ed. *Movement, Stability, and Lumbopelvic Pain*. 2nd ed. Edinburgh: Elsevier; 2007.

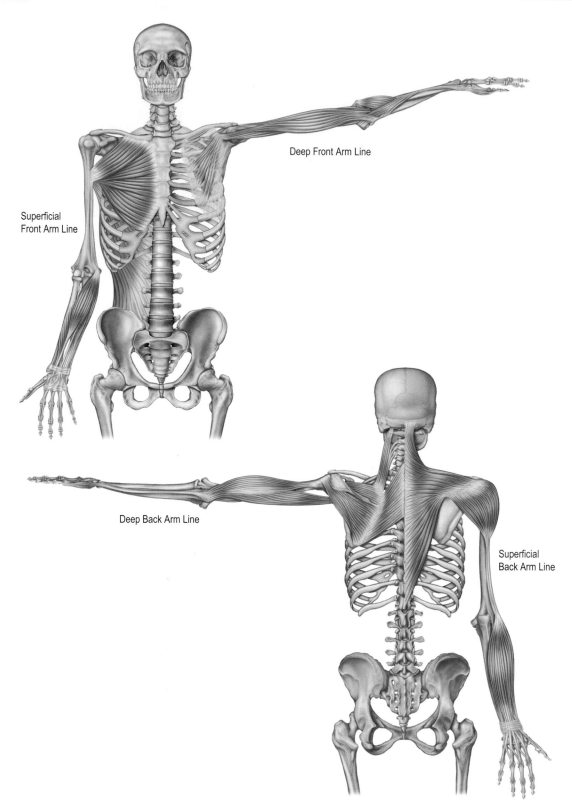

Deep Front Arm Line

Superficial
Front Arm Line

Deep Back Arm Line

Superficial
Back Arm Line

• **Fig. 7.1** The Arm Lines.

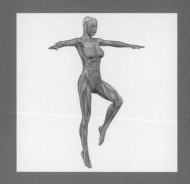

7

The Arm Lines

In this chapter we identify four distinct myofascial meridians that run from the axial skeleton through four layers of the shoulder, to the four quadrants of the arm and four 'sides' of the hand, namely the thumb, little finger, palm, and back of the hand (www.anatomytrains.com – video ref: Shoulders and Arm Lines, 13:05–14:35). Despite this apparently neat symmetry, the Arm Lines (Fig. 7.1) display more 'crossover' myofascial linkages among these longitudinal continuities than do the corresponding lines in the legs (see Discussion 7.2). Because human shoulders and arms are specialized for mobility (compared to our more stable legs), these multiple degrees of freedom require more variable lines of control and stabilization and thus more interline links.

Nevertheless, the arms are quite logically arranged with a deep and superficial line along the front of the arm, and a deep and superficial line along the back of the arm (Fig. 7.2/Table 7.1). The lines in the arm are named for their placement as they cross the shoulder (Fig. 7.3). (In Ch. 8 we look at the extensions of these lines that connect the shoulders contralaterally to the opposite pelvic girdle.)

Postural Function

Since the arms hang from the upper skeleton in our upright posture, they are not part of the structural 'column' as such. Thus we have included the appendicular legs in our discussion of the previous lines, but left the arms for separate consideration in a chapter of their own. Given their weight, and their multiple links to our daily activities like driving and digital interface, the Arm Lines do have a postural function: shoulder malposition can create significant drag on the ribs, neck, breathing function, low back, and beyond (Video 1.3). This chapter details the lines of pull on the axial skeleton from the arms when relaxed, as well as the tensile lines that come into play when using the arms in work or sport, supporting the body as in a push-up or yoga inversions, or in hanging from the arms, as in a chin-up or tree play (www.anatomytrains.com – video ref: Shoulders and Arm Lines, 03:01–09:33).

Movement Function

In myriad daily manual activities of examining, manipulating, responding to, and moving through the environment, our arms and hands, in close connection with our eyes, perform through these tensile continuities. The Arm Lines act across the 10 or so levels of joints in the arm to bring things toward us, push them away, pull, push or stabilize our own body, or simply hold some part of the world still for our perusal and modification. These lines connect seamlessly into the other lines, particularly the helical lines – the Lateral, Spiral, and Functional Lines (Chs 5, 6, and 8, respectively).

The Arm Lines in Detail

Common postural compensation patterns associated with the Arm Lines lead to all kinds of shoulder problems, as well as arm and hand problems, usually involving the shoulders being protracted, retracted, lifted, or 'rounded' (medial rotation and anterior tilt of the scapula). These compensations are often founded in the lack of support from the rib cage, which leads us to look to the cardinal lines as well as the Spiral and Deep Front Lines for a solution. Carpal tunnel, elbow and shoulder impingements, and chronic muscular or trigger-point pain emerge over time, apparently based on faulty postural support.

The Arm Lines are presented from the axial skeleton distally out to the hand. The order in which the lines are presented carries no particular significance.

❖ ♣ Orientation to the Arm Lines

The Arm Line anatomy shown in Table 7.1 is sufficiently complex to merit a simple way to orient to these lines and organize them in the reader's mind before setting off on this intricate journey. You can see the following for yourself in a mirror, or by observing a model (www.anatomytrains.com – video ref: Shoulders and Arm Lines, 16:01–17:19).

Position the arm out to the side, as in Fig. 7.2A, and arrange it so that the palm faces forward and the olecranon

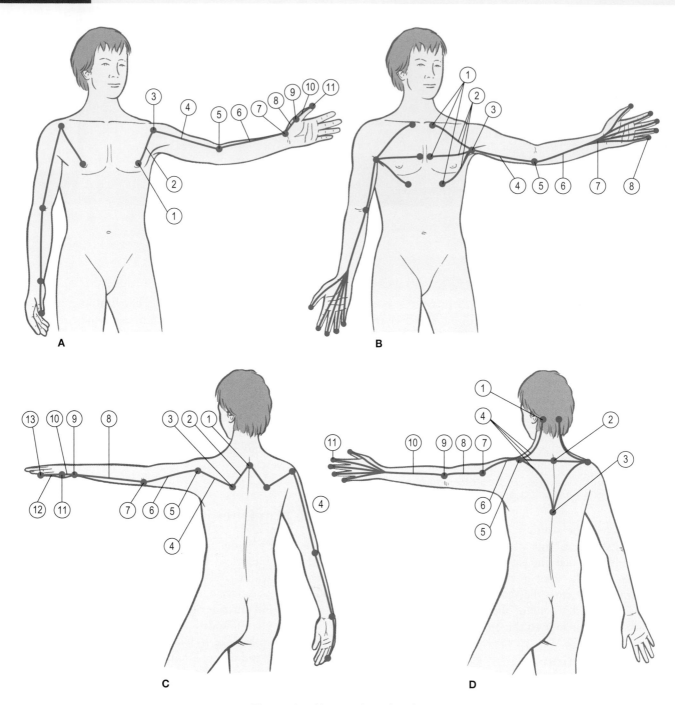

• **Fig. 7.2** Arm Lines tracks and stations.

of the elbow points down to the floor. The Superficial Front Arm Line (SFAL – Fig. 7.2B) is now arrayed along the front of your arm – palmar muscles, carpal tunnel, lower arm flexors, intermuscular septum, and pectoralis major. Turn around: the Superficial Back Arm Line (SBAL – Fig. 7.2D) is arrayed along the back side of the arm – trapezius, deltoid, lateral intermuscular septum, and extensors. Wipe a towel from your shoulder down to the back of your hand to cover this line.

Rotate your arm medially at the shoulder (no pronation at the radioulnar joint), so that the palm faces the floor and the olecranon of the elbow points back, as in Fig. 7.2C. In this position, the Deep Front Arm Line (DFAL – Fig. 7.2A)

is arrayed along the front – thumb, thenar muscles, radius, biceps, running under the major to pectoralis minor. The Deep Back Arm Line (DBAL – Fig. 7.2C) is arrayed along the back side of the arm – the hypothenar muscles, the ulna, the triceps, the rotator cuff, and (under the trapezius) the rhomboids and levator scapulae.

Keeping these 'sight lines' in mind when analyzing movement, especially movements where the arm plays a supporting role, will help distinguish which lines are being employed – and perhaps over- or under-employed – in a movement. Overuse of a particular structure 'downstream' (distally) will often precede strain injuries 'upstream' (proximally) in the given line (Video 2.6).

TABLE 7.1 Arm Lines: Myofascial 'Tracks' and Bony 'Stations' (Fig. 7.2)

Bony Stations		Myofascial Tracks	Bony Stations		Myofascial Tracks
A. Deep Front Arm Line			**C. Deep Back Arm Line**		
3rd, 4th and 5th ribs, inferior edge of clavicle	1		Spinous process of lower cervicals and upper thoracic, C1–4 TPs	1	
	2	Pectoralis minor, subclavius, clavipectoral fascia		2	Rhomboids major and minor, levator scapulae
Coracoid process	3		Medial border of scapula	3	
	4	Biceps brachii, coracobrachialis, brachialis		4	Rotator cuff muscles
			Head of humerus	5	
Radial tuberosity	5			6	Triceps brachii
	6	Pronator teres, supinator, radial periosteum	Olecranon of ulna	7	
				8	Fascia along ulnar periosteum
Styloid process of radius	7		Styloid process of ulna	9	
	8	Radial collateral ligaments		10	Ulnar collateral ligaments
Scaphoid, trapezium	9		Triquetrum, hamate	11	
	10	Thenar muscles		12	Hypothenar muscles
Outside of thumb	11		Outside of little finger	13	
B. Superficial Front Arm Line			**D. Superficial Back Arm Line**		
Medial third of clavicle, costal cartilages, lower ribs, thoracolumbar fascia, iliac crest	1		Occipital ridge, nuchal ligament, thoracic spinous processes	1, 2, 3	
	2	Pectoralis major, latissimus dorsi		4	Trapezius
Medial humeral line	3		Spine of scapula, acromion, lateral third of clavicle	5	
	4	Medial intermuscular septum		6	Deltoid
Medial humeral epicondyle	5		Deltoid tubercle of humerus	7	
	6	Flexor group		8	Lateral intermuscular septum
	7	Carpal tunnel	Lateral epicondyle of humerus	9	
Palmar surface of hand and fingers	8			10	Extensor group
			Dorsal surface of fingers	11	

🌼 The Deep Front Arm Line

The DFAL (Fig. 7.4) begins muscularly on anterior aspects of the 3rd, 4th and 5th ribs with the pectoralis minor muscle (Fig. 7.5). This muscle is actually embedded in the clavipectoral fascia (Fig. 7.6A) that runs underneath the pectoralis major from clavicle to armpit, and includes both the pectoralis minor and the subclavius muscles, with connections to the neurovascular bundle and lymphatic tissues in this area (Fig. 7.6B and www.anatomytrains.com – video

ref: Shoulders and Arm Lines, 29:56–32:28). The entire clavipectoral fascia, nearly as large as the pectoralis major, constitutes the initial track of this line; the pectoralis minor, however, provides the chief contractile structural tethering cord for the scapula, while the smaller subclavius stabilizes the clavicle[1] (Video 4.7).

The distal station for the pectoralis minor muscle is the coracoid process, a nub of the scapula which projects forward under the clavicle like a thumb or a 'crow's beak' (from whence it gets its name). Two other muscles proceed out to the arm from here, the short head of the biceps brachii and the coracobrachialis (see Fig. 7.5). There is clearly a myofascial continuity between the pectoralis minor and both these more distal muscles (Fig. 7.7), but by our Anatomy Trains rules, this connection would seem to be out of the running: in a relaxed standing posture, these arm muscles run in a radical change of direction from the pectoralis minor in this position (see Fig. 7.2A). When the arms are outstretched, however, at the horizontal or anywhere above (as in a tennis forehand), and especially in any hanging position (as in a swinging monkey or in a chin-up), these myofascial units link into a connected line (see Fig. 2.2). In normal 'arms down' posture, shortness in the proximal DFAL simply pulls the coracoid process down to create anterior tilt in the scapula, creating the rounded shoulders commonly commented upon by your mother.

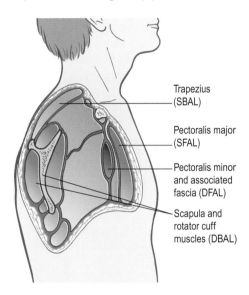

• **Fig. 7.3** The Arm Lines are named for their relative positions at the level of the shoulder. The four parallel planes that start the arm lines are clearly visible and divisible.

The DFAL is primarily a stabilizing line (comparable to the Deep Front Line in the leg), from the thumb to the front of the chest. In the quadruped, and in a rugby scrum or a yoga 'plank', this line would manage (restricting or allowing) side-to-side movement of the upper body. In the free arm in open chain movement, the DFAL controls the angle of the hand, principally via the thumb, and also the thumb's grip.

❖ ❖ ♣ The Pectoralis Minor

The pectoralis minor and the clavipectoral fascia are difficult to find and stretch in isolation from the over-lying pectoralis major. Excessive shortness in this myofascial unit can negatively affect breathing, neck and head posture, and, of course, the easy functioning of the shoulder and arm, especially in reaching upward. Hanging from a branch, or even putting the arm into hyperflexion (as in a deep 'Downward Dog' posture or kneeling before a wall and sliding the hands as far as possible up the surface), may result in creating a stretch in these tissues, but it is difficult for the practitioner to tell from the outside, as lifting the upper ribs by a backwards tilt of the rib cage (and thus avoiding the pectoralis minor stretch) is a common compensation. The following is a reliable way to manually contact this vital and often restricted structure at the proximal end of the DFAL.

Three indications for functional shortness in the pectoralis minor and clavipectoral fascia include: (1) restriction in upper rib movement in inspiration, such that the shoulders and ribs move in strict concert; (2) if the client has trouble flexing the arm and lifting the shoulder to reach the top shelf in the cupboard; and (3) if the scapula is anteriorly tilted or the shoulders rounded (see Fig. 7.35 and Discussion 7.1 at the end of this chapter). To determine the latter, view the client from the side: the medial border of the scapula should hang vertically, like a cliff. If it is sitting at an angle, like a roof, then a shortened pectoralis minor is likely pulling inferiorly on the coracoid process, tilting the

Trapezius (SBAL)

Pectoralis major (SFAL)

Pectoralis minor and associated fascia (DFAL)

Scapula and rotator cuff muscles (DBAL)

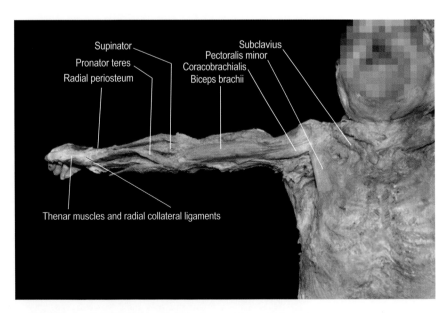

Supinator
Pronator teres
Radial periosteum
Subclavius
Pectoralis minor
Coracobrachialis
Biceps brachii

Thenar muscles and radial collateral ligaments

• **Fig. 7.4** The Deep Front Arm Line in dissection, *in situ*. The pectoralis major has been removed to show the line of myofascial force transmission between the pectoralis minor and the thumb.

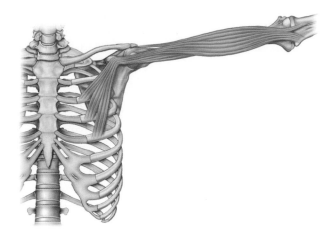

• **Fig. 7.5** The pectoralis minor clearly connects fascially to the short head of the biceps and coracobrachialis at the coracoid process, but they only function in an Anatomy Train fashion when the arm is nearly horizontal or above.

scapula. The longer, outer slips of the pectoralis minor – to the 4th and 5th ribs – will be implicated in this pattern. If the shoulders are rounded (medial rotation or strong protraction of the scapula – often seen when the client is supine and the tips of the shoulders are well off the table), the inner shorter slips to the 2nd (sometimes named as the costocoracoid ligament) and 3rd ribs are the ones that require lengthening.

Although a muscular pectoralis minor, especially the outer more vertical slips, may be felt through the over-lying and more horizontal pectoralis major, approaching from the axilla is to be preferred over treating the minor through the major. Position your client supine with her arm up, elbow bent, so that the back of her hand is resting on the table near her ear. If this is difficult, support the arm on pillows, or alternatively bring the arm down by the client's side so that it rests on your wrist.

Put your fingertips on her ribs in the armpit between the pectoralis and latissimus tendons. Kneeling beside the table

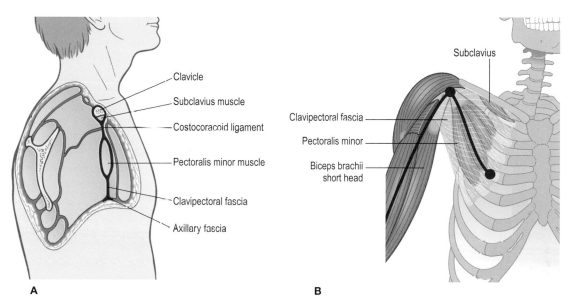

A

B

• **Fig. 7.6** (**A**) The beginnings of the Deep Front Arm Line include not only the pectoralis minor muscle, but also other structures in the same fascial plane from the clavicle down to the lower edge of the armpit. (**B**) This clavipectoral fascia which forms the proximal section of the DFAL is nearly as large as the overlying pectoralis major.

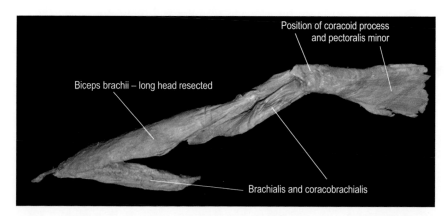

• **Fig. 7.7** The fascial 'fabric' connection between the pectoralis minor and the biceps is clear, even when removed from the coracoid process.

facilitates the proper angle of entry. Starting with the heel of your hand on the table to get the proper angle of approach, slide up slowly under the pectoralis major in the direction of the sternoclavicular joint, keeping your finger pads in contact with the front of the rib cage. It is vitally important to slide along the ribs, not into them or away from them. Pushing into the tissues overlying the ribs is a common error when first attempting this approach. Since the rib periostea are highly innervated, this pressure creates sharp and therapeutically useless pain. With the open client, the correct angle, and soft fingers, however, it is possible to go quite far underneath the pectoralis major, so a little practice is required to figure out how much skin to take with you – skin stretch is not the object (www.anatomytrains.com – video ref: Shoulders and Arm Lines, 30:12–36:00).

Draw an imaginary line down and slightly medial from the coracoid process to the outer and upper attachment of the rectus abdominis. You must go far enough under the pectoralis major to meet this line before you would have any expectation of encountering the outer edge of the pectoralis minor. When you do, it varies from a few skinny slips of muscle plastered to the wall of the ribs to a full, free, distinctly palpable muscle (the desired condition – though even in this condition it can still be muscularly or fascially short). In most cases no harm will come (and much benefit to shoulder mobility will arise) from going under the leading edge of the pectoralis minor, lifting the muscle away from the rib cage and stretching it toward its insertion at the coracoid. The client can help with a long slow inhale, or by lifting his arm toward the top of his head (Fig. 7.8).

Since the pectoralis minor muscle is embedded in the clavipectoral fascia, there is benefit in opening the tissue under the pectoralis major muscle even if the specific slips of the pectoralis minor are not felt. When the muscle can specifically be felt, be aware that the first slip you encounter is attached to the 5th rib. When this is freed or 'melted', the next slip further in will be attached to the 4th rib. In very open bodies, you can sometimes feel the slip attached to the 3rd rib (and most people will have an additional slip of fascia, some with muscle in it, on the 2nd rib as well). The outer slips pull the scapula into anterior tilt; the inner slips pull the scapula (not the humerus) into medial rotation.

The armpit is generally a little-touched area in our culture, so stay within the limits of your client's tolerance for sensation; return at another time if necessary. When working with women, be aware that lymphoid tissue connects the breast around the edge of the pectoralis to the armpit. By 'swimming' your fingers gently under the pectoralis major along the ribs you can avoid any problem with overstretching this tissue. It is also possible to contact this area with the client side-lying, so that gravity takes the breast away from you, although the instability of the shoulder in this position as well as the resulting malposition of the opposite shoulder against the table can present a disadvantage in some clients (www.anatomytrains.com – video ref: Shoulder and Arm Lines, 36:07–38:16).

In a few cases – especially those with mastectomy or radiation treatment – the pectoralis minor can be fastened fascially to the posterior surface of the pectoralis major. If the minor cannot be found by the methods above, supinate your hand so that the fingerpads face forward, using them carefully to strum along the posterior surface of the major. The minor presents itself as a series of fibers oblique to the direction of the pectoralis major fibers. When this condition is encountered, the minor can sometimes be teased away from the major by crooking your fingers and working slowly and carefully to make the separation between the fascial planes.

For movement therapists, you can contact these tissues by having your client kneel before a wall and slide his hands as far up the wall as possible while maintaining a straight back, or keeping the manubrium (not the xiphoid) of the sternum close to the wall. Kneel behind the client and slip your hands around the ribs under the pectoralis minor to find the same slips referenced above. Have the client allow his hands to slide down the wall while you find shortened tissues, and slide his hands back up the wall to assist and control the stretch.

In terms of movement homework, have the client link his fingers behind the lower back and slide them down toward his legs. His scapulae will then drop down the rib cage and come together toward the spine (Fig. 7.9). This will stretch the pectoralis minor and surrounding tissues (and strengthen the antagonistic lower trapezius), but the client should beware of resisting the temptation to arch his low back as he does it, as this will change the angle of the rib cage and negate the stretch.

❖ The Biceps Express

The short head of the biceps runs down from the coracoid to the radial tuberosity, thus affecting three joints: the gleno-humeral joint, the humero-ulnar joint, and the

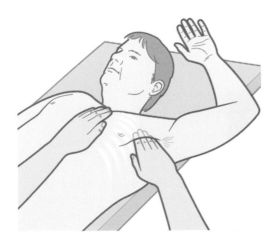

• **Fig. 7.8** The hand approaches the pectoralis minor from the axilla, under the pectoralis major, with the fingers heading in the direction of the sternoclavicular joint.

situation and the contraction of surrounding, assisting, or antagonistic muscles).

This biceps 'express' (see Ch. 2, p. 23, for a definition) has a series of 'locals' beneath it to help sort out its multiple functions. The coracobrachialis runs under the biceps from the coracoid process to the humerus, thus adducting the humerus (www.anatomytrains.com – video ref: Shoulders and Arm Lines, 38:17–42:25). The brachialis runs from the humerus, next to the coracobrachialis attachment, down to the ulna, clearly flexing the elbow (www.anatomytrains.com – video ref: Shoulders and Arm Lines, 43:48–45:47). Finally, the supinator runs from ulna to radius, supinating the forearm.

This provides a very clear example of an organizing, coordinating express arrayed over a series of differentiated locals. All of these muscles are included in the DFAL.

The practical point of this distinction is that postural 'set' is often more determined by the underlying locals than it is by the overlying express. Thus, while in extreme cases the biceps might have a role in chronic humeral adduction or elbow flexion, the therapist is far more likely to get results from addressing the underlying locals than from work on the superficial biceps.

The long head of the biceps, as well as its other 'foot', the tendon of Lacertus or bicipital aponeurosis, are examples of crossovers, and are dealt with in that discussion at the end of this chapter.

The Lower Arm

Both the short head of the biceps and the supinator attach to the radius. In the lower arm, we are inclined to include the pronator teres in this line because with the supinator it clearly controls the degree of rotation of the radius, and thus the thumb (see Figs. 7.4 and 7.11 – pronator and supinator form a 'V' converging on the radius), even though strictly speaking pronator teres is a crossover from the Superficial Back Arm Line. From all these radial attachments, we pass along the periosteum to the styloid process at the distal end of the radius on the thumb side of the wrist (www.anatomytrains.com – video ref: Shoulders and Arm Lines, 45:48–47:34). The fascial fabric below the distal ends of the two rotators is adherent to the periosteum of the radius, which is very reluctant to separate from the bone in dissection (see Fig. 7.4 distal to the 'V').

This long 'station' violates the spirit of the Anatomy Trains idea of longitudinal fascial continuities separable from their underlying bones (see the discussion of the 'inner and outer bags' in Appendix 1, p. 289). Spirit or not, such a fastening is a practical necessity when we consider the stabilizing function of this line for the thumb. The periosteum of the radius and ulna is of course continuous with the interosseous membrane spanning between them. The bones are nevertheless capable of sliding on one another (to reassure yourself of this, put the thumb and forefinger of your left hand on the radial and ulnar styloid processes at the wrist of your right hand. Ad- and abduct the wrist

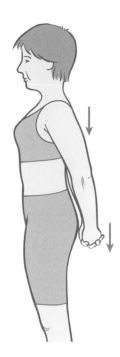

• **Fig. 7.9** Dropping the shoulder blades down the back and bringing them together while keeping the lumbars back will stretch and open the pectoralis minor and surrounding tissues.

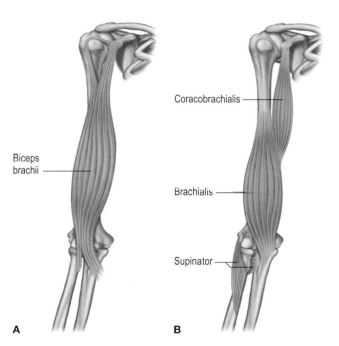

Coracobrachialis

Biceps brachii

Brachialis

Supinator

A   B

• **Fig. 7.10** The biceps brachii forms an express muscle (**A**), which covers three joints. Deep to the biceps lie three local muscles (**B**), each of which duplicates the biceps action on the individual joints. (Compare to the 4th hamstring, Fig. 6.20.)

radio-ulnar joint (the shoulder, elbow, and the spin of the lower arm) (Fig. 7.10 and www.anatomytrains.com – video ref.: Shoulders and Arm Lines, 42:25–43:47). Contracting it can thus have the effect of supinating the forearm, flexing the elbow, and diagonally flexing the upper arm (any or all of these movements, depending on the physics of the

• **Fig. 7.11** The DFAL runs down the periosteum of the radius and crosses over the inside of the wrist to join the thumb and its associated intrinsic thenar muscles (Video 3.14).

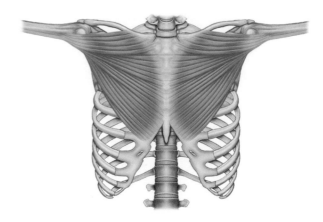

• **Fig. 7.12** The pectoralis major is the principal player in the start of the Superficial Front Arm Line.

(radially and ulnarly deviate if you prefer) to feel the limited slide of the radius on the ulna. In order to stabilize this movement, both of these lines must fasten to the periostea of these bones and (by implication) to the interosseous membrane.

If you get on your hands and knees and then feint left and right with your head and shoulders, like a lizard in a fight, you will feel this stabilizing strap of fascial webbing between the two bones, part of both the Deep Back and Deep Front Arm Lines – traditionally the stabilizers in our quadruped evolutionary history.

From the wrist, we traverse the radial collateral ligament over the thumb-side carpals, the scaphoid, and the trapezium, to the thumb itself (Fig. 7.11). Although the extensor pollicis brevis and abductor pollicis longus tendons accompany these tissues, these muscles arise from the ulna as part of the Deep Back Arm Line – one of the many examples of crossover between the lines discussed at the end of this chapter. The thenar muscles are included as part of the DFAL (www.anatomytrains.com – video ref: Shoulders and Arm Lines, 47:35–49:16).

❖ ❖ 🍀 The 'Thumb Line'

Practitioners of shiatsu or any other technique employing pressure through the thumb need to stay aware of the DFAL, which ends at the thumb. Good body mechanics for a long-term practice require that the DFAL stay open and lengthened, with the arms in a rounded position (elbows bent) while putting the pressure on the thumb (see Fig. 10.53, p. 205). Those practitioners who report pain as a result of this kind of pressure in the thumb itself or the saddle joint at its base will almost invariably show a collapsed DFAL, frequently at the area of the upper arm–coracoid or coracoid–ribs connections and frequently accompanied by elbows that are extended and locked. (See the section on the pectoralis minor above.)

🌸 The Superficial Front Arm Line

The Superficial Front Arm Line (SFAL) overlies the DFAL in the shoulder, beginning with a broad sweep of attachments, which in this line includes two very broad muscles. The pectoralis major, which has a broad set of attachments from the clavicle down onto the middle ribs, begins this line in the front (Fig. 7.12 and www.anatomytrains.com – video ref: Shoulders and Arm Lines, 18:25–25:03). The latissimus dorsi (which begins its embryological life as 'latissimus ventri', a muscle on the front with a firm attachment

to the anterior surface of the humerus, next to pectoralis, thus staking its tenuous claim to being part of the SFAL before it migrates around to our back later in development) sweeps up from the spinous processes of the lower thoracics, the lumbosacral fascia, the iliac crest, and lower lateral ribs (www.anatomytrains.com – video ref: Lateral Line, 43:58–48:40; Video 2.5). Between the pectoralis major and the latissimus, the SFAL has nearly an entire circle of attachments, reflecting the wide degree of control the SFAL exerts on movement of the arm in front of and to the side of the body (Fig. 7.13).

The latissimus picks up the teres major (yet another crossover muscle – see Discussion 7.2) from the lateral border of the scapula, and all three of these muscles twist and focus into bands of tendon which attach alongside each other to the underside of the anterior humerus (Fig. 7.14 – the old med school mnemonic is 'Lady Dorsi lies between two majors'). These bands surround and connect into the proximal part of the medial intermuscular septum, a fascial wall between the flexor and extensor group in the upper arm, which carries us down to the next bony station, the medial humeral epicondyle (Fig. 7.15 and www.anatomytrains.com – video ref: Shoulders and Arm Lines, 25:04–25:56; Video 3.15).

The track of the common flexor tendon continues down from the epicondyle, joining with the many-layered longitudinal muscles on the underside of the forearm (Fig. 7.16A and www.anatomytrains.com – video ref: Shoulders and Arm Lines, 25:56–27:40). The shorter of these muscles go to the carpal bones; the flexor superficialis muscles go to the middle of the fingers, and the profundus muscles reach to the tips of the fingers. This breaks, we should note, the usual pattern of having the deeper muscles be the shorter (Fig. 7.16B). These muscles to the fingers run through the carpal tunnel under the flexor retinaculum, to spread out over the ventral carpals to the palmar side of the fingers (Fig. 7.17 and www.anatomytrains.com – video ref: Shoulders and Arm Lines, 27:41–29:55).

As implied in our first paragraph, the SFAL controls the positioning of the arm in its wide range of motions in front

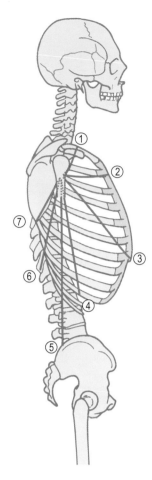

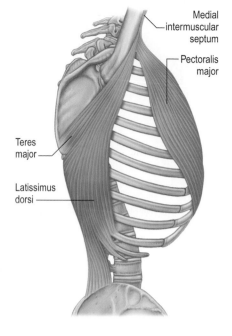

• **Fig. 7.14** The latissimus dorsi and teres major, even though they come from the back, are clearly connected into the same functional myofascial plane as the pectoralis major.

• **Fig. 7.13** Between the two triangular muscles – the pectoralis major and latissimus dorsi – the SFAL has a broad origin around the trunk from the clavicle (1) around the ribs to the pelvis (5) and the thoracic spine (7).

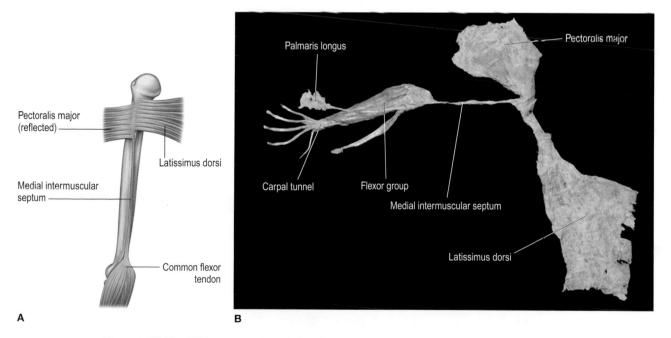

• **Fig. 7.15** (**A**) The SFAL connects from the medial humerus down the medial intermuscular septum to the medial humeral epicondyle on the inner side of the elbow. (**B**) A dissection of the entire SFAL intact as one myofascial meridian.

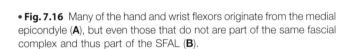

Flexor carpi
radialis

Flexor pollicis
longus

Palmaris
longus

Flexor
digitorum
superficialis

Flexor
carpi
ulnaris

Flexor digitorum
profundus

Flexor pollicis
longus

A   **B**

• **Fig. 7.16** Many of the hand and wrist flexors originate from the medial epicondyle (**A**), but even those that do not are part of the same fascial complex and thus part of the SFAL (**B**).

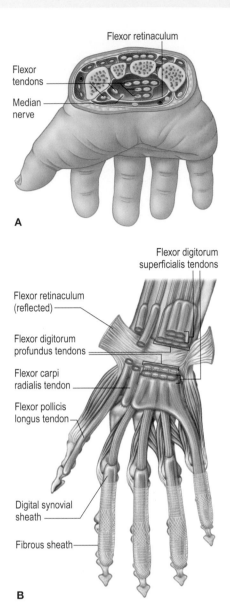

Flexor retinaculum

Flexor
tendons

Median
nerve

A

Flexor digitorum
superficialis tendons

Flexor retinaculum
(reflected)

Flexor digitorum
profundus tendons

Flexor carpi
radialis tendon

Flexor pollicis
longus tendon

Digital synovial
sheath

Fibrous sheath

B

• **Fig. 7.17** The SFAL passes through the carpal tunnel and out onto the palmar surface of the hand and fingers.

of and beside us. The large muscles of the pectoralis and latissimus provide the motive force for the large movements of adduction and extension, such as a swimming stroke or a tennis smash or a cricket bowl. By controlling the wrist and fingers, the SFAL participates with the DFAL in the grip (Video 4.8). Although the author is unfamiliar with avian anatomy in detail, in most birds the SFAL provides both the motive power of the wing beat, and the control of the 'ailerons' – the distal finger-like feathers. In a quadruped, the SFAL provides the forward motive power for the foreleg as well as control of the digits in those animals with 'hands'.

❖ ❖❖ *Stretch Assessment for the Superficial and Deep Front Arm Lines*

To feel or show the difference between the Superficial and Deep Front Arm Lines, lie supine near the edge of a treatment table or hard bed, and drop your arm, with the palm up and the shoulder abducted, off the edge. This is a stretch for the SFAL, and will be felt in the pectoralis major or somewhere along the SFAL track. Hyperextend the wrist and fingers to augment the stretch. To change the stretch to the DFAL, turn the thumb up, palm facing your feet, (medially rotating the shoulder to do it) and then stretch your thumb out along the other fingers, away from the shoulder as you let the arm drop off the table. You will feel the stretch track up the DFAL, all the way to the pectoralis minor.

Alternately, stand behind a model holding her wrists. Allow the model to lean forward from the ankles as if to begin a swan dive, with you counterbalancing the weight – assuring yourself and the model that you can easily hold her from falling forward. She is now both hanging from and leaning into both Front Arm Lines. Have the model laterally rotate the humeri (thumbs up), then take her wrists and have her lean forward, and report to you where the stretch is. She is likely to report feelings of stretch somewhere in the SFAL – from the pectoralis major on out through the hand flexors – and this can give you a good idea of where the tissues might be shortened or challenged (www.anatomytrains.com – video ref: Shoulders and Arm Lines, 17:20–17:52).

Then have the model medially rotate her humeri (thumbs down) and lean forward with you holding the wrists again. This time, the challenge is likely to come in some part of the DFAL – the pectoralis minor on out through the biceps and thumb, giving you some indication of where to work.

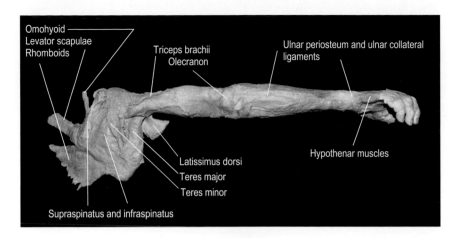

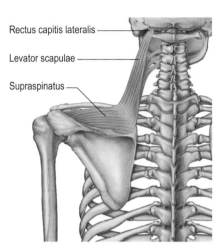

• **Fig. 7.18** The Deep Back Arm Line *in situ*, showing the connections from the rhomboids and scapula down to the little finger.

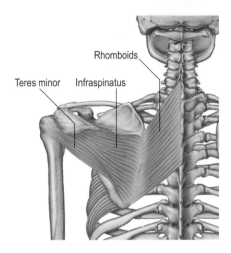

• **Fig. 7.19** The Deep Back Arm Line opens with the rhomboids, whose superficial layers of fascia pass across to the infraspinatus. This represents a switch, as we saw the rhomboids also connecting under the scapula to the serratus anterior in the Spiral Line (see Fig. 6.4, p. 96).

• **Fig. 7.20** An alternative branch line for the DBAL consists of the rectus capitis lateralis leading down onto the levator scapulae. Together, these two connect the head and neck to the supraspinatus over the apex of the scapula.

The qualification in these two statements comes from the abundance of crossover muscles that, in the variety of human arm usages, make blanket statements unwise.

The Deep Back Arm Line

The Deep Back Arm Line (DBAL) begins at the spinous processes of the upper thoracic and 7th cervical vertebrae, passing down and out with the rhomboid muscles to the vertebral border of the scapula (Fig. 7.18; www.anatomytrains.com – video ref: Shoulders and Arm Lines, 52:03–52:18; Video 2.8). The rhomboids are thus part of both the Spiral Line (Ch. 6) and the DBAL (Fig. 7.19 and www.anatomytrains.com – video ref: Shoulders and Arm Lines, 53:18–1:01:57). The fascial track splits here with a switch at the vertebral border: the Spiral Line continues deep to the scapula with the serratus anterior muscle (www.anatomytrains.com – video ref: Spiral Line, 16:00–20:28), while this DBAL continues around the scapula with the rotator cuff, specifically from the rhomboids to the infraspinatus, picking up the teres minor along the way (www.anatomytrains.com – video ref.: Shoulders

and Arm Lines, 1:04.21–1:08:10). These two muscles tack down to the next station on the posterior aspect of the humerus, on the greater tubercle, contiguous with the joint capsule.

Another branch line of the DBAL begins on the lateral lower surface of the occiput with the rectus capitis lateralis, continuing down with the levator scapulae from the posterior tubercles of the transverse processes of the first four cervical vertebrae (Fig. 7.20). The distal station of this line is the superior angle of the scapula, just above where the rhomboids join, but these fascial fibers link to the supraspinatus, which runs along the top of the scapula in the supraspinous fossa to the top of the ball of the humerus (www.anatomytrains.com – video ref: Shoulders and Arm Lines, 1:02:00–1:04:20). All three of these rotator cuff muscles go to the greater tubercle of the humerus.

The fourth of the rotator cuff set, the subscapularis covers the anterior surface of the scapula and goes to the lesser tubercle at the anterior aspect of the head of the humerus (Fig. 7.21; Video 6.18). The rhomboid myofascia pulls on both the subscapularis fascia and the infraspinatus fascia leaving the scapula as the thin slice of cucumber in the

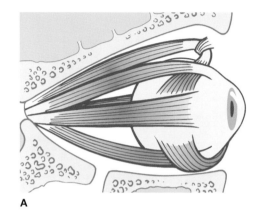

A
Subscapularis
Supraspinatus
Infraspinatus
Rhomboideus major and minor

B
Trapezius
Subscapularis
Supraspinatus
Infraspinatus
Teres minor
Teres major
Latissimus dorsi

• **Fig. 7.21** The second track of the DBAL is the entire rotator cuff complex that sandwiches the scapula, including the subscapularis (Video 6.18).

'scapular sandwich' made by the rotator cuff (Video 6.22). This whole complex of myofasciae surrounds the 'sesamoid' bone of the scapula. Subscapularis clearly plays a crucial role in the balance of the shoulder as part of the DBAL complex (www.anatomytrains.com – video ref: Shoulders and Arm Lines, 1:08:11–1:09:57).

These four muscles of the rotator cuff control the rounded head of the humerus in much the same way as the ocular muscles control the orbit of the eye (Fig. 7.22; Video 6.17). According to Frank Wilson, author of the delightful *The Hand*:[2]

> *The brain points the arm and finger as accurately as it points the eye. In the orbit and at the shoulder, the eye and the humerus are free to rotate (or swing) in front-to-back and side-to-side planes, and also around their long axes. And in both cases there is a precise arrangement of muscles aligned and attached to power each of these movements.*

From the shaft of the humerus near the ball where the rotator cuff attaches, and from the underside of the scapular glenum near the teres minor insertion, comes the longest of the three heads of the triceps brachii, the next track of this line (Fig. 7.23). In the hanging arm, similarly to the Deep Front Arm Line, the step from the rotator cuff to the triceps involves a radical change of direction, but with the shoulder abducted, as in a tennis backhand or the arm overhead, these two are fascially and mechanically linked. The triceps carries us down (including the anconeus along the way) to the tip of the elbow, the olecranon of the ulna (www.anatomytrains.com – video ref: Shoulders and Arm Lines, 1:09:58–1:11:16). We are stymied if we look for a muscular connection straight on from the point of the elbow, but not if we look for a fascial one: the periosteum of the ulna and adjacent layers pass down the entire length of the outside of the lower arm (www.anatomytrains.com – video ref: Shoulders and Arm Lines, 1:11:17–1:13:04). As with the DFAL, the DBAL is firmly fastened to the ulna for the distal half of the ulna, for the same reasons of stability discussed above.

When we reach the ulnar styloid process on the outside of the wrist, we can continue on the ligamentous capsule of the wrist, specifically the ulnar collateral ligament, outside

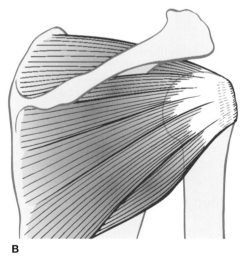

A

B

• **Fig. 7.22** There is an interesting muscular parallel between the control of the orb of the eye and the control of the rounded head of the humerus (Video 6.17).

the triquetral and hamate carpal bones and onto the periostea and ligaments that run up the little-finger side of the hand (see Fig. 7.23). The hypothenar muscles are part in this line (www.anatomytrains.com – video ref: Shoulders and Arm Lines, 1:13:04–1:13:48).

The DBAL, roughly equivalent to the Lateral Line in the leg, works with the DFAL to adjust the angle of the elbow, to limit or allow side-to-side movement of the upper body when in an all-fours position, and to provide stability from

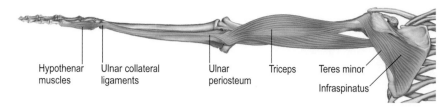

Hypothenar muscles | Ulnar collateral ligaments | Ulnar periosteum | Triceps | Teres minor | Infraspinatus

• **Fig. 7.23** The rotator cuff track of the DBAL connects to the triceps, with the proviso that the arm needs to be up at near horizontal or above for this connection to be active. The DBAL runs from the triceps attachment at the olecranon of the elbow down the periosteum of the ulna, across the outer edge of the wrist to the hypothenar muscles and the little finger. Compare to Fig. 7.18.

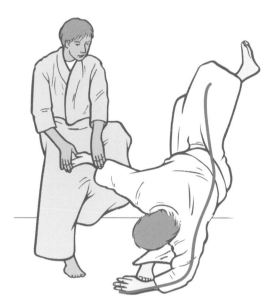

• **Fig. 7.24** A judo roll runs up the DBAL, from the outside of the little finger to the rotator cuff, before continuing on the Back Functional Line (see Ch. 8).

the outside of the hand to the back of the shoulder. This line is necessarily active in well-taught Pilates reformer work.

❖ A Judo Roll

An aikido or judo roll traces along the DBAL. It starts when the little-finger side of the hand makes contact with the mat, passing along the outside of the wrist, the shaft of the ulna, the triceps, and the back of the shoulder (Fig. 7.24). (A full roll will then continue along the Back Functional Line – see Chs 8 and 10.) It is important to keep this line strong, full, and round for a successful roll. Collapse anywhere along this line during a roll can lead to injury.

❀ The Superficial Back Arm Line

The Superficial Back Arm Line (SBAL) begins with the wide sweep of the trapezius's axial attachments, from the occipital ridge through the spinous process of T12. These fibers converge toward the spine of the scapula, the acromion of the scapula, and the lateral third of the clavicle (Fig. 7.25; www.anatomytrains.com – video ref: Shoulders and Arm Lines, 49:25–53:25; Video 6.2).

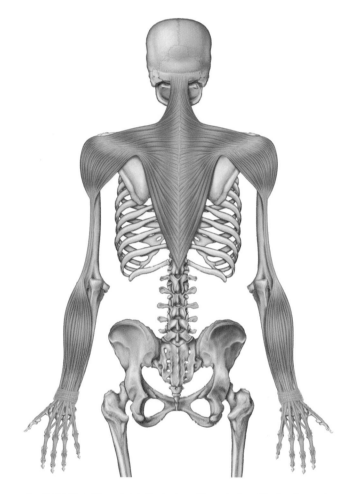

• **Fig. 7.25** The Superficial Back Arm Line starts with the trapezio-deltoid complex (Video 6.2).

In fact, the specific connections here are interesting: the thoracic fibers of the trapezius link roughly with the posterior fibers of the deltoid; the cervical fibers of trapezius link with the middle deltoid; and the occipital fibers of trapezius link to the anterior deltoid (Fig. 7.26; www.anatomytrains.com – video ref: Shoulders and Arm Lines, 53:27–54:55; Video 2.7). Draping Fig. 7.26 over a skeleton demonstrates that the SBAL sweeps from the back of the skull over the front of the shoulder and thence to the back of the arm, a situation that often causes confusion, tightness, and misuse across the anterior deltoid area and the underlying tissues if the shoulder is – and human shoulders often are – out of

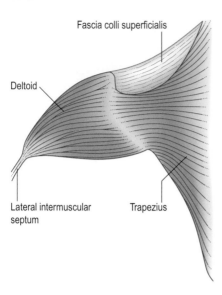

Fascia colli superficialis

Deltoid

Lateral intermuscular septum

Trapezius

• **Fig. 7.26** The trapezio-deltoid complex can be seen as one large triangular muscle that focuses down on the outside of the humerus from a broad attachment along the whole upper spine.

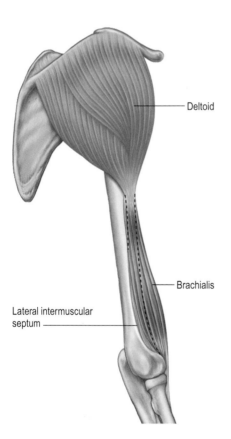

Deltoid

Brachialis

Lateral intermuscular septum

• **Fig. 7.27** The deltoid connects under the brachialis to the lateral intermuscular septum down to the lateral humeral epicondyle.

easy balance. Opening the anterior deltoid is an unexpected but essential component of easing forward head posture.

All these trapezio-deltoid lines converge onto the deltoid tubercle, where the fascial connection passes under part of the brachialis muscle to blend with the fibers of the lateral intermuscular septum (Fig. 7.27 and www.anatomytrains.com – video ref: Shoulders and Arm Lines, 54:56–55:53).

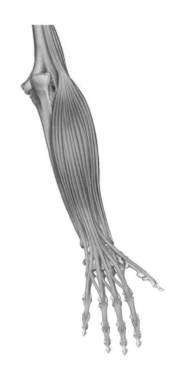

• **Fig. 7.28** From the lateral epicondyle, the common extensor tendon, along with the other deeper extensors, brings the SBAL down to the back of the hand.

The septum, which divides the flexors from the extensors (the 'front' and 'back' of the arm), passes down to its lower attachment at the lateral humeral epicondyle. From this station, the line continues directly onto the common extensor tendon, picking up the many longitudinal muscles that lie dorsal to the radius–ulna–interosseous membrane complex, passing under the dorsal retinacula to the carpals and fingers (Fig. 7.28 and www.anatomytrains.com – video ref: Shoulders and Arm Lines, 55:53–57:33).

The common extensor tendon, in addition to having a direct fascial connection to the intermuscular septum in the upper arm, arranges itself in a series of leaves or strips of fascia coming distally off the epicondyle, and the extensors, often shown as attached to the epicondyle, actually attach into these leaves, meaning that these muscles are incompletely separated at their proximal end by design. The superficial extensor muscles are suspended (as are all muscles, but these more than most) between their long tendons and their originating leaves.[3]

Similarly to the SFAL, the muscles show a reversal to the usual arrangement, with the superficial muscles controlling the carpals at the wrist, while the deep muscles reach all the way to the fingertips.

The SBAL is a single fascial unity from the spine to the backs of the fingers (Fig. 7.29A,B and www.anatomytrains.com – video ref: Shoulders and Arm Lines, 57:35–59:00). This line controls the arm for the limited amount of moving we do behind our lateral midlines, like a backhand tennis shot, or the obscured part of your child's magic trick. The SBAL also counterbalances the strong flexion tendency of the SFAL. The SBAL mostly controls the lifting (abduction)

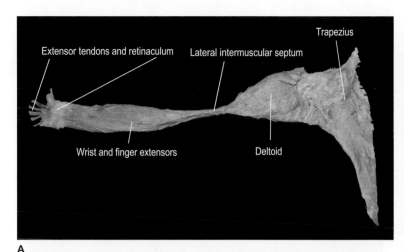

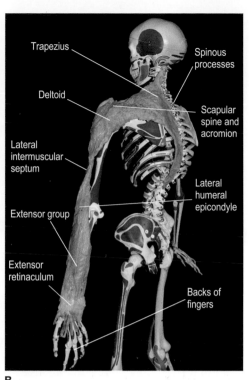

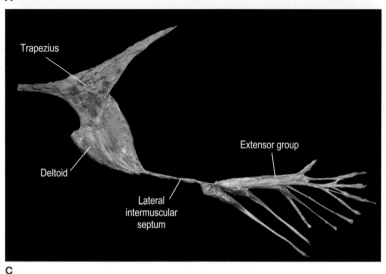

• **Fig. 7.29** The SBAL in dissection. In (**A**), the trapezius has been detached from the spinous processes and an unusually small attachment to the occiput (upper right). The fascial fabric connection over the scapular spine has been retained, as has the strong fascial connection from the deltoid to the lateral intermuscular septum, and finally the connection over the surface of the lateral epicondyle into the extensor group. The extensor retinaculum can be seen still covering these extensor tendons, which were cut shy of the fingers. In (**B**), this specimen has been laid over a classroom skeleton. (**C**) Untreated tissue dissection of the SBAL, showing the same clear connections, but with the forearm muscles separated out for clarity (www.anatomytrains.com – video ref: Anatomy Trains Revealed).

of the shoulder and arm, which can be held up in front of us for some time in daily activities, so it tends to get overworked and misused if the rib cage or spine collapses or slumps out from under the shoulder girdle (Video 3.13).

❖ ❖ Stretch Assessment for the Superficial and Deep Back Arm Lines

Face your client, take hold of her wrists, and have her lean back from the ankles into the 'sling' of her arms, while you support her weight. She is now hanging off and leaning into her two Back Arm Lines, as if water skiing. If you turn her wrists and arms in a lateral rotation (palms up), your client will generally feel the stretch (or restriction) in the SBAL, from the trapezius on out through the extensors. If you hold her wrists and arm in a moderately strong medial rotation (thumbs down), she will generally feel the stretch in the DBAL, through the rhomboids and rotator cuff and on out

that line (www.anatomytrains.com – video ref: Shoulders and Arm Lines, 17:53–18:27).

This exercise is full of 'generally' and 'probably' because of the number of crossover muscles within the arms (see Discussion 7.2, on crossovers, below). If a client does not feel the stretch in the areas suggested, it is worth noting where they do feel excessive stretch, as working to get more length in reported areas will – once again 'generally', because occupational or repetitive sport patterns can be very powerful in maintaining arm tensions – move the client toward the 'normal' pattern outlined above.

❦ Summary Overview 1 – the Bird's Wing

An easy and useful metaphor for understanding the four Arm Lines is to see them in relation to a bird's wing (Fig. 7.30). The Superficial Back Arm Line with the trapezius and

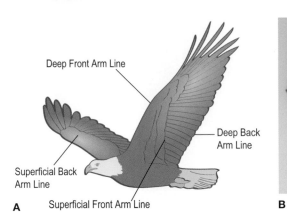
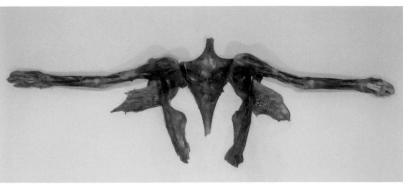

• **Fig. 7.30** (**A**) The Arm Lines can be compared to the four surfaces of a bird's wing. (**B**) The entire human 'wing' – the upper appendicular skeleton and all attendant muscles on both sides, hence all four arm lines – dissected off the axial 'fish body', seen in Ch. 5 as in Fig. 5.3 (Photo courtesy of the author.)

deltoid is the top of the wing – holding the wing out and lifting it when necessary – constantly active in isometric contraction while soaring, but pumping in concentric contraction when flapping. The Superficial Front Arm Line with the pectoralis major is the bottom of the wing – the motive power for flying, endurance-fiber 'dark meat' in ducks or geese, but phosphorus-rich, fast-twitch 'white meat' in the chicken or turkey, both of whom fly seldom, and then only for short frantic bursts.

The Deep Front Arm Line is the leading edge at the front of the wing, controlling the attitude – in our case, controlling the thumb's angle. Finally, the Deep Back Arm Line would be the trailing edge of the wing in a bird, giving the fine motor control to the 'ailerons' of the pin-feathers, or in our case, the fine adjustments of the little finger we use to good effect for precision in golf and racket sports.

🌸 Summary Overview 2 – Fascia/Muscle Alternation

Thus are the four arm lines arranged along the various aspects of the arm. In the shoulder, the lines are clearly arranged superficial and deep on the front and back of the rib cage, and it is from this cross-section that they derive their names (see Fig. 7.3).

In the upper arm, the four lines surround the humerus in a quadrant, the two superficial lines are represented fascially, and the two deep lines more muscularly (Fig. 7.31A).

In the lower arm and hand, the arrangement is still quadrate, but the expression is reversed: the two superficial lines include many muscles; the two deep lines are almost purely fascial (Fig. 7.31B). In the hand, the muscles of the two superficial lines become tendinous (although some intrinsic muscles of the hand could be included in our thinking here). The two deep lines include the thenar and hypothenar muscles covering the flexor retinaculum as indicated (Fig. 7.31C).

This alternation of predominant tissues is a metaphor that is too brittle to be pressed very hard, but is nonetheless useful to note. Both superficial lines, front and back, are muscular around the shoulder (traps, lats, pects, and delts), traded in for purely fascial septa in the upper arm, reverting to muscular flexors and extensors in the lower arm, and fascial tendons in the wrist and hand (www.anatomytrains.com – video ref: Shoulders and Arm Lines, 14:35–15:17).

Both Deep Arm Lines are more fascial than their superficial counterparts in the shoulder area (though with stabilizing muscles like the rotator cuff, levator scapulae, rhomboids, pectoralis minor, and subclavius). In the upper arm, these deep lines are highly muscular with the triceps and biceps. In the lower arm, these deep lines revert to fascial stability along the radius and ulnar bones, but in the hand they blossom into muscularity with the thenar and hypothenar muscles at the base of the hand.

This alternation generally corresponds to the alternation of joints in the arm between those of multiple degrees of freedom, like the shoulder and radio-ulnar joints, versus those with more limited, hinge-like motion, e.g. the elbow and wrists. Again, with the arm being designed for mobility over stability, this idea requires a host of qualifying adjectives and exceptions.

DISCUSSION 7.1

Scapular Position and Postural Balance

The mobility of the scapula (as compared with the more fixed hip bone) is crucial to the many services that our arms and hands provide. The clavicle has limited movement, and functions primarily to hold the arm away from the ribs in front (a uniquely primate need, since most quadrupeds prefer the shoulder joint close to the sternum under a proportionally narrower rib cage).

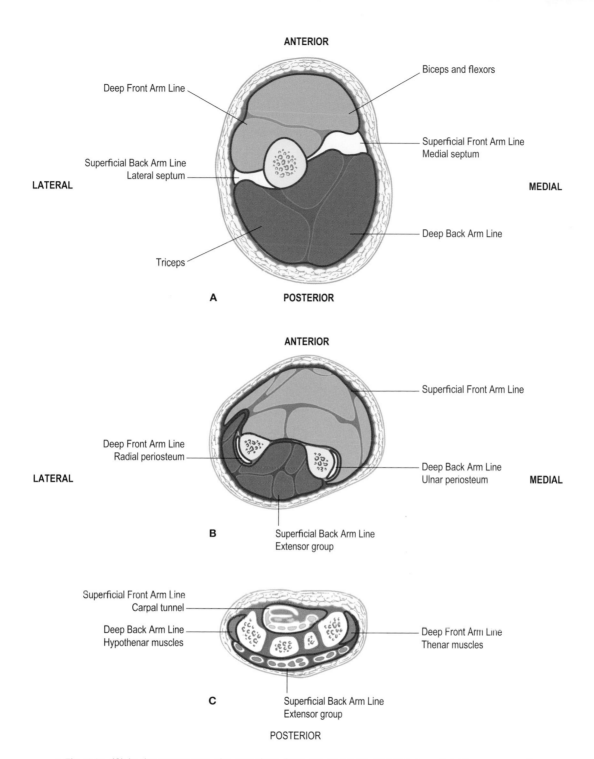

ANTERIOR

Deep Front Arm Line

Biceps and flexors

Superficial Front Arm Line
Medial septum

Superficial Back Arm Line
Lateral septum

LATERAL

MEDIAL

Deep Back Arm Line

Triceps

A   POSTERIOR

ANTERIOR

Superficial Front Arm Line

Deep Front Arm Line
Radial periosteum

Deep Back Arm Line
Ulnar periosteum

LATERAL

MEDIAL

B

Superficial Back Arm Line
Extensor group

Superficial Front Arm Line
Carpal tunnel

Deep Back Arm Line
Hypothenar muscles

Deep Front Arm Line
Thenar muscles

C

Superficial Back Arm Line
Extensor group

POSTERIOR

• **Fig. 7.31** (**A**) In the upper arm, the two deep lines are muscular and the superficial lines are purely fascial. (**B**) In the lower arm, the two superficial lines are heavily muscular, while the two deep lines are purely fascial. (**C**) In the hand, the deep lines have more muscular elements, and the superficial lines are almost purely tendinous.

While our clavicle is a fairly stable strut, our humerus, with its rounded head, maintains the widest range of possibilities. It is the scapula that must move the glenoid socket to keep the peace between the two and manage the arm's shifting positions while retaining some stability on the axial skeleton. Scapular stability is a tensegrity design problem, so soft-tissue balance is crucial. Finding the proper place for the scapula, a neutral position where it has the most possibility to move in response to our desires, is a worthy goal for manual and movement therapy.

Understanding the balance among the series of muscles that surround the roundhouse of the scapula will help us in this effort, especially concentrating on the scapular 'X'. Looking at the human scapula from behind, we see the array

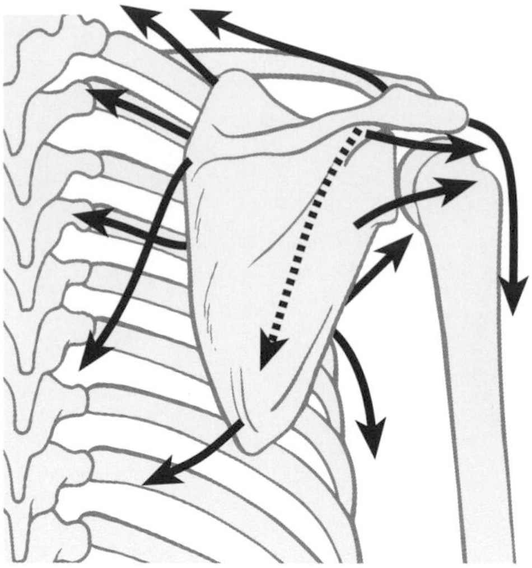

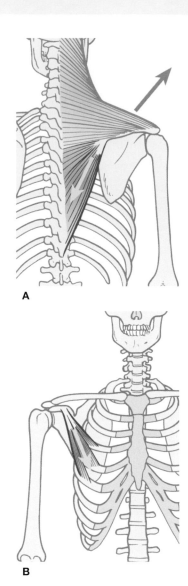

A

B

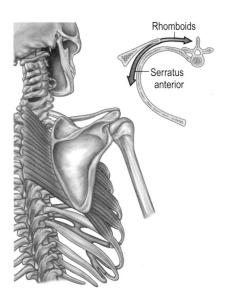

• **Fig. 7.32** The scapula is a roundhouse with many competing vectors of pull.

Rhomboids

Serratus anterior

• **Fig. 7.33** The reciprocal arrangement between the serratus anterior and the rhomboids gives them a crucial role in setting the postural position of the scapula along one leg of the scapular 'X'.

• **Fig. 7.34** The other leg of the scapular 'X' consists of a mechanical connection through the scapula between the lower part of the trapezius in the back and the pectoralis minor in the front (Video 4.6).

of vectors pulling it in nearly every direction (Fig. 7.32 or for a more detailed explanation: www.anatomytrains.com – video ref: Shoulders and Arm Lines, 06:22–12:59).

Of these, four stand out in providing scapular stability and determining postural scapular position, and these four form an 'X'. One leg of this 'X' is formed by the rhombo-serratus muscle, which we first saw in the Spiral Line (Ch. 6). While the rhomboids and the serratus anterior work together in the SPL, they work reciprocally as far as scapular position for the Arm Lines is concerned (Fig. 7.33). The serratus protracts the scapula inferiorly and laterally; the rhomboids retract it superiorly and medially. A chronically shortened ('locked short') serratus will pull the scapula wide on the posterior rib cage, causing the rhomboids to be

strained ('locked long'). This pattern frequently accompanies a kyphotic thoracic spine. When the rhomboids are locked short, which frequently accompanies a shallow thoracic curve (flat back), the serratus will be locked long, and the scapula will rest closer to the spinous processes than the angle of the ribs.

The other leg of the 'X' consists of the lower portion of the trapezius, which pulls medially and inferiorly on the spine of the scapula, and the pectoralis minor, which pulls down and in on the coracoid process, thereby pulling the scapula superiorly and laterally on the rib cage (Fig. 7.34). This antagonistic relationship most often appears with the pectoralis minor locked short and the lower trapezius locked long, resulting in an anterior tilt of the scapula on the ribs. Please note that this anterior tilt can often be disguised by a posterior tilt of the rib cage, leaving the appearance of a vertical scapula, but the underlying pattern remains the

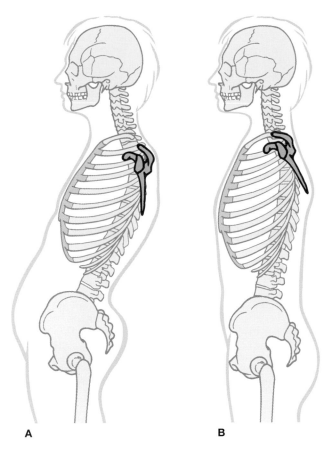

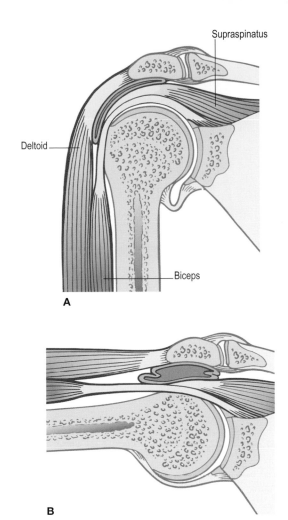

A

B

• **Fig. 7.35** The relative tilt of the scapula is better measured against the rib cage than the line of gravity. If the rib cage is posteriorly tilted (a common postural pattern in the modern world), the scapula may appear vertical to the floor but in fact be anteriorly tilted relative to the rib cage, involving a short pectoralis minor. Both (**A**) and (**B**) show an anteriorly tilted scapula relative to the rib cage; both need length in the pectoralis minor.

• **Fig. 7.36** There is a mechanical link between the supraspinatus and the long head of the biceps when the arm is abducted. This forges a crossover from the DBAL and the DFAL.

same, and lengthening work on the pectoralis minor is indicated for both Fig. 7.35A and B.

DISCUSSION 7.2

Crossovers

Though the lines we have described here are very logical, and certainly work usefully in practice, the extra rotational ability in the shoulder, lower arm, and hand requires a number of crossover 'switches' that muddle the neat precision of the Arm Lines, but provide additional possibilities for mobility and stability in movement (www.anatomytrains. com – video ref: Shoulders and Arm Lines, 15:18–15:38).

The two heads of the biceps brachii give us an instance of a crossover link between lines. So far, we have enunciated only the connection of the short head from the coracoid process to the radial tendon, which suited our purposes for the DFAL. The long head, however, passes through the intertubercular groove and onto the top of the glenum of the scapula, thus joining mechanically with the supraspinatus of the rotator cuff and on into the levator scapulae – or, in our language, connecting the DFAL to the DBAL (Fig. 7.36).

In addition to the two heads that give it its name, the biceps is also a biped with two 'feet', and this other foot provides another crossover. Aside from the radial tendon, the distal end of the biceps sports the odd bicipital aponeurosis weaving itself into the flexor group, thus linking the DFAL with the SFAL (Fig. 7.37). This structure, along with the oblique cord between the ulna and the radius, allows us to carry weight in the arms almost entirely through myofascial connection between the scapula and the fingers, without putting undue strain on the delicate elbow and radio-ulnar joints.

To expand this weight-carrying function, as it is yet another example of a crossover, when we carry an object like a suitcase by our sides, the weight is primarily carried by the fingers curled and held by the flexors of the SFAL (reinforced by the thumb gripped with the DFAL). This tensile weight is not carried to the medial epicondyle and on up the rest of the SFAL; however, it is intercepted by the

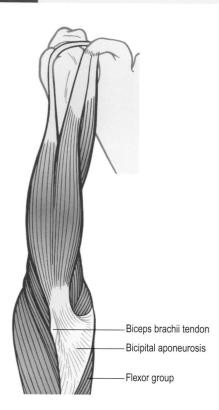

• **Fig. 7.37** The second tendon of the biceps brachii, which connects into the fascia of the forearm flexors, creates a link between the DFAL and SFAL.

bicipital aponeurosis and transferred to the biceps muscle, thus diverting strain from the vulnerable elbow and crossing over into the DFAL (Video 6.22). At the top of the short head of the biceps, the tension is transferred superiorly at the coracoid process to the coracoclavicular ligament and thus to the clavicle, where it is picked up by the clavicular portion of the trapezius (and thus transferred to the SBAL), which carries the tension to the occiput – a frequent site of headaches in those who venture out carrying a heavy object on one side (Fig. 7.38 and www.anatomytrains.com – video ref: Shoulders and Arm Lines, 15:39–16:05). (The need to counterbalance this pull on the other side can also lead to strain and pain in the opposite side of the neck or low back as well, especially for the unpracticed. Experienced carriers of asymmetrical loads, like mailmen, will have distributed the load, more or less successfully, over the whole structure.)

Releasing the upper structures of the DFAL is thus part of a strategy of relieving forward head posture or hyperextended upper cervicals, especially in those accustomed to carrying significant loads.

Other examples of crossovers include the distal attachment of the deltoid, which lies right up against the brachialis muscle. If we take this switch instead of the standard SBAL deltoid–lateral intermuscular septum connection, we have a link between the SBAL and the DFAL (Fig. 7.39).

The teres major muscle, which we included with the latissimus in the SFAL, is actually a crossover from the scapula (and thus the DBAL) into the SFAL, with its distal attachment on the anterior surface of the humerus (see Fig.

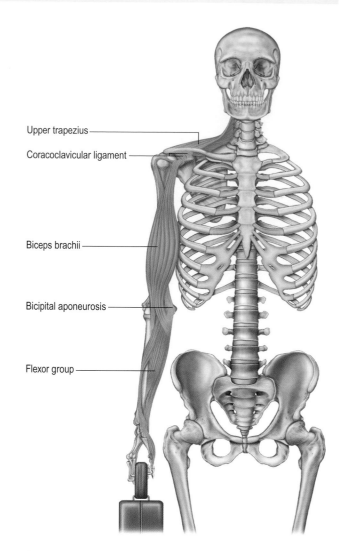

• **Fig. 7.38** When the arm is hanging, the myofascial continuity travels up from the hand to the short head of the biceps via the aponeurosis to the coracoclavicular ligament to the trapezius, terminating at the occiput.

7.14). Teres major has a distal attachment to the triceps as well as the humerus.

The brachioradialis arises from the lateral intermuscular septum and goes to the radius, thus making another connection from the SBAL to the DFAL (Fig. 7.40). The pronator teres could be said to make the same kind of connection from the DFAL to the SFAL.

Finally, the long pollicis muscles, abductor, and extensor longus and brevis, build from the periosteum of the ulna to the upper surface of the thumb, and could thus be said to connect the DBAL to the SBAL.

Other connections among the lines are made by the arms on a minute-by-minute basis to accommodate the varying movements and strains placed on the shoulder–arm complex – carrying a tray full of dishes, wielding a shovel, or attempting to put the hands together behind the back. These crossovers within the Arm Lines do not, however, alter the basic value of the connections we have detailed in the four formal longitudinal myofascial meridians.

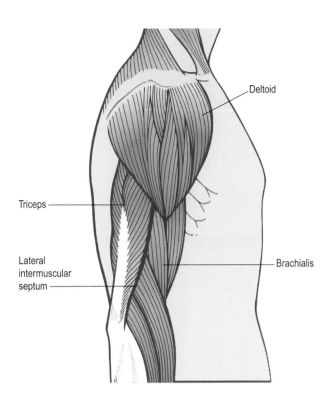

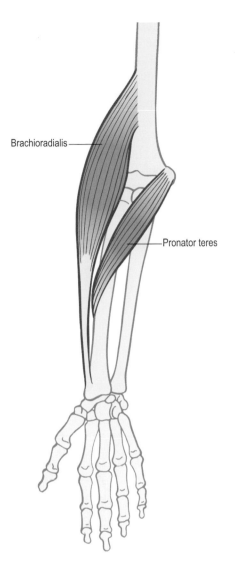

• **Fig. 7.39** The fascia of the deltoid is continuous with a portion of the brachialis, making a connection between the SBAL and the DFAL.

DISCUSSION 7.3

Arm and Leg Line Comparison

The alert reader will notice that the four arm lines bear some resemblance to four of the lines that course through the leg - the SBL, SFL, LL, and DFL. (A clinically useful correlate to the Spiral Line in the arm has not been found.) Although the leg and the arm are functionally different, the structural similarities beg for a comparison, and the results are quite astonishing.

The correspondence between the arm and the leg in the skeletal structure is unmistakable: both have a girdle arrangement close to the axial frame (hip bone and scapula), followed by a ball-and-socket joint, one bone in the upper limb, a hinge, two bones in the lower limb, three bones in the first tier of the outer limb, four bones in the second tier, and five digits with fourteen bones in toto.

Aside from the bony similarity (strange in itself when one considers that the arm and leg evolved at somewhat different times for different purposes), the muscles also display interesting correspondences, e.g. the hamstrings parallel the biceps, and the abductors have often been termed the 'deltoid of the hip'.[4]

In spite of these obvious correspondences, the tracks of the myofascial meridians fail spectacularly to provide direct parallels between arm and leg. On one level, the reason for this is developmental: all the limbs bud straight out from the side of the embryo, but in subsequent development, the

• **Fig. 7.40** The brachioradialis and pronator teres connect to the radial periosteum, creating crossover links from the SBAL and SFAL to the DBAL.

legs rotate medially on the trunk, while the shoulder rotates laterally. Thus when we adopt the fetal position, the elbows and knees tend to meet. You can demonstrate this for yourself by getting on your hands and the balls of your feet, and then bending both elbows and knees. The knees will go forward – maybe a little out or in, depending on your patterns, but primarily toward your arms. The elbows will bend in the opposite direction, toward the legs – again, maybe more outward, depending on your habit, but primarily toward your legs. Keep your hands on the floor and try to turn your elbows around so they look like knees to feel the impossibility of having your arms approach a parallel position to the legs.

On another level, the lack of correspondence is testimony to the malleability and plasticity of the fascial connections in the body. The parallels in the bones remain; the parallels in the muscles remain, but the longitudinal connections through the fascia have changed with the times.

The salamander's sidewards extensions of the spine have a different set of myofascial meridians from the loping forepaw and hind leg of the dog or the bear, which is again different from the unique upper limb of *Homo faber*.

Our own leg is quite similar to the quadruped hindlimb, with some allowances for the different attitude of the spine and hip, but the structure and function of mobility in the front and back lines, and stability in the inner and outer lines. The primate arm, however, went through some decisive changes, presumably during our ancestors' arboreal phase, which make its longitudinal connections unique. It is thus a useful exercise (though perhaps only for the anatomy nerds among us) to track the differences in each section of the two limbs.

Comparing the hand and foot first, we can see easy parallels side to side with the 'deep' lines, but the front and back are reversed (Fig. 7.41A). The Deep Front Arm Line connects on the inside to the thumb, as the Deep Front Line of the leg (yet to come, in Ch. 9) connects to the inner arch and big toe. The Deep Back Arm Line connects to the little finger as the Lateral Line connects to the outer arch and 5th metatarsal.

The Superficial Front Line of the leg, which involves toe and ankle extensors, corresponds easily to the Superficial

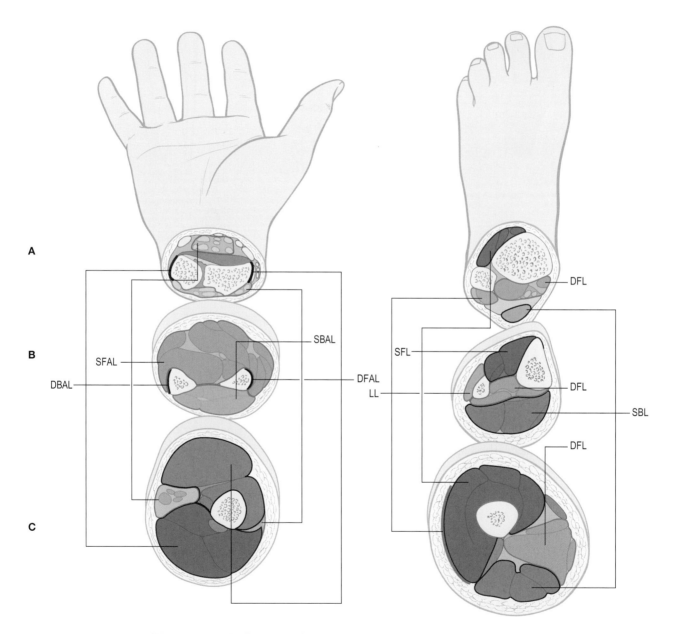

• **Fig. 7.41** (**A**) In the hand, the Deep Arm Lines correspond to the lateral and medial (Deep Front Line) lines of the foot, but the front and back lines are reversed. (**B**) In the lower arm, the reversal of the front and back lines continues, but the medial line goes to the 'fibula' of the arm, while the lateral line goes to the arm's 'tibia' – the ulna. (**C**) In the upper arm, the deep and superficial trade places – the quadriceps and hamstrings of the front and back lines of the leg (SFL and SBL) correspond to the deeper lines of the arm – the biceps of the DFAL and the triceps of the DBAL.

Back Arm Line, which contains finger and wrist extensors. The Superficial Back Line of the leg, flexing the toes and ankle, corresponds at this level to the Superficial Front Arm Line that curls the fingers.

In the lower arm, these parallels continue, with the exception that the Lateral Line in the leg connects via the peroneals to the fibula, while the Deep Back Arm Line connects to the tibia-equivalent ulna (Fig. 7.41B). In the leg, the Deep Front Line connects to the weight-bearing tibia, while the Deep Front Arm Line is tied inextricably to the more mobile radius. We can also note that in the lower leg, only the gastrocnemius, popliteus, and plantaris cross the knee; the rest of the foot-moving muscles are confined to the lower leg, whereas many of the muscles of both the SFAL and SBAL cross the elbow, though they are not designed to affect elbow movement very much.

By the time we get to the upper arm and upper leg, most of the parallels are spiraling out of control (Fig. 7.41C). We find that at this level, the Superficial Front Line of the leg (primarily the quadriceps) compares now with the Deep Back Arm Line (triceps). The Superficial Back Line (biceps femoris and the other hamstrings) now equates with the Deep Front Arm Line (biceps brachii and its underlying compadres). The Lateral Line of the leg (iliotibial tract) now parallels the Superficial Back Arm Line (lateral intermuscular septum), and the Deep Front Line (adductor muscles and associated septa) compares fairly easily to the Superficial Front Arm Line (medial intermuscular septum).

At the shoulder-to-hip level, the comparisons dim even more, but the Lateral Line (abductors) clearly continues the comparison to the Superficial Back Arm Line (deltoid). The Deep Front Line of the leg – the psoas and other flexors – might be compared with, strangely, the Superficial Front Arm Line, in that the pectoralis major and latissimus dorsi, like the psoas, both reach from the axial skeleton out across the ball and socket to the proximal limb bone, though under greater scrutiny the parallels begin to fade.

The Deep Back Arm Line (rhomboids to rotator cuff) can be usefully compared with the quadratus lumborum to iliacus connection – the iliacus paralleling the subscapularis, leaving the gluteus minimus as the infraspinatus of the leg. However, another argument can be made that the rotator cuff is similar to the deep lateral rotators of the leg (technically part of the Deep Front Line, and practically part of a non-existent 'Deep Back Line').

The Deep Front Arm Line (biceps–pectoralis minor) might bear comparison to the Superficial Back Line of the leg (biceps femoris–sacrotuberous ligament), though it also has elements of the Deep Front Line (proximity to the neurovascular bundle, and the clear parallel between adductor magnus and coracobrachialis).

The long and twisting road of evolution and the literal twisting of the arm and leg that takes place during fetal development have both served to blur easy one-to-one comparisons among the arm and leg lines, as differing kinetic connections have been made in each. That said, the Lateral Line corresponds to the Superficial Back Arm Line above the elbow, and the Deep Back Arm Line below. The Deep Front Line compares to a combination of the Deep and Superficial Front Arm Lines above the elbow, and the Deep Front Arm Line below. The Superficial Front Line compares to the Deep Back Arm Line above the elbow, and to the Superficial Back Arm Line below. The Superficial Back Line compares to the Deep Front Arm Line above the elbow, and the Superficial Front Arm Line below.

Given the similarities of skeletal and muscular structure, the differences created by the variation in longitudinal fascial connections are quite striking. And strikingly complex – congratulations to any reader who actually made it through this morass to the end of this chapter. In the following chapter, we turn our attention to the vastly simpler extensions of the Arm Lines across the trunk.

References

1. Myers T. Treatment approaches for three shoulder 'tethers'. *J Bodyw Mov Ther.* 2007;11(1):3–8.
2. Wilson FR. *The Hand.* New York: Vintage Books/Pantheon Books; 1998.
3. Van der Wal J. Architecture of the connective tissue in the musculoskeletal system. *Int J Ther Massage Bodywork.* 2009;2(4): 9–23.
4. Myers T. *Hanging around the shoulder.* Massage Magazine 2000 (April–May). *Also available in* Body³, *self-published in 2004 and available via* www.anatomytrains.com.

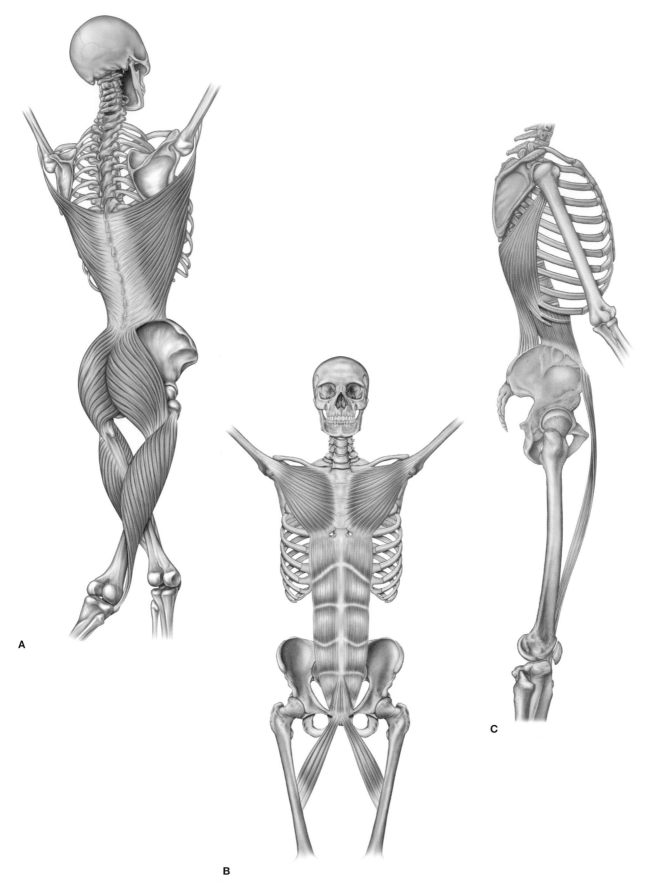

• **Fig. 8.1** The Back, Front, and Ipsilateral Functional Lines.

8

The Functional Lines

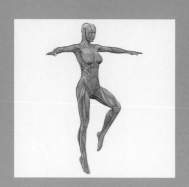

The Functional Lines (Fig. 8.1) extend the Arm Lines across the surface of the trunk to the contralateral pelvis and leg (or up from the leg to the pelvis across to the opposite rib cage, shoulder, and arm, since our meridians transfer force in either direction). One of these lines runs across the front of the body, one across the back, so that the right and left lines together form an 'X' across the torso (Fig. 8.2/Table 8.1). A third line in this group, the Ipsilateral Functional Line, runs from the shoulder to the inside of the same knee. These lines are called the 'functional' lines to emphasize that they are rarely employed, as the other lines are, in modulating standing posture. They immediately come into play during athletic or other activity where one appendicular complex is stabilized, counterbalanced, or powered by its contralateral complement. An example is in a javelin throw or a baseball pitch, where the player powers up through the left leg and hip to impart extra speed to an object thrown from the right hand (Fig. 8.3).

Postural Function

The Functional Lines form stabilizing 'X's, crossing at the pubic symphysis in the front and across the sacrolumbar junction in the back. As mentioned, these lines are less involved in compensating standing posture than others under discussion in this book. For the most part, they involve superficial tissues that are so much in use during day-to-day activities that their opportunity to stiffen or fascially shorten to maintain posture is minimal. If they do distort posture as a whole, their action is to bring one shoulder closer to its opposite hip, either across the front or across the back. Though that pattern is common – especially closing across the front – the myofascial source for it usually resides in the Spiral Line or in deeper layers described in Ch. 9 (or in the cranial or visceral fasciae). Once these other myofascial structures have been balanced, these Functional Lines generally accept the new pattern without requiring further work.

These lines do, however, have strong postural stabilizing functions in positions outside the resting standing posture. In almost all loaded lifts, or yoga inversions that require stabilizing the upper girdle to the trunk (or, vocationally, those electricians and painters who often work above their head), these lines distribute strain downward or provide the stability upward to fix the base of support – from pelvis to ribs to shoulders – for the upper limb.

Less frequently, they can be used to provide stability or counterbalance for the work of the lower limb in a similar way, as in a football kick.

There is one common postural compensation pattern associated with the Functional Lines and that is a preference rotation usually associated with handedness or a specific asymmetrical activity such as a sport, where one shoulder draws closer to the opposite hip repetitively. This can affect the tonus and coordination of all six Functional Lines, but, again, the Spiral, Lateral, or Deep Front Lines are usually more salient to the pattern shift.

Movement Function

These lines enable us to give extra power and precision to the movements of the limbs by lengthening their lever arm through linking them across the body to the opposite limb in the other girdle (Video 3.16). Thus the weight of the arms can be employed in giving additional momentum to a kick, and the movement of the pelvis contributes to a tennis backhand. While many applications to sport spring to mind when considering these lines, the mundane but essential example is the contralateral counterbalance between shoulder and hip in every walking step.

The Functional Lines appear as spirals on the body, and always work in helical patterns. They could be considered as appendicular supplements to the Spiral Line, or, as stated, the trunk extensions of the Arm Lines. In real-time activity, the lines of pull change constantly, and the precision of the lines detailed below is a summary of a central moment in the sweep of forces (see Discussion 8.1).

137

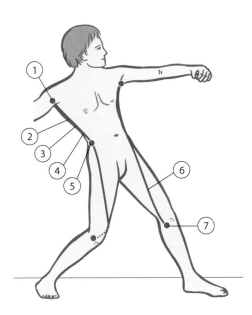

• **Fig. 8.2** Functional Lines, tracks and stations.

TABLE 8.1	Functional Lines: Myofascial 'Tracks' and Bony 'Stations' (Fig. 8.2)	
Bony Stations		**Myofascial Tracks**
Back Functional Line		
Shaft of humerus	**1**	
	2	Latissimus dorsi
	3	Lumbodorsal fascia
	4	Sacral fascia
Sacrum	**5**	
	6	Gluteus maximus
Shaft of femur	**7**	
	8	Vastus lateralis
Patella	**9**	
	10	Subpatellar tendon
Tuberosity of tibia	**11**	
Front Functional Line		
Shaft of humerus	**1**	
	2	Lower edge of pectoralis major
5th rib and 6th rib cartilage	**3**	
	4	Lateral sheath of rectus abdominis, semilunar line
Pubic tubercle and symphysis	**5**	
	6	Adductor longus
Linea aspera of femur	**7**	
Ipsilateral Functional Line		
Shaft of humerus	**1**	
	2	Latissimus dorsi, anterior edge
End of ribs 10–12	**3**	
	4	External oblique
Anterior superior iliac spine	**5**	
	6	Sartorius, pes anserinus
Medial tibial condyle	**7**	

The Functional Lines in Detail

The Back Functional Line

The Back Functional Line (BFL) begins (for analytic purposes; in practice it connects in with the Superficial Front or Deep Back Arm Lines, depending on the particular action) with the distal attachment of the latissimus dorsi (see Fig. 8.1A; Video 2.10). It runs down a little inferior to the approximate center of that muscle's spread, its aponeurotic attachment comprising the superficial laminae of the thoracolumbar fascia.

The BFL crosses the midline approximately at the level of the sacrolumbar junction, passing through the sacral fascia to connect with the lower (sacral and sacrotuberal) fibers of the gluteus maximus on the opposite side.

The lower fibers of gluteus maximus pass deep to the posterior edge of the iliotibial tract (ITT), and thus under the Lateral Line, attaching to the posterolateral edge of the femur, about one-third of the way down the femoral shaft. If we continue on in the same direction, we find fascial fibers linking the gluteus at the top of the linea aspera to the beginning of the vastus lateralis muscle, which in turn

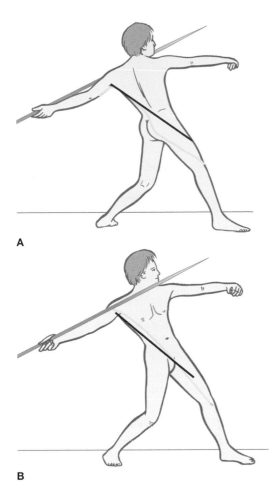

A

B

• **Fig. 8.3** The Functional Lines add the impetus of the trunk momentum, fascial elasticity, and muscle power to the strength of the limbs, stabilized around the axis of the contralateral girdle. In this instance, as the arm is drawn back to throw the javelin, the right Back Functional Line is contracted or at minimum passively shortened, while the right Front Functional Line is stretched and readied for contraction. The left FFL is lightly shortened as the non-dominant shoulder approaches the contralateral hip. The left BFL is correspondingly lightly stretched during this maneuver. When the javelin is thrown, all these conditions reverse – the right FFL contracts, the right BFL is stretched, and their left-side complements exchange stabilizing roles.

links us down through the quadriceps tendon to the patella, and via the subpatellar tendon to the tibial tuberosity. We end the line here (though, having reached the tibial tuberosity, we could continue this line down to the medial arch by means of the tibialis anterior and the anterior crural fascia as discussed in Ch. 4 on the SFL).

Fascially, another 'attachment' of the gluteus runs down the lateral intermuscular septum between the biceps femoris hamstring and the vastus lateralis muscle. This septum joins the iliotibial tract at the surface, but attaches to the linea aspera along the femur. Its lowest attachments are to the lateral tibial condyle and fibular head. The twisting motions of the heavy upper body (which could be augmented by a racquet or kettlebell) are anchored, via this line, to the spine, pelvis, femur, and even down into the lower leg – all to provide a good foundation and to distribute the strain over many accommodating structures.

The Front Functional Line

The Front Functional Line (FFL) begins at about the same place as its complement, with the distal attachment of the pectoralis major on the inner humerus, passing along the lowest fibers of that muscle to their origin on the 5th and 6th ribs (Fig. 8.1B; Video 2.9). Since the clavipectoral fascia containing the pectoralis minor also connects to the 5th rib, the FFL could be said to be an extension of both the Superficial and Deep Front Arm Lines.

These pectoral fibers form a fascial continuity with the abdominal aponeurosis that links to the external oblique and rectus abdominis muscles, and the line passes essentially along the outer edge of the rectus or inner edge of the oblique fascia to the pubis, a strip of fascia known as the semilunar line. Passing through the pubic bone and fibrocartilage of the pubic symphysis, we emerge on the other side with the substantial tendon of the adductor longus – the round tendon easily felt and seen in the groin – which passes down, out, and back to attach to the medial aspect of the linea aspera on the posterior side of the femur.

From the linea aspera we can imagine a link to the short head of the biceps, and thus to the lateral crural compartment and the peroneals/fibularii (Spiral Line, Ch. 6, p. 101). This, however, would involve passing through the intervening sheet of the adductor magnus, which is not allowed by the Anatomy Trains rules. We will therefore end the FFL at the end of the adductor longus on the femur (see Fig. 2.6).

The Ipsilateral Functional Line

The Ipsilateral Functional Line (IFL) follows the most lateral fibers of that most lateral muscle, latissimus dorsi which attaches to the outer portion of the lower three ribs (Fig. 8.4; Video 4.9), with a strong fascial fabric connection to the posterior fibers of the external oblique, the same fibers employed in the Lateral Line in Chapter 5. If we follow the external oblique we arrive at the anterior iliac crest, where fibers connect fascially over the ASIS to the sartorius muscle. The sartorius takes us down to the pes anserinus, on the medial epicondyle of the tibia.

This line can be felt when supporting the body in an open chain via the latissimus – as on the rings, or a circus performer aloft on silks, or in swimming when pulling the hand down through the water in a crawl stroke. Hanging from a chinning bar or a tree branch and twisting the pelvis and legs will also bring this line into your awareness.

❖ ❖ Palpating the Functional Lines

For both the Front and Back Functional Lines, we begin in almost the same place: in the armpit, on the underside of the humerus, where the tendons of the pectoralis and the latissimus come together. With your model standing with his arm straight out to the side, pressing down on your shoulder, it is easy for you to trace both these tendons from

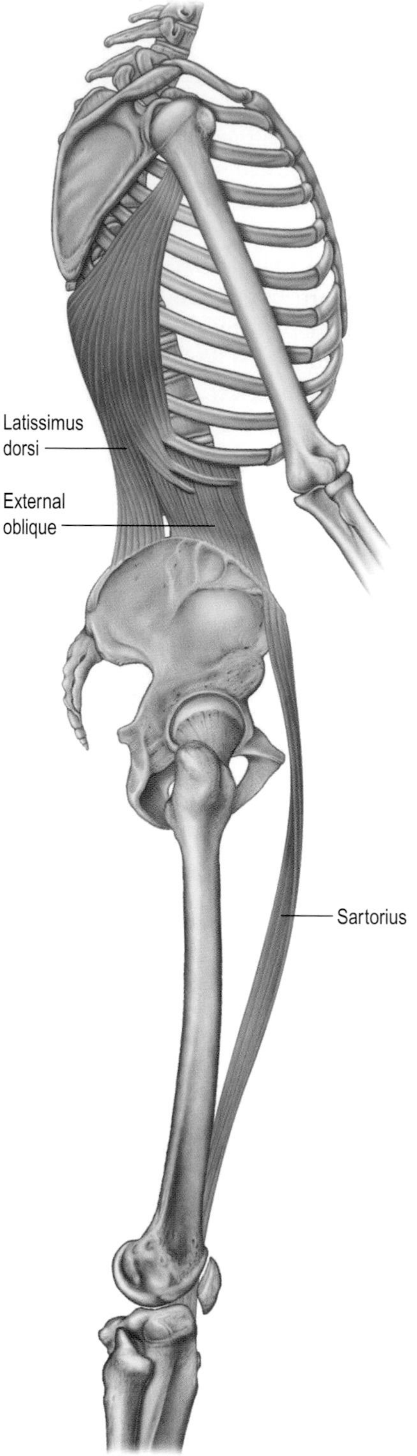

Latissimus
dorsi

External
oblique

Sartorius

• **Fig. 8.4** The Ipsilateral Functional Line is a third stabilizing line, tracing the most lateral fibers of the latissimus dorsi to the lower outer ribs, thence onto the posterior external oblique over the ASIS onto the sartorius to the tibial condyle in the inside of the knee (Video 4.1, Video 3.15). This line is used in stabilizing an athlete on the rings, and to stabilize the torso during the pull down of the crawl stroke in swimming.

either side of the armpit up onto the antero-inferior aspect of the humerus.

Taking the BFL first, we can trace it from this attachment across the lower third of the latissimus directly to the midline at about the sacrolumbar junction. Have your model press an elbow down against resistance to feel this lateral part of the latissimus, though the line itself runs a bit medially from the lateral edge (www.anatomytrains.com – video ref: Functional Lines, 19:19–22:39). The main sheet of the muscles runs around and down the back into the lumbodorsal fascia (www.anatomytrains.com – video ref: Functional Lines, 22:40–26:03). The sacral fascia comprises many layers; the BFL passes through the most superficial layers, which may not be separately discernible (www.anatomytrains.com – video ref: Functional Lines, 26:04–29:45). If you stand behind your model with one hand on the sacrum while the model pushes back into your other hand with his lifted elbow, you will feel the sacral fascia tighten to stabilize.

Across the sacrum, we pick up the line with the lower edge of the gluteus maximus where it is attached to the sacrum just above the tailbone (www.anatomytrains.com – video ref: Functional Lines, 29:45–35:18). The BFL includes the lower 5 centimeters/2 inches or so of this muscle. Track this section of the muscle below the gluteal fold (which is not muscular but lies in the superficial fascial layer) down to the next station, the readily discernible lump of connective tissue where the gluteus attaches to the back of the femoral shaft about one-third of the way between the greater trochanter and the knee.

From here, the vastus lateralis can be felt as the muscular part of the lateral aspect of the thigh, diving under the iliotibial tract of the Lateral Line, joining with the rest of the quadriceps at the patella to link through the subpatellar tendon to the tibial tuberosity, clearly palpable at the front-top of the tibial shaft.

The FFL is easier to palpate on oneself. Follow the lower edge of the pectoralis major, which forms the front wall of the armpit, down and in to where it ties into the ribs (www.anatomytrains.com – video ref: Functional Lines, 04:58–8:15). The underlying pectoralis minor could be seen to connect into this line as well at the 5th rib (www.anatomytrains.com – video ref: Functional Lines, 08:16–12:24). The next track runs down along the outer edge of the rectus abdominis, which can be felt in most people by actively tightening the rectus and feeling for its edge (www.anatomytrains.com – video ref: Functional Lines, 12:25–15:50). Follow these semilunar lines, a sealed seam of several abdominal layers, down as they narrow down to the outer-upper edge of the pubic symphysis.

The tiny pyramidalis muscle, if present, runs obliquely up from the pubic bone and can thus be included as part of this line. The line crosses through the pubis (which may be a bit of a touchy palpation for some clients) but re-emerges in the tendon of the adductor longus on the opposite side (www.anatomytrains.com – video ref: Functional Lines, 15:51–18:58). This tendon is readily palpable and usually visible when one sits cross-legged in a bathing suit or underwear. Follow this tendon distally into the thigh and you can approach, but usually not reach, the final station where it inserts into the linea aspera on the posterior side of the femur, about halfway down the thigh. Although this is the anatomical end of the muscle according to anatomy atlases the world over, the functional fascial attachment clearly links down to the medial femoral epicondyle, readily palpable a few centimeters above the medial knee. Palpate this bone from above while your model stands and turns strongly away from you and towards you to convince yourself that the functional base for *all* the adductors is this large tendinous attachment above the knee.

DISCUSSION 8.1

❖ Forces in Motion

Our description of these lines required several approximations, not only because of individual differences but also because forces along these lines often sweep across fans of muscle and sheets of fascia. In other words, bringing back a javelin for a throw will pass through the precise BFL only for an instant as the force sweeps from the lateral outer edge of the latissimus around to its upper inner edge. Hurling the javelin a second later will likewise occasion a sweep of force across the fans of the FFL in the pectoralii, abdominal obliques, and inner thigh muscles (see Fig. 8.3).

Let us illustrate the versatility of these lines with a tennis volley. The serve involves a sharp pull directly along the FFL involving principally the pectoralis major, but perhaps also the pectoralis minor in a connection to the abdominal muscles, whose sharp contraction adds to the force and the expulsion of air and sound that often accompanies the serve, and finally the adductor longus or its neighbors who act to keep the abdominals from pulling the pubic bone up (Fig. 8.5).

The return shot a moment later might be a straight forehand shot, with the arm out relatively horizontally from the shoulder. In this case the linkage would go up the Superficial Front Arm Line from the palm that holds the racquet, to pass from one pectoralis across the chest to the pectoralis and Superficial Front Arm Line on the opposite side (Fig. 8.6). This connection can be felt across the chest in such a shot, or observed in the movement of the opposite arm forward to help stabilize the working shoulder and impart additional momentum to the ball.

The backhand required a moment later could pass across from one latissimus to the other along their upper edges (Fig. 8.7). A forehand to the opposite corner might be

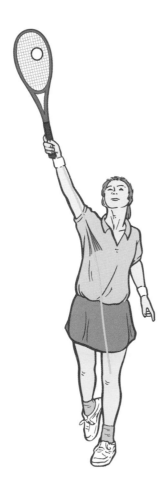

• **Fig. 8.5** The Front Functional Line in a tennis serve. The stronger and more vertical the serve, the more the Superficial Front Line will also participate in driving the ball.

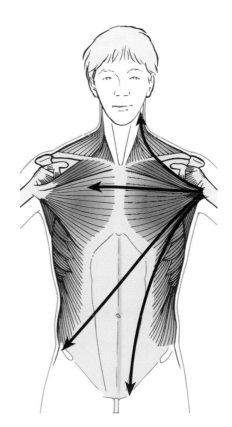

• **Fig. 8.6** A tennis forehand connects the Superficial Front Arm Line to its partner directly on the opposite side – one of several angles that the arms can transmit force to the front of the torso.

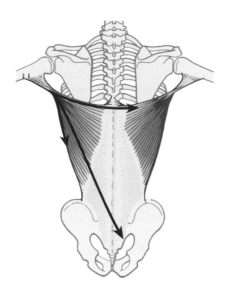

• **Fig. 8.7** A backhand shot could similarly join the latissimus to its opposite partner as well as down the torso to the pelvis and beyond.

carried across the body, essentially on the Spiral Line, to the opposite anterior spine of the hip. Alternatively, Fig. 8.8 shows another route crossing over from the Spiral Line to the FFL. A high backhand to return a lob might require the entire latissimus. The rest of the volley might go diagonally down and across as we have detailed with the BFL, or straight down the Superficial Front Line for a point-winning slam right at the net.

For another example, imagine a vaulter levering off the pole: the force flickers across the entire triangular field of the pectoralis or the latissimus, linking and anchoring to various tracks and stations in all three of these lines from second to second. In this example, the stability–mobility equation is reversed, with the shoulder stabilizing the body on the pole, and the hips and legs imparting momentum over the bar. If we add the deltoid–trapezius connection from the Superficial Back Arm Line to the latissimus–pectoralis ring of attachments, we see an entire circle of stabilization around the shoulder joint, any piece or all of

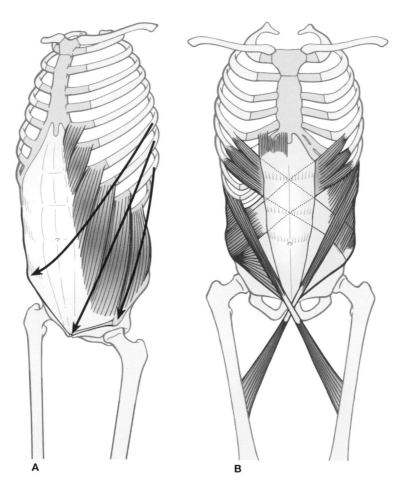

A   **B**

• **Fig. 8.8** Consider the sheet of the external oblique (**A**), whose upper fibers all start from the ribs, but with a sweep lower attachments. The lateral fibers go to the ipsilateral hip bone (part of the Lateral Line as well as the Ipsilateral Functional Line), the middle fibers go to the pubic bone (and on into the adductors on the opposite side), essentially a branch of the Functional Line as shown in (**B**), while the upper fibers cross via the contralateral internal oblique to attach to the opposite hip bone (Spiral Line). Thus two Functional Lines, the Spiral Line, and the torso portion of the Lateral Line all lay claim to part of the external oblique. All these could be grouped as the 'helical' lines, as opposed to the Superficial Front and Back Lines, and the Lateral Line taken as a whole, which constitute the 'cardinal' lines.

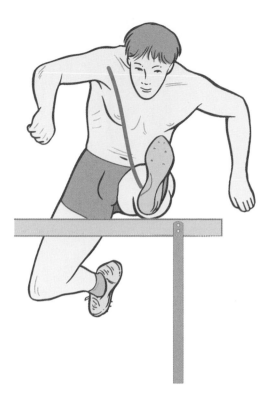

• **Fig. 8.9** The forces going through the hurdler's body cross the Front Functional Line only at one moment during the leap, but a connection between the forward leg and the opposite shoulder is maintained throughout the movement.

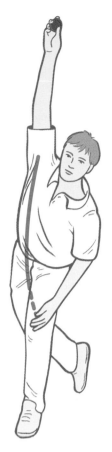

• **Fig. 8.10** The cricket bowler uses the Front Functional Line to add impetus to the power of the arm. See Ch. 10 for further discussion of the Anatomy Trains in movement.

which may be called upon during the vault (see Fig. 7.13, p. 120).

The lower end of these Functional Lines works in the same way. In a hurdler, the forces approaching the roundhouse of the pubic bone from above sweep around the fan of abdominal muscle, and from below along the fan of adductors.[1]

Depending on his relation to the hurdles, and how much he abducts his leg to go over them, the line of pull from pubis to leg might travel on the pectineus, or any of the adductors, more than likely sweeping through all or most of them during each leap. In this case, the anteriority of the opposite shoulder works through this line to give added impetus to the leading leg (Fig. 8.9).

From this, we hope the reader grasps the idea that while the Functional Lines present the idealized line, the actuality of moment-to-moment movement flickers across the body from motor unit to motor unit on a multiplicity of connections combining the Functional, Spiral, and Lateral Lines.

❖ Engaging the Lines

Pitching a baseball or bowling at cricket are perfect ways to engage these lines: the wind-up involves a shortening of the BFL and a stretching of the FFL on the dominant side, while the pitch itself reverses that process, shortening the FFL and stretching the BFL (Fig. 8.10) – and the same for the javelin thrower in Fig. 8.3. In the final act, the BFL acts as a brake to keep the strong contraction along the FFL and the momentum of the arm from going too far and damaging joints involved in the movement. Baseball pitchers frequently turn up with damage to the rotator cuff tendons, particularly the supraspinatus and infraspinatus, or SLAP (superior labrum from anterior to posterior) tears to the joint labrum. While remedial work on these muscles or their antagonists may be helpful, long-term relief depends on reinforcing the strength and precise timing of the BFL in acting as a whole-body brake to the forward motion of throwing, rather than asking the small muscles of the shoulder joint to bear the entire burden. Such injuries may be preventable with increased training for medial rotation of the non-dominant hip.[2]

While precise and individual coaching is required to effect coordination changes, the foundation can be laid by teaching the client to engage the line as a whole. Have the client lie prone on the floor or treatment table. Have them lift one arm and the opposite leg at the same time – this will engage the BFL. Most clients, however, will engage the muscles to lift one limb slightly before the other. Laying your hand gently on the humerus and opposite femur in question will allow you to feel with great precision which set of muscles is being engaged first (www.anatomytrains.com

– video ref: Functional Lines, 35:20–40:09). Use verbal or manual cues to elicit a coordinated contraction. Once the coordination is achieved, you can build strength by applying equal pressure to both your hands so that the client works against that resistance. Be sure to strengthen both the dominant and non-dominant side for best results.

The FFL can be similarly engaged as a whole with the client supine by using your hands on their upraised arms and thighs to help them coordinate the engagement of the contralateral girdles (www.anatomytrains.com – video ref: Functional Lines, 43:44–48:17).

Both the Triangle and Reverse Triangle pose of yoga stretch the BFL on the side of the hand reaching for the ground (see Fig. 6.22, p. 105 and www.anatomytrains.com – video ref: Functional Lines, 40:10–43:41). The FFL can be easily stretched from a kneeling position by reaching up and back with a slight rotation toward the reaching arm (www.anatomytrains.com – video ref: Functional Lines, 48:18–50:36 and Fig. 1.24).

The act of paddling a kayak or paddleboard engages the stabilizing element of these two lines (Fig. 8.11). The paddling arm connects from the Deep Back Arm Line, pulling from the little-finger side through to the BFL, and thus stabilized to the opposite leg. The upper arm pushes through the Deep Front Arm Line to the thumb, stabilizing via the FFL to the opposite thigh. If the knee is not fixed against the hull of the kayak, the push will be felt passing from foot to foot, almost in imitation of a walking movement (Video 6.4).

Movement and strain pass easily and evenly along these lines (www.anatomytrains.com – video ref: Functional Lines, 50:38–1:04:54). Excess strain or immobility at any track or station along the line could lead to a progressive 'pile-up' elsewhere on the line that could lead to problems

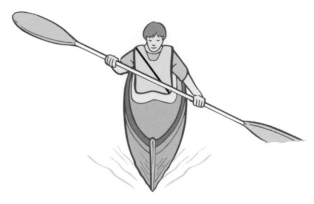

• **Fig. 8.11** The kayaker uses the opposite hip to stabilize his paddling – the lowered pulling arm via the BFL, and the lifted pushing arm via the FFL.

over time. We have found it useful to accompany a sports enthusiast on an outing, whether it be for a run, a climb, a scull, or a practice, to determine where along these and other lines there may be some 'silent' restriction that is creating 'noisy' problems elsewhere. The client who is made aware of these lines and the desire for easy flow along them can sometimes do self-assessment when engaged in the sport. In practice, the limitations become especially evident when the client is tired or at the end of a long stint.

References

1. Myers T. Fans of the hip joint. *Massage Magazine No. 75*; 1998. Also available in Body[3], *self-published in 2003 and available via: www.anatomytrains.com.*
2. Wolf Chuck. *Insights Into Functional Training.* Aptos, California: On Target Publications; 2017.

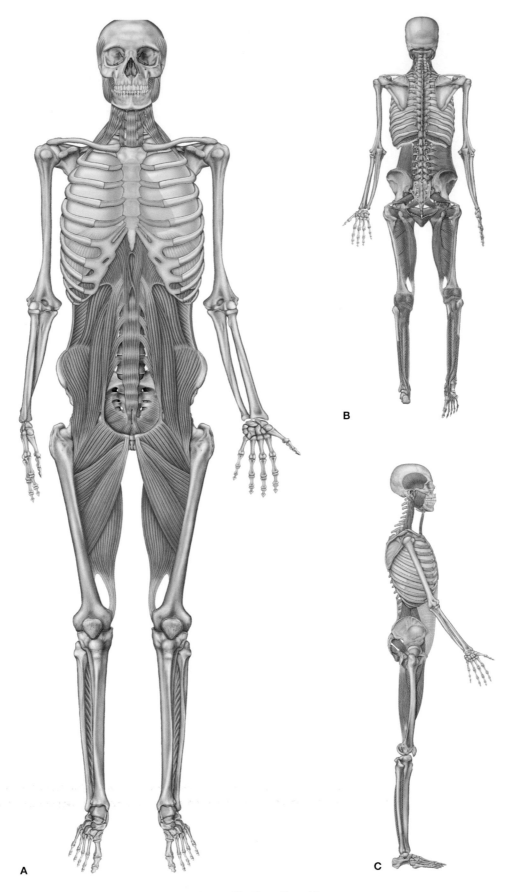

A

B

C

• **Fig. 9.1** The Deep Front Line.

9

The Deep Front Line

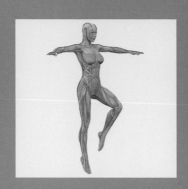

OVERVIEW

Interposed between the left and right Lateral Lines in the coronal plane, sandwiched between the Superficial Front Line (SFL) and Superficial Back Line (SBL) in the sagittal plane, and latticed by the helical Spiral and Functional Lines, the Deep Front Line (DFL) (Fig. 9.1; Video 2.11) comprises the body's myofascial 'core'. Beginning from the bottom, the line has roots deep in the underside of the foot, passing up just behind the bones of the lower leg and knee to the medial quadrant of the thigh. From here the major track passes in front of the hip joint, pelvis, and lumbar spine, while an alternate track passes up the back of the thigh to the pelvic floor, with the two tracks in effect gripping the hip joint fore and aft. The two tracks rejoin beside and at the front of the lumbar spine, where the psoas complex and diaphragm overlap. From the psoas–diaphragm interface, the DFL continues up within the rib cage along several paths conjoined around and through the thoracic viscera, ending on the underside of both the neuro- and viscerocranium (Fig. 9.2/Table 9.1; Video 4.10).

Compared to our other lines in previous chapters, this line demands definition as a three-dimensional space, rather than as a line. All the other lines are volumetric as well, of course, but they are more easily diagrammed as lines of pull. The DFL very clearly occupies a three-dimensional space. Though fundamentally fascial in nature, in the leg the DFL includes many of the deeper and more obscure supporting muscles of our anatomy (Fig. 9.3). Through the pelvis, the DFL lies in intimate relation with the hip joint, and relates the wave of breathing to the rhythm of walking. In the trunk, the DFL is poised, along with the autonomic ganglia, between our neuromotor 'chassis' and the more ancient organs of that support our 70 trillion cells within the ventral cavity. In the neck, it provides the counterbalancing lift to the downward pull of both the SFL and SBL. A dimensional understanding of the DFL is necessary for successful application of nearly any method of manual therapy or movement education.

Postural Function

The DFL plays a major role in the body's support:
- lifting and managing the responsiveness of the inner arch
- stabilizing each segment of the legs, up to, and down from, the hip
- supporting the lumbar spine from the front
- surrounding and lacing in the abdominopelvic balloon
- stabilizing the chest while allowing the rhythmic expansion and relaxation of breathing
- balancing the fragile neck and heavy head atop it all.

Lack of support, balance, and proper tonus in the DFL (as in the common pattern where short DFL myofascia does not allow the hip joint to open fully into extension) will produce overall shortening in the body and encourage collapse in the lumbo-pelvic core. This lays the groundwork for negative compensatory adjustments in all the other lines previously described.

Movement Function

Aside from hip adduction and the breath wave in the diaphragm, there is no movement that is strictly the province of the DFL, yet neither is any movement outside its influence. The DFL is nearly everywhere surrounded or covered by other myofascia, which duplicate the roles performed by the muscles of the DFL. The myofascia of the DFL is infused generally with denser fascia and more slow-twitch, endurance muscle fibers, reflecting the role the DFL plays in providing stability and subtle positioning changes to the core structure, enabling the more superficial structures and lines to work easily and efficiently with the skeleton. (This also applies to the DFL's first cousins, the Deep Arm Lines; see Ch. 7.)

Thus, failure of the DFL to work properly does not necessarily involve an immediate or obvious loss of function, especially to the untrained eye or to the less than exquisitely sensitive perceiver. Function is usually transferred to the outer lines of myofascia – but with slightly less elegance

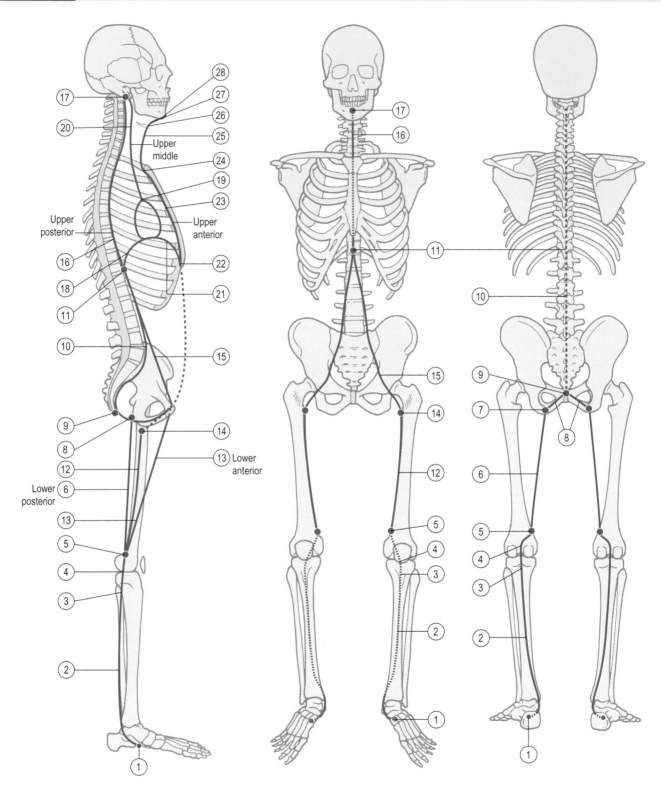

• **Fig. 9.2** Deep Front Line tracks and stations.

and grace, and slightly more strain to the joints and peri-articular tissues, which can set up the conditions over time for injury and degeneration. Thus, many difficult-to-fix injuries are predisposed by an earlier failure within the DFL which is only revealed later when the precipitating incident takes place and exposes the core deficiency.

'A Silken Tent'

The following sonnet by Robert Frost summarizes clearly the role of the Deep Front Line and its relationship to the rest of the Anatomy Trains, and the ideal of balance among the tensegrity system of the myofascial meridian lines:

TABLE 9.1 Deep Front Line Myofascial 'Tracks' and Bony 'Stations' (Fig. 9.2)

Bony Stations		Myofascial Tracks
Lowest Common		
Plantar tarsal bones, plantar surface of toes	1	
	2	Tibialis posterior, long toe flexors
Superior/posterior tibia/fibula	3	
	4	Fascia of popliteus, knee capsule
Medial femoral epicondyle	5	
Lower Posterior		
Medial femoral epicondyle	5	
	6	Posterior intermuscular septum, adductor magnus and minimus
Ischial ramus	7	
	8	Pelvic floor fascia, levator ani, obturator internus fascia
Coccyx	9	
	10	Anterior sacral fascia and anterior longitudinal ligament
Lumbar vertebral bodies	11	
Lower Anterior		
Medial femoral epicondyle	5	
Linea aspera of femur	12	
	13	Medial intermuscular septum, adductor brevis, longus
Lesser trochanter of femur	14	
	15	Psoas, iliacus, pectineus, femoral triangle
Lumbar vertebral bodies and TPs	11	
Upper Posterior		
Lumbar vertebral bodies	11	
	16	Anterior longitudinal ligament, longus colli and capitis
Basilar portion of occiput	17	
Upper Middle		
Lumbar vertebral bodies	11	
	18	Posterior diaphragm, crura of diaphragm, central tendon
	19	Pericardium, mediastinum, parietal pleura
	20	Fascia prevertebralis, pharyngeal raphe, scalene muscles, medial scalene fascia
Basilar portion of occiput, cervical TPs	17	
Upper Anterior		
Lumbar vertebral bodies	11	
	21	Anterior diaphragm
Posterior surface of subcostal, cartilages, xiphoid process	22	
	23	Fascia endothoracica, transversus thoracis
Posterior manubrium of sternum	24	
	25	Infrahyoid muscles, fascia pretrachialis
Hyoid bone	26	
	27	Suprahyoid muscles
Mandible	28	

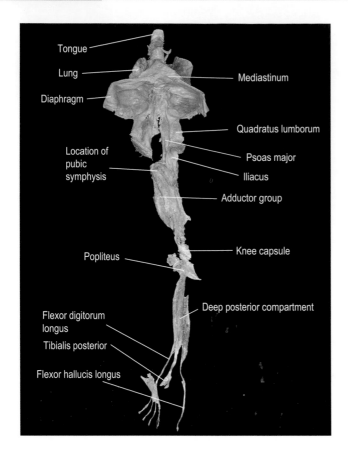

• **Fig. 9.3** An early attempt to dissect out the Deep Front Line shows a continual soft-tissue connection from the toes via the psoas to the tongue.

She is as in a field a silken tent
At midday when a sunny summer breeze
Has dried the dew and all its ropes relent,
So that in guys it gently sways at ease,
And its supporting central cedar pole,
That is its pinnacle to heavenward
And signifies the sureness of the soul,
Seems to owe naught to any single cord,
But strictly held by none, is loosely bound
By countless silken ties of love and thought
To everything on earth the compass round,
And only by one's going slightly taut
In the capriciousness of summer air
Is of the slightest bondage made aware.

('THE SILKEN TENT' FROM THE BOOK THE POETRY OF ROBERT FROST EDITED BY EDWARD CONNERY LATHEM. COPYRIGHT © 1969 BY HENRY HOLT AND COMPANY, COPYRIGHT © 1942 BY ROBERT FROST, COPYRIGHT © BY LESLEY FROST BALLANTINE. REPRINTED BY PERMISSION OF HENRY HOLT AND COMPANY, LLC.)

The Deep Front Line in Detail

The Foot and Leg: the Lowest Common Track

With a reminder that both function and dysfunction in any of these lines, but this one especially, can travel either up or

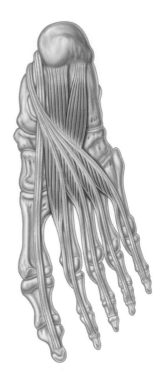

• **Fig. 9.4** The lower end of the DFL begins with the tendons of the flexor hallucis longus and flexor digitorum longus.

down the tracks or out from the middle, we will begin once again at the bottom and work our way up.

The DFL anchors itself deep in the sole of the foot with the distal attachments of the three muscles of the deep posterior compartment of the leg: the tibialis posterior and the two long flexors of the toes, the flexor hallucis and digitorum longus (Fig. 9.4).

The tissue between the metatarsals can also be included in this line – the dorsal interossei and accompanying fascia. This connection is a little hard to justify on a fascial level except via the link between the tibialis posterior tendon and the ligamentous bed of the foot. The lumbricals clearly link fascially and functionally with the SFL, but the interossei and the space between the metatarsals both feel and react therapeutically as part of the 'core' structure of the foot.

Depending on how you wield the scalpel, the tibialis posterior has multiple and variable tendinous attachments to nearly every bone in the tarsum of the foot except the talus, and to the middle three metatarsal bases besides (Fig. 9.5). This tendon resembles a hand with many fingers, reaching under the foot to support the arches and hold the tarsum of the foot together.

The three major tendons pass up inside the ankle behind the medial malleolus (see Fig. 3.13 – their lubricating tendon sheaths are colored blue). The tendon of the flexor hallucis (the tendon from the big toe) passes more posteriorly than the other two, beneath the sustentaculum tali of the calcaneus and posterior to the talus as well. This muscle–tendon complex thus provides additional elastic recoil support to the medial arch during the push-off phase of walking (Fig. 9.6). The tendons of the two toe flexors cross

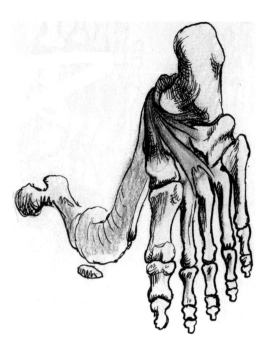

• **Fig. 9.5** Deep to the long toe flexors are the complex attachments of the tibialis posterior, also part of the DFL. (Reproduced with kind permission from Grundy 1982.)

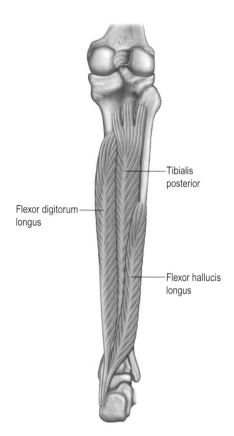

Tibialis posterior

Flexor digitorum longus

Flexor hallucis longus

• **Fig. 9.7** The three muscles of the deep posterior compartment of the leg, deep to the soleus, comprise the DFL.

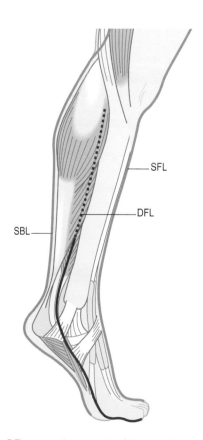

SFL

DFL

SBL

• **Fig. 9.6** The DFL passes between the SBL and SFL tracks, contracting during the push-off phase of walking to support the medial arch.

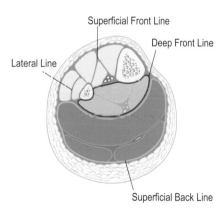

Superficial Front Line

Deep Front Line

Lateral Line

Superficial Back Line

• **Fig. 9.8** The deep posterior compartment lies behind the interosseous membrane between the tibia and fibula. Notice that each of the fascial compartments of the lower leg ensheathes one of the Anatomy Trains lines.

in the foot, helping to ensure that toe flexion is accompanied by prehensile adduction.

The three join in the deep posterior compartment of the lower leg, filling in the area between the fibula and tibia behind the interosseous membrane (Fig. 9.7).

This line employs the last available compartment in the lower leg (Fig. 9.8). The anterior compartment serves the Superficial Front Line (Ch. 4), and the lateral fibularii/ peroneal compartment comprises the Lateral Line (Ch. 5). Just above the ankle, this deep posterior compartment is completely covered by the superficial posterior compartment with the soleus and gastrocnemii of the Superficial Back Line (Ch. 3) (Fig. 9.9). Access to this deep compartment for manual and movement therapy is discussed below.

❖ General Manual Therapy Considerations

Piecemeal experimentation with the myofascia of the Deep Front Line can produce mixed results. The myofascial structures of the DFL accompany the extensions of the viscera into the limbs – i.e. the neurovascular bundles – and are thus studded with endangerment sites and difficult points of entry. Practitioners familiar with working these structures will be able to make connections and apply their work in an integrated way. If these DFL structures are new to you, it is recommended that you absorb these methods from a class, where an instructor can assure your placement, engagement, and intent. With that in mind, we offer a palpation guide to structures in the DFL, but not to particular techniques in detail. References to the Anatomy Trains technique videos (www.anatomytrains.com), and the cited videos linked from this book where techniques are presented visually, are provided when appropriate.

Common postural compensation patterns associated with the DFL include chronic plantarflexion (or resistance to dorsiflexion), high and fallen arch patterns, pronation and supination, genu valgus and varus, anterior or posterior pelvic tilt, pelvic floor insufficiency, lumbar malalignment, thoracolumbar rotations, breathing restriction, flexed or hyperextended cervicals, temporomandibular joint (TMJ) syndrome, swallowing and language difficulties, and the general core collapse which accompanies depression or defeat.

❖ ❖ Palpation Guide 1: Deep Posterior Compartment

Although it is next to impossible to feel the tendons of the flexor digitorum longus or the tibialis posterior on the bottom of the foot, the flexor hallucis longus can be clearly felt. Extend (lift) your big toe to tighten the tendon around the windlass of the metatarsal head, and it will be clearly palpable along the medial edge of the plantar fascia, under the medial arch (see Fig. 9.4 and www .anatomytrains.com – video ref: Deep Front Line, Part 1, 23:46–26:18).

The tendons can be more easily felt along the medial side of the foot and ankle, in roughly the same way the peroneal tendons run on the outside of the foot (Video 6.3). Place a finger directly under the medial malleolus, and invert and plantarflex the foot; the large tendon that pops under your finger is the tibialis posterior. The flexor digitorum runs about one finger width posterior to the tibialis posterior, and can be felt when the smaller toes are wiggled.

The big toe flexor lies posterior and deep to these two. To find the flexor hallucis at the ankle, put a thumb or finger into the space in front of the medial side of the Achilles tendon and press into the posteromedial aspect of your ankle (taking care not to press on the nerve bundle). Flex

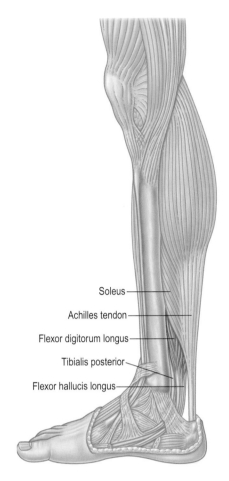

Soleus

Achilles tendon

Flexor digitorum longus

Tibialis posterior

Flexor hallucis longus

• Fig. 9.9 A medial view of the lower leg with the DFL structures highlighted. They can only be directly palpated just above the ankle.

and extend the big toe – the substantial tendon of flexor hallucis longus will slide under your finger (www.anatomytrains .com – video ref: Deep Front Line, Part 1, 08:05–09:18).

These three muscles are covered completely by the soleus about three inches (7 cm) above the malleolus as they pass up into the deep posterior compartment (see Fig. 9.9), just behind the interosseous membrane between the tibia and fibula (Fig. 9.10). Reaching this myofascial compartment manually is difficult. It is possible to stretch these muscles by putting the foot into strong dorsiflexion and eversion, as in the Downward-Facing Dog pose or by putting the ball of your foot on a stair and letting the heel drop. It is, however, often difficult for either practitioner or client to discern whether the soleus (SBL) or the deeper muscles (DFL) are being stretched.

It is possible to feel the state of the compartment in general by feeling through the soleus, but only if the soleus can be relaxed enough to make such palpation possible. In our experience, trying to work these muscles through the soleus is either an exercise in frustration or a way to damage the soleus by overworking it – almost literally poking holes in it – in the attempt to reach these muscles deep to it (www.anatomytrains.com – video ref: Deep Front Line, Part 1, 20:11–23:45). An alternative way to reach this hidden layer is to insinuate your fingers close along the

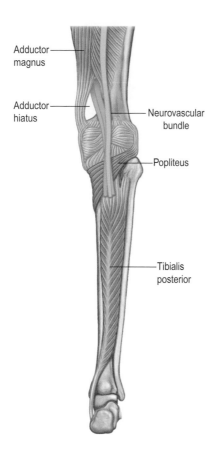

• **Fig. 9.10** The DFL passes behind the knee, in a deeper plane of fascia than the Superficial Back Line, with the popliteus, neurovascular bundle, and fascia on the back of the knee capsule.

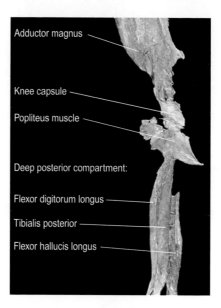

• **Fig. 9.11** The fascia surrounding the popliteus and the posterior surface of the ligamentous capsule of the knee links the tibialis posterior to the distal end of adductor magnus at the medial femoral epicondyle.

medial posterior edge of the tibia, separating the soleus from the tibia in order to get to the underlying (and often very tense and sore) muscles of the deep posterior compartment (Fig. 9.11 and www.anatomytrains.com – video ref: Deep Front Line, Part 1, 09:20–15:03).

Another hand can approach this compartment from the outside by finding the posterior septum behind the fibularii, and 'swimming' your fingers into this 'valley' between the fibularii and the soleus on the lateral side. Your goal is the lateral edge of the fibula, which is easier to feel in some than in others, and easier to feel on most closer to the malleolus. When in this position, you have the fascial layer of the deep posterior compartment between the 'pincers' of your hands (see Fig. 9.10 and www.anatomytrains.com – video ref: Deep Front Line, Part 1, 15:03–20:10). Couple this firmly held position with client movement, dorsi- and plantarflexion, and you can help bring mobility to these deeper tissues. Multiple repetitions may be necessary as the leg becomes progressively softer and more accessible, and movement more differentiated between the superficial and deep compartments.

These lower DFL tissues are very useful in easing stubborn arch patterns, both 'fallen' and 'high' arch patterns (www.anatomytrains.com – video ref: Deep Front Line, Part 1, 26:26–30:33), as well as bunions (www.anatomytrains.com – video ref: Deep Front Line, Part 1, 30:33–32:26). More subjectively, these muscles are associated with anxiety patterns – the result of a chronic 'be on your toes' somato-emotional attitude.

🌸 The Thigh – Lower Posterior Track

At the top of the deep posterior compartment, we pass over the back of the knee with the fascia which comprises the anterior lamina and tendon of the popliteus, the neurovascular bundle of the tibial nerve and popliteal artery, and the outer layers of the strong fascial capsule which surrounds the back of the knee joint (see Figs. 9.10 and 9.11). The next station of this line is at the medial side of the top of the knee joint, the adductor tubercle on the medial femoral epicondyle.

The fascia surrounding the adductors is a unitary bag that ties all the adductors to the linea aspera of the femur at the deepest aspect (Video 6.21). Nearer the surface of the inner thigh, it presents us with a switch or choice point as we move up, as the heavy fascial walls on the front and back of the adductors head off in different directions, which will not rejoin again until the lumbar spine (Fig. 9.12). We will term these two fascial continuities the lower posterior and lower anterior tracks of the DFL.

The posterior track consists of the adductor magnus muscle and the accompanying fascia between the hamstrings and the adductor group (Fig. 9.13). If we run behind the adductor group from the epicondyle, we can follow this posterior intermuscular septum up the thigh to the posterior part of the ischial ramus near the ischial tuberosity (IT), which is the attachment point of the posterior 'head' of adductor magnus (Fig. 9.14).

From the ischium, there is a clear fascial continuity up the buttock deep to the gluteus maximus onto a group of muscles known as the deep lateral rotators (Fig. 9.15 and

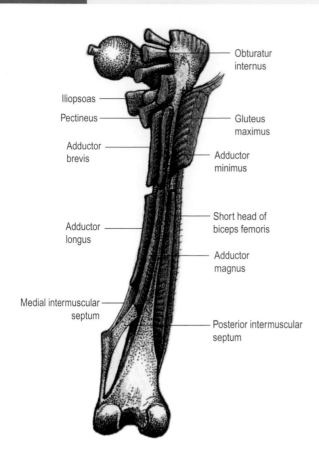

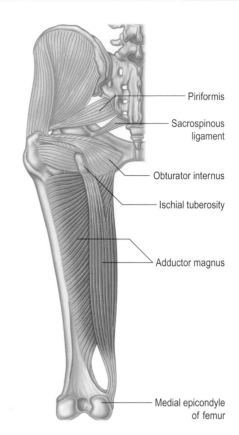

• **Fig. 9.12** From the medial epicondyle, two fascial planes emerge, one carrying up and forward with the adductor longus and brevis (the lower anterior track of the DFL), and another with the adductor magnus and minimus (the lower posterior track). Both ultimately surround the adductors, and both are connected from the fascia lata at the surface to the linea aspera, but each leads to a different set of structures at the superior end. (Reproduced with kind permission from Grundy 1982.)

• **Fig. 9.14** The adductor group from behind, showing the lower posterior track of the DFL up to the ischial tuberosity. This lies in the same fascial plane as the deep lateral rotators, but the transverse direction of the muscular fibers prevents us from continuing up into the buttock with this line.

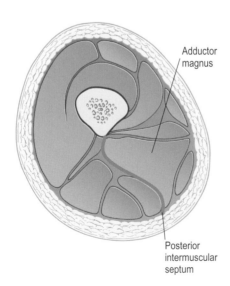

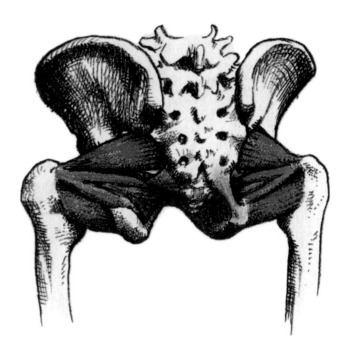

• **Fig. 9.13** The lower posterior track of the DFL follows the posterior intermuscular septum up the posterior aspect of the adductor magnus muscle.

• **Fig. 9.15** The deep lateral rotators, although they are crucial to the understanding and optimization of human plantigrade posture, do not fit easily into the Anatomy Trains schema. (Reproduced with kind permission from Grundy 1982.)

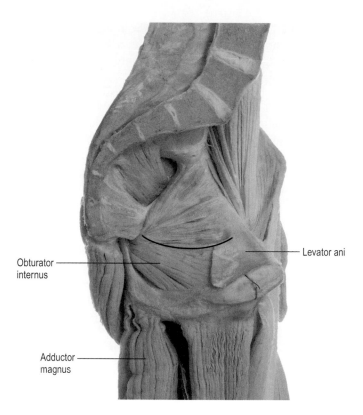

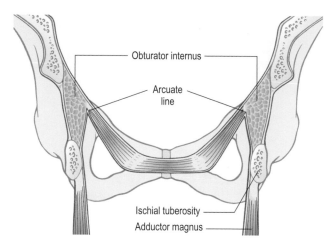

• **Fig. 9.17** From the posterior intermuscular septum and adductor magnus, the fascial track moves up inside the ischial tuberosity on the obturator internus fascia to contact the pelvic floor (levator ani).

• **Fig. 9.16** Although all overlying fascia has been removed in this dissection, there is a connection from the adductor magnus (and the posterior intermuscular septum represented by the dark slit just posterior to it) across the ischial tuberosity and the lower obturator internus fascia to the arcuate line (black line) where the levator ani joins the lateral wall of the true pelvis. (© Ralph T. Hutchings. Reproduced from Abrahams, et al. 1998.)

www.anatomytrains.com – video ref: Deep Front Line, Part 1, 1:23:27–1:35:54). Thus if we were going to include the deep lateral rotators in the Anatomy Trains system, they would be, strangely, part of this lower posterior track of the DFL (see also the section on the 'Deep Back Line', Ch. 3, p. 50). In fact, however, even though there is a fascial connection between the posterior adductors and the quadratus femoris and the rest of the lateral rotators, the muscle fiber direction of these muscles is nearly at right angles to the ones we have been following straight up the thigh. Thus, this connection cannot qualify as a myofascial meridian by our self-imposed rules, though they are clearly tied to this fascial plane up the back of the thigh. These important muscles are most usefully seen as part of a series of muscular fans around the hip joint, as they simply do not fit into the longitudinal meridians we are describing here (see 'Fans of the Hip Joint'[1] in *Body*[3], published privately and available from www.anatomytrains.com; Video 3.18).

We will have an easier time finding our myofascial continuity if we run inside the lower flange of the pelvis from the adductor magnus and its septum up onto the medial side of the IT–ischial ramus (Fig. 9.16). We can follow a strong fascial connection over the bone onto the dense outer covering of the obturator internus muscle, connecting with levator ani of the pelvic floor via the arcuate line (Fig. 9.17).

This is an important line of stabilization from the trunk down the inner back of the leg.

The pelvic floor is a complex set of structures – a muscular funnel, surrounded by fascial sheets and visceral ligaments – worthy of several books of its own.[2] For our purposes, it forms the bottom of the trunk portion of the DFL with multiple connections around the abdominopelvic cavity. We have been following the lower posterior track listed in Table 9.1. This track takes us from the coccygeus and iliococcygeus portions of the levator ani onto the coccyx, where we can continue north with the fascia on the front of the sacrum. This fascia blends into the anterior longitudinal ligament running up the front of the spine, where it rejoins the lower anterior track at the junction between the psoas and diaphragmatic crura (Fig. 9.18).

The complex sets of connections here are difficult to box into a linear presentation. We can note, for instance, that the pelvic floor, at least the central pubococcygeus, also connects to the posterior lamina of the rectus abdominis reaching down from above (described later in this chapter – see Fig. 9.31).

❖ *Palpation Guide 2: Lower Posterior Track*

The area of the DFL behind the knee is not easily amenable to palpation or manual intervention due to the passage of the neurovascular bundle and fat pad superficial to these tissues. The next station, the medial femoral epicondyle on the inside just above the knee, is easily felt if you run your thumb along the medial side of your thigh with some pressure until you find the knob of the epicondyle a couple of inches (5 cm) above the knee.

This station marks the beginning of a division between the posterior septum that runs up the back of the adductors, separating them from the hamstrings, and the anterior (medial intermuscular) septum dividing the adductors from the quadriceps. Taking the posterior septum first, place your model on his side, and find the medial femoral epicondyle (see Fig. 9.14). You will find a finger's width or more of

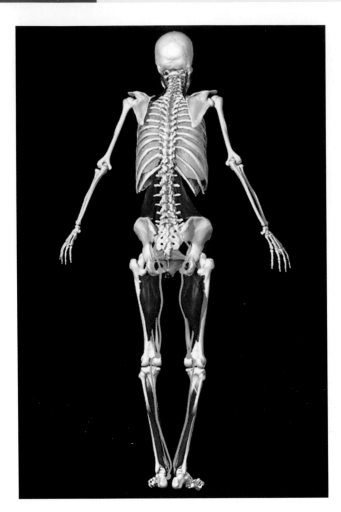

• **Fig. 9.18** Deep Front Line, lower posterior tracks and stations view as imaged by Primal Pictures. (Image provided courtesy of Primal Pictures, www.primalpictures.com.)

space between this condyle and the prominent medial hamstring tendons coming from behind the knee. This valley is the lower margin of the septum.

Follow this valley upward as far as you can toward the IT. In some people, it will be easy to follow, and you can work your way more deeply into this septum in its slightly 'S'-shaped course toward the linea aspera (see Fig. 9.13). In those where the adductor magnus is 'married' to the hamstrings, however, the septum and surrounding tissues may be too bound to find any valley very far up the thigh. Indeed, the septum may feel instead like a piece of strapping tape between the muscles, or a string of bead-like structures which may be calcium lactate crystals in the septum. Having space between these muscle groups so that the septum is open and movement is free is the desired state. Fingers insinuated into this division accompanied by flexion and extension of the knee can lead to freer gliding between the hamstrings and posterior adductors – important for any athlete, or, conversely, for any duck-footed walker.

The upper end of this valley will emerge at the postero-inferior point of the ischial tuberosity. You can usually orient yourself at this point by placing your fingers in the

lower posterior corner of the IT with your model side-lying, and having her adduct (lift the whole leg toward the ceiling). Adductor magnus, attaching to the bottom of the IT, will 'pop' your fingers in this movement.

To isolate the hamstrings, alternate this movement with knee flexion (leg relaxed on the table while pressing the heel against some resistance you can offer with your other hand or outer thigh). The hamstrings attach to the posterior aspect of the IT; you will feel this attachment tighten in resisted knee flexion (see Fig. 9.16). Place your fingers between these two structures and you will be on the upper end of the posterior adductor septum. The septum runs in a straight line between the femoral epicondyle and this upper end. In cases where the valley is impenetrable, work to spread the fascial tissues laterally and relax surrounding muscles will be rewarded with the valley appearing, and, more to the point, differentiated movement between pelvis and femur, and between hamstrings and adductor magnus (www.anatomytrains.com – video ref: Deep Front Line, Part 1, 43:25–44:59).

The adductors themselves are amenable to general spreading work along their length (www.anatomytrains.com – video ref: Deep Front Line, Part 1, 36:20–42:00), and to specific work up on the medial area of the hip joint near the ischial ramus, especially for correcting a functionally short leg (www.anatomytrains.com – video ref: Deep Front Line, Part 1, 45:00–52:20).

From the adductor magnus, there is connecting fascia from the IT along its medial surface to the obturator internus fascia, and from this fascial sheet onto the pelvic floor sheets via the arcuate line (see Fig. 9.18). Palpating in this direction is not for the faint of heart and should initially be practiced with a friend or tolerant colleague, but it is a rewarding and not very invasive way of affecting the pelvic floor, the site of so many insults to structure, especially for women. On your side-lying or prone model, place your hand on the inside posterior edge of the IT. Keep your index finger in contact with the sacrotuberous ligament as a guide, to avoid going too far anterior on the ischial ramus. Begin to slide upward and forward in the direction of the navel, keeping your fingerpads in gentle but direct contact with the bone. A little practice will teach you how much skin to take – stretching skin is not the object (Fig. 9.19).

Beyond the IT/ramus you will feel the slightly softer tissue of the obturator internus fascia under your fingerpads. Care must be taken to stay away from the anal verge, and some verbal reassurance is often helpful. Continue upward along the obturator fascia until you encounter a wall ahead of your fingertips. This wall is the pelvic floor, the levator ani muscle.

No words can substitute for the experiential 'library' of assessing the state of the pelvic floor in a number of subjects. We have found that many pelvic floors, especially in the male of the species, will be high and tight, meaning that your fingers will have to run deep into the pelvic space before encountering a solid-feeling wall. Fewer clients – more female, and often post-partum – will present with a

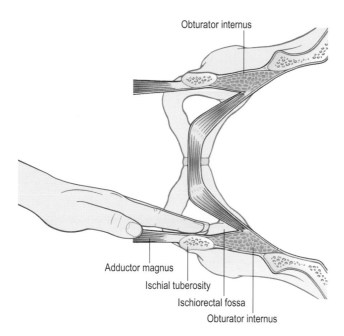

• **Fig. 9.19** A difficult but highly effective technique for contacting the posterior triangle of the pelvic floor involves sliding into the ischiorectal fossa along the ischial tuberosity in the direction of the navel until the pelvic floor is felt and assessed. Depending on its condition, manual therapy can be used to either lower both the tone and the position of the posterior pelvic floor, or encourage its increased tone.

lax pelvic floor, which you will encounter much lower in the pelvis, and with a spongy feel. Only occasionally will you find the converse patterns – a low pelvic floor that is nonetheless highly toned, or the spongy pelvis floor that is nonetheless located high in the pelvis.

For those clients with the common pattern of a high, tightened levator ani, it is possible to hook your fingers into the obturator fascia just below the pelvic floor, and bring that fascia with you as you retreat toward the IT (see Fig. 9.19). This will often relax and lower the pelvic floor. For those with a toneless or fallen pelvic floor, pushing the fingertips up against the pelvic floor while calling for the client to contract and relax the muscles will often help the client find and strengthen this vital area. This is a simple palpatory introduction into an area that is complex anatomically, neurologically, and psychologically, where care, sensitivity, experience, and skill are required to unravel the thousand ills to which this particular flesh is heir.

The Thigh – Lower Anterior Track

Returning to the inside of the thigh just above the knee, we can take the other track of the DFL in the thigh, the lower anterior track, which is the more primary line of the DFL in our myofascial meridians approach. This fascial line penetrates the adductor magnus through the adductor hiatus with the neurovascular bundle, to emerge on the anterior side of this muscle, in the intermuscular septum between the adductor group and the quadriceps group (Fig. 9.20; Video 4.11).

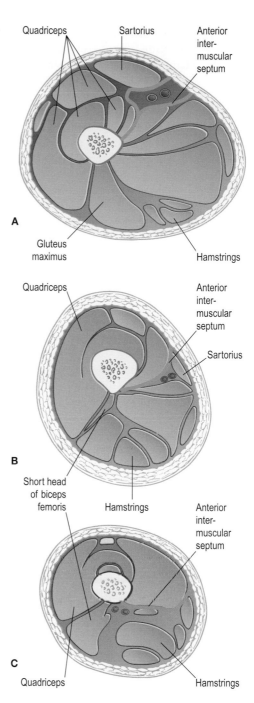

• **Fig. 9.20** The lower anterior track of the DFL follows the anterior intermuscular septum between the adductors and the hamstrings. (**A**) is closer to the hip; (**C**) is closer to the knee.

This septum lines in the sulcus that underlies the sartorius muscle. Although we keep to our tradition in depicting this as a line, it is especially important here to expand one's vision to see this part of the DFL as a complex curvature in a three-dimensional fascial plane. It sweeps up in a sail shape: at the surface, its 'leech' (outer edge) runs up under the sartorius from just above the inner part of the knee to the front of the hip and the femoral triangle (with the sartorius acting as a 'leech line' – adjustably tightening the edge of this fascia where it interfaces with the fascia lata).

The 'luff' (inner edge) is firmly attached to the linea aspera on the 'mast' of the femur from the medial posterior knee up the back of the femur to the lesser trochanter (Fig. 9.21). The 'foot' of the sail is tied to the 'boom' of the ischiopubic ramus.

From here the main track of the DFL continues up on the psoas muscle complex and its associated fasciae, which climb forward and up from the lesser trochanter. The psoas major passes directly in front of the hip joint and rounds over the iliopectineal ridge, only to dive backward behind the organs and their enfolded peritoneal bag to join to the lumbar spine (Fig. 9.22). Its proximal attachments are to the bodies and transverse processes (TPs) of all the lumbar vertebrae, frequently including T12 as well. Each psoas fills in the gully between the bodies and TPs in the front of the spine, just as the transversospinalii fill in the laminar grooves between the TPs and spinous processes behind the spine (Fig. 9.23).

In the groin, the anterior intermuscular septum opens into the femoral triangle, or the 'leg pit', bordered on the medial side by the adductor longus, on the lateral side by the sartorius, and superiorly by the inguinal ligament (Fig. 9.24). Within the femoral triangle we find the femoral neurovascular bundle, a set of lymph nodes, and the continuation of the DFL myofascia – the iliopsoas on the lateral side and the pectineus on the medial side, all covering the front of the hip joint and head of the femur, all attaching to the lesser trochanter.

While the pectineus is confined to the femoral triangle, both the psoas and the iliacus extend above the inguinal ligament into the trunk. The iliacus is a one-joint flexor of the hip, equivalent in some ways to the subscapularis in the shoulder. The iliacus is definitely and obviously a hip flexor, though there is some controversy over whether it is a medial or lateral rotator of the hip (see 'The Psoas Pseries'[3]).

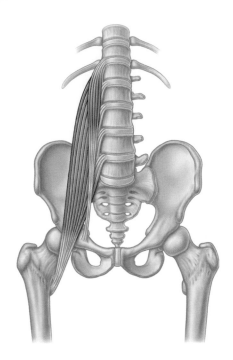

• **Fig. 9.22** The psoas major is the principal supporting guy-wire between the spine and the leg, joining upper to lower, breathing to walking, and acting with other local muscles in complex ways for steadying various movements.

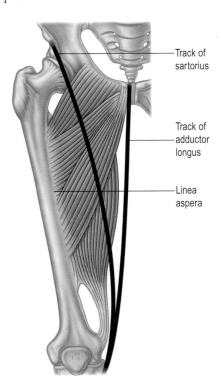

• **Fig. 9.21** The anterior septum of the thigh presents a complex curve not unlike a sail that sweeps from the linea aspera out to the sartorius.

Track of sartorius

Track of adductor longus

Linea aspera

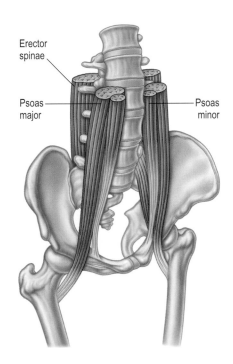

Erector spinae

Psoas major

Psoas minor

• **Fig. 9.23** There are four 'gullies' around the spine; the erector spinae muscles in the back and the psoas in the front fill in these gullies and support the lumbar vertebrae.

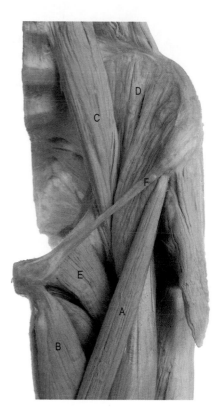

• **Fig. 9.24** The femoral triangle, the leg's equivalent to the armpit, opens from the anterior septum between the sartorius (**A**) and the adductor longus (**B**). It passes, with the psoas (**C**), iliacus (**D**), pectineus (**E**), and neurovascular bundle (not pictured), under the inguinal ligament (**F**) into the abdominal cavity. The psoas, iliacus, and pectineus form a fan reaching up from the lesser trochanter to the hip bone and lumbar spine. Length and balanced tone in this complex is essential for structural health and freedom of movement. The ability of the hip joint to open – either in the first year of life or the thirtieth, depends on these tissues' ability to lengthen. (© Ralph T. Hutchings. Reproduced from Abrahams, et al. 1998.)

The psoas muscle, also clearly a hip flexor and also variously described as a medial or lateral (or, as this author has been persuaded, a non-) hip rotator, is even more mired in controversy in terms of its action on the spine (Fig. 9.25).[4] This author is convinced, through clinical experience, that the psoas should be considered as a triangular muscle, with differing functions for the upper psoas, which can act as a lumbar flexor, and the lower psoas, which clearly acts as a lumbar extensor. If this differentiation of function is valid, the lumbars can be fully supported by balancing the various slips of the psoas with the post-vertebral multifidi, without reference to the tonus of the abdominal muscles (again, see 'The Psoas Pseries'[3]). Understanding this differentiation allows us to see the psoas as at least four separate muscles. If we get down to being segmentally specific in the lumbars with rotations and spondylolisthesis, we have to work with each of the ten neuromotor units within each psoas on either side of the spine. The psoas is simply not one fusiform string, it is an entire harp for the lumber spine – its power, and its relationship to the sacrum, pelvis, and leg (Video 3.17).

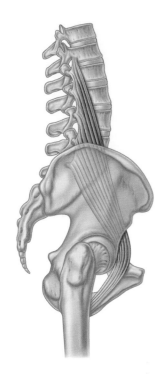

• **Fig. 9.25** The human psoas muscle makes a unique journey around the front of the pelvis – forward and up from the trochanter to the iliopectineal ridge, then back and up to the lumbar spine. No other animal makes use of such a course for the psoas. In most quadrupeds, the psoas does not even touch the pelvis unless the femur is extended to its limit, whereupon most quadrupeds reflexively retract their leg.

❖ ❖ 🌼 Psoas Express and Locals

We have said that multi-joint express muscles often overlie other monarticular locals. In the case of the psoas muscle, there are two sets of locals that serve the same area, but here they lie on either side of the express instead of underneath (Fig. 9.26). While there is controversy as to exactly what functions the psoas performs,[2,4–8] there is not about the territory it covers, which is from the lesser trochanter to the bodies and TPs of all the lumbar and often the 12th thoracic vertebrae.

We can cover the same territory in two other ways, one medial and the other lateral to the psoas major itself. On the medial side, we could follow the pectineus from the lesser trochanter (and the linea aspera just below it) over to the iliopectineal ridge (Fig. 9.27). From here, with the connecting fascia of widespread lower end of the lacunar ligament and only a slight change in direction, we can pick up the psoas minor (which is expressed as a muscle in about 51% of the population, but is expressed as a fascial band in a much higher percentage.[9] The psoas minor runs on top of the fascia of the psoas major to insert, or reach its upper station, at the 12th thoracic vertebra.

On the lateral side, we begin with the iliacus, widening up and laterally from the lesser trochanter to attach all along the upper portion of the iliac fossa (Fig. 9.28). The fascia covering the iliacus is continuous with the fascia on the anterior surface of the quadratus lumborum,

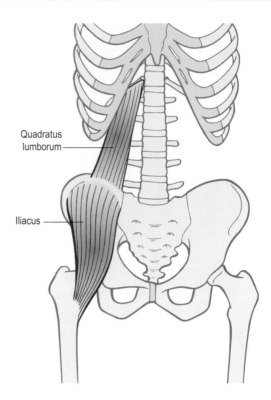

Quadratus lumborum

Psoas minor

Psoas major

Pectineus

• **Fig. 9.26** The DFL attaches the inner femur to the core structures in front of the spine and lowest rib, including the diaphragm and mesentery (not pictured). In the center of these connections lies the psoas major express, flanked by two sets of locals.

Quadratus lumborum

Iliacus

• **Fig. 9.28** The outer line of hip–spine locals comprises the iliacus, linking into the quadratus lumborum.

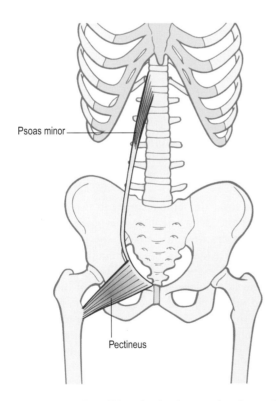

Psoas minor

Pectineus

• **Fig. 9.27** The inner line of hip–spine locals comprises the pectineus, linking via the lacunar ligament with the psoas minor.

which takes us up to the TPs of the lumbar vertebrae, just behind the psoas attachments, as well as to the 12th rib (www.anatomytrains.com – video ref: Anatomy Trains Revealed: Deep Front Line).

Thus, when either the lower lumbar vertebrae or the thoracolumbar junction (TLJ) are being pulled down and forward toward the front of the pelvis, any or all three of these pathways could be involved, and all three should be investigated in dealing with a lower lumbar lordosis, compressed lumbars, an anteriorly tilted or even a posteriorly tilted pelvis.

In the misty past, when this author began teaching manual therapy, few practitioners knew much about the psoas or how to find and treat it. In the past 20 years, its role has been more widely recognized and sometimes to the exclusion of these important more-or-less monarticular accompanying muscle groups, which, to be effective in changing patterns in the groin area, should draw practitioners' attention.

A lunge, a Thomas test, or those asanas in yoga known as the 'warrior poses', are common ways to induce a stretch in the psoas, which works well as long as the lumbars are not allowed to fall too far forward in the lunge, and the pelvis is kept square to the leg in front (see Fig. 4.17A, p. 62). One can explore these two local complexes from this position (Fig. 9.29). To engage the outer iliacus–quadratus complex, let the knee of the extended leg turn medially toward the body, letting the heel fall out. Moving the ribs

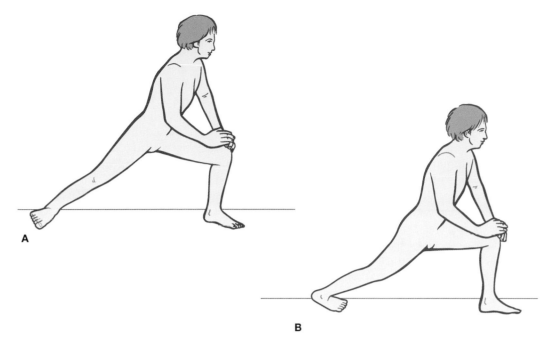

• **Fig. 9.29** Positions for emphasizing stretch in (**A**) the inner set of locals and (**B**) the outer set of locals.

away from the hip on the same side will emphasize this stretch. To engage the inner pectineus–psoas minor complex, let the extended leg turn out, with the heel going in and the weight coming onto the inner big toe. Drop the hip toward the floor a little and this inner line through the groin will be felt in sharper relief.

🌸 *The Thoracolumbar Junction (TLJ)*

The upper end of the psoas blends fascially with the crura and other posterior attachments of the diaphragm, particularly with the arcuate line between the body and transverse process of T12, all of which blend with the anterior longitudinal ligament (ALL), running up the front of the vertebral bodies and discs.

The connection between the psoas and diaphragm – just behind the kidneys, adrenal glands, and celiac (solar) plexus, and just in front of the major spinal joint of the thoracolumbar junction (TLJ: T12–L1) – is a critical point of both support and function in the human body (Fig. 9.30). It joins the 'top' and 'bottom' of the body, it joins breathing to walking, assimilation to elimination, and is, of course, via the celiac plexus, our second largest after the brain itself, and a center for the 'gut reaction'.

❖ *Palpation Guide 3: Lower Anterior Track*

The anterior septum of the adductors, or medial intermuscular septum, runs under the sartorius muscle, and you can usually gain access to this valley by feeling for it just medial to the sartorius (see Fig. 9.20). Like the sartorius, the septum is medial on the thigh on the lower end, but lies on the front of the thigh at its upper end. As with the posterior septum, different clients will allow you in to various depths, although this valley is more evident than the posterior

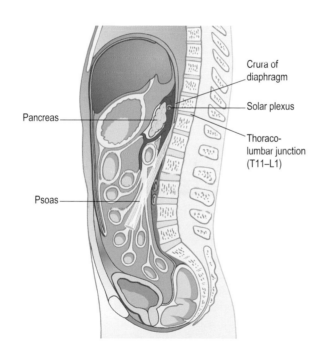

• **Fig. 9.30** The meeting place between the upper and lower tracks of the DFL is the front of the upper lumbar vertebrae, where the upper reaches of the psoas mingle with the lower aspects of the diaphragm, where walking meets breathing. It corresponds closely to the location of an essential spinal transition (T12–L1), as well as the adrenal glands and solar plexus, our 'abdominal brain'.

septum in most people, and is evident in the lean client when he or she simply holds the entire leg up off the table in a laterally rotated position. As you palpate the septum for depth and freedom, alternate the client's movements of adduction with full knee extension (which will activate the quadriceps under your fingers) to help you be clear about where the line of separation lies (www.anatomytrains.com – video ref: Deep Front Line, Part 1, 42:00–43:24).

At the top of this septum, it widens out into the femoral triangle, bounded by the sartorius running to the anterior superior iliac spine (ASIS) on the outside, the prominent tendon of adductor longus on the medial side, and superiorly by the inguinal ligament (see Fig. 9.24). Within the femoral triangle, medial to lateral, are the pectineus, psoas major tendon, and iliacus. The femoral neurovascular bundle and lymph nodes live here also, so tread carefully, but do not ignore this area vital to full opening of the hip joint.

Have your model lie supine with her knees up. Sit on one side of the table facing her head, with one of her thighs against the side of your body. Reach over the knee, securing the leg between your arm and your body, and put your entire palmar surface onto the medial aspect of the thigh, fingers pointing down. Drop your fingers slowly and gently into the opening of this leg pit, with your ring or little finger resting against the adductor longus tendon as a guide, so that the rest of your fingers are just anterior and lateral to it. Watch out for stretching the skin as you go in. It sometimes helps to reach in with your outer hand to lift the skin of the inner thigh before placing your palpating inner hand in the groin, so that you drop both the skin and your fingers into the femoral triangle at the same time (www.anatomytrains.com – video ref: Deep Front Line, Part 1, 52:22–54:40).

Once into the space, if you extend your fingers, the fingernail side will contact the lateral side of the pubic bone. Ask your model to lift her knee toward the opposite shoulder (combining flexion and adduction) and, if you are properly placed, you will feel the pectineus pop into your fingers – a band an inch or more ($\approx$3 cm) wide near the pubic ramus. The muscle can be best worked in eccentric contraction while the client either slides the heel out to full leg extension, or pushes down on her foot, creating a pelvic twist away from you.

To find the psoas at this level, move your fingers just anterior and a little lateral of the pectineus. Avoid putting any pressure or sideways stretch on the femoral artery. On the lateral side of the artery (usually; it can vary which side of the artery affords easier access) you will find a slick and hard structure lying in front of the ball of the hip joint. Have your model lift her foot straight off the table, and this psoas tendon should pop straight into your hands, feeling about like a slippery clothesline. There is little that can be done with it at this level in most people, as it is so tendinous, but this is the place where the psoas rests nearest the surface. What is useful here is to ease and dissolve any extra bands around the attachment at the lesser trochanter (if you can reach it) that are adhering the psoas tendon to surrounding structures. This often occurs in patients with pelvic torsions or scoliosis in the spine.

The iliacus is adjacent to the psoas in the femoral triangle, just lateral to it, and is chiefly and usually distinguished from the psoas by being a bit softer (because it is still more muscular as opposed to the tendinous psoas at this level). It can be followed (skipping over the inguinal ligament) up to its anterior attachment inside the lip of the anterior iliac crest.

The iliacus and psoas can both be reached above the inguinal ligament in the abdominal area as well. Standing beside your supine model, have her bend her knees until the feet are standing, heels close to the buttocks, and place your fingers in the superior edge of the ASIS (www.anatomytrains.com – video ref: Deep Front Line, Part 1, 59:15–1:02:03). Sink down into the body, keeping your fingerpads in contact with the iliacus as you go. Keep the fingers soft, and desist if you create painful stretching in the model's peritoneal structures (anything gassy, searing, hot, or sharp). The psoas should appear in front of the tips of your fingers at the bottom of the 'slope' of the iliacus (www.anatomytrains.com – video ref: Deep Front Line, Part 1, 1:02:05–1:12:30). If the psoas remains elusive, have your model gently begin to lift her foot off the table, which should immediately tighten the psoas and make it more obvious to you. At this point, you are on the outside edge of the psoas, and these fibers come from the upper reaches of the psoas – the T12–L1 part.

Although you can follow these outside fibers up, it is not recommended that you work the psoas above the level of the navel without a detailed understanding of the kidney's attachments and blood supply.

Having found this outside edge, keep a gentle contact with the 'sausage' of the psoas (the client needs to keep her foot in the air for this), staying at the level between a horizontal line drawn between the two ASISs and another drawn at the level of the umbilicus. Move up and across the top of the muscle until you feel yourself coming onto the inside slope. It is important not to lose contact with the muscle as you do this (remember, foot off the table if you are in any doubt), and important not to press on anything that pulses. You are now on the inside edge of the psoas, in contact with the fibers which come from L4–L5 (and are thus more responsible, when short, for lumbar lordosis).

The psoas minor is only present as a muscle in about half the population, and, for this author, is often difficult to isolate from psoas major, except as a tight band across its anterior surface. With the client supine and the knees bent, you can sometimes feel the small band of the psoas minor tendon on the surface of the major by having the client do a very small and isolated movement of bringing the pubic bone up toward the chest. The problem is that this movement may produce contraction in the larger psoas, and may also produce contraction in the abdominals, which can obscure your appreciation of the tiny psoas minor.

The final part of the psoas complex, the quadratus lumborum (QL), is best reached from a side-lying position. It is nearly impossible to affect this muscle approaching it posteriorly, as is commonly taught in manual therapy schools. A posterior approach may do wonders for the thoracolumbar fascia or the iliocostalis, but the QL is far too deep to reach from the back. Instead, walk your fingers along the inside of the iliac crest from the ASIS toward the back, and you will encounter a strong fascial line going superior and posterior toward the end of the 12th rib. This is the outer edge of the QL fascia, sometimes termed the lateral fascial raphe, and access to this outer edge, or the front surface just anterior to the edge, will allow you to lengthen this crucial structure. The use of a deep breath to facilitate release can be very helpful (www.anatomytrains.com – video ref: Deep Front Line, Part 1, 1:12:31–1:18:26).

🌸 🌼 A Branch Line: the 'Tail' of the Deep Front Line

From the medial arch to the psoas, the DFL follows the tradition of the other leg lines in having a right and left half, two separate myofascial guy-wires proceeding from the inner foot to the lumbar spine. These are presumably equal (though due to injury, postural deviation, or at minimum handedness and 'footedness', they seldom are). At the lumbar spine, the DFL more or less joins into a central line, which, as we move into the upper reaches of the DFL, we will parse as three separate lines from front to back, not right and left.

It is worth noting, however, that we have a possible third 'leg', or more properly 'tail' on the DFL, which we will describe here before proceeding upward. If we track down the DFL from the skull on the ALL, and instead of splitting right and left on the two psoases, we simply kept going on down the front of the spine (Fig. 9.31), we would pass down the lumbars between the two psoas complexes that initiate

the legs, and pass instead onto the front of the sacrum and to the anterior surface of the coccyx.

From here, the fascia keeps going in the same direction by means of the pubococcygeus muscle that passes forward to the posterior superior surface of the pubic tubercle and pubic symphysis in close proximity to the suspensory ligament of the bladder (Fig. 9.32). We have found this continuity in dissection.

Since the rectus abdominis is the deepest of the abdominal muscles at this point, fascially speaking, the fascia from the pelvic floor runs up to the posterior lamina of the rectus abdominis fascia so that our 'tail' is carried right up the ribs. On its way, it includes the umbilicus, thus linking into the many myofascial and visceral connections that radiate from there.

◆ ◆ The Pelvic Floor

Relative to this branch line, a second approach to the pelvic floor (the first appears above, in 'Palpation guide 2: lower posterior track', p. 155; techniques that involve entering body cavities are not included in this book) can be made from the pubic bone. Have your model lie supine with his knees up, and with a recently emptied bladder. This

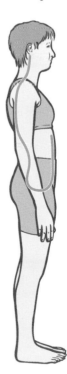

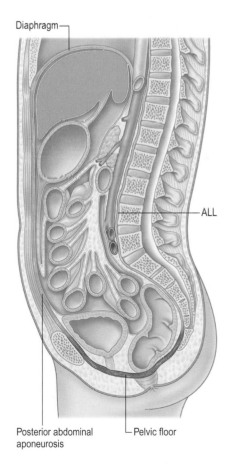

• **Fig. 9.31** The DFL passes down the mid-sagittal line as the anterior longitudinal ligament (ALL), which extends along the front of the sacrum and coccyx onto the pubococcygeus, the longitudinal muscle of the pelvic floor, a myofascial tail on the spine.

• **Fig. 9.32** If we follow the anterior longitudinal ligament down the midline to the tailbone we can continue onto the central raphe of the pelvic floor, across the levator ani to the back of the pubic bone and on up onto the posterior abdominal fascia behind the rectus.

palpation requires that we reach the posterior side of the pubic bone, and by an indirect route. Place the fingertips of both hands on the belly about halfway between the top of the pubis and the navel. Sink gently down into the abdomen toward the back. Desist in the face of any visceral pain.

Now curl your fingertips down toward the model's feet to come behind the pubic bone. Have your client gently bring the pubic bone up over your fingertips toward his head, pushing from the feet to avoid the use of the abdominal muscles (which, if used, will push you out). Then flex your fingertips up gently to come into contact with the back of the pubic bone (Fig. 9.33). Your fingers are now curled in a half circle, as if you are holding a suitcase handle. When you can find this spot properly, especially in someone whose body is open enough to allow you to get there easily, you can almost lift the 'suitcase' of the pelvis off the table by this 'handle'.

When you have contact with this aspect of the pubic bone, have your model squeeze the pelvic floor, and you and he both should be able to feel the contraction where the pelvic floor attaches to the posterior superior edge of the pubis. The connection between the pelvic floor and the rectus abdominis is also clear in this position. This access can be used to loosen the too tight anterior pelvic floor, or to encourage increased tone in those with a weak pelvic floor or urinary incontinence (www.anatomytrains.com – video ref: Deep Front Line, Part 2).

To attain the proper placement, it is important to start high enough in the belly. The direct approach – starting at the pubic hair level and trying to dive directly behind the bone – will not work. In clients with a tough layer of fat, overdeveloped abdominals, or in those not accustomed to intra-abdominal work, successive tries and reassuring words may help achieve this contact.

NOTE: Even this palpation (let alone work) is contraindicated in anyone with a bladder or any lower abdominal infection.

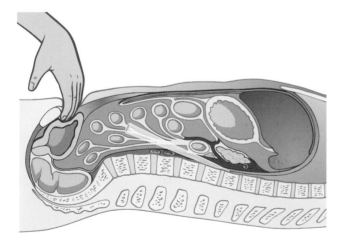

• **Fig. 9.33** The fascial connection between the abdominal fasciae and the pelvic floor behind the pubic bone is a potent spot for structural change, but must be approached with caution and sensitivity.

The Umbilicus

The umbilicus is a rich source of emotional connections as well as fascial ones, being the source of all nourishment for the first nine months of life (Fig. 9.34). Although the umbilicus is easily reached on the front of the abdominal fascial planes, the holding and adhesions are most often in the posterior laminae of the abdominal fascia, so we must find our way behind the rectus abdominis. This layer is in contact with the peritoneum, and therefore has many connections into the visceral space, including connections to the mesocolon, bladder, and the falciform ligament dividing the liver.

To reach these layers, position your model supine with the knees up, and find the outer edge of the rectus. If it is hard to feel in a relaxed state, having your client lift the head and upper chest to look at your hands will bring the edge into relief. Position your hands with elbows wide, palms down, and the fingertips pointing toward each other under the edges of each rectus. Bring your fingers slowly together, being sure that the rectus muscle – not just fat tissue – is ceilingward of your fingers. (If you have very short fingernails, you can do this palpation and technique in the supinated, palms up position, which is easier. If you do not have short fingernails, know that fingernail marks in the abdominal tissues take a long while to fade, so be advised.)

When you feel your fingertips in contact with each other, the fascia of the transversus and peritoneum on the inner aspect of the umbilicus will be between your fingers. Gauge your pressure – even minimal pressure can be painful or emotionally challenging to some clients. Getting truly informed consent from and staying engaged with the client, lift the umbilicus toward the ceiling and/or toward the client's head. Again, this stretch can be distressing, so go slowly, letting

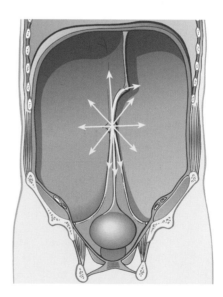

• **Fig. 9.34** A view looking forward at the posterior of the belly wall. The umbilicus, not surprisingly, since it is the fundamental source of nourishment for our first 9 months of life, has numerous fascial connections in all directions.

the tissue release gradually before moving more into the stretch. Having the client maintain their breathing is very important during this move (www.anatomytrains.com – video ref: Deep Front Line, Part 2, 27:30–32:26). Although challenging, the results in increased breath or even a flood of relieved tears are worth it.

The Upper Posterior Track

From each psoas and quadratus lumborum, we could track up to their respective domes of the diaphragm, and even up into the pleural fascia around each lung, which leads to the scalene group on the left and right sides of the neck. This was explored at the end of Ch. 5 as a deep track within the Lateral Line (p. 85). In this chapter, we focus on the structures closer to the midline.

Once we have reached the thoracic level, the diaphragm offers us the opportunity to continue upward through the thoracic cavity on any of three alternate lines: anterior, middle, and posterior. The most posterior of these lines is the most simple and profound, and can be easily traced anatomically, but not manually. Keep following the anterior longitudinal ligament all the way up the front of the spine to the occiput. This posterior line would include the two muscles that attach to the ALL, the longus capitis and longus colli, as well as the tiny rectus capitis anterior (Fig. 9.35).

Also associated with this upper posterior track are the scalene muscles, especially the fascia on their profound side, near the thoracic inlet. Before (see Ch 5.), we looked at the scalenes in their role in rib and lung support. Here we look at them as part of neck and head stabilization.

The middle and posterior scalenes, which are incompletely separated in most people) act more like a 'quadratus cervicorum': stabilizing the head in lateral flexion much as the quadratus lumborum does for the lumbar spine. The anterior scalene, however, is angled forward and can join in the 'forward head' club, pulling the TPs of the middle and lower cervicals closer to the 1st rib, creating or maintaining the conditions for lower cervical flexion/upper cervical hyperextension (or rotation, if the shortness is one-sided) (www.anatomytrains.com – video ref: Deep Front Line, Part 2, 50:41–58:17 and see also Fig. 5.17, p. 84). Work done to free the sternocleidomastoid (SCM) and suboccipital muscles should precede and be accompanied by work with the anterior scalene.

The top of this posterior track of the DFL joins into the 'topmost vertebra', the occiput, on its basilar portion just in front of the body of the atlas and the foramen magnum.

The Longus Capitis, Longus Colli, and Scalene Muscles

The longus capitis and colli are unique among the muscles of the neck in their ability to counteract neck hyperextension. Both the SBL (obviously) and the SFL (through the common but improper use of the sternocleidomastoid muscle) have the tendency to produce hyperextension in the upper cervicals (Fig. 9.36) (www.anatomytrains.com – video ref: Deep Front Line, Part 2, 58:18–1:02:49). Though the infrahyoid muscles (see Fig. 9.45) could conceivably be used to counteract this tendency, they are too small and too involved in the fluctuating movements of speaking and swallowing to counteract the steady postural pull of such large muscles. Thus it falls to the DFL, and the longus capitis and longus colli in particular (with support from below, of course), to take a large role in maintaining the proper alignment of the head, neck, and upper back. And thus it falls to the manual practitioner or somatic educator

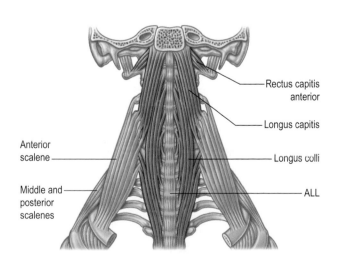

• **Fig. 9.35** The upper posterior track of the DFL is the simplest – just follow the anterior longitudinal ligament up the front of the vertebral bodies all the way to the basilar portion of the occiput. Along the way, this track includes the longus capitis, longus colli, and the rectus capitis anterior muscles.

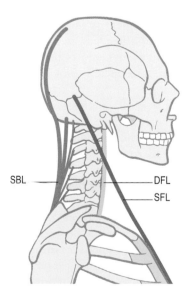

• **Fig. 9.36** The SFL and SBL can both be involved in postural hyperextension of the upper cervicals. It falls to the DFL to restrain this common postural tendency by providing a counterbalancing flexion to the upper cervicals.

to reawaken and tonify these muscles in the client with hyperextended upper cervicals, or to loosen them in the less common case of the 'military neck', or over-flexed upper cervicals.

The longus capitis and longus colli may seem beyond reach, but by carefully following the directions given here, it is possible to affect them. With your model lying on her back with the knees up, and you sitting at the head of the table, put your fingertips on the back edge of the SCM, in the triangle between the anterior edge of the trapezius and the posterior edge of the SCM. Gently lift the SCM forward and up with the fingernail side, and contact the outer fascia of the harder 'motor cylinder' – the scalene fascia in this instance. Slide your fingerpads forward and medial along the front of the scalene fascia until you reach the TPs of the cervical vertebrae. Pressing is not required. Any nerve referral from the brachial plexus or color change in the client's face is reason enough to desist and seek hands-on guidance. The fingers simply slide forward and in from behind the SCM up onto the front of the TPs, if the client's openness allows it (www.anatomytrains.com – video ref: Deep Front Line, Part 2, 58:18–1:01:27).

From the front of the TPs, these muscles can be loosened in those with a military, overly straight cervical curve, or encouraged into action for those with hyperlordotic upper cervicals (www.anatomytrains.com – video ref: Deep Front Line, Part 2, 1:01:27–1:02:39). Lifting the head will obviously engage these muscles, but a more subtle, postural toning comes from lifting both feet off the table.

To counter hyperextended cervicals, simply ask the client to slowly flatten their neck to the table, not lifting their head but sliding the back of it up the table toward you. This can be assisted by the client's pressure on her feet, flattening the lumbar and cervical curves. Your fingers follow the neck vertebrae down toward the table, keeping your client aware of these muscles and this area. Verbal encouragement is fine, but manual encouragement is not – pushing of the neck vertebrae is not recommended, as this can create serious problems. It is the client's efforts here that produce the results; the therapist is merely providing awareness of a long-disused area.

As elsewhere, stay off anything with a vascular pulse in it. This method is designed to take you into the front of the cervical spine and its fascial layers, but behind the carotid artery, jugular vein, and vagus nerve imbedded in the alar fascia. Moving slowly and cautiously, and without pressure, will help assure your adherence to the Hippocratic Oath.

The middle and posterior scalenes are easily accessible to you through this same window between the trapezius and the SCM. The middle scalene is a prominent, and usually the most lateral, guitar string to be felt on the lateral midline of the bottom of the neck. The posterior scalene tucks into the pocket behind and medial to this middle scalene. These muscles are often incompletely separated in any case, and so can be treated as one – the quadratus lumborum of the neck, so to speak.

The posturally important anterior scalene – more like the psoas of the neck – can be reached by placing your fingertips close to the clavicle, and again lifting both heads of the SCM forward, out of the way, and sliding your fingertips underneath. Once again, nerve referral from the brachial plexus is a distinct possibility here when the fasciae are bound together, so move slowly and without pressure (www.anatomytrains.com – video ref: Deep Front Line, Part 2, 46:32–50:38), easing the adventitia away from the dense covering of the anterior scalene.

The anterior scalene is a band approximately half an inch wide, underneath and parallel to the clavicular head of the SCM. You should be able to feel it contract under your fingertips at either the beginning or end (depending on your model's breathing pattern) of a moderately deep inhale (www.anatomytrains.com – video ref: Deep Front Line, Part 2, 50:39–58:16). Once contacted the anterior scalene fascia can be 'hooked' toward the occiput in conjunction with the client's breath, using the same movement we used to engage the longus muscles above.

The Upper Middle Track

The middle track of the upper DFL follows the fibers of the diaphragm half-way up to the central tendon that spans between the high points of the two domes (Fig. 9.37). The central tendon blends with the pericardial sac around the heart and the accompanying tissues of the mediastinum, including the parietal pleura of the lungs, and the tissues surrounding the esophagus and pulmonary vasculature (Fig. 9.38). These tissues, like the diaphragm itself, also pass all the way back to join the ALL on the anterior surface of the thoracic vertebrae, but these middle tissues form a visceral line of pull worthy of separate consideration (Fig. 9.39).

As the fasciae which surround all this tubing emerge from the top of the rib cage at the thoracic inlet, they split to the left and right, following the neurovascular bundles into the Deep Front Arm Lines on each side (Fig. 9.40). The Deep Front Arm Lines are thus the expression of the DFL in the arms, such that axillary access to these tissues can lead to release in the thoracic tissues of the DFL.

Tissues from the dome of the pleura of the lungs reach up and back to hang from the TPs of the lower cervical vertebrae, associated with the inner aspect of the scalene muscles (scalenus minimus, or suspensory ligament of the lung), bringing this line once again in contact with the ALL/longus capitis part of the posterior line described above (see Fig. 9.35).

The major part of this middle line, however, passes up with the esophagus into the posterior side of the pharynx, including the pharyngeal constrictors, which can clearly be seen hanging from the median raphe of connective tissue in Fig. 9.41. This line also joins the occiput (and the temporal via the styloid muscles, see below), slightly more anterior than the upper posterior track, attaching to a small

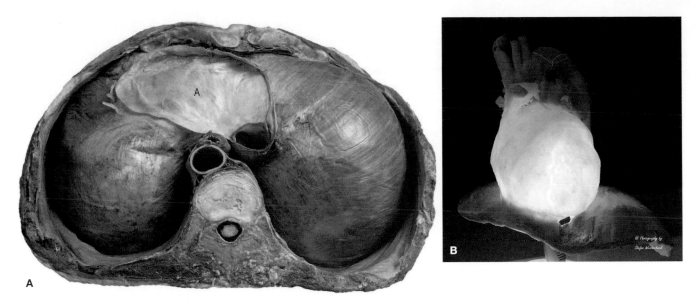

A

• **Fig. 9.37** (**A**) Viewing the diaphragm from above, we see how the pericardium, A, is firmly attached to the central tendon. The 'tubing' of the esophagus and vena cava would also be associated with this track. (**B**) A recent plastination showing the blending of the pericardium with the diaphragm, both of which arise from the septum transversum area in the embryo. (A, © Ralph T. Hutchings. Reproduced from Abrahams, et al. McMinn's color atlas of human anatomy, 3rd edn. Mosby; 1998. B, Photo courtesy of the Fascial Net Plastination Project/Fascia Research Society, photographer Stefan Westerback.)

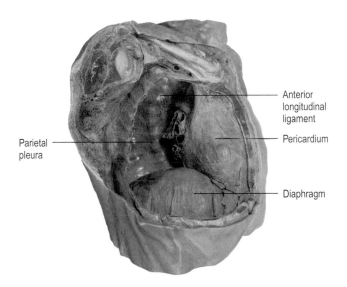

Parietal pleura — Anterior longitudinal ligament

— Pericardium

— Diaphragm

• **Fig. 9.38** From the central tendon of the diaphragm, the fascial continuity travels up the pericardium and parietal pleura of the lungs (here the left lung is removed), forming sheaths and supporting webbing around all the nerves and tubes of the pulmonary and systemic circulation. (© Ralph T. Hutchings. From Abrahams, et al. 1998.)

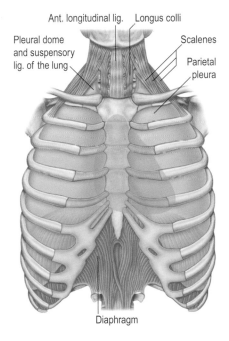

Ant. longitudinal lig.   Longus colli

Pleural dome and suspensory lig. of the lung   Scalenes

Parietal pleura

Diaphragm

• **Fig. 9.39** Seen from the front, the mediastinum between the heart and lungs connects the diaphragm to the thoracic inlet.

protuberance known as the clivus of the occiput, or pharyngeal tubercle. The posterior fascia of this middle branch of the DFL (the buccopharyngeal or visceral fascia) is separated from the posterior line (the anterior longitudinal ligament and prevertebral layer of cervical fascia) at this point by a sheet called the alar fascia that joins the right and left neurovascular sheaths (Fig. 9.42).

The Upper Anterior Track

The third and most anterior track of the DFL in the upper body follows the curve of the diaphragm all the way over to its anterior attachment at the xiphoid process at the bottom of the sternum (see Fig. 9.2, side view, upper anterior track, and www.anatomytrains.com – video ref: Deep

Front Line, Part 2: 32:29–38:37). This fascia connects to the fascia on the deep side of the sternum, although it requires a fairly sharp turn by Anatomy Trains standards from the nearly horizontal anteromedial portion of the diaphragm to the vertical endothoracic fascia on the posterior aspect of the sternum. We emphasize once again that all three of these tracks through the thorax are joined as one in the living body, and are being separated here for analysis only.

This fascia includes the serrated fan of the transversus thoracis muscle and by extension the entire plane of endothoracic fascia in front of the viscera but behind the costal cartilages (Fig. 9.43).

This line emerges from the rib cage just behind the manubrium of the sternum. This myofascial line clearly continues from this station with the infrahyoid muscles – the sternohyoid express covering the sternothyroid, thyrocricoid, and cricohyoid locals – up to the suspended hyoid bone itself (Fig. 9.44; Video 4.11).

This group is joined by that odd leftover from the operculum, the omohyoid, which functions in speaking, swallowing, and also to form a protective tent around the jugular vein and carotid artery during strong contractions of the surrounding neck muscles.

From the hyoid, the stylohyoid connects back to the styloid process of the temporal bone. The digastric muscle manages to go both up and forward to the chin as well as up and back to the medial aspect of the mastoid process. It even manages to avoid dirtying its hands by touching the hyoid at all – two slings of fascia reach up from the hyoid,

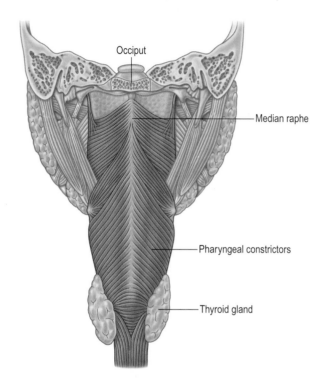

• **Fig. 9.41** A posterior view of the upper middle track of the DFL – the back of the throat, including the pharyngeal constrictors supported by the median raphe which hangs from the clivus of the occiput.

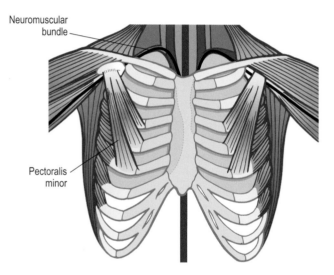

• **Fig. 9.40** The DFL connects to the myofascia of the Deep Front Arm Line, following the path of the neurovascular bundle.

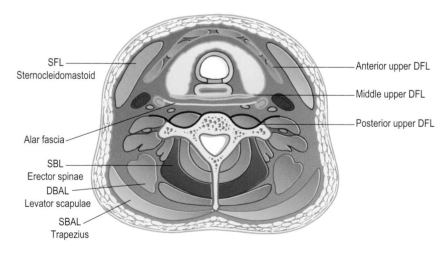

• **Fig. 9.42** A cross-section through the neck reveals the related but still distinct posterior, middle, and anterior tracks of the DFL.

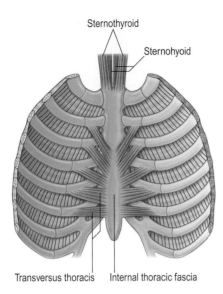

Sternothyroid

Sternohyoid

Transversus thoracis   Internal thoracic fascia

• **Fig. 9.43** This upper anterior track includes the transversus thoracis, that odd and variable muscle on the inside of the front of the ribs which supports the costal cartilages and can contract the chest when we are cold.

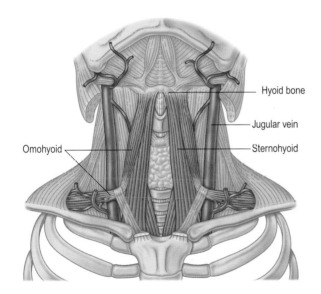

Hyoid bone

Jugular vein

Sternohyoid

Omohyoid

• **Fig. 9.44** The infrahyoid muscles emerge from behind the sternum, joining the inside of the ribs to the front of the throat and the hyoid bone (Video 4.11).

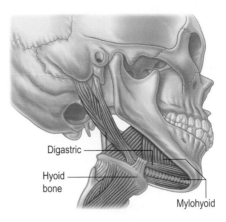

Digastric

Hyoid bone

Mylohyoid

• **Fig. 9.45** From the hyoid bone, there are connections both forward to the jaw and back to the temporal bone of the cranium.

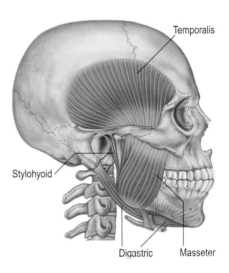

Temporalis

Stylohyoid

Digastric   Masseter

• **Fig. 9.46** Though the case for a direct connection from the delicate suprahyoid muscles to the strong jaw muscles is difficult to make, there is definitely a mechanical connection from the floor of the mouth to the jaw muscles to the facial and cranial bones. (www.anatomytrains.com – video ref: Anatomy Trains Revealed: Deep Front Line.)

allowing the digastric to pull straight up on the whole tracheal apparatus when swallowing. By these two muscles, this most anterior branch of the DFL is connected to the temporal bone of the neurocranium (Fig. 9.45).

Two muscles, the mylohyoid and geniohyoid, accompany the digastric in passing up and forward to the inside of the mandible, just behind the chin. These two form the floor of the mouth under the tongue. (It is interesting to note the parallel between the construction of the floor of the mouth and that of the floor of the pelvis, in which the geniohyoid equates with the pubococcygeus, and the mylohyoid equates with the iliococcygeus.)

From these hyoid muscles, we could claim a mechanical connection through the mandible (though a direct 'fibers in the same direction' connection is a little harder to justify) with the muscles that close the jaw (Fig. 9.46). The masseter, which lifts up from the zygomatic arch, and the medial pterygoid, which lifts up from the underside of the sphenoid, together form a sling for the angle of the jaw (Fig. 9.47), thus connecting with the floor of the mouth. The temporalis has only a mechanical connection with the rest of the line through the mandible, pulling straight up on the coronoid process of the mandible from a broad attachment on the temporal bone. The temporalis fascia runs across the skull coronally under the galea aponeurotica, the scalp

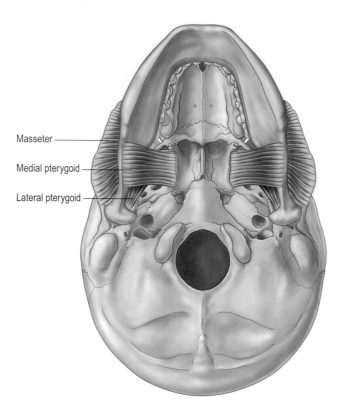

• **Fig. 9.47** Seen from below, the essential sling for the ramus of the mandible created by the two masseters acting in concert with the two medial pterygoids is unmistakable.

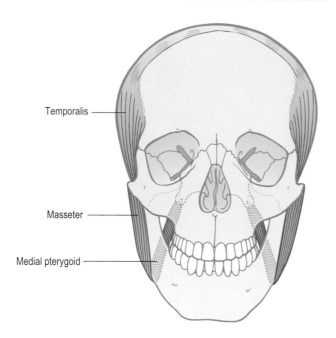

• **Fig. 9.48** The upper reaches of the DFL includes the sling created by the masseter on the outside and the medial pterygoid on the inside, and the fascia from the temporalis which loops up over the head beneath the galea aponeurotica of the SBL.

fascia that was involved in the SFL, SBL, LL, and SPL (Fig. 9.48).

Thus we see the complex core of the body's myofascia, snaking up the 'hidden' places in the inner legs, passing through the leg pit into the trunk to join the tissues in front of the spine. From here, we have seen it split (at least for analysis) into three major routes: behind the viscera directly in front of the spine, up through the viscera themselves, and up in front of the viscera to the throat and face.

DISCUSSION 9.1

❖ ❖ ❖ ❖ The Deep Front Line and Stability in the Legs

In the posture of the lower leg, the DFL structures tend to act as counterbalance to the Lateral Line structures (Fig. 9.49). The fibularii (peroneals), when locked short, tend to create an everted, or pronated ankle, or a laterally rotated forefoot. While the tibialis anterior has been seen to counterbalance the fibularis longus in the Spiral Line, so does the tibialis posterior. If the muscles of the deep posterior compartment are over-shortened, they tend to create an inverted or supinated ankle, or a medially rotated forefoot. Together, these myofascia help to stabilize the tibia–fibula over the ankle, and maintain the inner arch.

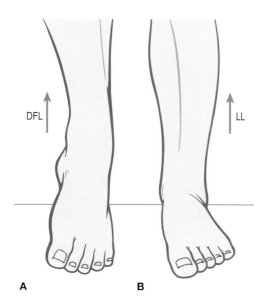

• **Fig. 9.49** In the lower legs, the Lateral Line and DFL are antagonists: when the DFL is too short, the feet tend toward supinated and inverted (**A**); when the Lateral Line becomes chronically short, the feet tend toward the pronated and everted (**B**).

At the knee, the DFL and LL counterbalance each other like bowstrings on either side of the leg (Fig. 9.50). When the legs are bowed ('O' legs, laterally shifted knees, *genu varus*), the DFL structures in the lower leg and thigh will be found to be short, and the LL structures, the iliotibial tract and fibularii, will be under tensile strain, with fascia in the locked long position. In the case of knock knees ('X' legs, medially shifted knees, *genu valgus*), the reverse will be true: the lateral structures will be locked short, and the DFL structures will be strained, or locked long. Pain will tend to occur on the strained side, but the side that needs work is that with the short bowstring. In short, work with the fascia on the outside of the knocked knees and open the inner line to ease bowed legs.

In the thigh, the adductor muscles enclosed by the anterior and posterior septa also act to counterbalance the abductors of the LL, and any imbalance can often be seen by checking the relative position of tissues on the inside and outside of the knee, including the tissues of the thigh above the knee (Fig. 9.51). In terms of directionality, with knock-knee patterns the adductor fascia tends to be pulled down toward the knee, and with bow-legged patterns the DFL tends to be pulled up the inseam of the leg into the hip – but these are generalities, not hard-and-fast rules, so you must look.

In regard to pelvic position, it is helpful to consider the septa themselves as structures worthy of consideration (Fig. 9.52). In an anteriorly tilted pelvis, the front septum is often short and glued down to both adjacent muscle groups, and requires lengthening along with adductor longus and brevis. In this case, the posterior septum is under strain and lifted, and its fascial plane should be induced to come caudally (Video 6.24). In a posteriorly tilted pelvis, the reverse is true: the anterior plane often needs to be brought inferiorly; the posterior septum needs to be free from the pelvic floor as well as from the deep lateral rotators and other adjacent muscle groups. In this way, the anterior septum can be thought of as an extension of the psoas, and the posterior septum an extension of the deep lateral rotators, the piriformis specifically, and pelvic floor, associated with the adductor magnus muscle.

DISCUSSION 9.2

❖ ✿ ✿ The Middle of the Deep Front Line and Visceral Manipulation

The endothoracic tissues of the DFL, from the diaphragmatic crura to the thoracic inlet, are not available to be

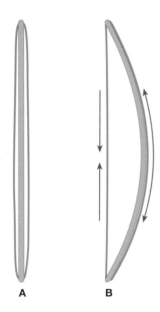

• **Fig. 9.50** When the tensile tissues on the inside or outside of the legs are tightened, the skeletal structure of the leg responds like the wooden bow, bending away from the contracture, and causing strain to the tissues on the convex side. The type of interaction between the DFL and the LL is active in knock-knees and bow legs (genu varus and valgus).

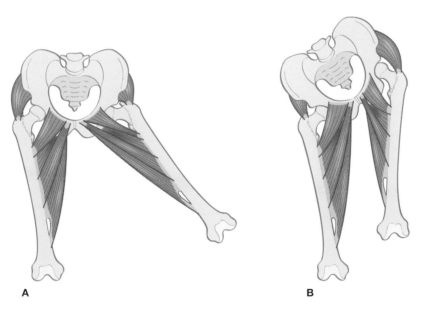

• **Fig. 9.51** The adductors balance the abductors in side-to-side issues in the thigh and hip. In this diagram, notice how the abductors are shorter on the side with the lower iliac crest. Somewhat counter-intuitively, the adductors of the DFL tend to be shorter on the high hip side.

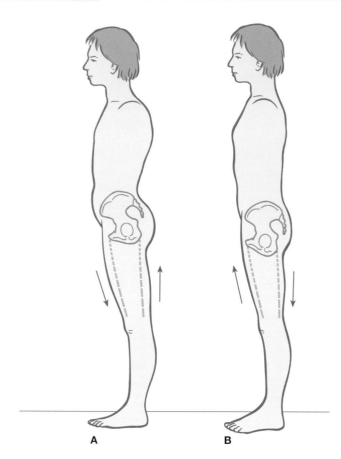

A   **B**

• **Fig. 9.52** In assessing the relative tilt of the pelvis, it is worthwhile considering the anterior (medial) and posterior intermuscular septa of the thigh as guy-wires that can exert a restriction on the flexion–extension excursion of the pelvis.

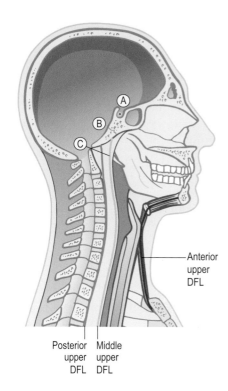

Anterior upper DFL

Posterior upper DFL   Middle upper DFL

• **Fig. 9.53** At the upper pole of the DFL, we see a close approximation among important structures deriving from the three germ layers.

reached by direct manipulative work. The entire rib cage forms a box in which there is always a negative pressure, pulling the tissues out against the ribs and attempting to pull the ribs in. These areas are amenable to indirect work, however, via the scalenes and neck fasciae from above, or via the peritoneum, the lower edge of the rib cage, or the psoas from below.

They may also be affected by the techniques of Visceral Manipulation. These techniques are found in some Asian abdominal methods, and ably set forth in several books by the developer of Visceral Manipulation, the French osteopath Jean-Pierre Barral.[10,11]

DISCUSSION 9.3

✿ The Upper Pole of the DFL and the Ecto-, Meso-, Endodermal Connection

The very top of the DFL is a fascinating physiological crossroads. The posterior track of the anterior longitudinal ligament joins just anterior to the foramen magnum, the middle track of the pharynx joins just anterior to that, and the anterior track of the laryngo-hyoid complex joins, among other attachments, to the lower extensions of the sphenoid via the medial pterygoid.

It is tempting to note the proximity of these points to central structures deriving from the embryonic ectoderm, mesoderm, and endoderm. Sitting literally in the saddle of the sphenoid (sella turcica), the hypothalamus–pituitary axis is a central junction box of both the fluid and the neural body, of primarily ectodermal derivation (Fig. 9.53A). This so-called 'master gland' sits below the circle of Willis, acting as the sommelier of our fluid system, tasting the blood delivered fresh from the heart and adding its powerful hormonal spices and autonomic motor responses to the mix.

Just behind and below this lies the synchondrosis of the sphenobasilar junction, a central fulcrum of the craniosacral rhythm, itself a central feature of the fibrous body, the mesodermal body – the collagenous net and all the vascular pulses that produce the fluid waves (Figs. 9.53B and 9.54).[12–14]

Just behind and below this (but all within a couple of centimeters) lies the top of the pharynx, the central and original gullet of the endodermal tube, where the pharyngeal raphe joins the occipital base (see Fig. 9.53C). Humans are uniquely situated so that the direction of the gut (basically vertical from mouth to anus) and the direction of voluntary movement (basically horizontally forward) are not the same. In our human faces, 'bite' has been subordinated to 'sight', and the gut hangs from this crucial center at the bottom of the skull. Few other animals have so

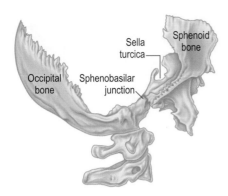

• **Fig. 9.54** The sphenobasilar junction (SBJ) is a crucial hinge of the craniosacral pulse, where the 'bodies' of the occipital and sphenoidal 'vertebrae' meet.

completely divorced the line of sight and motion from the line of direction of the spine and gut. This is at least possibly one source of our psychosomatic split from the rest of the animal world.[15]

One wonders about the communication among these anterior 'junction boxes'. Can pursing the lips for receiving a kiss or a strawberry, or the tensing of the tongue that accompanies 'disgust' be felt in the sphenobasilar junction, or perceived by the pituitary? One can at least imagine an inter-regulatory function among these three major systems proceeding from this point of proximity down the entire organism via the central nervous system, the submucosal plexus, the cranial pulse, or the long myofascial continuity we have traced here from face and tongue to inner ankle.

References

1. Myers T. Fans of the hip joint. *Massage Magazine*. 1998;75:38–43. Or in Body³, *privately published 2003 and available at*: www.anatomytrains.com.
2. Schleip R. *Lecture Notes on the Adductors and Psoas*. Rolf Lines: Rolf Institute; 1988:14–17. www.somatics.de. 11/88.
3. Myers T. The psoas pseries. *Massage and Bodywork*. 1993. Mar–Nov. *Also in* Anatomist's Corner, *self-published in 2007 and available via*: www.anatomytrains.com.
4. Morrison M. *Further Thoughts on Femur Rotation and the Psoas*. Rolf Lines: Rolf Institute; 2002:8–11. www.anatomytrains.net. M 4/01.
5. Bogduk N. *Clinical Anatomy of the Lumbar Spine and Sacrum*. 3rd ed. Edinburgh: Churchill Livingstone; 1997:102.
6. Rolf I. *Rolfing*. Rochester, VT: Healing Arts Press; 1989:170.
7. Murphy M. *Notes for a Workshop on the Psoas*. 1992. Unpublished.
8. Myers T. Poise: psoas-piriformis balance. *Massage Magazine*. 1998. (Mar/Apr). *Or in* Body³, *privately published 2003 and available at*: www.anatomytrains.com.
9. Simons D, Travell J, Simons L. *Myofascial Pain and Dysfunction: The Trigger Point Manual*. Vol. 1. 2nd ed. upper half of body. Baltimore: William & Wilkins; 1998.
10. Barral JP, Mercier P. *Urogenital Manipulation*. Seattle: Eastland Press; 1988.
11. Schwind P. *Fascial and Membrane Technique*. Edinburgh: Churchill Livingstone; 2006.
12. Upledger J, Vredevoogd J. *Craniosacral Therapy*. Chicago: Eastland Press; 1983.
13. Milne H. *The Heart of Listening*. Berkeley: North Atlantic Books; 1995.
14. Meert G. *Venolymphatic Drainage Therapy*. Edinburgh: Churchill Livingstone; 2012.
15. Kass L. *The Hungry Soul*. New York: Macmillan; 1994.

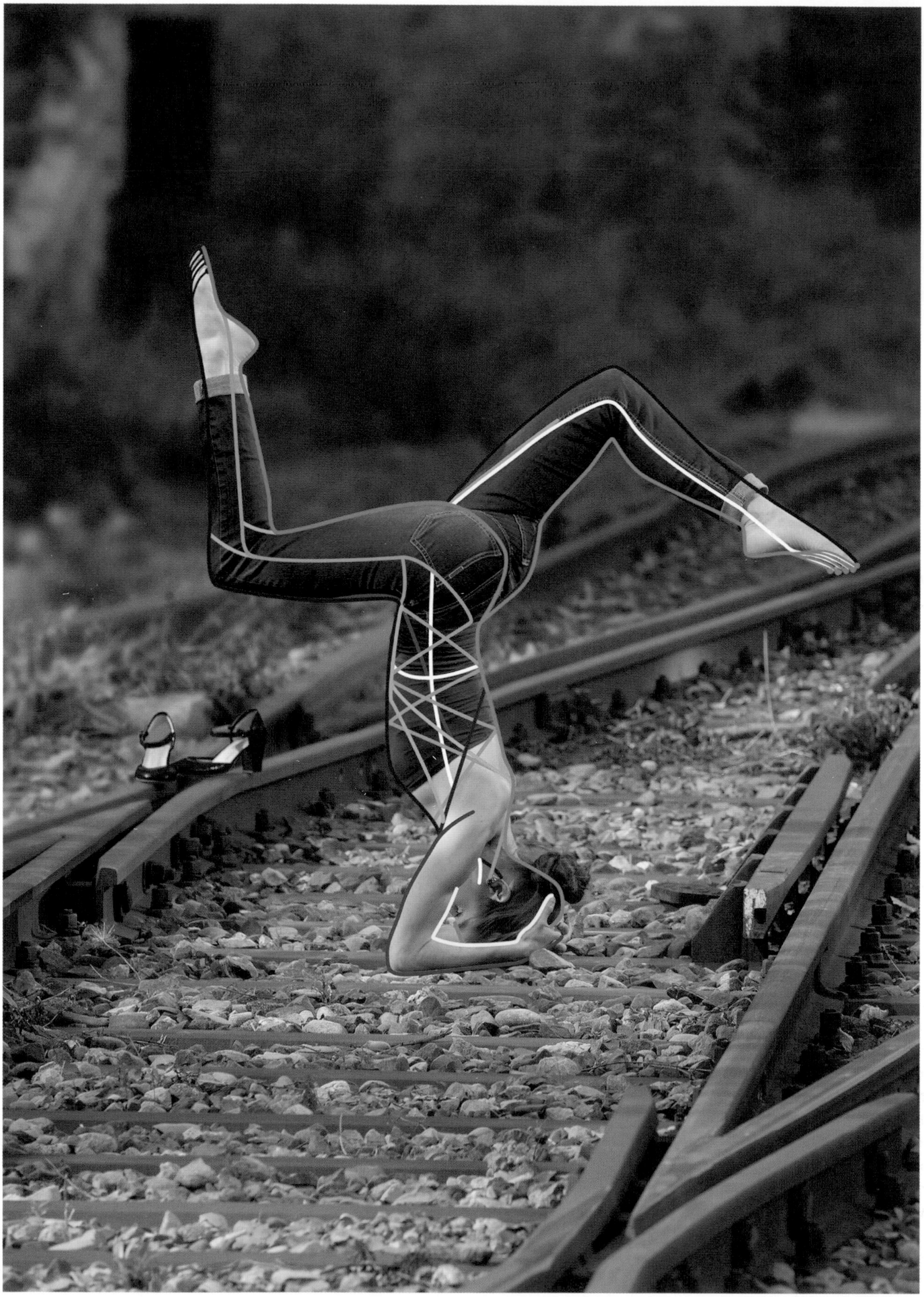

• **Fig. 10.1** Anatomy Trains in motion

10
Anatomy Trains in Movement

WITH CONTRIBUTIONS BY JAMES EARLS AND KARIN GURTNER

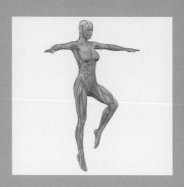

With the entire suite of 12 myofascial meridians delineated, this chapter outlines some of the applications and implications of the Anatomy Trains scheme in movement training and therapy.

Given that movement is now recognized as a form of medicine, or even an essential 'nutrient' contributing to our health, movement education has leverage in three primary social areas:[1]

- physical education for the young, early and in school
- the wide spectrum of rehabilitation (anything that turns a negative into a neutral)
- performance enhancement, which in turn parses into:
  - sports and athletics on one side;
  - artistic expression (dance, theater, music) on the other (Fig. 10.1).

Each of these sectors contributes to the health of the populace. Given the impoverished state of movement education worldwide, improvement in each arena is vitally important to active longevity.[2] Across the world, body usage, movement integration and postural faults are widely ignored, yet change could be easily effected within existing institutions.

Most educational systems focus on visual and auditory learning, with few resources left over to expand a curriculum of 'kinesthetic literacy'.[3] We are familiar with building and testing IQ, and we are becoming ever more familiar with 'EQ' – emotional intelligence. A similar effort needs to be made with 'KQ' – somatic intelligence. What is the topology of movement skills? Which of those are necessary to a long and successful life? What do our clients/students/patients need as basic movement literacy to negotiate their inner and outer environment? A likely but unfortunate event these days is that we often emerge from the educational system with more knowledge about external subjects than we have about our most proximate, ever-present, and intimate tool – our bodies in motion.

A few coins per child given toward better physical education could yield a large benefit in terms of reduced medical costs and higher levels of health and performance. A few dollars per patient could improve integration of rehabilitation and prevent relapses for all manner of physical injury or post-surgical recovery. Where the dollars are being spent – in athletics – insights are being gained that could be applied more widely in education and rehabilitation if there were improved cross-pollination and means of dissemination this new information.

We can all benefit from more coordination among movement professionals, from orthopedists to the more 'mindful' preventive practices. Too many practitioners rely on only one point of view, either blindly believing in received oral lore, or insisting on 'evidence base' over clinical experience at the other. Differing professions use the same word for different events, or conversely different terms for the same event – e.g., ask different professional groups to define the word 'stretch'.[4] A 'unified field' – a coherent theoretical basis – in the movement therapies would do much to advance all the modalities within it.

The intent of Anatomy Trains is to provide a platform for dialogue, the basis of a common language of wholeness within which to examine human structure and functional movement.

Although Anatomy Trains was developed out of the author's experience of mapping global patterns of postural compensation (see Ch. 11 and the appendices which follow, aimed more at structurally oriented manual therapy), many movement-based therapies and training methods such as physiotherapy, rehabilitative exercise, Pilates, yoga, and performance-based personal and team training have found value in using the Anatomy Trains map to reveal the inner workings of the stability/mobility equation.

Accordingly, here we explore some simple applications of Anatomy Trains to common foundational movement patterns. This chapter also includes a section on walking from our path-forging colleague James Earls[5] and another on contemporary movement from Karin Gurtner, the strongest of willows. Additional material from earlier editions and supplementary videos are available via the accompanying eBook at www.expertconsult.com and www.anatomytrains.com.

Additionally, movement professionals will find applicable research information in Appendix 1, especially the sections on fascial properties in fitness training, sensory neurology in skill acquisition, and remodeling responses to intervention or injury.

Applications of Anatomy Trains in Movement

Although applications for both movement and manual therapy have been interspersed throughout the preceding chapters, the specific sequencing of soft-tissue releases or movement education strategies is left to in-person training.[6] This book is primarily designed to aid the reader in observing these body-wide myofascial patterns, so that currently held skills and treatment protocols can be applied globally in novel ways.

None of the forays that follow is intended to be in any way exhaustive, but merely to guide the reader a little way down the road toward the variety of possible uses for the scheme, both as self-help and in the healing/performance/rehabilitation professions.

Still photographs are a frustrating way to go about assessing movement, but are necessitated by the form of a book. Assessing clients in standing is explored more deeply in the next chapter, and in-person classes. (Digital courses in motion assessment are available: www.anatomytrains.com, www.astonenterprises.com) (www.anatomytrains.com – video ref: BodyReading, 101).

Anatomy Trains is not primarily a theory of movement, but simply a map of how stability is maintained and strain distributed across the body during movement. Few movements are made with a myofascial meridian as a whole, but most movements require stabilization throughout an entire line (Video 6.25).

For instance, put one foot on top of the other as you sit, and attempt to lift the lower foot against the upper by lifting the knee. Although the rectus femoris and psoas major may be the muscles primarily responsible for attempting to move the leg, the entire Superficial Front and Deep Front Lines, of which these muscles are part, will tense some muscles to 'pre-stress' the fascia from toes to hip. This can be felt by the discerning into the belly, sternum, and neck. This kind of stabilizing isometry and strain distribution goes on mostly under the radar of conscious awareness, but is vitally necessary for the effective 'anchoring' in one part that forms the basis of successful movement for another.

Similarly in standing, let your weight shift forward into your forefoot to feel the Superficial Back Line stiffen fascially as a whole, no matter which muscles are actually involved in the movement. Stand on a single foot to feel the interplay between the Lateral Line and the Deep Front Line – both of which will be immediately 'denser' to the touch all the way to the hip and beyond – as they manage the inside–outside balance of the leg as the weight shifts second-by-second on the medial and lateral arches of the foot.

You can use your knowledge of the lines to see how compensations or inefficient postures are inhibiting integrated movement or effective strength in the moving body. In general, one wants to see:

- Each line and 'track' within the line able to either lengthen or contract from its resting length, i.e. the line should be neither concentrically nor eccentrically overloaded when at rest.
- Even tone along the length of the lines. Structural isolation is the opposite of integration, so areas of hypertone or hypotone should be evened out through stretching, bodywork, or strength work.
- Each line should be able to stabilize segmental arrangement in a neutral position while the action is being performed, e.g. in a lateral kick in football (soccer), the abdominals in the Lateral Line should have sufficient tone on both sides to keep the rib cage in place so that the force of the kick is not robbed by rotation or sideshift of the ribs.

To get our eyes used to seeing this way, let us begin with some fairly simple analyses of some classical sculpture, before moving on to more functional applications.

Classical Sculpture

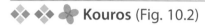 ### Kouros (Fig. 10.2)

Aside from the modern and extraordinarily functional example of Fred Astaire, this pre-classical sculpture represents, to this author's eye, the most compelling example of poise and balance among the Anatomy Trains lines – better even than the Albinus figure that served for many years as the Anatomy Trains 'brand' (see Fig. 1.1A). This Kouros (lad) – one of many such sculptures from the pre-classical period – presents a balanced tensegrity between the skeletal and myofascial structure rarely seen today; in fact rarely seen in art after this period. The muscles and bones are represented a bit massively for modern taste, but the whole neuromyofascial web 'hangs together' with a calm ease that nevertheless manages to convey a total readiness for action – in other words, ideal balance in the autonomic nervous system expressed in the shape of the neuromyofascial web.

Notice the length and support through the core Deep Front Line (DFL) that imparts support up the inner line of the leg and throughout the trunk. Notice the balance of soft-tissues between the inside and outside of the knee. See the ease with which the head sits on the neck, and the shoulders drape over the upright rib cage. There is distinct muscle definition, but the connection along the lines is not lost or overcome. We could do worse, as a culture, than to work toward a physical education system that would generate bodies approaching this functional ideal.

Bronze Zeus (Fig. 10.3)

This sculpture shows the body beautifully poised for martial action. Though it is probably blasphemous to reduce Zeus to a lines analysis, we will risk the thunderbolt he looks ready to hurl to note how he stabilizes his body for maximum effect. The improbably long left arm is held out along the line of his sight, suspended by the Superficial Back Arm Line, counterbalancing the weight of the right arm held behind. The right arm grips the bolt or spear with

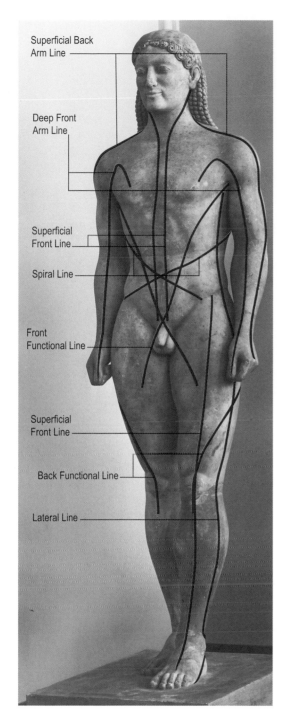

• **Fig. 10.2** Kouros. The pre-classical Kouroi series of sculptures shows close to ideal 'coordinated fascial tensegrity' – balance and proper placement for the Anatomy Trains lines. (Reproduced with kind permission from Hirmer Fotoarkiv.)

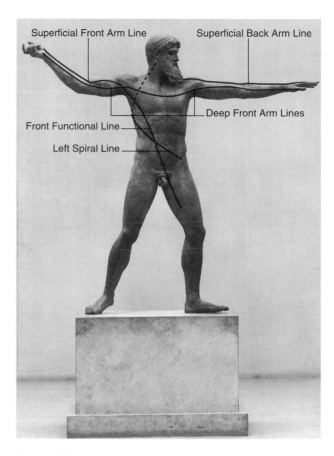

• **Fig. 10.3** Zeus. Most martial or sportive actions involve connecting the arm to the opposite leg to increase leverage. (Reproduced with kind permission from Hirmer Fotoarkiv.)

The right leg is contracting along the Superficial Back Line, pushing onto the ball of the foot and extending the hip to start the body on its forward path, pushing the weight onto the stable left leg. The left leg is planted firmly, the knee slightly bent, with stabilizing tension along all four leg lines, so that the left Spiral Line and right Front Functional Line, which are both anchored to the left leg, can assist the two front Arm Lines in imparting forward momentum to the right shoulder and arm.

Because he is clearly throwing along the horizontal plane, the two Lateral Lines are quite balanced with each other. By this we can infer that it is being thrown for accuracy over a short distance (compare to the 'Hail Mary' throw in Fig. 8.3, where the Arm Lines are also strongly assisted by the Spiral and Functional Lines). Were it to be thrown earthward from heaven, the left Lateral Line would necessarily shorten and the other lines adjust to angle the bolt downward.

Heracles (Fig. 10.4)

Here we see a weary Hercules, leaning on his club and resting from his labors, so it may be unfair to subject him to a critical lines analysis. This representation, however, is typical of classical art, and it provides a clear contrast with the pre-classical Kouros and Zeus.

both thumb and fingers, engaging both the Superficial and Deep Front Arm Lines, thus linking into both the pectoralis major and minor across the front of the chest to the opposite side. This connection allows the front of the outstretched arm to counterbalance and provide a base for the throw; they will reverse their position but stay connected during the throw itself.

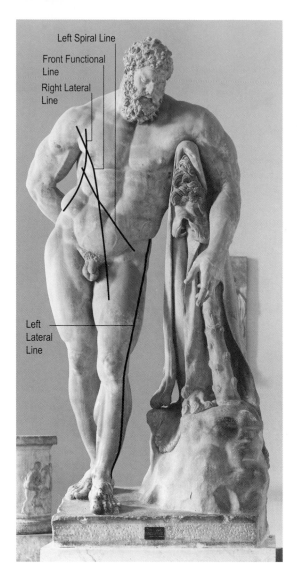

Left Spiral Line

Front Functional Line

Right Lateral Line

Left Lateral Line

• **Fig. 10.4** Herakles (Heracles, Hercules). The classical Herakles shows a shortening of the core and asymmetrical imbalance among the lines. (Reproduced with kind permission from Hirmer Fotoarkiv.)

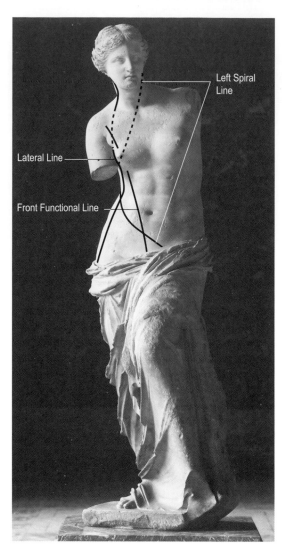

Left Spiral Line

Lateral Line

Front Functional Line

• **Fig. 10.5** Aphrodite de Melos (Venus de Milo). Any seductive pose will involve asymmetrical shortening of the helical lines. (Reproduced with kind permission from Hirmer Fotoarkiv.)

Blessed with fabled strength though he may be, notice that Heracles' body shows the characteristic hip-hiked, off-center *contrapunto* pose that can be found in most classical art. This involves a commonly seen pattern: shortness in the lower left Lateral Line (LL), and the upper right Lateral Line. This is accompanied by a retraction or collapse in the core or Deep Front Line, demonstrated in several ways. There is a twist in the core supporting the lower thoracic spine, i.e. in the psoas complex with both sides shortening to accommodate it. The chest, though massive, seems slightly collapsed toward an exhalation pattern. The lack of inner length can also be seen in the 'girdle of Adonis' spilling over the edge of the pelvis (that is not fat, but rather a result of core shortening). It extends to the legs, where the shortness of the DFL in the adductor group and deep posterior compartment of the lower leg pulls up on the inner arch and helps to shift the weight onto the outside of the foot.

The collapse can be read in the tissues of the knee, where the tissues on the inner knee (DFL) are lower than the tissues on the outer knee (LL). Contrast this with the core support found in any of these examples, even the asymmetrical and unathletic Venus.

Aphrodite de Melos (Fig. 10.5)

We are, of course, unable to comment on Venus's Arm Lines, but the charm of her seductive pose is surely enhanced by shortening the left Spiral Line (SL) and the right Front Functional Line (FFL). Someone standing straight is not nearly as inviting (compare this pose to most of the statues of Athena – i.e. 'Justice' or the Statue of Liberty – who generally stand foursquare, inviting respect but not familiarity). The straight pose calls for maximum stability in the cardinal lines: front, back, sides, and core (Deep Front) lines. Any sinuous pose such as seen here or in the fashion magazines will involve an asymmetry in the helical lines: the Lateral, Spiral, and Functional Lines.

Notice how the shortening of the left SL shifts her head to the right, protracts the right shoulder, and gives a left rotation to the rib cage relative to the pelvis. The shortness in the right FFL further contributes to all of these and also to her modesty, as the adductor longus on the left side, the lower track of the right FFL adducts the left hip across the body.

Additional shortening in the right LL is necessary to bring sufficient weight back onto the right leg. Even so, we are left with the impression of impending movement, in that she seems not quite securely balanced on her right leg. Some have surmised that in the original she was holding the baby Eros in her right arm, which would help counter-balance her weight, or perhaps she is about to take a step into the pool that will once again render her virginal.

Discobolus (Fig. 10.6)

The discus thrower of Praxiteles is the consummate representation of the lines in service of an athletic skill. The trim young fellow holds the discus with the Superficial Front Arm Line (SFAL) of his right arm from the flexed fingers to the pectoralis major, stabilizing his hold with the pressure from his thumb, which connects up the Deep Front Arm Line through the biceps to the pectoralis minor. This tension is balanced by a similar engagement in the two front Arm Lines on the left side, and the two are connected across the pectoral muscles in the chest down the arm to his left hand, which is clearly fully involved in the throw.

He has 'coiled the spring' of his body by shortening the right Spiral Line, which is clearly pulled in from the right side of the head (the splenii muscles) around the left shoulder (rhomboid and serratus anterior) across the belly (left external and right internal oblique) to the right hip. This tension carries beyond the hip to the tensor fasciae latae, iliotibial band, and down the front of the shin via the tibialis anterior to the inner arch of his supporting right foot. The Front Functional Line from his left shoulder to his right femur is likewise short. The left Lateral Line is shorter than the right, which is extended.

He has been like this for over 2000 years, but any moment now he will 'rise and cast' the discus. The obvious power will come from the right SFAL bringing the discus forward across his body, but the coordination with the other lines will really make the difference in the distance he achieves. Shortening the right SL in preparation stretches and potentiates the left, which he will now shorten strongly, bringing his eyes and head to the left and the right shoulder forward working off the left hip. As he turns this will bring his weight onto the left leg and foot, which will become the fulcrum for the remainder of the movement. At the same time, he will shorten the Back Functional Line from the left shoulder to the right femur, pulling the left shoulder back and rotating the whole trunk to the left. Shortening the right LL will help stabilize the platform of the shoulder and

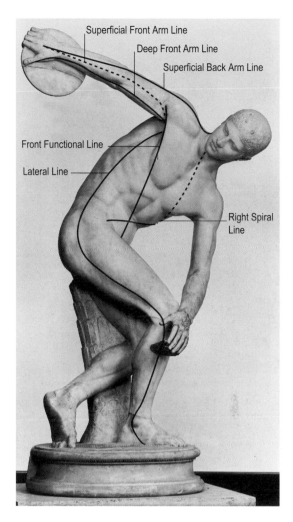

• Fig. 10.6 Discobolus. The great athletes involve all the lines, distributing the strain evenly across the body. (Reproduced with kind permission from Hirmer Fotoarkiv.)

add a little more impetus to the throw. Finally, the erectors of the Superficial Back Line will straighten the flexion in his body, leaving his back extended and his head lifted to follow the flight of the discus. The right Back Functional Line, from right shoulder to left femur, will contract at the end of the movement to save his right rotator cuff from overstrain, allowing him to stay healthy for future contests.

❖ ❖ ❖ Athletics

Space allows for only a few examples of the exertion and stability required across the world of sport. The first two photos show airborne use of the lines, mostly in sagittal movement, the second two show differing rotational movements.

Tennis (Fig. 10.7)

We can imagine our tennis server is short, so she leaps to get the highest advantage on the ball. Spiking into a serve or a short return when up in the air involves shortening the

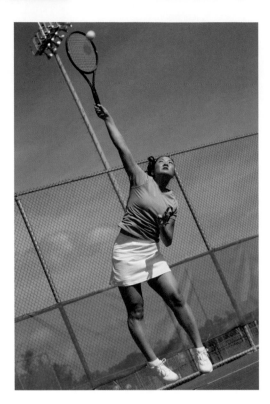

• **Fig. 10.7** Tennis player. (© iStockphoto.com, reproduced with permission. Photograph by Michael Krinke.)

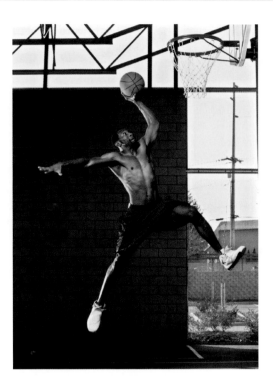

• **Fig. 10.8** Basketball player. (© iStockphoto.com, reproduced with permission. Photograph by Jelani Memory.)

front lines from end to end against each other to get the force in the right direction. The obvious lines for the power of the stroke are provided by both the Superficial and Deep Front Arm Lines that grip and power the racket, arrayed along the visible surface of the right arm in this picture. Notice how the left Front Arm Lines have contracted in against the body to provide stability for more height and stretch to the right side.

In the torso, the power is passed to three lines in the trunk. Firstly, the Front Functional Line continues the power in a straight line from the pectoralis major and the rectus abdominis through the pubic symphysis to the left adductor longus, which in this open chain pulls the left thigh forward to counterbalance the right arm. Secondly, the right Spiral Line is shortened, turning the head to the right, pulling the left shoulder around the rib cage, and shortening the distance from the left ribs to the right hip. The left Spiral Line is conversely stretched or lengthened – a pre-stretch prior to forceful closing of this line in the stroke. Thirdly, these two are assisted by the Lateral Lines, where the left is shortened for stability, and the right is fully lengthened for reach. During the shot and follow through, the right Lateral Line and left Spiral Line will shorten along with the right Front Functional Line to provide more power.

When one is airborne, the only counterbalance to the weight of the racket and ball is the inertia of the body itself. We have seen how the weight of the arm is playing against the inertia of the left leg, but it is also working against the inertia of the core – the weight of the pelvis and legs

themselves. This drawing on the stability of the core, represented in our scheme by the Deep Front Line, can be seen here in the supination of the feet, adduction of the thighs, and the pulling of the DFL structures up the inner line of the leg into the underside of the pelvis. This 'gathering' in the core is essential to the power and precision of the shot when out of contact with the ground.

Basketball (Fig. 10.8)

In the service of 'nothin' but net', we are once again airborne and open chain, though here the desire to get the ball up to the hoop, rather than down, means that the front lines are open and the back lines are tensed, leaving the body in a bit of a bow that keeps his eyes on the prize. At the same time, notice how active the leading leg is – muscles bulging, foot dorsiflexed – the left leg is as important as the right arm in 'aiming' and guiding the body toward the hoop.

The right Superficial Front Arm Line from pectoral to splayed fingers is coming down, like a wing lifting the body to counterbalance the throw with the left. The left Superficial Front Arm Line is providing the power, while the Deep Front Arm Line (see that thumb?) is doing the fine guiding of the ball for precision delivery.

The left Front Functional Line is stretched prior to contracting for the dunk, while the right FFL stabilizes from the flexed left hip to outstretched right arm. The left Back Functional Line is contracted right now, but will have to relent in a second or two. The right BFL is stretched around the trunk from right shoulder to left hip. The left Spiral

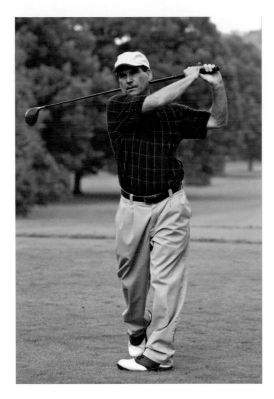

• **Fig. 10.9** Golfer at the end of a drive. (© iStockphoto.com, reproduced with permission. Photograph by Denise Kappa.)

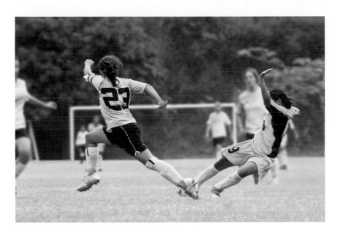

• **Fig. 10.10** Football players. (© iStockphoto.com, reproduced with permission. Photograph by Alberto Pomares.).

Line is more contracted, locating the head on the torso, and the right SL is more stretched.

Finally, we note the difference between the left and right Deep Front Line in the legs, where the right DFL is fully stretched and open, but the definition in the adductors on the left side shows how essential this line is, as for the tennis player, in providing core support for the balance of the trunk, even when the foot is not on the ground.

Golf (Fig. 10.9)

This golfer, caught at the final moment of follow-through from a fairway shot, demonstrates a pleasing integration of the helical lines in motion. Golf engages the entire Spiral and Functional Line complex evenly, but for the head that counter-rotates to follow the path of the ball. The right SL is fully engaged; the left is conversely contracted, right down to the supinating left foot. These lines were in opposite states of length at the beginning of the swing.

The only quarrel we might pick is with the height of the right shoulder, which is being restricted by the (out of sight) rotator cuff of the Deep Back Arm Line, causing the shoulder to lift slightly at this phase of the swing.

In the follow-through the Superficial Front Line is for the most part opened and stretched, especially on the right side, with the Superficial Back Line shortened, creating a bow upon which the spirals are laid. The swing starts with the SFL short and the SBL long, so this SBL contraction lifts the head and rib cage during the latter part of the swing.

The weight on the legs has shifted to the inner part of the right foot (and right on past, at the moment of this picture) and onto the outside of the left foot. This involves a contraction of the Deep Front Line on the left leg (in addition to the contraction in the SPL already noted) and a stretch in the Lateral Line on the outside of the left leg. This balance between the Deep Front Line on the inner line of the leg and the Lateral Line on the outer aspect of the leg is crucial to remain centered on the legs while the Spiral Lines roll the weight through to the inside of the following foot and the outside of the leading foot. If these lines do not maintain a coordinated tension through the myofascia, the upper lines cannot easily coordinate the precision swing.

The right Front Functional Line, from right shoulder to left hip, is fully contracted; its complement from right hip to left humerus is fully stretched. The left Back Functional Line is contracted, pulling the left shoulder back, and its complement, running from the right shoulder across the back and around the outside of the left thigh to the knee, is fully stretched. These have likewise traded roles from the moment of greatest backswing to this moment of follow-through when the picture was taken.

Football (Fig. 10.10)

In this photo of school athletics, we see rotation with reaching, in contrast to the pulling in on closed chains seen in a golf stroke. Here we can comment on both number 23 and number 9, seemingly successful in stealing the ball from her competitor even as she falls. The player in blue shows a very even-toned stretch along the left Lateral Line coupled with a beautiful reciprocal motion: the closing twist from the right Spiral Line, and concomitant stretch of the left Spiral Line.

The Functional Lines, as above and as in most sportive moves, are likewise fully engaged, though here the movements of the arms are in the service of the coordination of the legs, not vice versa. The left Front Functional Line and right Back Functional Line are participating with the

Spiral Line in generating the torso twist, while the two complementary lines are stretched into stabilizing straps. Notice how her arms attempt to stabilize the leg, with the left arm up and out in front, and the right arm back, wrist and elbow flexed to connect the arm to the chest.

The defender in yellow has her (left) wrist extended, helping to tighten the back as her right leg works off her own body's inertia to hook the ball with her right foot, even in mid-fall. While we need not repeat the litany of helices in the Spiral and Functional Lines, we do note the interplay between the Lateral Lines and the Deep Front Lines in her legs: the LL on the outside of her right leg must relent and stretch to allow the DFL on the inside to pull the ball toward her. Conversely, the DFL on the left leg is lengthening, allowing the foot to stay on the ground until the last possible moment. Such interplay can be seen in skiing, skateboarding, or any sport where side-to-side motion necessitates that these normally stabilizing lines become part of the movement and work reciprocally.

❖ ❖ ❧ Musicians

Musicians the world over are among those who manifest intense concentration around an object which cannot change shape. The tendency for the body to shape itself around the solid instrument is very strong in all types of music. So strong in fact, that, during a time when I enjoyed a vogue with London's orchestral musicians in my practice, I could often accurately anticipate the player's instrument before being told, just on the basis of body posture. The accommodation to the flute, or violin (or guitar or saxophone) was so clear that the instrument could almost be 'seen' still shaping the body, even when it was still in its case. So let this section serve for anyone who builds themselves around an unmalleable piece of their environment – potters, jewelers, bicyclists, and postmen among them.

Through cross-fertilization from the world of dance concerning body use, and the proliferation of the Alexander Technique and other forms of re-patterning the use of the self, musicians and their teachers as a class have become more aware of postural and movement issues. Paying attention to self-use can certainly affect both the quality of playing and the longevity of the professional player.

Here are a few examples from the classical repertoire, though the same problems and the same principles would apply to rock, jazz, and traditional musicians. In the following examples, we presume right-handed players, as the pictures show. Many of the assessments would obviously switch sides with a left-handed player and instrument.

Cellist (Fig. 10.11)

Although this player demonstrates fairly good body use, we can see that the Superficial Front Line is significantly shortened, pulling the head down toward the pubic bone. This will negatively affect breathing during playing, as well as putting long-term strain into the lower back.

Secondly, the left Lateral Line is shortened, pulling the head to the left, and shortening the distance between the left armpit and the side of the left hip. This pattern is likely, over time, to pull on the core line, the Deep Front Line, and require compensations there that could have negative long-term structural and even physiological effects, as in a fascial shortening of the quadratus lumborum right behind the kidney.

The sets of Arm Lines are used differently, of course, between fingering and bowing. In both cases, the arm is held abducted by the coordination of the Superficial and Deep Back Arm Line, and the playing depends on the opposition of the thumb and fingers – the Superficial and Deep Front Arm Lines. The fact that the bowing arm is held further away from the body, both to the front and out to the side, contributes toward the tendency to counterbalance by shortening the left LL. Slightly dropping the right elbow and lifting the left while playing can help to counterbalance this tendency. Pressing into the left foot a bit more could also help center his body relative to the chair and the cello.

Violist (Fig. 10.12)

The tendencies of the cellist are magnified in the violist, owing to the necessity to clamp the instrument between the left shoulder and the left side of the jaw. Although the photograph shows trained good use, the shortening of the left Lateral Line is still clear, and it extends into, and is often sharply present in, the neck. This chronic shortness can sometimes lead to impingement problems through soft-tissue tightening around the brachial plexus or actual stenosis at the cervicals, either of which can adversely affect the ability of the left hand to finger properly. This problem can be ameliorated, if not solved, by adding an extension to the chin rest to make the two sides of the neck more equal in length.

In addition, the player of the smaller stringed instruments adds a rotational component, bringing the right shoulder across the body with the right Front Functional Line, while, counter-intuitively, the right Spiral Line brings the left shoulder and ribs closer to the right hip. This combination often leads to shortening of the Superficial Front Line along the front of the torso, along with a widening or weakening of the tissues of the Superficial Back Line.

The siren beauty of the strings have lured many a musician to a host of structural problems because of the ability of the body to bend around the instrument, while the instrument is unable to return the favor. The shortness in this player's SFL causes his pelvis to be posteriorly tilted on the chair, putting the tailbone perilously near the seat. Note how this particular player has broadened his base of support by tucking his right foot back, thus ensuring more movement through his pelvis, despite its bad position. Good sitting will support both better playing and a longer career. Though it is hard to see with the bulky trousers, the anterior lower Spiral Line of the right leg will be strained in this

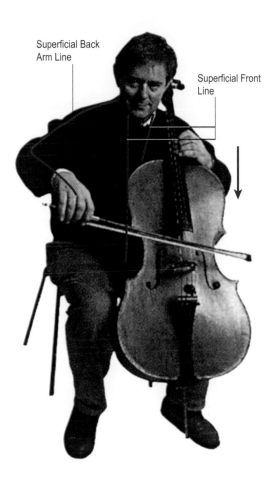

• **Fig. 10.11** A cellist. (© Phil Starling http://www.philstarling.co.uk. Reproduced with kind permission.)

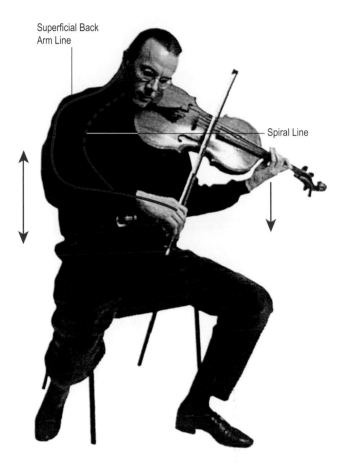

• **Fig. 10.12** A violist. (© Phil Starling http://www.philstarling.co.uk. Reproduced with kind permission.)

posture, leading sometimes to medial collateral or iliolumbar ligament problems for the tucked-back leg.

Flautist (Fig. 10.13)

The flute and many woodwinds, like the violin family, requires serious asymmetrical accommodation, but to the opposite side. The right Lateral Line, the right Front Functional Line, and the left Spiral Line are all commonly shortened in flute playing. The Superficial Front Line also commonly shortens, but interestingly, because the head is turned to the left, the right Superficial Front Line, running from the pubic bone up through the sternocleidomastoid, is often more affected than the left part of that line.

The conflict between the lifted right arm (Superficial Back Arm Line) and the left rotated head can make for a confused area in the right shoulder and neck of many flute players, while the left arm, having to reach around the front of the body for the fingering, often puts eccentric strain on the upper left shoulder muscles – particularly the levator scapulae and supraspinatus of the Deep Back Arm Line.

The characteristic cock of the head, the shift of the rib cage toward the left, and the consequent right tilt of the shoulder girdle are dead giveaways of the flute player.

Trumpeter (Fig. 10.14)

Our previous examples all involve an asymmetrical relationship to the instrument; there is of course an entire class of instruments held more or less symmetrically, such as the trumpet, the clarinet, oboe, and the like.

In these cases, any Spiral, Lateral, and Functional Line imbalances are less likely to be due to the instrument, but there is one imbalance common to these players. Since the arms and the instrument must be held in front of the body, the tissues of the Superficial Back Line tend to get short, especially the deep muscles of the spine. Given that the brass or woodwind player is more dependent than others on the breath, this shortness in the back forces the player to concentrate the breath in the front of the lungs and the front of the body. This trumpet player ably demonstrates the common result – the SBL is short, but the Superficial Front Line is long, so that the chest and belly are expended in front.

Despite ill-fitting jeans, this player has fairly good pelvic position but is still chronically hyperextended in the lumbars. He could learn to counterbalance the weight of the trumpet and arms at less cost to his back.

Since approximately 60% of the lungs lie behind the mid-coronal line of the body, it is often beneficial to work

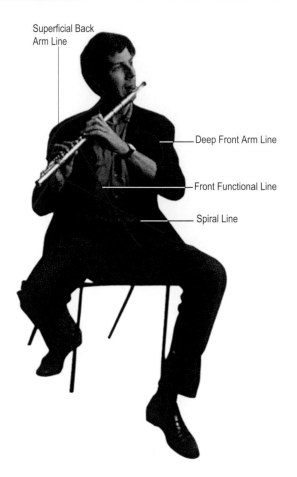

• **Fig. 10.13** A flautist. (© Phil Starling http://www.philstarling.co.uk. Reproduced with kind permission.)

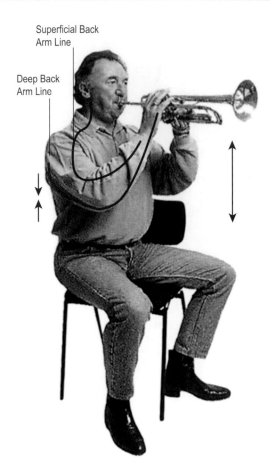

• **Fig. 10.14** A trumpeter. (© Phil Starling http://www.philstarling.co.uk. Reproduced with kind permission.)

with pelvic position for these players, to see whether a different positional support can result in release of some of the muscles of the back, so that more breath movement occurs in the back part of the rib cage and the posterior diaphragm.

❖ ❖ Sitting

Sitting, as common as it is in the Western world, is a fraught and dangerous activity (Fig. 10.15)! Sitting with the myofascial meridians in balance is a rare event (Fig. 10.16). The principles included here are applicable to driving or flying, to basic office ergonomics, to authors at the end of a long season of book writing – to anyone who must sit for significantly long periods.

Sitting more or less eliminates the legs from their support function, leaving the pelvis as the major base of support for the segmented tentpole of the human spine. In sitting, then, we can see the pure interplay among the myofascial meridians in the trunk. From front to back, we all must find balance among the Superficial Front Line, the Deep Front Line, and the Superficial Back Line. With asymmetrical sitting, we can involve the Lateral or Spiral Lines, and we will touch upon that before we leave the subject. Our main concern, however (because it is a ubiquitous postural

problem), is with sagittal flexion–extension balance, and thus with the three lines arrayed along the sagittal plane – the Superficial Front Line in front of the ribs, the Deep Front line in front of the spine, and the Superficial Back Line behind the spine.

The proper balance for the spine in sitting approximates the proper balance for standing: easy, full extension with the major body weights of head, chest, and pelvis poised one atop the other over the anterior ischial tuberosities, more or less on the same coronal plane as the top of the acetabulum. As we have noted in their previous respective chapters, the SFL generally creates trunk flexion (except at the upper neck), the SBL generally creates extension, and the DFL is capable of adjusting either way at various levels of the spine. Easy alignment in sitting can be created by balancing these three lines, though at first attempt this balance may not seem so 'easy' because of the necessity of moving beyond the neuromuscular and connective tissue habitus.

It is extraordinarily easy, in fact, to fall into a habit of sitting that allows one or more of the following to happen:
1. the head to come forward by flexing the lower cervicals
2. the upper neck to go into hyperextension
3. the chest and front of the rib cage to fall
4. the upper lumbars to move posteriorly and into flexion

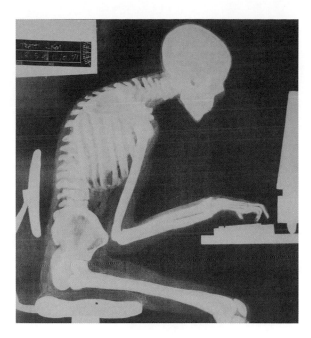

• **Fig. 10.15** Serious spinal damage at 0 miles per hour! (© BackCare. Reproduced with kind permission, www.backcare.org.uk.)

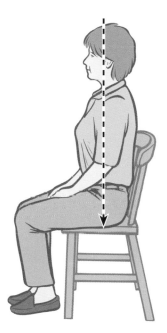

• **Fig. 10.16** Balanced upright sitting.

5. the pelvis to roll back so that the weight goes onto the posterior aspect of the ischial tuberosities (i.e. the pelvis tips toward the tailbone).

This necessarily involves a shortening of the SFL as well as parts of the DFL. Depending on the particular pattern of sitting displayed, allowing the body to come up often involves lengthening and lifting tissues along the trunk portion of the SFL (the fascial planes associated with the rectus abdominis, for example). When the tissues in the front pull down, the tissues of the SBL (the erectors and their fascia) often widen as they go into eccentric loading,

so it will also ease the client's passage toward supported sitting to bring the tissues of the SBL medially and inferiorly to correct the widening (Fig. 10.17).

It is also often essential to get the client to 'engage' (create more standing tonus in) the DFL. Specifically, the psoas muscle needs to be deployed to steady the lumbars forward to lift the chest, and the deep longus capitis and longus colli muscles on the anterior longitudinal ligament of the cervical bodies must be employed to counteract the tendency of both the SFL and SBL tissues to hyperextend the upper cervicals, pushing them forward. Restoring standing tonus in these muscles just in front of the spine and just behind the throat is as much a requirement for 'core competency' as tonus in the transversus abdominis (www.anatomytrains.com – video ref.: Pelvis DVD or the sitting webinar).

The next section describes a spinal integration exercise for sitting that is helpful in bringing all these desirable ends to happen at once. (Of course, more detailed mobilization work tailored to the individual is often also required.) Once balanced sitting is achieved, it needs to be practiced assiduously for some days or weeks until both the nerves and their minions, the muscles, have adjusted to the change. After this initial period of conscious attention, this kind of sitting will be able to be nearly effortlessly maintained for hours without diminishing breathing or attention, nor creating structural pain. (The research, however, still points to the advisability of changing position frequently.[7])

❖ Integrating the Spine in Sitting

(The author is grateful to Judith Aston (www.astonkinetics.com) for having conveyed the basis for this spinal integration exercise in sitting, but notes that he learned the following sequence from her in 1975. By now it may not accurately represent her current approach, and, memory being what it is, additions or omissions have likely crept in – but she deserves credit for the original idea.)

Nearly everyone's schooling involved the postural adjustment to standard issue desks. The author's experience is echoed by many of his clients: curled into whatever desk fell to the alphabetical roll call, our thoracic spines bent over our work, and when called upon, we raised only our heads, putting a hyperextended neck over the flexed spine, as in Fig. 10.15. Desks that are adjustable to the children, like posturally efficient orthopedic seats, would be wonderful, but are unlikely to arrive soon, given current school budgets. A brief lesson in adjusting yourself to the chair and desk – finding the comfortable seated posture, and using the spine as a whole in moving in a chair – is a cheaper alternative which might divert a lifetime of bad habit, deoxygenated lack of focus and creeping pain.

In such a sedentary culture, so married to its computers and its cars, the lack of generalized training in sitting lies somewhere between silly and sinful. The basis of the following exercise is that postural adjustments in sitting are best thought of as adjustments of the entire spine, not

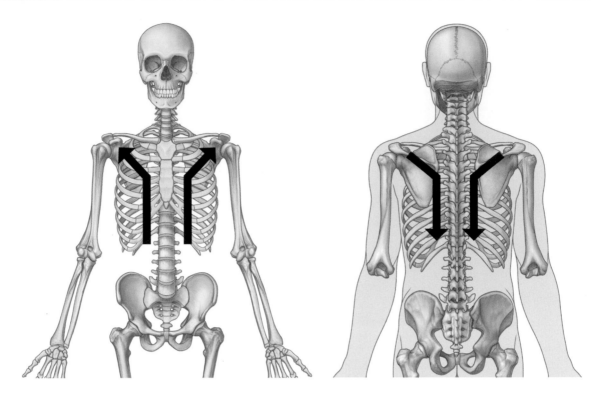

• **Fig. 10.17** With sitting patterns that resemble Fig. 10.15, a strategy of lifting and spreading the anterior tissues while dropping and centering the posterior tissues – with a combination of manual therapy, ideo-kinesis, or training – is a necessary prelude to strengthening the core for an easy but mechanically sound approach to prolonged sitting.

any single body segment. The exercise is intended to evoke a spring-like, integrated motion of the spine for postural adjustments in sitting, to correct the 'school desk' problem.

Sit on a stool or forward on a chair; do not touch or lean into the back of the chair during this exercise. A hard or lightly padded seat is better in order to feel exactly where you are on the ischial tuberosities (ITs). Sit tall, and rock your pelvis forward and back a bit to center yourself so that you are at your tallest, and there is a comfortable lumbar curve.

Very slowly let yourself roll back on your ITs, letting your body respond to the change in pelvic posture. Your tailbone comes slowly toward the chair and the lumbar curvature reduces and reverses. Keep the movement slow and small; stay sensitive to your response. If you let the rest of your body respond rather than holding a postural position, you will feel that as the pelvis tilts posteriorly the chest begin to lower in the front.

Move back and forth, slowly within small range of movement, between these two positions, and notice the relationship: rock the pelvis back, the chest falls or flexes a little; rock the pelvis forward, the chest is lifted again without effort.

Continue the movement, turning your attention to your neck: if you do not hold the head steady in relation to the horizontal, but let it go with the rest of the spine, the head will start to incline forward as the neck naturally begins to flex, and the line of sight falls toward the floor. We are so

inclined to separate the head from the rest of the body that this is the most difficult connection for most of us to get. We are accustomed to keeping our head oriented to our right-angled rooms' horizontal, not letting it respond to the inner whispering of the rest of the spine. Persist and the connection will be felt.

Move from upright sitting to full flexion of the spine. At full flexion, the tailbone is close to the stool, your sternum is closer to your pubic bone, and you are looking into your lap (Fig. 10.18). Making sure to initiate from the pelvis, reverse the movement, letting the pelvis start a wave that moves the lumbars, which in turn moves the thorax, which in turn extends the neck and lifts the head. Move through this sequence a few times until the entire spring of the spine feels easy with this movement.

It is important that you do not let the chest fall behind the pelvis as you go into this movement (Fig. 10.19). The center of gravity of the chest and head taken together stay over the pelvis, even in full flexion. If, as you move into flexion, your breathing and organs feel cramped for space, you are perhaps letting the weight of the upper body fall behind the pelvis. Check by doing the exercise beside a mirror; the movement should be easy, and the fully flexed position physiologically tenable.

Now, still initiating from the pelvis, continue the movement from flexion to upright, and then through upright toward hyperextension. At this end of the spine's range, the pubic bone moves toward the chair seat, the lumbar

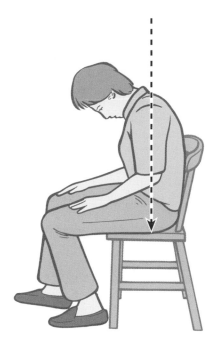

• **Fig. 10.18** Full-flexion phase.

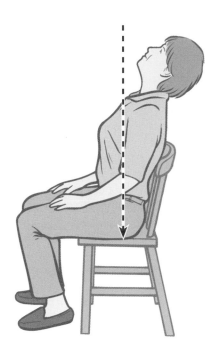

• **Fig. 10.20** Improper hyperextension phase with head hyperextended beyond the rest of the spine.

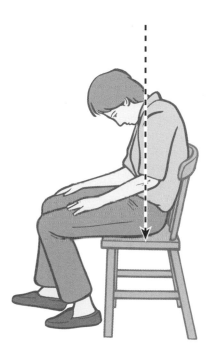

• **Fig. 10.19** Improper full flexion pose with chest falling behind pelvis.

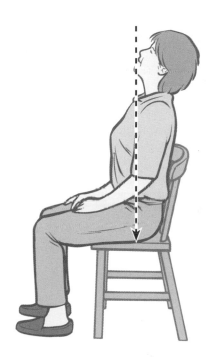

• **Fig. 10.21** Proper hyperextension phase.

curve is exaggerated, and the sternum lifts. Be attentive to let the angle of the head follow the dictates of the rest of the spine; do not let it lead the movement (Fig. 10.20). If you do the movement properly and let the head and neck coordinate with the rest of the spine, the neck will not reach full hyperextension in this movement; there will be some ability to hyperextend 'left over' (Fig. 10.21).

Let the body return to upright, passing through neutral toward flexion, and allow the spine to move through its entire range from flexion to hyperextension and back again,

until the full movement is familiar. Initiate the movement at all times from the pelvis, feeling the slow shift of the weight from the back to the front of the ITs, stopping and moving more slowly if the head rebels and tries to take over control of the movement. For best effect, it is important to remain cognizant of the spine at all times, cultivating the image of the spine as a spring moving easily and evenly from full flexion to full extension with a resting neutral in the middle. Although children and impatient adults will want to run through the full range quickly, slower movement is better in getting the initial completeness into the spinal movement, and in integrating it into everyday activity.

Once the integrated movement is familiar, come from the hyperextended end of the movement with your eyes open, and stop when the eyes reach horizontal as in Fig. 10.16. Feel the position the rest of your body has taken. Feel the ease in your breathing. Perhaps you have found a new sitting position for yourself. Check it by moving on down into flexion, and then back up until your eyes are level, being careful to let the eyes be passive, allowing the initiation to come from the pelvis. The more you practice this exercise, the easier it becomes to make this new position your own, rather than an imposition of 'good posture'.

By these lights, we could hope that from now on, any change of your head position involves a change of the whole integrated spring of your spine to support your head in the new position. To look down at your desk, or this book, or your knitting, let your pelvis roll back a bit to automatically and coherently carry your chest and eyes to the task. To look up, let the pelvis roll forward a little, biomechanically supporting the lift of the body and the eyes. To follow that bird above you, let the pelvis roll forward even more so that the spine operates as a coordinated whole, not in disjointed pieces where one section moves a lot and another section not at all.

It is quite easy to add rotation to this pure flexion and extension by pushing on one foot and letting the body follow. If the bird flew off to your left, let the pelvis roll forward as you increase the pressure on your right foot. To look down and left, roll your pelvis back while lifting a little on the left foot (and letting the hips respond). Move in this way for a while and it will become reflexive, and you will engender a habit that will delight your spine for the rest of your life.

In this conception sitting up straight like a Victorian and dropping your head to read is just as silly as flexing your back and hyperextending your neck to look at the teacher or your screen. Both of these movements involve 'breaking' the functional integrity of the spine, which is designed to act as a unified spring.

Since sitting in this way projects a natural authority as well as ease, you may find that people in a group are naturally turning to you to see if you will speak. If this is uncomfortable, or not what you want to project, it is possible to let your thoracic spine find the chair back while still maintaining pelvic support from the ITs, rather than letting your chest fall behind the pelvis, which leaves you sitting on your tailbone but apparently assuming a subservient sitting posture.

If you guide clients into these movements, be sure they are initiating from the pelvis. A hand on their lower back will usually tell you where their movement is coming from. Sometimes another hand on the head is necessary to keep the head connected with the rest of the spine. Be sure to let the client perform the full motion entirely solo several times before the session ends, and reinforce the idea for several sessions running. Investment on their part is required, but an integrated spine is your (and their) reward.

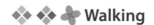 **Walking**

As stated in Chapter 2, Anatomy Trains is not especially useful as a way to parse movement as a whole. Nevertheless, a simplified analysis of walking may prove useful – although walking is of course not so simple.[8]

Taking a step forward, whether it is initiated from the hip flexors of the DFL, such as the psoas and iliacus, or by release of the hip extensors and spinal muscles, certainly involves flexion at the hip, extension of the knee, and dorsiflexion at the ankle and metatarsophalangeal (ball of the foot) joints necessary to walking forward, all of which are created by the shortening of the myofascia of the SFL. The muscles may fire or engage in a sequence, but the leg portion of the SFL is also engaged as a fascial whole throughout the 'reaching forward', swing phase.

As the leg travels forward, its entire myofascia prepares to receive the weight of the body and the ground reaction. Motor units tense within the fascial web to handle the precise amount of force expected. One has only to step from one room into another in the dark with an unexpected drop or rise of no more than a couple of inches (5 cm) to realize how little is required to upset this preparation, and how much shock is sent through the unprepared musculoskeletal system when it is surprised in this way.

Once the heel strikes and the roll over the foot begins, the SBL myofascia takes over the stabilizing role as the back of the standing leg engages into hip extension and plantarflexion. Again, no matter what the firing sequence of the muscles, the entire lower section of the SBL is engaged fascially from lower back to toes throughout this phase. During all these phases, movement should be tracking through the four 'hinges' of the leg in more or less a straightforward fashion. The hip, of course, does some rotation during walking, and the weight falls from lateral to medial across the metatarsophalangeal joint, but in general, contradictions in the vectors among these joints will result in joint wear, ligamentous overstrain, and myofascial imbalance (Fig. 10.22).

The Lateral Line (LL – abductors, ITT, and lateral compartment of the lower leg) provide stability that prevents the hip falling inward into adduction, while the adductor group and the other tissues of the DFL assist the flexion/extension motions and provide stability from the inner arch up the inside of the leg to the medial side of the hip joint, guiding it and preventing excess rotation of the hip.

It is important to understand that the pendulum of the leg starts not at the hip but at the 12th rib and 12th thoracic vertebra, with the upper reaches of the psoas and quadratus lumborum (see Fig. 9.26). In the light of this, the movements of the innominate bones in walking become understandable, combining a simultaneous pelvic rotation around the vertical axis in the horizontal plane, a lifting (side shift or side tilt) of each innominate in the coronal plane around the A–P axis, and a tilt in the sagittal plane around the left–right axis in which the flexion or extension of the innominate mirrors that of the femur in walking

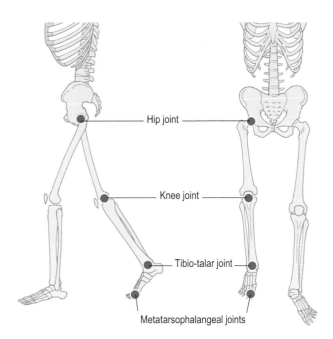

• **Fig. 10.22** Each step involves movement through four 'hinges' of the leg, around which the soft tissue must be balanced for joint longevity and efficient walking.

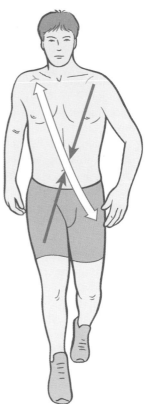

• **Fig. 10.24** The winding and unwinding of the torso in walking involves the Functional Lines (pictured) in alternating contraction, and the Spiral Lines and Lateral Lines as well.

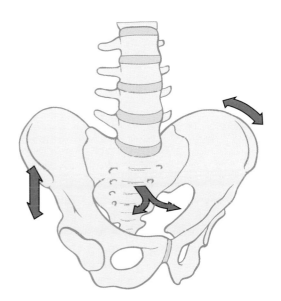

• **Fig. 10.23** The pelvis has movement in all three Euclidian planes in proper walking – side-to-side around the A–P axis, rotating around the vertical axis, and each innominate tilts not-quite-sagittally around the left–right axis. Too little movement in one plane often results in excessive movement in another plane.

(Fig. 10.23). With this in mind, one can see that for the pelvis, proper initiation of walking is a DFL coordination, whereas the line that has to move through the most range and provide the most adjustment and stability is the LL.

Different patterns of walking mix differing amounts of each of these three axial motions. Lack of one motion will usually require an increase in one or more of the others in compensation. Learning how to read these motions in the walking pattern of your clients will make your work more efficient (www.anatomytrains.com – video ref: BodyReading, 101).

In the upper body, the Lateral Lines alternate in shortening on the weighted side to keep the torso from falling away from the weighted leg. The common contralateral pattern of walking also involves the Functional Lines and Spiral Lines bringing the right shoulder and rib cage forward to counterbalance the left leg when it swings forward and vice versa (Fig. 10.24).

Beneath this outer, appendicularly oriented movement, the torso winds like a watch spring, countering the twist that the metronome of the legs produces in the pelvis. This rotational energy, working through the myofascia of the intercostals in the ribs and the abdominal obliques, is stored and released with each step. When this small inner rotation of the ribs is stopped for any reason, the movement is exported outward and can be seen in excessive motion of the arms or side-to-side shift of the upper body during walking.

Lack of coordination or excessive myofascial binding in any of these tissues sets up characteristic patterns of walking, some of which are simply personal and idiosyncratic, while others are downright inefficient, and can lead to joint or myofascial stiffness problems.

Our colleague James Earls improves this simplistic planar analysis by integrating the lines with contemporary gait theory.

Anatomy Trains in Gait, by James Earls[9]

Anyone who has taken the time to coach a child to pitch a baseball or bowl a cricket ball has observed that gradual transition of body use from a more Alpha motor neuron 'single-muscle' style movement to the more Gamma-based smooth recruitment of coordinated motor units within long kinetic chains. When performing complex movements such as throwing, running, or jumping, reliance on individual muscles results in underpowered movement, with reduced accuracy and repeatability of the task at hand. Even the casual observer can see the difference when the full body becomes involved in a performance – the difference between Fred Astaire's elegant grace and the clumsy efforts of your favorite uncle on the ballroom floor.

Who has not felt the difference between taking a long, brisk walk along forest paths or city streets – one feels as if one can go on forever – versus having a slow amble around an exhibition, where 'museum feet' often turn a pleasant afternoon into a painful and tiring experience? These two conditions of 'walking' may be given the same name but the mechanics involved are vitally different. We propose that the difference is that the former makes efficient use of stored elasticity in the myofascial meridians compared to the stop-and-start inelastic nature of the latter, which, by its nature, requires more of a 'single-muscle' isolated type of body use.

African women have almost the same energy costs walking with 20% of their bodyweight on their head as when they took a normal stroll along the road.[10] The question physicist and bodyworker Zorn and the rest of us are left to ponder: how do these women manage to maintain the same metabolic cost when the actual work they are performing increases?[11]

The Stretch–Shortening Cycle

To answer this conundrum we first have to explore the nature and role of the myofascia in absorbing, storing and releasing energy back into the moving system. Using the fascial tissue's stored energy to facilitate movement is much more efficient than muscular contractions which require the ratcheting of actin and myosin and the increased expenditure of calories. (Calories are expensive in the evolutionary sense. The cost/benefit equation must weigh strongly on the side of benefit, as we cannot afford to 'spend' more calories in the search for food than we receive from consuming them.) If we are to match the efficiency of the African bearers our body must seek a metabolically cheap method of propulsion.

Walking is often described as controlled falling; with each step we have to prevent ourselves from accelerating toward the floor. To stay aloft and keep moving forward, we use the skeleton's limited stability (with its 'inner bag' of ligaments, see Appendix 1, p. 244) against the downward pull of gravity. The interaction between gravity and ground reaction force at heel strike creates a number of 'folds' through the body at each successive joint and in almost

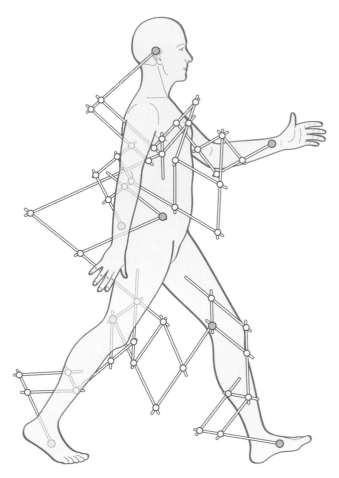

• **Fig. 10.25** This simplified side view shows the natural instability of the joints that sends the forces into the surrounding soft tissue. The alignment of the joints acts to deliberately channel these forces in the appropriate direction, i.e. to the myofascia that can deal with and decelerate the potential for collapse. (Courtesy of the Max Planck Institute.)

every plane of movement (Fig. 10.25).[12] This adaptation at the joints guides the forces into the body's soft tissue that lengthens as it decelerates our 'fall' to the floor.

Traditional anatomy has sometimes taught us that the absorption of the force was performed through eccentric contraction of the associated muscles that then concentrically contracted to create the recovery movement.[13,14] Recent research demonstrates the preference for certain muscles to take up the myofascial slack in isometric contraction during repetitive movements such as walking – even as their accompanying tendons are absorbing the energy as they are elongated.[12,15,16] There are many benefits to this utilization of the elastic nature of the myofascia (see Appendix 1 section on fascial training).

The viscoelastic response of the myofascia – pre-stress, stiffening under load, characteristic of tensegrity structures, see Appendix 1 – is the first in a sequence of events summarized together as the stretch shortening cycle (SSC). Veteran researchers Komi and Blazevich have both separately described this combined mechanism as being the 'way humans prefer to move'.[17,18] Our bodies like it, presumably, because it is efficient. This efficiency is due to the utilization of elastic energy absorbed by the fascial tissues and a resultant increase in muscle power output.

We step, the joints adapt, tissues lengthen. The viscous and elastic response of the extracellular matrix (ECM) in the lengthened tissues absorbs the energy and slows the lengthening. The tissue stretch also triggers a proprioceptive response to signal to the muscles to contract isometrically. Force transmission is thus effected from the moving joints to the soft tissue, and from there around the body via the myofascial meridian lines, as we will see.

This neural part of the SSC is most commonly explained using the stretch or myotatic reflex – the lengthening of the muscle spindle stimulates a muscle contraction automatically via the spinal cord.[12] While this is possible, it seems to be an oversimplification: the reflex arc is simply too slow (it is initiated approx. 40 milliseconds after the onset of stretch[12]) to create the necessary response during faster activities such as running or jumping. It may be that the muscle contraction occurs prior to the stretch based on previous experience, or that the reflex muscle contraction relies on a local exchange of proprioceptive information between the mechanoreceptors or a direct link through the fascial web – but this is not yet fully understood.[19]

The muscle fiber's isometric contraction stops the muscle from deforming, further transferring the deceleration of downward movement into the surrounding elastic fascial tissues. Like bouncing on a trampoline, the downward push will eventually be met by the upward pull of the increasing tension on the elastic tissue until the point at which the two are in balance. As the deceleration stops and the return movement begins, it is initiated by elastic recoil, not concentric contraction. However, when concentric contraction is added following this type of preparatory countermovement in the SSC, the force of the contraction is transferred more effectively and efficiently into directed movement, as its force is not absorbed willy-nilly by the elastic tissues because they have already been prestretched (and thus aligned, see Appendix 1, p. 244) along the direction of the contraction.

The body has thereby transferred kinetic energy (the downward 'fall') into potential energy (the energy stored in the elastic fascial tissue) back into kinetic energy in the opposite direction (elastic recoil) – the full stretch shortening cycle.

Dynamic Anatomy: Walking

Dynamic anatomy must be mapped in function rather than in the anatomical position – the body is designed to move, not stand still. Hunting, climbing, carrying, going downhill – these complex actions require significant variations of kinematics. Gravity, ground reaction force, momentum and the structure of the joints will all interact to create myriad directions of force through the body which must be adapted to and recovered from, preferably with as little energy expenditure as possible. The three qualities of the SSC

– viscoelasticity, isometric contraction and elastic loading – give us a highly energy-efficient system with which to walk and run. For our analysis we posit a repetitive stride rhythm of walking on an even flat surface. Variations in tempo, gradient or camber will require extra muscular work; however, we still use many of these fundamental dynamics below under a wide variety of conditions.

Of the four influences on movement listed above, gravity is the most predictable constant. Ground reaction force and momentum will alter depending on the task, terrain, footwear, and limb length, along with many other variables. While individual anatomy differs, the overall angulation of the joints will be within certain ranges, which allows us to predict certain propensities in the interactions of these four main factors.

On impact with the walking surface there is a sudden deceleration starting with the contact of the calcaneus. Though heel strike angle varies (and therefore the ground reaction force angles vary also), the sudden halting of the calcaneus sets off a chain of events through the joints between the foot and the spine that will be determined by the natural inclinations of the bony articulations and limited by the relatively unyielding ligaments.

The first link in the chain is the talus, which, due to its precarious position on the sustentaculum tali, continues a groundward journey after the heel has hit the ground. At heel strike the calcaneus's shape causes it to medially tilt and medially rotate. The talus follows the calcaneus, also tilting and rotating medially, until the downward force is absorbed by the soft tissues in the plantar surface of the foot and the tendons coming down from the lower leg.

The talus is held in a mortise and tenon joint between the tibia and fibula, a design that allows dorsi- and plantarflexion but limits rotation. Thus the rotation of the talus on heel strike turns the bones of the lower leg medially, almost like the turn of a screwdriver in its slot (Fig. 10.26). The rotation of the tibia is transferred through the ligaments to encourage the femur to follow, creating a medial rotation from the knee up to hip joint.

At the moment of heel strike and shortly after, the hip is flexing (and requiring the extensors to resist further flexion) and the weighted hip is also adducting to bring the body's center of gravity over the forward foot. As the hip joint of the forward limb is adducting, the opposite (extended) limb will be abducting, producing a tilt of the pelvis and therefore an adaptation of side flexion through the spine to dampen the frontal plane deviation before it reaches the head.

Returning to the foot for a moment and going distally instead of proximally from the talus, it is the reaction of the talus and calcaneus which unlock the midtarsal joints, allowing the distal bones of the foot to adapt to the surface and also to disperse the forces involved at heel strike into the myofascial tissues.[20] We must come back from this pronation and get the foot re-supinated prior to toe-off in order for the bones and joints to re-engage and create a more stable base in anticipation of the push-off

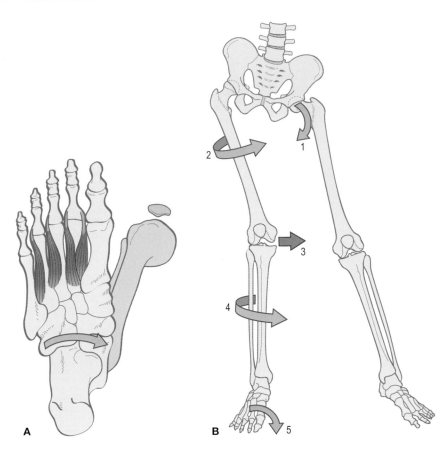

A

B

• **Fig. 10.26** The calcaneus and talus rotate medially on heel strike, and like a screwdriver turning a screw (**A**), this medial rotation within the tibio-talar joint is sent up the leg to the hip (**B**). (B, Adapted with permission from Götz-Neumann K. Gehen Verstehen: Ganganalyse in der Physiotherapie. Düsseldorf, Germany: Thieme-Verlag, Inc.; 2002.)

phase and its imminent energy release as we propel ourselves forward.[12,20] Failure to supinate fully increases strain of the plantar tissues that must compensate for the reduced stability from the bony structures that should have re-locked.

As this sequence of events flows upward, the body can take further advantage of the many inherent qualities of the myofascial tissues. The initial deceleration that must occur across each of the joints can be partially absorbed by the natural non-Newtonian viscoelastic reaction in the mucopolysaccharides of the ECM. The degree to which this happens is difficult to quantify at this time, we simply know that it does occur and that the degree of stiffening is likely to vary among individuals or even from place to place within an individual.

After the initial learning period of our first year or two of walking life, the interaction between gravity, ground reaction force, momentum and the joint angles sets up a characteristic pattern of adaptation. The joints channel the mechanical forces into the web of soft tissue, affecting the myofascial tensions and positions, which in turn stimulate the mechanoreceptors embedded within (see Appendix 1).

Stretch, load, pressure, and shear in the fascial system registers in the mechanoreceptors, to be weighed in the central nervous system and transferred into neuron signals to the motor units in the musculature, which adjust tissue stiffness to match the demands of the situation. It is this recursive process – mechanics, sensing, assessing, sending

motor signals which in turn adjust the mechanics – happening over and over again, step after step, day after day, that creates the characteristic pattern of movement we can recognize in a friend from far away. Over time, the relative strength of muscles, facility in neural pathways, the tonicity of the fascia, and even the shapes of the bones and joints will 'build into' this pattern.[21]

Mapping Dynamic Anatomy

The Anatomy Trains Myofascial Meridians provide a map with which to analyze the functioning (or less than optimal functioning) of these patterns of movement.

Although all the lines are involved, the Spiral Line is especially significant in the dynamic anatomy of walking, as walking is very much a movement derived from rotational forces. The transverse plane element begins at heel strike with the need to decelerate the plantarflexion and pronation in the foot, the internal rotation of the lower limb and further flexion at the hip. In Chapter 6 (Discussions 6.3–6.6, pp. 107–111) we saw the connection between the foot and pelvic position, with hip flexion/anterior tilt tending to create pronation and hip extension/posterior tilt bringing the foot toward supination. However, this was performed from a neutral anatomical position; in other words, it was about standing posture. Looking dynamically, at heel strike with the hip already flexed and the leg medially rotated, the increased force along the anterior portion of the Spiral Line will load the ITB behind the greater trochanter, switching on the upper gluteus maximus (Fig. 10.27). The gluteal muscle can then be used to 'brake' some of the internal rotation of the lower limb as well as the flexion occurring at the hip.

As we saw in the Lateral Line (Ch. 5), both the TFL and gluteus maximus are encased within the same fascial

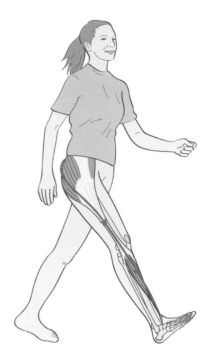

• **Fig. 10.27** The sequence of rotations initiated at heel strike is due to the offset of the talus on the calcaneus (see Fig. 10.25 and Fig. 5.5). The medial rotation that accompanies foot pronation and knee and hip flexion all have to be decelerated to give control to the foot and to the knee (see Fig. 10.26). The force created by the interaction between gravity, ground reaction, and the natural alignment of the joints needs to be decelerated by the appropriate soft tissue – in this case, the upward pull of the tibialis anterior connecting to the ITB to the superior fibers of the gluteus and on into the lumbar fascia. In this way the joints act like riverbanks, channeling force into these myofascial tissues.

layer and thus this modified Spiral Line connection remains true to the Anatomy Trains 'Rules of the Game' (Ch. 2). By recruiting gluteus maximus at heel strike we also bring in the Back Functional Line through the gluteal continuity with the thoracolumbar fascia (TLF) and the contralateral latissimus dorsi. This relationship has been well documented by Vleeming (posterior oblique sling) and investigated as part of the 'Swingwalker' mechanism by Zorn as it creates a sling across the back of the pelvis.[12,22] This contralateral arrangement of joining the lower limb to the opposite upper limb uses a superficial layer of myofascia, allowing the inner layers of the trunk to rotate differently from this outer later.

Once the forces at heel strike have been successfully negotiated the limb progresses through weight acceptance and eventually to toe-off. The external rotation of the stance leg (created by the swing of the other limb) assists with the correction back to a supinated position, giving a stable base for the forces involved. A thorough description of all the joint and ligament events is beyond our scope here, but if we track the progression of forces through the soft tissue we can clearly see the tension moving through hip abductors, from the gluteus maximus at heel strike to the gluteus medius at weight acceptance and then the tensor fasciae latae as the hip comes into extension (Fig. 10.28). This progression through the fan of the abductors/pelvic stabilizers brings us from the Back Functional Line (G. Max.) which decelerates the pronation to the anterior Spiral Line (TFL) which can then assist with foot supination.

The body's forward momentum, like the force of gravity, will also be decelerated by heel strike and so, as the skeleton progresses over the foot and comes into extension the anterior tissues are stretched (Box 10.1). The elastic load will be encouraged into much of the Superficial Front, Deep Front and anterior Spiral Lines as the body is held back by the foot's contact with the floor, which is eventually released as we progress through the rockers of the foot and come to toe-off (Fig. 10.29).

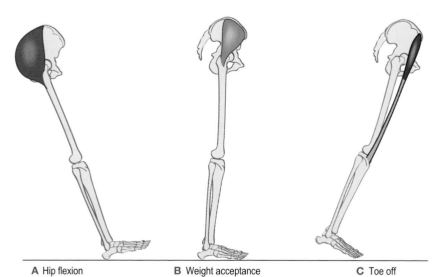

A Hip flexion   B Weight acceptance   C Toe off

• **Fig. 10.28** As the body progresses from heel strike (**A**) to weight acceptance (**B**) and finally toward toe-off (**C**), the line of tension progresses through the muscular 'fan' of the hip abductors.[4] The hip extension created prior to toe-off will tension all of the anterior flexors which act within various myofascial meridian lines. When the 'express' (see Ch. 2) myofascial units are engaged across multiple joints, the elastic tissue exploits the dynamics of the SSC to minimize the work of the 'local', individual muscles.

BOX 10.1

Exercise 1 – Stand tall, with your feet in a comfortable position. Reach back with one foot to lightly touch the floor behind you, keeping your standing leg straight. Once the toes have touched, let your limb relax and return. Experiment with different distances (do not strain or over-reach).

What creates the return? Some of you may say gravity; others will list the many hip flexors. So, repeat the exercise but this time with your head in a slightly protracted position. Do you feel a difference? Most people performing the experiment notice a considerable loss of force in the return movement yet gravity has remained constant and we did nothing directly to the many hip flexors. However, we did alter the tension of the SFL and DFL and lost some of their elastic contribution. Thus can a small adjustment in one segment affect the efficiency of elastic recoil many segments distant.

Exercise 2 – Begin with one leg extended behind and in toe-off position – big toe and ball of the foot in contact with the floor. Release the back foot's contact with the ground to unleash the leg and feel the force of its flexion. Compare the power of this 'automatic' flexion when you release the toes with varying degrees of thoracic and cervical extension.

Exercise 3 – Compare the force produced when you first reach back with one leg and positioning your foot in toe extension. Let your thorax tip forward as your leg goes back to comfortably maximize your extensional reach. Gradually bring your trunk back up, keeping the ball of your foot in place to feel the tension spread through the lines on the front of the body – SFL, DFL, and FFL.

Again release your foot at various degrees of thoracic extension to feel the relationship between the upper body position and the elastic power across the front of the hip.

In these exercises we begin to feel how the foot's contact with the ground acts as a lock to let the tissue be tensioned by the progression of the upper body over it that brings the limb into extension. Any limit in the ability to extend (which may be in the hip or the thorax, but could also be caused by restrictions elsewhere – for example, the inability to extend the knee, dorsiflex the ankle, or extend the toes will limit the hip) will reduce the loading ability and therefore also reduce the elastic contribution from the anterior tissues of the Superficial and Deep Front Lines and the anterior Spiral Line.

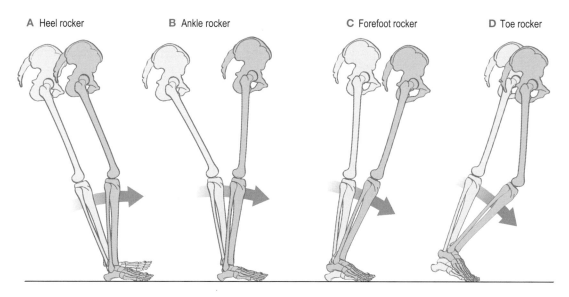

A Heel rocker   **B** Ankle rocker   **C** Forefoot rocker   **D** Toe rocker

• **Fig. 10.29** The progression of the body over the limb uses four so-called 'rockers' on the foot: (**A**) the roll around the calcaneus, (**B**) the dorsiflexion at the ankle over the top of the talus, (**C**) the rock over the metatarsal heads and, finally, (**D**) toe extension. During this sequence the plantarflexors of the Superficial Back Line, Lateral Line, and Deep Front Line are loaded, triggering the catapult that brings us forward into the next step. (Discussed fully in 'Born to Walk', Earls 2013). (Republished with permission of Slack Incorporated, from Gait analysis: Normal and Pathological Function, Perry J, Burnfield JM, 2nd edition, 2010; permission conveyed through Copyright Clearance Center, Inc.)

Most readers of this book will be aware of the tensional relationships that run throughout the body. By moving the head forward (a very common postural fault), we alter the ability of the leg movements described above to load elastic energy through a greater portion of the Superficial Front and Deep Front Lines.

As mentioned above, when the limb comes into extension the line of tension moves to the hip flexors including the tensor fasciae latae as part of the Spiral Line (see Fig. 10.28C). The tensioning created by the forward momentum can therefore assist with the foot's correction toward supination prior to toe-off via the anterior lower Spiral Line, i.e. the ITB linked to the tibialis anterior. This is further enhanced by the contralateral arm swing. When seen from the front of the body the opposite shoulder is rotating away from the extended leg side, creating tension through the

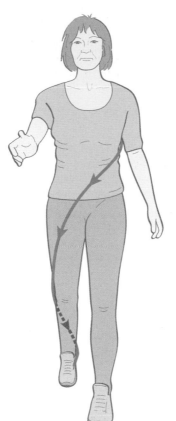

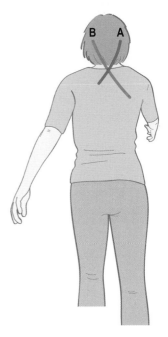

• **Fig. 10.30** As the lower limb goes into extension and relative rotation occurs from the pelvis to the rib cage to the opposite shoulder, the anterior portion of the Spiral Line will be tensioned by this momentum, assisting first with supination of the foot prior to toe-off and then with hip flexion and pelvic rotation as the foot leaves the floor into the swing phase.

• **Fig. 10.31** When the shoulder and arm swing back on the opposite side from toe-off, it tensions the whole of the anterior portion of the Spiral Line but eases the upper posterior portion (**A**). The upper portion of the complementary Spiral Line is tensioned by the forward swing of the opposite shoulder (**B**). This keeps the eyes headed forward throughout the gait cycle.

serratus/external/internal oblique line that adds more supportive tension in preparation for the propulsion at toe-off (Fig. 10.30).

The swing of the arm creates an apparent paradox in the upper Spiral Line – the splenii, rhomboids, and serratus anterior – which cannot be consistently shortened throughout – either serratus anterior or the rhomboids will be long or short, since they cannot both be in the same state on the same side (Fig. 10.31). As the arm swings forward the serratus anterior will be passively shorter (or at least under less tension) and the adjoining rhomboids will be lengthened (or under more tension). This makes sense when we look at the trunk and head prior to toe-off. In Fig. 10.30 we can see that the pelvis is rotated to the right and will therefore encourage the spine and head to the same direction. This tendency will be reduced by the forward swing of the right arm and rib cage that tensions the right rhomboids and left splenii to produce force of counter-rotation.

When we consider these rotational forces acting through the body in walking, we can overlay the map of the Anatomy Trains to see how the long cooperative chains assist for overall stability and ease. The abduction and adduction tendencies are dealt with by the Lateral Line that includes the ability of the lateral obliques to control the rotational relationship between the pelvis and rib cage (Fig. 10.32).

If we overlay the Deep Front Line we see that it is in an ideal position to tension through its entire length prior to toe-off. Ideally the ankle can dorsiflex while the toes and knee fully extend as the hip is extended, internally rotated

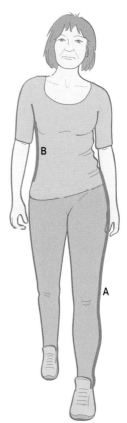

• **Fig. 10.32** In walking, the Lateral Line primarily decelerates the required side to side sway of the body that creates hip ab/adduction (**A**), with the lengthening swapping sides above the pelvis as the ilium drops away from the ribs on the opposite side of the adducting hip (**B**). The 'X' pattern of fibers in the Lateral Line (see Ch. 5) also assists with the ability to stabilize in various degrees of rotation.

and abducted while the thoracics maintain extension. If all this takes place in a coordinated fashion then a myofascial connection can be transmitted through the length of the DFL, a force that also assists with the correction to supination and hip flexion in preparation for the next step (Fig. 10.33).

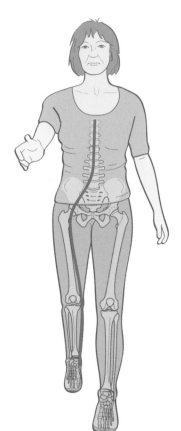

• **Fig. 10.33** The position of the lower limb prior to toe-off should be ideal for engaging the entire DFL. The combination of toe extension, ankle dorsiflexion, knee extension, and hip extension/internal rotation/abduction will combine to produce force transmission through the tissues of the entire Deep Front Line (provided that the joints can successfully move into those positions).

Including joint kinematics and the recoiling nature of the myofascial tissue leads to a deeper understanding of how to correct dysfunction of this complex. We can be informed by, but not rely on, the electrical activity measured by EMG readings as these measurements only tell us about the electrical activity with the muscle–tendon unit but not about its length or the amount of stored elastic tension in the collagenous part of that unit.[12]

If we want to develop an understanding of whole-body movements we need to leave behind the 'single muscle' analyses and parsing the body into 'locomotor' and 'passenger' sections. We need to appreciate the holistic nature of ingrained patterns within our myofascial system and understand the (sometimes quite distant) reasons for their presence. The continuities of the myofascia act to transfer force, to communicate necessary information to the mechanoreceptors, but also to control and capture mechanical force and work most efficiently when a countermovement is involved.[18,23,24]

Expand your view to include these long cooperative chains of tissues that are our transmission lines of preference. We can use our bodies more efficiently when they are coordinated body-wide to work together in time and space. As therapists, we can use these connections to ensure our clients' bodies utilize correct range of motion at each joint. As with the rest of the examples in this book, malalignment or bad timing in one segment can create problems either up or down the chain from the offending part. In assessing and treating gait anomalies, we need to see the whole system in context. The Anatomy Trains provides a map to make practical sense out of these whole-body pattern assessments. (Here, James Earls' contribution ends.)

❖ ❧ An 'Awareness Through Movement' Lesson

The short and simple movement exercise in the next section ('Rolling over') is inspired by the work of Dr Moshe Feldenkrais,[25] who devised hundreds of movement explorations he termed 'Awareness Through Movement' (ATM) lessons. The specifics of the lesson and the analysis of the myofascial meridians related to the lesson are the author's own interpretation, but the general approach and the principles are drawn from the Feldenkrais work.

This particular lesson was chosen for its simplicity and for its application to a number of common somatic restrictions. Perhaps more importantly, it is an example of primal movement, representative of developmental movements (see next section) that are primary building blocks of our daily movement repertoire. It is the contention of many movement therapists that missing or eliding over any of the phases of developmental movement can predispose the subject to structural or movement idiosyncrasies at best, difficulties at worst. While such a claim is hard to prove, clinical experience confirms that primary developmental movements have been tremendously useful in discovering underlying dysfunctional patterns that lead to surface difficulty or tendency toward specific injury.

❖ Rolling Over

The following lesson is absolutely designed to be experienced; just reading it over will not convey its essence. You can read the lesson, then follow it on the floor, or have someone read it to you, or record the text and play it back to yourself as you move. Each suggested movement should be repeated again and again, gently and slowly, exploring the feelings they create in every part of the body (Video 6.4).

Many such lessons (and far more sophisticated ones) are available on tape and in print from a number of sources in the world of Feldenkrais ATM teachers (www.feldenkraisresources.com, www.feldenkrais.com, www.feldenkraisinstitute.org).

Lie on your back with your knees up, so your feet are standing on the floor (Fig. 10.34). Begin by bringing both knees toward the floor to your right, and then come back to where you started. Do this a number of times, staying within the bounds of easy motion, not trying to stretch or strain. Let the knees slide past each other so that both feet stay on the floor, although eventually the left foot will perforce leave the floor. You will feel the weight shifting over to the side of the right hip as you move, and coming back to center as you bring your knees back up.

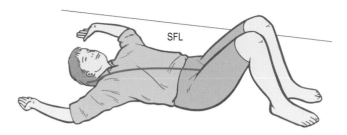

• **Fig. 10.34** Begin by lying comfortably on your back and letting your knees go to the right. The right Front Functional Line will be the prime mover, but all the lines will soon be involved.

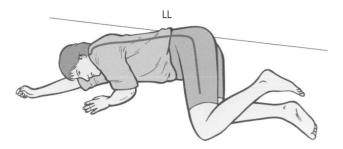

• **Fig. 10.35** When you reach side-lying, which Lateral Line feels longer and less toned? You can continue rolling by taking your knees and elbows away from each other.

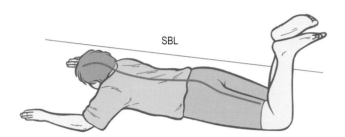

• **Fig. 10.36** After you reach the prone position, you are free to activate the SBL in a variety of ways, mostly to lift your eyes and other senses into the world. You can continue on around the roll by taking your knees to the left and letting the rest of your body follow.

What is the response further up your body? Do you feel the ribs lifting off the floor on the left side, or feel some response in the shoulder girdle? Rest a moment.

Put your arms beside or above your head, palms up. Find the easiest comfortable place, again without stress or stretch. If this is too difficult or stressful, put your hands on your chest and adapt the next set of instructions to your comfort. Begin once more to let your knees fall to the right, but this time add another movement: each time you move your knees to the right, extend your right hand or elbow further up over your head. It does not have to go very far; the important part is to coordinate it with the knees, so that the arm is extended as the knees go right, and the arm comes back down as the knees return to upright.

As you repeat this motion, begin to extend it so that the ribs and your head follow the knees. Let the arm extend out more and you will find that you will eventually roll onto your side. Do this motion a number of times, moving from your back to your side and back again, coordinating the arm and the knees. If it is more comfortable, let your head roll onto your right arm as you come to side-lying.

As you do this motion, you can let your left arm cross to the right, either across your chest or over your head, your choice. Either way, let it arrive on the floor in front of your face. So now you are lying on your side, with your knees up (hips flexed) and your left arm in front of you (Fig. 10.35). Now begin to take your knees and elbows away from each other and then back toward each other. Most bodies will respond to this movement in such a way that as the knees and elbows move apart from each other, you will tend to go from your side to your belly. As the knees and elbows approach each other, you will tend to move toward lying once more on your side, and eventually your back. Experiment with this movement, going from full flexion on the back to relaxed extension on your belly (Fig. 10.36).

Be slow – do not throw yourself through the movement. Beware of the tendency to fall as you move toward the belly; see if you can relax the muscles of your torso enough so that you can ease toward the floor without falling. Can you reverse the motion at any time, change your mind and go back to the side? Can you move from the back to the side to the belly by just moving your arms and knees?

Now that you are lying on your belly, turn your head so your face is to your right. Bring your feet up so that your knees are bent at a right angle, and begin to take your feet over to your left, as if to take the outside edge of your left foot to the ground. As before, let your legs slide on each other, so that your right knee comes off the ground only toward the end of the movement. Make sure the movement is comfortable, and repeat it several times until it is easy, even elegant.

As you do the movement, you may find that once again, your body is following the movement, that the right side of the ribs is beginning to lift up to follow the hips. Your head will probably be comfortable rolling onto your extending left arm. As you roll onto your left side, bring your knees and elbows together once again and you will find it easy to roll onto your back. Again, do this movement – from the belly over the left side to the back – several times until it feels easy and coordinated.

At this point you have completed a 360° roll of the body. If you have room, you can continue going in the direction you have started. If not, you can go back the way you came. Notice whether going one way is easier than the other. Practice rolling in both directions until it is easy and effortless either way. Do it more slowly rather than more quickly – doing it quickly is not an indication of movement mastery. If you can do it slowly, without falling or skipping over places, and without throwing yourself through the movement via momentum, then you can say you have mastered the movement.

As you perform this movement in a coordinated way, you can feel the accordion-like folding and unfolding of the myofascial meridian lines.

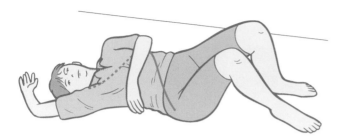

• **Fig. 10.37** The right Spiral Line is the primary rotator of the trunk, assisted in this movement by the left Front Functional Line bringing the left arm toward the right hip.

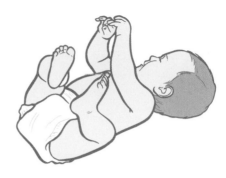

• **Fig. 10.38** Lying on the back, a baby's first postural preference, supports all three axial weights – head, chest, and pelvis – and all four appendicular weights – arms and legs – when the baby relaxes its SFL.

ATM Lesson Lines Analysis

Looking at this lesson with an Anatomy Trains lens, the obvious part of this lesson is in the line doing the spiral movement necessary to rolling. Since we initiated the movement in the limbs, the helical Functional Lines (see Ch. 8) are key to creating the movement. As we lie on our backs and begin to take the knees to the left, the left Back Functional Line (BFL) initiates the movement, and the left Lateral Line and right BFL are stretched until they begin to pull the body on along with it, like a string around a top. The right Spiral Line and the left Front Functional Line (FFL) also begin to pull as the right hip bone turns to the right, pulling the left rib cage along with it, but the primary line of pull is through the BFL (Fig. 10.37). The left FFL continues the pull from side to belly, and the right BFL completes the pull onto side and back, all coordinated with the two Spiral Lines.

Looking into the lesson a little more subtly, however, we can notice that in each phase of the movement, the cardinal lines open to the floor. When we are lying on the back, the Superficial Back Line opens and the Superficial Front Line subtly closes or shortens (see Fig. 10.34). We move to the right side by opening the right Lateral Line, whether we think of it that way or not. By the time we are lying on our right side, the right LL is more open overall, and the left LL more closed (not necessarily contracted, perhaps just passively short – see Fig. 10.35).

As we roll from the right side onto our ventral surface the SFL opens to the floor and the SBL closes behind us (see Fig. 10.36). We see it in babies, rocking on their bellies to lift the head and strengthen the SBL, and we can feel the closing of the line closest to the ceiling in ourselves, even if it is not so marked in the adult body. To continue onto the left side, we must open the left LL and close the right. Once the movement is mastered and we are rolling freely, we can feel the lines opening to the floor as we approach them, and we can feel (as the student) or see (as the teacher or practitioner) where the body is holding or restricted in its ability to open, thus restricting other places in their ability to move. It is this opening to the floor that is really the key to an easy accomplishment of this primal movement, not the spiral pulls that initiate the movement (which in any case vary widely in their point of initiation). Looking for where

the cardinal lines are blocked and working with those restrictions will very often bring more ease into this sequence than working with the Functional or Spiral Lines.

The point here is that subtle and underlying neurologic accommodations in the meridians as a whole are keys to adaptive movement. These underlying adjustments to movement are fundamental, and established in our earliest, pre-verbal experiments with our bodies. They are harder to see than some of the obvious movements we looked at earlier in this chapter, but they are often key to unlocking and resolving a pattern.

❖ ❖ 🍀 Developmental Movement Stages

The previous section dealt with rolling over, which is the first postural change a baby makes on its own, but not the last. In this section, we expand our view to take in the whole progression from lying to standing that each of us must either make or find a way around if we are to successfully negotiate standing up and walking through this world. Running yourself or your clients through this sequence is a marvelous self-help exercise that calms the mind and organizes the body through deep remembering of these primal and foundational movements (www.anatomytrains.com – video ref: Functional Lines, 50:40–1:05:27).

Almost all of us, even the youngest or most infirm, can easily lie on our backs, since the large body weights (head, chest, pelvis, and, if so desired, arms, and legs: totaling seven) are all supported by the floor in this position (Fig. 10.38). As suggested in the last section, in this position, the SBL tends to relax into the floor, while the SFL, open to the 'sky' where danger may lurk, tends to carry more protective tone.

After some months of ossification and muscle building, a baby, through experimentation (chiefly through trying to follow Mom with his eyes), will eventually turn from back to side to belly, much as we did in the previous section, where the SBL gains more tone and the SFL snuggles to the floor (Fig. 10.39). In this position, the baby has supported one of the large weights – the head – up in the air, giving

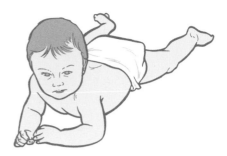

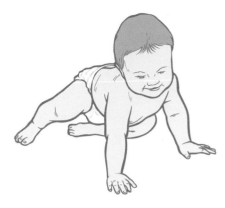

• **Fig. 10.39** Lying on the belly, a baby's first real postural change, achieves support for the head, allowing greater movement, and sets the stage for its first automotivation, creeping.

• **Fig. 10.41** Crawling liberates the last of the axial weights – the pelvis – from the floor, but requires support from all four, or at least three of the four, appendicular limbs.

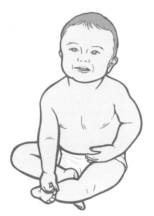

• **Fig. 10.40** Sitting supports two of the heavy axial weights above the pelvis, and allows the baby more manipulative freedom.

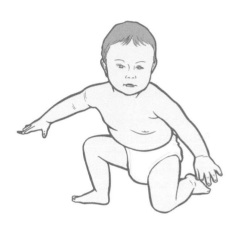

• **Fig. 10.42** The increased precision in balance involved in kneeling can only be built on the skills in the previous stages.

the eyes greater range and allowing greater freedom in creeping around. The muscles of the SBL strengthen in lifting up the head, and the secondary cervical curve is strengthened and set into place.

By looking over his shoulder (on the side of the cocked leg – babies almost always have one leg flexed and the other extended) the baby employs the helical lines (Spiral, Functional, and Lateral) to twist around to sitting (Fig. 10.40). The weight must shift in the pelvis from the ASIS to the ischial tuberosity, which happens by the weight rolling out over the greater trochanter and onto the bottom of the pelvis. Sitting on the floor requires the same balance among the three sagittal lines as was described above in the section on sitting in a chair – the SBL, SFL, and DFL. In sitting, the child has managed to raise and support two of the body's heavy masses – the head and the chest – off the ground. The child's freedom of movement and reach of both hands and eyes are increased (and you are busy child-proofing the house).

The next developmental stage involves the baby reaching around and forward to pass onto hands and knees, into crawling (Fig. 10.41). Once this stage is reached, it requires yet more strength from the cardinal lines, and yet more coordination between the limbs via the Functional Lines. Greater strength in the SFL is also necessary to keep the trunk aloft and not allow the lumbars to fall into extreme lordosis. Notice that the baby has now managed to get three of the heavy weights into the air: head, chest, and pelvis.

Now the question becomes – how do we get all this centered over the small base of support the feet provide?

The next stage, usually accomplished with the help of furniture or a parental leg, involves coming to kneeling, by rolling one foot on the floor from the dorsal to the plantar surface (Fig. 10.42). At this stage, all the leg lines must strengthen and develop in their coordination to support the body's entire weight through the hips. Through the previous stages of creeping and crawling, the primary weight was borne through the shoulders, but now the primary weight must stabilize through the pelvis down through the hips.

When the legs are strong enough, the child spirals up from kneeling to precarious standing, which usually manifests as walking (Fig. 10.43). Although some parents would disagree and development is malleable and differs among individuals, most children can walk before they can comfortably stand, as momentum is easier to maintain than the stasis (as in riding a bike). In the walking or running position, the body is supported primarily on one foot, with a part of the other – the heel or the ball of the foot – providing some balance as the child moves.

True standing – and an approach to the balance of the lines approaching Fig. 10.2 – requires all this prior

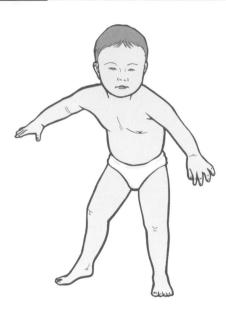

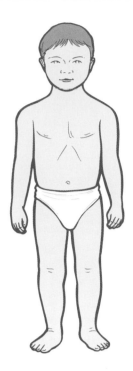

• **Fig. 10.43** As the baby gets on top of the second foot, with 1.5 feet's worth of support, the seemingly precarious act of walking provides a momentum that makes this motion easier to maintain at first than the really precarious act of standing.

• **Fig. 10.44** The act of standing – human plantigrade posture on two full feet – is the end-product of many stages of evolution, both phylogenetically and ontogenetically.

developmental movement, which has strengthened and aligned bones, developed joints, and brought fascial strength and elasticity as well as muscular strength and coordination to these longitudinal lines of stability and support, all in the service of easy, balanced standing and marvelously efficient walking (Fig. 10.44).

All complex human activities rest in the cradle of this basic sequencing of perception and movement that leads the baby from a passive lying on the back to active standing in the world. Since you cannot talk a baby in and out of clothes, car seats, etc. during that first year, a great deal of what is communicated to the baby during this sequence is conveyed kinesthetically. This suggests that anyone who interacts with babies could be learning basic handling skills to facilitate these patterns and alleviate movement problems in later life.

All parents and all therapists would benefit from being familiar with both this sequence, and with understanding the consequences when this sequence is interrupted or diverted. Children and this process are resilient, so even badly handled children arrive at standing and walking, but missing pieces can nevertheless affect movement in profound ways, including biomechanics, perception, and the ability to respond to certain situations.

The story goes (and the author got this verbally from Moshe Feldenkrais before his death, so cannot otherwise attest to its accuracy) that Moshe Feldenkrais was sat down at a dinner table next to anthropologist extraordinaire Margaret Mead. Mead, who said:

'Oh, yes, Feldenkrais – you're the movement man. I have a question I've been meaning to ask you: Why can't the Balinese men learn to hop? They are good dancers, ride bikes, and are otherwise quite coordinated, but I cannot teach them to hop from one leg to the other.'

'It sounds as if they are missing a stage of creeping', mused Feldenkrais.

'Of course', said Mead, smacking her forehead, 'The Balinese don't let their babies touch the ground for the first "rice year" (seven months), so they never get to creep on their bellies.'

Watch a baby in the initial stages of motivating its belly across the floor at about six months or so, and you will see where the underlying movement for transferring the weight from foot to foot, and thus hopping, lies. The baby thrusts one foot as the other retracts, building from reflex movement to the coordination that will later allow the transfer of the weight of the upper torso to each leg – in Anatomy Trains terms, running all the trunk lines into one set of leg lines, and then running them all into the other, alternating in turn. Without this stage grooved into their brains, the Balinese men could still walk, run, and dance, but not directly and specifically hop from one foot to the other. Whatever the veracity of the vignette or the concept, it serves to illustrate how underlying 'missing' patterns can manifest in subtle but specific alterations to the ability to move.

The practiced eye can see into movement to determine which lines are underperforming, and which stages of development might have been missed or skewed. Easy familiarity with the patterns of changing posture in movement as outlined above are a prerequisite for this kind of seeing.

Some Examples From Asian Somatics

Yoga Asana

Although we have used several yoga poses to illustrate stretching or engaging the various individual lines in each of their respective chapters, more complex poses engage

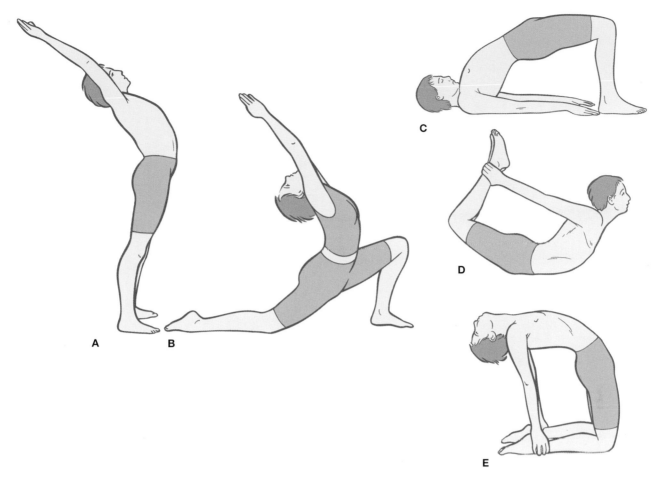

• **Fig. 10.45** Superficial Front Line stretches. In each of the following illustrations, each pose may stretch or challenge multiple muscles or lines, or have other intentions than mere stretch. We include these here for a simplified understanding of how the continual fascia within a line continuity may be stretched, as well as the individual structures. In all but (**C**), the upper cervical hyperextension is a common pitfall.

parts of multiple lines. Using the simple line drawings we include here (which are not refined enough to be accurate in any particular yogic approach), we can assign some asanas or postures to each individual line. These poses are named variously in different traditions; the names here are in common use.

Stretching of the Superficial Front Line (and consequent contraction along the Superficial Back Line) can be seen in the reach that begins the Sun Salutation sequence (Fig. 10.45A), or the basic warrior poses such as the Crescent Moon (Fig. 10.45B). The Bridge pose is a basic regulated stretch for the SFL (Fig. 10.45C), as is the more advanced Bow pose (Fig. 10.45D). The Camel also provides a strong stretch for the entire SFL (Fig. 10.45E). The Wheel, or backbend, pictured in Fig. 4.7A, is a strong stretch for the SFL. Many of these poses are nearly the same somatic configuration, simply with different orientations to gravity.

Stretching the Superficial Back Line is a primary action of the Downward Dog (Fig. 10.46A) and the Forward Bend poses (Fig. 10.46B). The Child's pose stretches the upper part of the SBL while allowing the knees to flex, which eases the stretch on the lower part (Fig. 10.46C). The Plow pose is also a strong stretch for the upper SBL (see Fig. 4.7B).

Although the Boat pose (Fig. 10.46D) is clearly a stretch to the SBL (as if the Downward Dog were turned upside down) and a muscle strength challenge for the SFL across the front of the legs and torso, this pose is actually a core strengthening pose which reaches into the psoas and other hip flexors of the Deep Front Line.

The Lateral Line is stretched by the Gate pose shown in Fig. 10.47 – showing a stretch of the left side – as well as the Triangle pose (see Fig. 4.17B or Fig. 10.51). The LL is also strengthened (a good thing for what is primarily a stabilizing line) by holding the body straight supported on one hand as in the Side Plank pose of Fig. 10.47B, where the Lateral Line closest to the floor prevents the body from collapsing from ankle to ear. The Half Moon pose (not pictured) requires work from the Lateral Line closest to the ceiling.

The upper Spiral Line is stretched by the simple Sage pose and any of a number of complex twisting poses

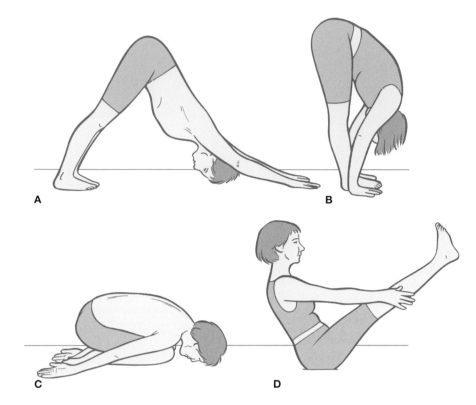

• **Fig. 10.46** Primary Superficial Back Line stretches.

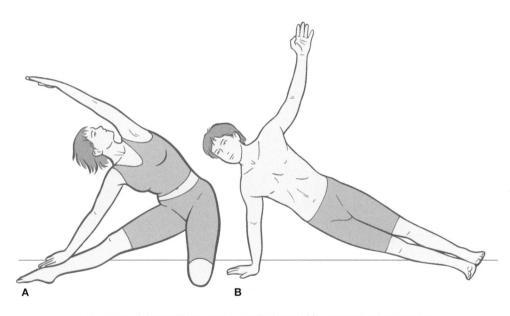

• **Fig. 10.47** A Lateral Line stretch, and a Lateral Line strengthening exercise.

(Fig. 10.48A and see also Fig. 6.22). Such poses strengthen one side of the Spiral Line while challenging its complement. Of course, such poses also offer challenges to the pelvic and spinal core, as well as the more superficial Spiral and Functional Lines. The Pigeon pose challenges the deep lateral rotators (a branch of the Deep Front Line) and the lower outer Spiral Line (biceps femoris and the peroneals – Fig. 10.48B). The anterior lower Spiral Line (tensor fasciae latae and tibialis anterior) can be stretched in the lunges and deep warrior poses by turning the stretched back foot out (laterally rotating the leg – see Fig. 9.29).

All the Arm Lines are challenged by the shoulder-and-arm focused poses. The Cow pose challenges primarily the Superficial Front and Back Arm Lines, whereas the Eagle pose challenges primarily the Deep Front and Back Arm Lines (Fig. 10.49 A and B).

Poses such as the Tree (Fig. 10.50) are primarily balance-promoting poses, passing all the lines from the upper torso

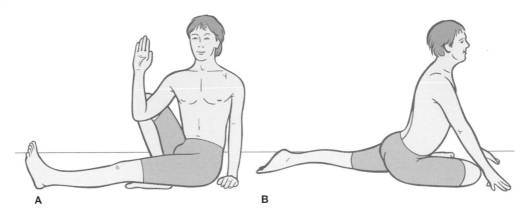

• **Fig. 10.48** Spiral Line stretches.

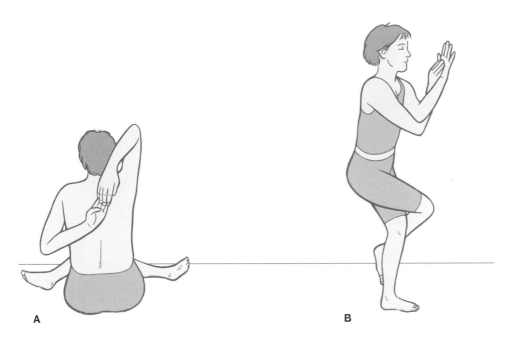

• **Fig. 10.49** Arm Line stretches.

down through one leg, and promoting tonal and neurological balance between the Lateral Line on the outer leg and the Deep Front Line on the inner leg. The Headstand pose (Fig. 10.50B) calls for balance among all the torso lines – SBL, SFL, LLs, and SPLs, as well as the DFL and Functional Lines, while using the arms and shoulders as temporary 'legs', i.e. as compressional support for much of the rest of the body's weight.

Progress in yoga or similar systems can be assessed by tracing the length in individual tracks or changes in the angles of the curves of the lines in asana. Figs. 10.51 and 10.52 show two poses – *Trikanasana* and *Parivrtta Parsvakonasana* – performed by an experienced teacher (A), a middling student (B), and a neophyte (C). Compare the lines to trace the progress. A detailed comparison of the photos is available in the eBook.

Shiatsu, Acupressure, or Thumb Work

The practice of shiatsu, acupressure, and some other forms of pressure-point work such as finding and eradicating trigger points involve placing significant pressure through the thumbs. The thumb, we remember, is the end point of the Deep Front Arm Line. To 'give weight' and create sustained pressure through the thumb requires using many of the muscles of the arm – all four lines, in fact – as fixation muscles to steady the limb. We have noted that myofascial continuities can only pull, they cannot push. Given that the pressure is coming down through the thumb, one might expect that the DFAL was the least important of the lines, being in a curved position and relatively relaxed for this motion compared to the other stabilizing lines of the arm. But because of the connection from the thumb to the ribs along the DFAL, it is very important.

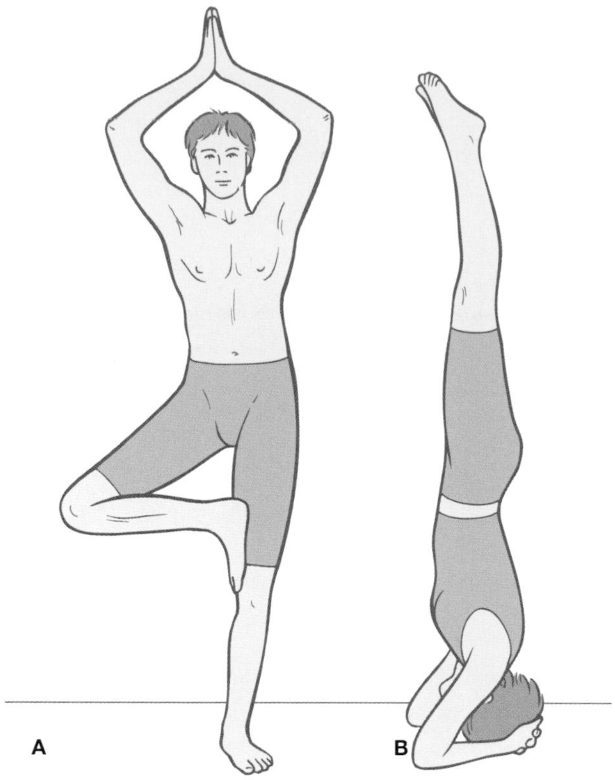

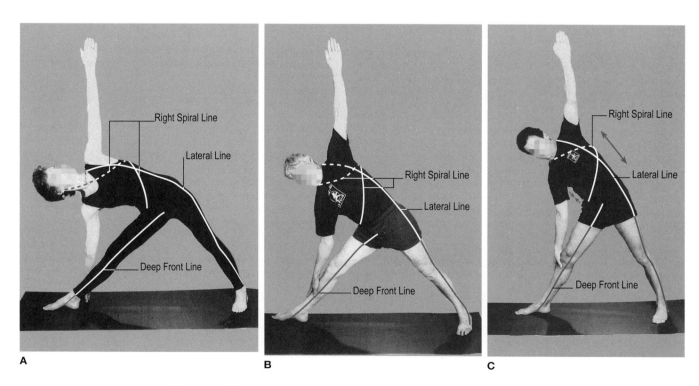

• **Fig. 10.50** Balancing poses.

Practitioners of these arts frequently have presenting problems in their shoulders or neck. When we have these practitioners mock up how they work, universally they are collapsing somewhere along the DFAL – in other words, along the myofascial meridian that runs from the ribs out through the pectoralis minor and the inside curve of the arm to the thumb. When this line shortens, the rest of the lines, and most usually one of the back lines of the arm, must take up the flag and end up overworking (Fig. 10.53A). For the shiatsu worker to stay healthy and pain-free in both joints and soft tissues, it is necessary to keep the DFAL open and lengthened, so that tension and pressure are distributed evenly around the tensegrity of the arm (Fig. 10.53B). In this way, the pressure is taken by the skeleton from the thumb to a balanced axial complex, not distributed sideways through the soft tissues of the Arm Lines.

Aikido or Judo Roll

Although our limbs are bony and angular, practitioners of martial arts can often make it look as if the body is made of India rubber as they roll effortlessly along legs, arms, and trunk. There are many rolls in Asian martial arts. Here we discuss a forward roll common to both aikido and judo.

In terms of the Anatomy Trains, we can see that in a forward roll the little finger is the first edge of the body to make contact with the floor or mat, bringing our attention to the Deep Back Arm Line (Fig. 10.54A). The body

• **Fig. 10.51** Trikanasana (Triangle pose) as performed by (**A**) an experienced teacher, (**B**) an experienced student, and (**C**) a neophyte student.

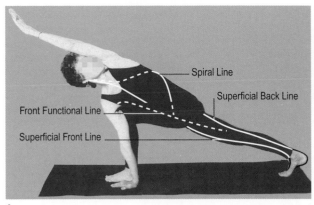

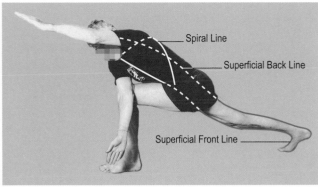

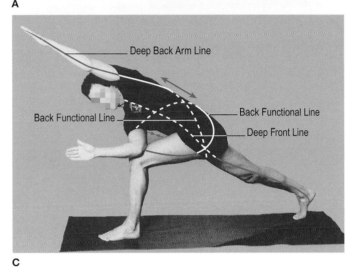

• **Fig. 10.52** Parivritta Parsvakonasana (Revolved Lateral Angle pose) as performed by (**A**) an experienced teacher, (**B**) an experienced student, and (**C**) a neophyte student.

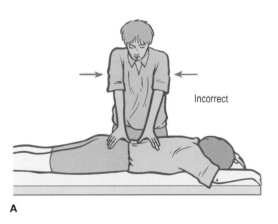

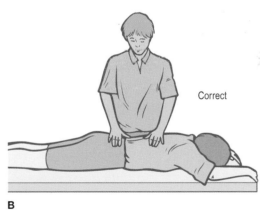

• **Fig. 10.53** Anyone relying on his thumbs to create pressure should take care to keep the Deep Front Arm Line open and round. Collapsing in the upper part of the DFAL is a reliable way to ensure subsequent hand, elbow, shoulder, or neck problems.

supports or guides itself on this line (although in an actual roll, little weight is placed on the arm), moving up the surface of the ulna and onto the triceps.

As the roll reaches the back of the shoulder, the baton is passed from the triceps to the latissimus, or in Anatomy Trains terms from the DBAL to its extension, the Back Functional Line. The body rolls on the diagonal of the BFL, by now supporting the weight of the entire body, crossing

the midline of the back and onto the opposite hip (Fig. 10.54B). From here the Lateral Line of the leg supports the body, passing down the iliotibial tract and the fibularii as the opposite foot hits the floor and begins the process of standing up again (Fig. 10.54C).

A roll also requires proper balance between the Superficial Front and Back Lines, as over-contraction of the SBL will interfere with obtaining a smoothly rounded shape for

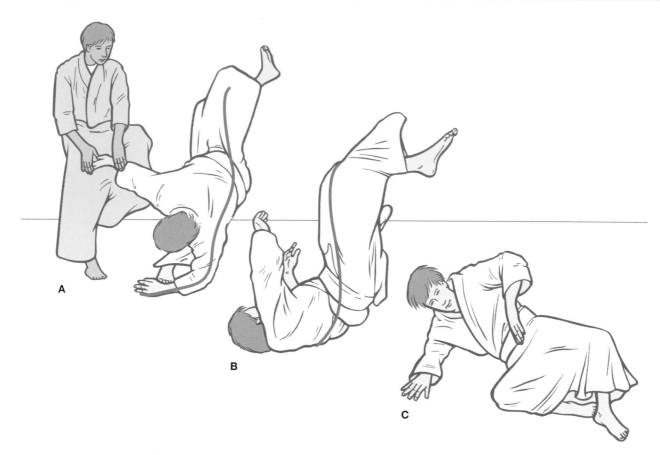

• **Fig. 10.54** An aikido forward roll travels along the Deep Back Arm Line, the Back Functional Line, and the Lateral Line.

the trip across the lumbars, and over-contraction of the SFL, which is very common in the early stages of learning, causes hyperextension of the upper cervicals, making it hard to tuck the head out of the way and coordinate the back muscles.

Staying strong, open, and aware of these lines as you pass through the roll will make it smoother and safer. Conversely, shortening, tightening, or retracting these lines when attempting a roll will result in a bumpy ride.

Karate Kick

Fig. 10.55A, a karate kick to the front, involves contraction of the Superficial Front Line to create the kick, and lengthening along the Superficial Back Line to allow the kick to happen. Restrictions in either of these lines could affect the ability of the student to perform this action.

Notice also how the arms counterbalance the flexed leg. The two front Arm Lines on the left flex the arm and bring it across the chest, while the two Back Arm Lines abduct the right arm and extend the elbow. The left leg and right arm are stabilized across both front and back via the Functional Lines to provide a base for the action of the left arm and right leg. The Front Functional Line adds to the force of the kick, and the Back Functional Line must lengthen to allow it while maintaining core support between the two.

Less obviously, the Deep Front Line is involved in the ability to make this kick work for the whole body. The posterior adductors and posterior intermuscular septum must lengthen to allow the hip to flex fully without tilting the pelvis posteriorly. More to the point, the iliopsoas is active in flexing the hip and holding the femur in flexion. Either of these factors can create a downward pull compressing the spine. In Fig. 10.55B, a similar kick from the side, we can see this effect in action. The tissues of the SFL remain long, but the core is nevertheless pulled down. The front of the spine is clearly shortened from the anterior cervicals to the pelvic floor.

Some years ago it was my privilege to work with an Olympic contender on the British karate team. Long of limb (and very fast), this gentleman was set fair to bring home the gold, but for one problem – kicking caused an increasingly sharp and debilitating pain in his lower back. My first line of inquiry was in the SBL, reasoning that the tension of the hamstrings was being passed around through the sacrotuberous ligament to the sacrum and the sacrolumbar fascia, thus causing some kind of radicular compression. When this avenue proved fruitless, I watched him kicking once again and saw what I should have seen in the first place, what we see in Fig. 10.55B, a slight shortening in the core of the trunk when he kicked. By examining the structures of the DFL, I determined that the upper-outer fibers

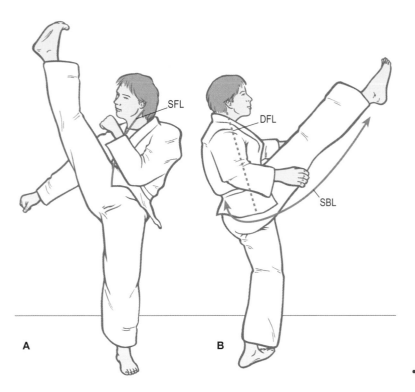

A   B

• **Fig. 10.55** Karate kicks to the front.

of the psoas muscles were overworking, causing a compression of the lumbar spine (and thus some kind of impingement) when he kicked. By working to even out the load over the entire iliopsoas, we were able to reduce the compression and increase the springiness of the lumbar spine – and yes, he went on to capture a medal.

In Fig. 10.56, we see a side kick. Here we can note the upper body leaning off the SBL of the grounded leg. The left Lateral Line is shortened all the way from the side of the head to the side of the foot to fix the body in a 'Y' shape. The height of the kick thus depends on the ability of the SBL to lengthen in the standing leg, the strength of the LL and its abduction ability, and the ability of the inner arch of the kicking leg to stretch away from the ischiopubic ramus and lumbar spine – in other words, the extensibility of the DFL, particularly in the adductors. This particular kicker seems also to be supporting the torso with the upper left Spiral Line, looping under the right ribs from the left side of the head to the left hip. Notice that very little kicking power is provided by the LL, which is primarily a line of stabilization. The power in the kick, as with a horse, comes from the combination of the sagittal lines – the extensors of SBL and SFL.

Summary

These examples serve to show a few of the directions where the Anatomy Trains scheme can be applied in action. Obviously, these applications could be expanded and filled in with more detail – for original movement skills acquisition, for personal and athletic training, for rehabilitation, and in artistic enhancement – but we have chosen width over

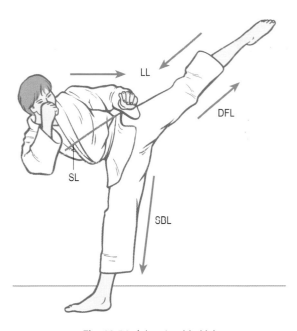

• **Fig. 10.56** A karate side kick.

depth in this introductory volume. Further application in various modalities are offered in the videos on the accompanying site, and via the online and in-person classes Anatomy Trains offers worldwide.

The principles, however, are the same for all applications: look for the areas where fascial or muscle shortening are limiting motion, and then check out the full extent of the lines in which these specific structures live and have their being. On the other side of the coin, areas that have laxity or too much movement/too little stability can be identified and strengthened. What is commonly identified as a 'weak gluteus medius' is often better dealt with as a coordination problem of the Lateral Line. Strengthening through a line – so that the line as a whole responds in coordinated fashion rather than just a specific muscle – can improve functional stability in the young athlete or the older veteran alike.

When doing a functional assessment of a client or student such as FMS (Functional Movement Screen) or SFMA (Selective Functional Movement Assessment), it is obviously useful to observe and assess which specific structures might be involved in an action or in its restriction.[26] The examples in this chapter will perhaps have convinced the reader of the value in also doing a more global myofascial meridian assessment as part of this process.

View clients as they perform an action, preferably from a bit of a distance so that the entire body is within your foveal vision. Assessing movement from your peripheral vision – originally developed, after all, to detect movement – can also be helpful, and is sometimes more revealing than staring right at them. See whether one or more of these lines is not restricting the overall movement. Working with the entire line will often bring an increased freedom that working on only the obviously affected part will miss.

One more time we emphasize: the body does not think, as we commonly do, in terms of individual muscles as the actuators of movement. The body thinks in terms of individual neuromotor units of ten to several hundred muscle fibers, recruited in coordinated fashion based on remembered patterns in the cerebellum, regardless of the muscle to which they ostensibly belong. The current generation is stuck with the concept of individualized muscles – even after 30 years of trying to eradicate this way of thinking, the author still thinks in terms of muscle names – but the coming generations will see movement differently.

Anatomy Trains is simply a more global way to map the movement/stability interplay. Practicing assessment in this way expands your training and treatment options by letting you see the organismic movement picture, not just the machine 'parts'.

To conclude this chapter, we are pleased to include this new contribution by Karin Gurtner on 'Anatomy Trains in Motion', a programme built on fascial properties and myofascial meridians principles, now offered worldwide. We find value in nearly all movement methods – the ones referred to in this book as well as the myriad others not specifically mentioned.

We are often asked: 'What is the best form of movement?' Since the real answer depends on a multifactorial blend of age, psychology, physiology, movement capacity, and goals, the snappy but pertinent answer is: 'The one you'll actually do!' Any movement is better than no movement, and any method that gets us – especially the younger 'us' – up off the couch and moving our bum is to be preferred to the latest craze or even the absolutely 'correct' class we seldom attend.

The process outlined and illustrated here (for the fully developed version, go to www.art-of-motion.com) is a program of mindful, strengthening, and integrating movements that are readily adaptable. They can be progressed for the athlete, or regressed for the differently abled, and would be a sound basis for a schools-based program of physical education or, if you prefer, 'movement hygiene'. We referred to this at the beginning of the chapter as 'KQ' – kinesthetic intelligence or movement literacy; the Anatomy Trains in Motion library of interconnected movement explorations are a significant contribution to KQ.

Anatomy Trains in Motion – Structural Integration Through Movement, by Karin Gurtner

Alongside the role fascia plays in force transmission, morphogenesis, immunity, and wound healing, as well as its multiple responses to exercise in general, can we specifically bring the body toward structural integration through movement?

Structural Integration (see Appendix 2, p. 323) describes bodywork modalities that seek to deliberately alter fascia and habit to enhance easy postural alignment, function and dynamic vitality. If structure refers to the organization of elements within a system, then a well-integrated structure operates coherently, with all elements cooperating in unitary intent.

Fascia itself, of course, has been with us since before our ancestors crawled out of the sea, and since humans first started to motivate purposefully. Without naming it, the ancient dancers, athletes, fighters, therapists, and yogis utilized the properties of fascia in their training regimes that we are now supporting (and sometimes refuting) through research.

If we add recent scientific insights to these ancient understandings, can we apply a safer, more long-term, and more comprehensive approach to neuromyofascial training?

The sequences below expand the concept of how to train fascia in a way that supports the goals of Structural Integration – alignment, ease, and coherence.

Training Fascial Properties

The question is not whether fascia contributes to or is engaged in movement: all voluntary movement involves myofascial force transmission. Not all movements, however, train the same fascial properties or to the same degree or with the same efficiency.

In the previous decades of muscle-focused training, actual exercise sequences have varied depending on the goals – strength, endurance, power, speed, stability or flexibility – for each of which we needed to understand the properties and workings of muscle tissues and neuromotor patterning. Even as we continue to learn more about the cybernetics of movement, we are now embarked on a similar research and practice-based journey: What movements or exercises for which populations enhance which of the protective properties of fascia?

The Anatomy Trains concept, the Fascial Fitness* explorations, and applications of recent research in physiotherapy – all the new information on fascial sensing leading to new understandings in self-regulation – are early scouting parties in mapping the topology of training fascia with the same specificity we have mapped muscles and joints. The following Anatomy Trains in Motion and Myofascial Slings sequences are offered in the same spirit of building coherence in the entire neuromyofascial web.

Training fascia intentionally means knowing why you do what you do and what it is you aim to achieve. Before engaging the Anatomy Trains in Motion, let's review foundational principles:

- Your body, mind and emotions are inseparably part of you.
- Movement is (at least) a neuro-myo-fascial-skeletal-psycho-emotional-perceptual synergy that is linguistically and socially influenced and imponderable in its wholeness.
- Fascia is the body-wide, collagenous connective tissue system in which all other physical tissues and systems are embedded, held, and spatial relationships maintained.
- With an estimated 100,000,000 nerve endings in its interstitium, fascia is likely the richest and arguably the most influential sensory organ of kinesthesia, including both proprioceptive and interoceptive endings.[27,28]

Anatomically, the myofascial meridians are continuities of muscles and fascia. Functionally, they are kinesthetic slings that have proprioceptive and interoceptive (psychobiologic) functions – as well as tensile strength, active and passive tone, and elastic resilience. These lines are adaptable yet stabilizing. They transmit force in-series over long distances and contribute to the tensegral balance of the body. In other words, the myofascial meridians inherit all of the fascial qualities, and add the flickering or blazing neuromuscular adjustments required by moment-to-moment adaptation and loading.

In this section, five fascial qualities are linked to specific practice. To make this of tangible practical value, two exercise examples follow each description, each linked to videos. (Of course, the exercise examples may engage or enhance other fascial qualities in addition to the one they represent here). A lesson planning guide follows. These examples represent a small part of the repertoire of Anatomy Trains in Motion and Slings Exercises, to be found at www.art-of-motion.com.

1. Force Transmission

The collagenous network transmits force; in other words, fascia facilitates and modulates mechanical communication across all the body tissues. The myofascial meridians chart in-series tensional force transmission. Force distribution also travels in parallel, between adjacent myofascial structures.[29]

Force transmission increases movement efficiency by decreasing strain on individual parts and increasing communication between the involved muscles and fascia. For force to be transmitted in an efficient and healthy manner, fascial cells are constantly remodeling the network to balance the need for sufficient tensile strength, without creating movement-reducing adhesions to neighboring tissues or shutting down perfusion to local cells.

In practice, linear movement – with clearly aligned dynamic exercises, using body weight and actively sustained stretches – fosters more in-series force conduction. Multi-dimensional movements performed in a generous and fairly slow manner lead to more widespread distribution of forces.

Roll Down & Forward Fold Leg Stretch
Force transmission experienced in the Superficial Back Line (Fig. 10.57)

Lunge & Side Bend
Force transmission experienced in the Back Functional Line (Fig. 10.58):

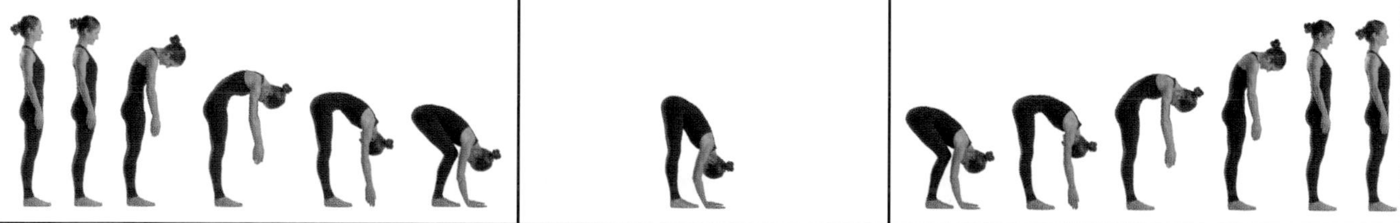

Rolling down	Forward fold leg stretch	Rolling up
Upper portion actively lengthening and strengthening:	Lower portion lengthened actively or passively:	Lower portion gently and upper portion actively strengthened:
Muscles eccentrically strengthened (actively lengthened)	Muscles lengthened (actively or passively)	Muscles concentrically strengthened
Fascia tensioned	Fascia tensioned	Fascia tensioned

• Fig. 10.57

Lunge with side bend and single arm circle

Active lengthening and strengthening:

Muscles eccentrically strengthened (actively lengthened) and concentrically strengthened

Fascia tensioned

Video Force Transmission: anatomy-trains-in-motion.com

• **Fig. 10.58**

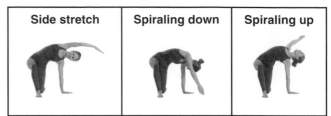

Side stretch	Spiraling down	Spiraling up

Glide within and between the myofascial structures of the thorax:

Muscles actively lengthened and gently strengthened

Fascia gliding

• **Fig. 10.59**

2. Glide

The multidimensional fiber organization supports structural integrity though progressive stabilizing layers, while enabling relative motion between them in more fluid fascia. Perifascial membranes between structures and perimysial glide within each muscle also enables differentiated fascicle activation and fascial tensioning in adjacent myofascial structures, which is essential for efficient core stabilization, movement functionality, and tissue hydration.

Common features of glide-enhancing exercises are a moderate intensity, generous range of movement and perceptible tension changes between adjacent layers. Frequently spiraling, arching, curling, and wave-like movements, as well as domino (bone-by-bone or myofascial layer-by-layer) sequences, are incorporated to enhance glide from the outside in. Also used are self-massage exercises in which the massaged body part is relaxed, and the skin and superficial fascia are slowly 'rolled' or 'dragged' to create shear and resultant hydration in the underlying myofascial structures.

Side Stretch & Spiraling
Glide experienced within and between all of the myofascial meridians in the upper portion (Fig. 10.59):

Sit Back With Curl Up & Arch
Glide experienced within and between the Superficial Front Line, Lateral Line, Spiral Line and the Functional Lines as well as the Deep Front Line from knees to chest (Fig. 10.60):

3. Elasticity

Helical collagen architecture gives tissue its elastic property. Key features of resilient fascia are the collagenous double-lattice pattern (especially in the myofascia) and crimp formation (especially in the tendinous portion).

In rhythmical or oscillating motions, substantial fascial structures such as ligaments, tendons and aponeuroses absorb tension and release it in recoil. This kinetic mechanism contributes to efficiency and spring, giving a sense of light-footedness when walking, double the satisfaction when running and athletic ease when swinging the golf club. Inelastic walking can be seen sometimes in the old or the differently abled, but inelasticity can be experienced by us all in the tired feet that follow a couple of hours of 'walking' through a museum.

Elastic recoil still requires muscle contraction to enhance or dampen these energies as required, but resilient fascia reduces the muscles' expenditure to a minimum.[30]

To utilize the elastic storage capacity of fascia, the tissue needs to be loaded appropriately and rhythmically. The good news is that elasticity can be (re)trained in an enjoyable and safe manner. Enhance tissue resilience gradually and in well-measured doses, considering individual factors. Exercises employed to train elastic recoil include rhythmical bounces and jumps, swinging movements, dynamic spiraling of the spine and domino motions.

Dynamic Knee Bend & Arm Pendulum
Elasticity experienced in the lower portion of the body-wide myofascial meridians and the Back Functional Line, with momentum added by the Arm Lines (Fig. 10.61):

Dynamic Hip Release & Spiraling
Elasticity experienced in the Spiral Line and Front Functional Line as well as the Deep Front Line and BFL, empowered by the SBL lowest portion (Fig. 10.62):

4. Plasticity

Fascial plasticity refers to the tissue's ability to take on a new shape more permanently, which happens in morphogenesis and growth, as well as in wound healing – and in specifically applied manual therapy or exercise.

In practice, we focus on the shape-changing behavior, specifically lasting length changes. Variables either permit or inhibit plasticity changes, including collagen density and

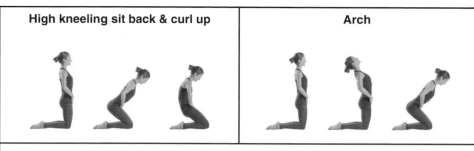

High kneeling sit back & curl up	Arch

Glide within and between the myofascial structures of the thighs and within the myofascial origami of the abdomen:

Muscles eccentrically strengthened (actively lengthened) and concentrically strengthened

Fascial gliding

Video Glide: anatomy-trains-in-motion.com

• **Fig. 10.60**

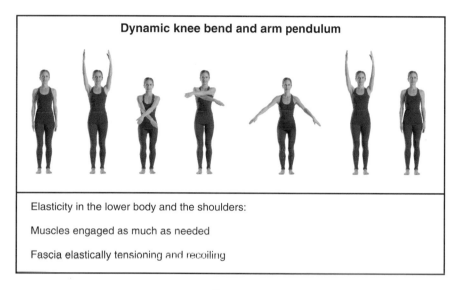

Dynamic knee bend and arm pendulum

Elasticity in the lower body and the shoulders:

Muscles engaged as much as needed

Fascia elastically tensioning and recoiling

• **Fig. 10.61**

ground substance viscosity. To attain a useful lengthening response, a relaxed stretch is required, generally for one to five minutes. Attempting fascial lengthening at high speeds results in tearing, then scarring, then shortening – not lengthening.

Neural plasticity can accompany fascial plasticity. A 'sense of melting' and actual fascial webbing change are both beneficial. Putting awareness into relaxation promotes parasympathetic nervous system activity. Relaxed ('restorative') poses, where muscles and fascia can gradually lengthen, lend themselves to fascial melting.

Another way of facilitating fascial pliability is through slow (e.g., Tai Chi) or sustained self-massage exercises. Time frames can vary considerably with the density of the fascia being challenged, ranging from ten to twenty seconds, up to a few minutes.

Melting exercises or sustained stretches may temporarily compromise tissue integrity during remodeling – i.e., a strong stretch session just before a football game might not

be the best strategy. Here, to assure a healthy degree of myofascial responsiveness, long-held melting poses or massages are complemented in these sequences with invigorating motions, in which the previously lengthened muscles and fascia are gently engaged to more quickly restore normal tissue integrity.

Melting Deer Pose

A sense of melting and lengthening experienced in the central portion of the Lateral Line and Deep Front Line (Fig. 10.63):

Neck Massage & Nodding

A sense of softening and opening experienced in the neck portion of the Superficial Back Line (Fig. 10.64)

5. Kinesthesia: Proprioception and Interoception

Anatomy Trains in Motion exercises make use of kinesthesia, both its proprioceptive and interoceptive aspects.

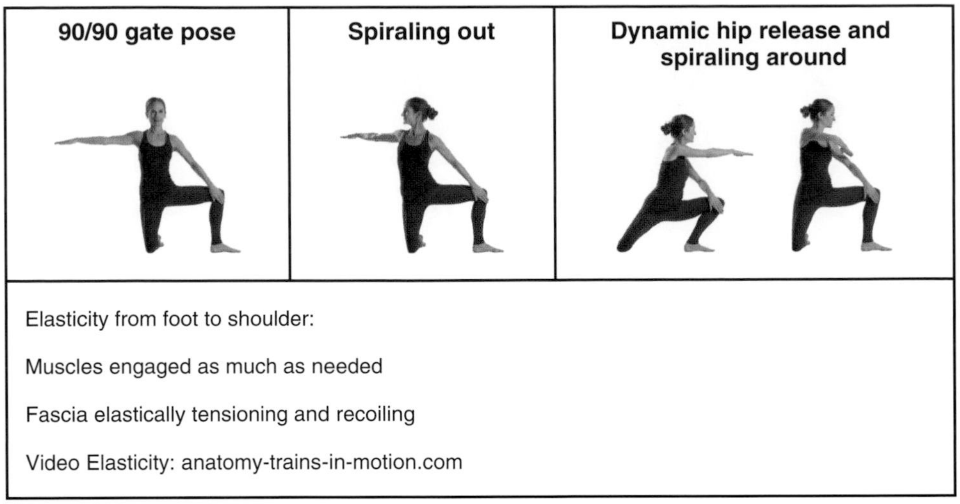

90/90 gate pose	Spiraling out	Dynamic hip release and spiraling around

Elasticity from foot to shoulder:

Muscles engaged as much as needed

Fascia elastically tensioning and recoiling

Video Elasticity: anatomy-trains-in-motion.com

• **Fig. 10.62**

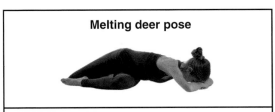

Melting deer pose

Relaxed lengthening:

Muscles passively stretched

Fascia passively tensioned

• **Fig. 10.63**

Proprioceptors give us a sense of our position in space and its progression in movement. Interoceptors – and we have found this out only recently – extend into the myofasciae to give us a sense of the condition of the physiology there. These signals, which go to the anterior insula not the parietal cortex like proprioception, give rise to homeostatic motivations, guiding adaptive behaviors with a strong affective quality that prod us to regain and sustain equilibrium.

Although both are intimately woven into our kinesthetic intelligence, it is worthwhile to differentiate proprioception and interoception, i.e. training proprioceptive finesse and interoceptive clarity.

Proprioception lets us know where we are in space, without judgment. Proprioception promotes joint centering, overall alignment, as well as smoothly coordinated, well-timed execution of the movements we repeat.

Interoception is the unconscious or conscious ability to sense how the body feels about what it feels – the effects of movement on emotional states, which motivates behavior changes geared toward well-being. Interoceptive clarity is intangible, personal and interpretive. In practice,

interoceptive learning requires mindful movement that brings awareness to the perception of bodily sensations and to our emotional responses to what is felt.

In terms of exercise selection, unusual variations, active and melting lengthening of muscles and fascia, differentiated strengthening, and stimulating self-massages benefit proprioception and interoception alike when done in a mindful manner. Cueing the breath is a powerful tool to convert negative into positive interoceptive feelings, fostering a sense of joy in movement.

Leg Float Up & Pelvic Tilt

Proprioceptive coordination and interoceptive awareness experienced in the DFL, SFL and SBL (Fig. 10.65):

Pelvic Curl

Proprioceptive coordination and interoceptive awareness experienced in the DFL, SFL and SBL (Fig. 10.66):

Slings in Motion Strategy

Even simple and small movements tend to employ all of the myofascial meridians in at least a stabilizing role. It is as difficult to isolate a myofascial meridian as it is to isolate a muscle. What is attainable – and of practical value – is to focus in both assessment and treatment on individual lines and their role in dynamic stabilization and coordinated motion.

Lesson Planning

There is no such thing as a 'one size fits all' sequencing of exercises. There are, however, ways of creating sequences that facilitate dynamic stability, strength and agility along with overall resilience, which have proven successful in practice.

The lesson planning guide for a Slings in Motion class is illustrated in Fig. 10.67 (and see Table 10.1).

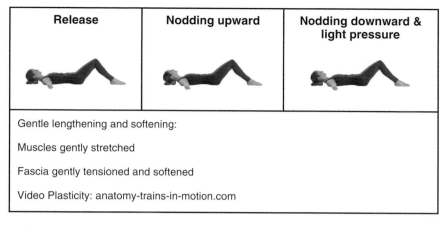

Release	Nodding upward	Nodding downward & light pressure

Gentle lengthening and softening:

Muscles gently stretched

Fascia gently tensioned and softened

Video Plasticity: anatomy-trains-in-motion.com

• Fig. 10.64

Centering on balls	Leg float up	Pelvic tilt	Table top	Leg float down

Inside-out dynamic stabilization and outside-in movement:

Muscles deliberately engaged for core stabilization and movement ease

Sensory feedback from fascial receptors

Video Kinesthesia: anatomy-trains-in-motion.com

• Fig. 10.65

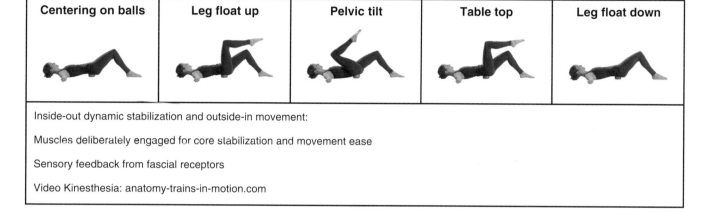

Centering	Pelvic Tilt	Hammock	Shoulder Bridge	Curling Down

Dynamic stabilization and inside-out movement:

Muscles deliberately engaged for core and movement control

Sensory feedback from fascial receptors

• Fig. 10.66

Slings in Motion Experienced

Video Lesson: anatomy-trains-in-motion.com

Any movement is better than no movement – but how much better is a mindful and versatile movement practice that speaks in a specified and deliberate manner to the interconnected complexity of our holistic nature? Structurally integrating the body through motion can be applied to physical education and rehabilitation, as well as in athletic or artistic performance enhancement.

We want a movement practice that engages a diverse spectrum of fascial qualities, using the Anatomy Trains body map to navigate the holistic intricacy of our myo-fascial-skeletal anatomy with clear intention and precise instructions.

Structural Integration is a state of consistent engagement with your movement, not an end-result that, once achieved, makes you feel fine forever. While moving coherently comes with immediate and abundant benefits – from improved stability and injury resistance to feeling at home in your

TABLE 10.1 **Slings in Motion Lesson Planning Guide: 60 Minutes**

Theme	Timing	Direction	Body Focus	MM(s): Primary	MM(s): Assisting	Energetic Quality
1. **Arriving:** Getting moving	15–20	Outside in	Feeling movement	Various	Various	Awakening
2. **Centering:** Sense of balance		Inside out	Core awareness	DFL	SBL	Grounding
3. **Easy flow:** Warming up		Outside in	Global pliability	SBL	DFL, SFL	Gently energizing
				LL, ALs	DFL	
				SFL	DFL, SBL	
4. **Contrasting flow:** Body of lesson	25–30	Inside out Outside in	Expanding movement scope and diversity	SPL DFL, LL FLs SBL, SFL	DFL, ALs ALs DFL, ALs DFL	Energizing, challenging, satisfying, grounding
5. **Gentle flow:** Winding down	5–10	Inside out	Rebalancing	SBL, SFL DFL	ALs	Calming
6. **Absorption & Invigoration:** Feeling relaxed and awake	5	Inside Inside out	Stillness Awakening	DFL SBL, SFL SPL SFL, SBL	DFL DFL, ALs DFL, ALs	Rejuvenating, inward focus Gently vitalizing, opening outward

ALs, Arm Lines; DFL, Deep Front Line; FLs, Functional Lines; LL, Lateral Line; MM, myofascial meridian; SBL, Superficial Back Line; SFL, Superficial Front Line; SPL, Spiral Line.

Primary Movement Dimension(s)	Primary Exercise Type	Included Primary Movements
Sagittal plane body motion, multidimensional arm movements	Mobilizing	Centered body alignment and/or trunk and leg flexion Multidimensional arm and shoulder movements
Stillness	Core activation	Centered body alignment Expansive breath
Sagittal plane slow motion Frontal plane slow motion Sagittal plane slow motion	Mobilizing, active lengthening, strengthening	Segmental spine flexion Hip flexion Dorsiflexion and plantar flexion Lateral spine flexion Generous arm and shoulder movement Segmental spine extension Hip extension
Multidimensional motion in all planes, at different rhythms and with various intensities	Diverse blend of rhythmical dynamic exercises, grounding poses and mellow motions	Whole-body movement including three-dimensional motion of the: • spine, including spiraling • hip joints, including rotation of the pelvis over the femur • shoulders, including movement of stabilized scapula over the humerus Dynamic stabilization of the: • spine • pelvis • shoulder girdle and shoulder joint
Sagittal plane slow motion	Gentle mobilizing, balanced lengthening and toning, core stabilization	Flexion and extension of the: • spine • hip joints • knees • feet Dynamic stabilization of the: • spine • pelvis
Stillness Sagittal plane and transverse plane motion	Back massage followed by gentle spinal spiraling followed by upper body flexion, extension, centering	Most comfortable supine position Spine flexion Gentle, multidimensional spinal movement Spine flexion, extension and centering

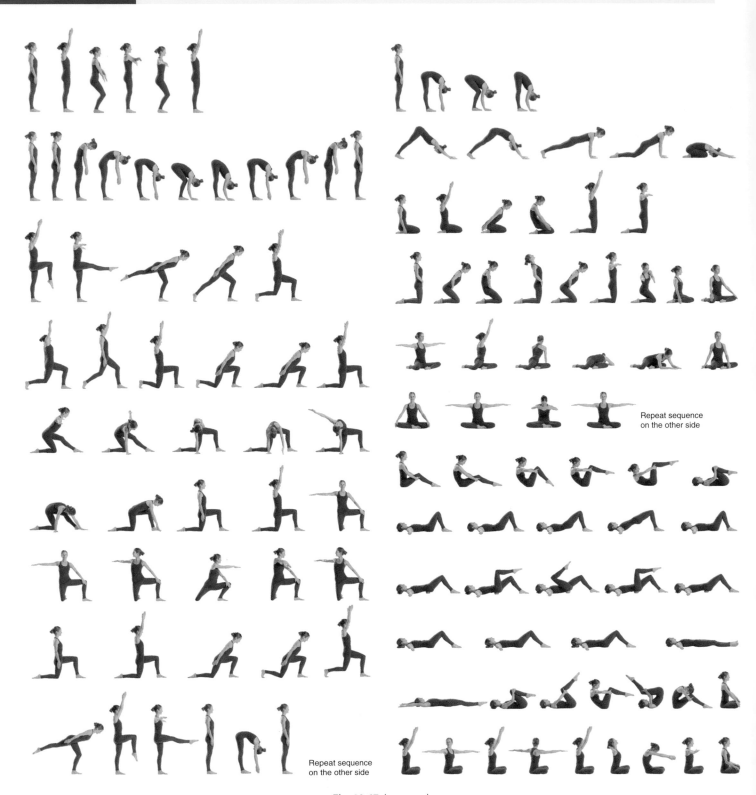

Repeat sequence on the other side

Repeat sequence on the other side

• **Fig. 10.67** Lesson plan

body – the process of structural integration through motion is a lifetime commitment to yourself. As important as it is to give the time to engage in intelligent exercise, it is even more important how you move in your life around your practice.

Movement, being active with joy, can be considered among the most health-promoting and mood-lifting 'nutrients'. Learn to love movement – it strengthens your resilience and somatic trust. It is the most effective medicine on the planet with the fewest side effects. To sustain your structural integrity, go the extra step every day, take the stairs instead of the elevator with a smile, stretch out with pleasure for no reason at the airport, and jump over a puddle or towards a friend, just because it's fun!

References

1. Bowman K. *Move Your DNA*. Carlsborg, WA: Propriometrics Press; 2017.
2. Young D, Reynolds K, Sidell M, et al. Effects of physical activity and sedentary time on the risk of heart failure. *Circ Heart Fail*. 2014;7:21–27.
3. Myers T. Kinesthetic dystonia. *J Bodywork Mov Ther*. 1998;2(2): 101–114.
4. Myers T, Frederick C. Stretching and fascia. In: Schleip R, Findley TW, Chaitow L, et al, eds. *Fascia: The Tensional Network of the Human Body*. Edinburgh: Churchill Livingstone; 2012: 433–439.
5. Earls J, Myers T. *Fascial Release for Structural Balance*. London: Lotus, Berkeley: North Atlantic; 2010.
6. Anatomy Trains courses. Online. Available: www.anatomytrains .com/courses. Accessed August 31, 2019.
7. Owen N, Healy G, Mathews C, et al. Too much sitting: the population-health science of sedentary behavior. *Exerc Sport Sci Rev*. 2010;38(3):105–113.
8. Perry J, Burnfield JM. *Gait Analysis*. 2nd ed. Thorofare, NJ: Slack Inc.; 2010.
9. Earls J. *Born to Walk*. Berkeley: North Atlantic; 2014.
10. Alexander RM. Making headway in Africa. *Nature*. 1986;319: 623–624.
11. Zorn A, Hodeck K. Walk with elastic fascia. In: Dalton E, ed. *Dynamic Body*. Oklahoma City: Freedom From Pain Institute; 2011.
12. Perry J, Burnfield JM. *Gait Analysis*. 2nd ed. Thorofare, NJ: Slack Inc.; 2010.
13. Premkumar K. *The Massage Connection: Anatomy and Physiology*. Baltimore: Lippincott, Williams & Wilkins; 2004.
14. Musculino J. *Kinesiology: The Skeletal System and Muscle Function*. St Louis: Mosby; 2006.
15. Fukunaga T, Kawakami Y, Kubo K, et al. Muscle and tendon interaction during human movements. *Exerc Sport Sci Rev*. 2002;30(3):106–110.
16. Sawicki GS, Lewis CL, Ferris DP. It pays to have a spring in your step. *Exerc Sport Sci Rev*. 2009;37(3):130–138.
17. Komi P, ed. *Neuromuscular Aspects of Sport Performance*. Chichester: Blackwell Publishing; 2011.
18. Blazevich A. The stretch-shortening cycle. In: Cardinale M, Newton R, Nosaka K, eds. *Strength and Conditioning: Biological Principles and Practical Applications*. Oxford: Wiley-Blackwell; 2011:209–218.
19. Oschman J. *Energy Medicine in Therapeutics and Human Performance*. Edinburgh: Butterworth Heinemann; 2003.
20. Michaud T. *Human Locomotion: The Conservative Management of Gait-Related Disorders*. Newton: Newton Biomechanics; 2011.
21. Wolff J, Wessinghage D. *Das Gesetz Der Transformation Der Knochen*. Berlin: Hirschwald; 1892.
22. Vleeming A, Pool-Goudzwaard AL, Stoeckart R, et al. The posterior layer of the thoracolumbar fascia: its function in load transfer from spine to legs. *Spine*. 1995;20:753.
23. Kawakami Y, Muraoka T, Ito S, et al. In vivo muscle fiber behavior during countermovement exercise in humans reveals a significant role for tendon elasticity. *J Physiol*. 2002;540(2):635–646.
24. Kjaer M, Langberg H, Heinemeier K, et al. From mechanical loading to collagen synthesis, structural changes and function in the human tendon. *Scand J Med Sci Sports*. 2009;19(4): 500–510.
25. Feldenkrais M. *The Potent Self*. Berkeley: Frog Books; 2002.
26. Cook G. *Movement: Functional Movement Systems: Screening, Assessment, and Corrective Strategies*. Aptos, CA: On Target Publications; 2010.
27. Craig AD. *How Do You Feel?: An Interoceptive Moment With Your Neurobiological Self*. Princeton: Princeton University Press; 2015.
28. Grunwald M. *Homo Hapticus*. München: Droemer Verlag; 2017.
29. Huijing PA. Intra-, extra-, and intermuscular myofascial force transmission of synergists and antagonists: effects of muscle length as well as relative position. *Int J Mech Med Biol*. 2002;2:1–15.
30. Reeves ND, Narici MV, Maganaris CN. Myotendinous plasticity in aging and resistance exercise in humans. *Exp Physiol*. 2006;91(3):483–498.

11

BodyReading® – Structural Analysis

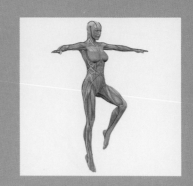

Can we usefully compare postural and structural relationships in terms of these myofascial meridians? Can this information be developed into unambiguous treatment strategies for unwinding and resolving body-wide patterns of compensation?

Attempts at objective and inter-operator reliable visual analysis of overall postural patterns are fraught with difficulty, with few norms having been established scientifically.[1,2] Yet, useful clinical information can be gleaned from an analysis of the standing client. This chapter puts forward one method for obtaining such information and putting it to use (Video 6.25). In this chapter, we refer only to still photos of standing posture; in practice, such information would and should be corroborated with a carefully taken history, palpation, and gait or other movement assessments such as those detailed in the previous chapter.

The Anatomy Trains map was first developed as just such a postural visual assessment tool for Structural Integration clients (see Appendix 3 on our Structural Integration method). This chapter describes the language and method of 'BodyReading' that we employ in our training seminars, where we systematically expand this introductory overview to standing assessment. Although this process is most easily assimilated when taught in person, attentive readers will be able to utilize this tool with their own clients, patients, or students, to apply various therapeutic protocols in a global and progressive manner. A 'Visual Assessment' video course based on these same principles is also available (www.anatomytrains.com – video ref: BodyReading, 101).

Of course, many have tried to parse posture before us. From the bio-mechanical side, Florence Kendall and her kin paved the way in understanding lumbopelvic relationships, leading to Janda's upper crossed syndrome.[3,4] The somato-emotional point-of-view was first articulated by the awesome and difficult Wilhelm Reich, followed by the bioenergeticists and body-centered psychologists.[5–7] On a physiological level, the somatotyping work of William Sheldon – measuring ectomorphy, mesomorphy, and endomorphy – sought to connect shape to specific physiologies and psychological tendencies. Sheldon's work generated controversy on several levels, but this author still gets value from noticing the

dosha, as these somatotypes are called in Ayurveda, and adapting the treatment plan accordingly.[8]

Our assessment tool rests on the concept of 'tensegrity' put forth at the end of Appendix 1. Practitioners seeking bio-mechanical alignment and other forms of movement efficiency, as well as kinesthetic literacy (an accurate sensing of where our body is in space and how position is changing), or even psychosomatic ease, will do well to consider the unique properties tensegrity geometry shares with the human body. These include tensegrity's unique ability to 'relax into length' as well as its distributive properties, accommodating local strain or trauma by dispersing it via small adjustments over the entire system (see Fig. A1.81, p. 307).

As clients resolve dysfunctional patterns, they more closely approach a 'coordinated fascial tensegrity' balance among the lines, creating a resilient and stable 'neutral' around which movement occurs.[9] When accumulated strain is unwound into the desired efficiency and ease, the struts of the bones seem literally to float within a balanced array of tensile collagenous tissues, including the more closely adherent ligamentous bed, as well as the parietal myofascial system arranged in the longitudinal meridians that are the subject of this book.

The process of modeling the human frame in this way is just getting underway, but already a certain sophistication is available in the tensegrity models of Tom Flemons (www.intensiondesigns.ca – Fig. 11.1). The relationship between the bones, myofasciae, and ligaments is more closely approximated when the common tensegrity icosahedron is modified to approach that of Fig. 11.2, which is the same set of relationships, just shifted in their points of attachment, a process we can see happening to the connective tissue network *in vivo* in the films of Dr J-C Guimberteau (see Figs A1.98–A1.100, pp. 316–317) (www.anatomytrains.com – video ref: Interior Architectures).

Fascial tensegrity implies evenness of tone – with allowances for differences of muscle fiber type and density variations from superficial to deep – along each line and among the lines (Video 1.2). Anecdote and informal clinical observation suggest that inducing this even tone produces

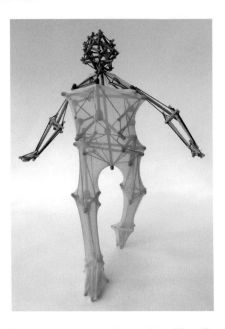

• **Fig. 11.1** The wonderful and varying models of Tom Flemons (www. intensiondesigns.ca) demonstrate clear similarities to human postural response and compensation patterns. With each iteration, these models get more sophisticated, and more closely approach human movement.

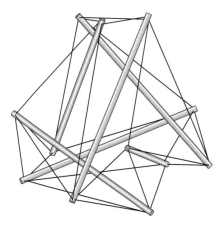

• **Fig. 11.2** The tensegrity icosahedron shown in Figure A1.80A (p. 306) is commonly used by advocates of tensegrity as a simple demonstration model. Here we picture the same model, only with the end points of the dowels slid closer to each other so that the same construction shifts into a truncated tetrahedron. Our body works more like this still very simplified model. This results in (1) a more stable, less deformable structure; (2) the long part of the elastics parallel the dowels, just as most of our myofasciae parallel the bones, especially in the limbs; and (3) the short elastics that are tying the end of the bones together resemble the joint ligaments. Jolt one of the bones, as in an accident, and the strain is transferred strongly to these ligaments.

increased length, ease, generosity of movement, and injury-preventing adaptability for the client in both somatic and psychosomatic terms. To gain these heights for ourselves and our subjects, we must first have an accurate reading of where the skeleton literally stands in terms of its sometimes very small but telling aberrations from vertical symmetrical balance. This will allow us to accurately map the meridians

and soft-tissue components necessary to improve the state of balance and support.

The first section of this chapter sets out the procedure to assess any given posture using the myofascial meridians, with emphasis on the accurate description of skeletal position. The main body of the chapter analyzes the standing posture of several 'clients' using this procedure to generate a single- or multi-session strategy. The final part of this chapter sketches in some of the more subjective elements of the 'BodyReading' or Anatomy Trains mapping process.

Global Postural Assessment Method

Many forms of structurally oriented manipulation use an analysis of standing posture as a guide in forming a treatment strategy. Osteopaths, chiropractors, physiotherapists, soft-tissue practitioners, and movement educators such as Alexander and yoga teachers have used various grids, plumb lines, and charts to help assess the symmetry and alignment of the client.[8,10–12] Our own approach and vocabulary emphasize the interrelationships within the person's body, rather than their relation to anyone else or any platonic ideal. For this reason, the photographs herein are devoid of such outside reference – except of course the line of gravity as represented in the orientation of the picture.

It is important to 'expose', not 'impose' proper body use. That there are benefits to an easy, upright alignment within the strong and shadowless gravitational field of the earth is a generally inescapable idea. The advisability, however, of in any way compelling left/right symmetry or even a 'straight' posture on a client is far more dubious. Alignment and balance are dynamic and neurologically adaptive, not static and biomechanically fixed. Postural reflexes and the emotional connection to muscle tension lie fairly deep in the brain's movement structure. Efficient structural relationships must thus be exposed and adopted within the clients, not imposed upon them. The idea is to assist the client in the process of 'growing out of the pattern', not to box someone into a particular postural ideal. The former eases tension and leads to new discoveries; the latter piles more tension onto what is already there.

The goal of making such an analysis is to understand the pattern – the 'story', if you will – inherent in each person's musculoskeletal arrangement, insofar as such a task is possible using any analytical method. The use of such an analysis merely to identify postural 'faults' for correction will severely limit the practitioner's thinking and the client's empowerment.

Once the underlying pattern of relationships is grasped, any (or several) treatment methods may be employed to resolve the pattern. Applying the Anatomy Trains myofascial meridians to standing posture is a vital step in this process of understanding structural patterns of collapse and shortness, but not the first step. The next section outlines a five-step method of structural analysis:

1. Describe the **skeletal geometry** (where is the skeleton in space, and what are the intra-skeletal relationships?)

2. Assess the **soft-tissue pattern** creating or maintaining that position (individual muscles, fasciae, or myofascial meridians)
3. Synthesize an **integrating story** that accounts for as much of the overall pattern as possible
4. Develop a short- or long-term **strategy** to resolve undesirable elements of the pattern
5. **Evaluate and revise** the strategy in the light of observed results and palpatory findings.

Step 1: a Positional Vocabulary

Terminology

To describe the geometry of the skeleton – the position of the skeleton in space – we have developed a simple, intuitive but unambiguous language that can be used to describe any position in space, but which, in this chapter, we use to describe interosseous relationships in standing posture. The vocabulary derives from our former colleague Michael Morrison.[13] This language has the dual advantage of making sense to (and thus empowering) clients, students, and patients, while also being capable of bearing the load of sufficient detail to satisfy the most exacting practitioner-to-practitioner or practitioner-to-mentor dialogue. It has the disadvantage of not conforming to standard medical terminology (e.g. 'varus' and 'valgus', or a 'pronated' foot). Because these terms are often used in contradictory or imprecise ways, this disadvantage may prove an advantage in the long run.

The four terms employed here are: 'tilt', 'bend', 'rotate', and 'shift'. The terms describe the relationship of one bony portion of the body to another or occasionally to the gravity line, horizontal, or some other outside reference. They are modified with the standard positional adjectives: 'anterior', 'posterior', 'left', 'right', 'superior', 'inferior', 'medial', and 'lateral'. These modifiers, whenever there is any ambiguity, refer to the top or the front of the named structure. 'Left' and 'right' always refer to the client's left and right, not the observer's.

As examples, in a left lateral tilt of the head, the top of the head would lean to the left, and the left ear would approach the left shoulder. A posterior shift of the rib cage relative to the pelvis means that the center of gravity of the rib cage is located behind the center of gravity of the pelvis – a common posture for fashion models. In a left rotation of the rib cage relative to the pelvis, the sternum would face more left than the pubic symphysis (while the thoracic spinous processes might have moved toward the right in back). Medial rotation of the femur means the front of the femur is turned toward the midline. This use of modifiers is, of course, an arbitrary convention, but one that makes intuitive sense to most listeners (Fig. 11.3).

One strength of this terminology is that these terms can be applied in a quick overall sketch description of the posture's major features, or used very precisely to tease out complex intersegmental, intrapelvic, shoulder girdle, or intertarsal relationships.

Compared to What?

Because the terms are mostly employed without reference to an outside grid or ideal, it is very important to clarify exactly *which* two structures are being compared. To look at one common example that leads to much misunderstanding, what do we mean by 'anterior tilt of the pelvis' (sometimes termed in physiotherapy an 'anterior rotation' of the pelvis, but for consistency will be an 'anterior tilt' here)?

Imagining that we share a common understanding of what constitutes an anterior tilt pelvis, we are still open to confusion unless the question 'Compared to what?' is answered. If we consistently compare the tilt of the pelvis to the horizontal line of the floor, for instance, this reading will not lead us to useful treatment protocols of femur-to-pelvis myofascia since these tissues relate the pelvis to the femur, not pelvis-to-floor (Fig. 11.4). Since the femur can also be commonly anteriorly tilted, the pelvis can easily be (and often enough is) anteriorly tilted compared to the ground while at the same time being posteriorly tilted compared to the femur (see Fig. 11.4C). Both descriptions are accurate as long as the point of reference is agreed – but in practice, confusion often reigns on this point.

When employing the following terms, be careful to specify, especially as you start, the two elements that are being compared.

Definitions: Tilt, Bend, Shift, and Rotation

- **Tilt.** 'Tilt' describes simple deviations from the vertical or horizontal, in other words, a body part or skeletal element that is higher on one side than on another. Although tilt could be described as a rotation of a body part around a horizontal axis (left–right or A–P), 'tilt' has a readily understood common meaning, as in the Tower of Pisa.

  'Tilt' is modified by the direction to which the top of the structure is tilted. Thus, in a left side tilt of the pelvic girdle, the client's right hip bone would be higher than the left, and the top of the pelvis would point toward the client's left (Fig. 11.5A). An anterior tilt of the pelvic girdle would involve the pubic bone going inferior relative to the posterior iliac spines, and a posterior tilt would imply the opposite (Fig. 11.5B). In a right side tilt of the head, the left ear would be higher than the right, and the planes of the face would tilt down to the right (Fig. 11.5A). In a posterior tilt of the head, the eyes would look up, the back of the head approaches the spinous processes of the neck, and the top of the head moves posteriorly (Fig. 11.5B). In Fig. 11.4C, the legs as a whole are anteriorly tilted, and the pelvis is posteriorly tilted relative to the femurs. The head in this diagram is anteriorly tilted – looking down – which is an equivalent position to the pelvis in Fig. 11.4B. Our terminology is thus applied consistently throughout the entire body.

  Tilt is commonly applied to the head, shoulder girdle, rib cage, pelvis, and tarsi of the feet. Tilt can be used

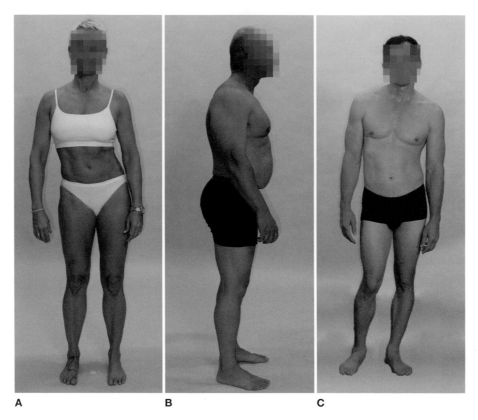

A   B   C

• **Fig. 11.3** These deliberately exaggerated postures show (**A**) a left shift of the pelvis relative to the feet, right shift of the ribs relative to the pelvis, and left shift of the head relative to the ribs. Notice that the head is not shifted relative to the pelvis. Although we cannot directly see them, we can presume multiple bends in the spine. The pelvis has a right tilt, and the head and shoulders have a left tilt. In (**B**), we see an anterior shift of the head relative to the ribs, and an anterior shift of the ribs relative to the pelvis. This involves posterior bends in both cervical and lumbar curves, as well as lateral rotations in all four limbs. The pelvis appears to have an anterior tilt, but neither the ribs nor the head are tilted relative to the ground. In (**C**), we can see a left tilt of the pelvis, a right tilt of the rib cage and shoulder girdle, and a left tilt of the head, with a concurrent left bend of the lumbars and right bend in the thoracics. The right femur shows a lateral rotation while the left demonstrates a medial rotation relative to the tibia.

broadly, such as 'a right side tilt of the torso relative to gravity', or very specifically, such as 'an anterior tilt of the left scapula relative to the right' or 'a posterior tilt of the right innominate bone relative to the sacrum' or 'a medial tilt of the navicular relative to the talus'. Once again, for clarity in communication and accuracy in translating this language into soft-tissue strategy, it is very important to understand to what the term being used is related: an 'anterior pelvic tilt relative to the femur' is a useful observation, a simple 'anterior pelvic tilt' opens the door to confusion.

• **Bend.** A 'bend' is simply a series of tilts resulting in a curve, usually applied to the spine. If the lumbar spine is side bent, this could be described as a series of tilts between each of the lumbar vertebrae, but we usually summarize these tilts as a bend – either side, forward or back. In the right bend in Fig. 11.5A, the top of L1 faces more the client's right than the top of L5.

The normal lumbar curve thus has a back bend, and the normal thoracic spine a forward bend. A lordotic spine could be generally described as an 'excess posterior

bend in the lower lumbars', or could be specified in more detail. A low but strong lumbar curvature might parse out on investigation as: 'the lumbars have a strong posterior bend from L5–S1 to about L3, but have an anterior bend from L3–T12.'

In the spine, the essential difference between a tilt and a bend is whether the deviation from 'normal' is a single-segment or multi-segment event – and it is usually the latter. If the rib cage is tilted off to the right, we can presume that either the pelvis is likewise right tilted so the lumbars run straight, or more likely, as in Fig. 11.5A, the lumbar spine has a right side bend. Further, spinal mechanics dictates that the left bend in the lumbars very likely involves the tendency toward a right rotation of some of those vertebrae. The spine can have one uncompensated bend, but commonly has two bends that compensate each other, and more complex spinal patterns, e.g. scoliosis, can have three or even four bends over the two dozen vertebral segments.

• **Rotation.** In standing posture, rotations usually occur around a vertical axis in the horizontal plane, and thus

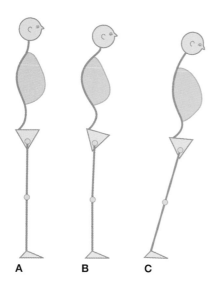

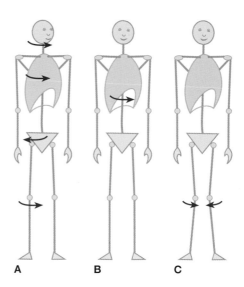

• **Fig. 11.4** In (**A**), 'neutral' posture, more or less, is depicted diagrammatically. If for a few pages we accept the convention of these diagrams, we can see that in (**B**), the pelvis is anteriorly tilted – the top of the pelvis tilts toward the front – relative to both the femur *and* the ground. In (**C**), we see the common but commonly mis-assessed situation of the pelvis being anteriorly tilted relative to the ground but *posteriorly* tilted relative to the femur. 'Compared to what?' is a meaningful question.

• **Fig. 11.6** Rotations all take place in the horizontal plane around a vertical axis, and are therefore modified only with left or right (for axial structures – (**A**)) or medial and lateral (for paired structures – (**C**)). Rotations frequently counter each other from the ground up (**A**). One rotation in the middle, as in (**B**) (or mocked up in Fig. 11.3A), is not as simple as it looks to unwind.

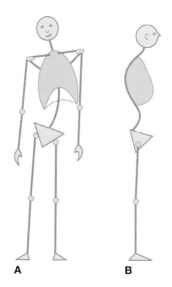

• **Fig. 11.5** In (**A**), the pelvis is tilted left, due to a short left leg. This has resulted in a compensatory right bend of the spine, right tilt of the shoulder girdle, and left shift of the rib cage relative to the pelvis. In (**B**), we see an anterior tilt of the pelvis, with a posterior bend of the lumbars and an anterior shift of the head due to an anterior bend in the upper thoracic spine. The neck is thus anteriorly tilted, and only by a sharp posterior bend in the upper cervicals can this fellow keep his eyes looking forward horizontally – compare to Fig. 11.3B.

often apply to, for example, the femur, tibia, pelvis, spine, head, humerus, or rib cage. Rotations are named for the direction in which the front of the named structure is pointing. For instance, in a left rotation of the head (relative to the pelvis), the nose or chin would face

to the left of the pubic bone (Fig. 11.6A). In Fig. 11.6A, *both* the head and rib cage are right rotated relative to the pelvis. The head and the rib cage are neutral to each other, relative to rotation. Making this observation is crucial to strategy: attempting to de-rotate the head of this person via the neck muscles would fail; it is the structures between the ribs and pelvis that govern this rotational pattern.

Notice that, if the rib cage were left rotated relative to the pelvis, the head could be right rotated relative to the rib cage and still be neutral relative to the pelvis or feet (Fig. 11.6B). In this case, therapeutic strategy would need to consider the twist/rotational imbalance in both the cervical and lumbar tissues (as well as shoulder-to-axial structures) to resolve this more complex pattern.

In paired structures, we use medial or lateral rotation (Fig. 11.6C). While this is in common use as regards femoral or humeral rotation, we extend this vocabulary to all structures. What is commonly called a 'protracted' scapula would, in our vocabulary, be a 'medially rotated' scapula, since the anterior surface of the scapula has turned to face the midline. A medially rotated calcaneus often accompanies what is commonly called a 'pronated' foot (which we would call, and not just to be confusing, a 'medially tilted' foot).

• **Shift.** 'Shift' is a broader but still useful term for displacements of the center of gravity of a part (right–left, anterior–posterior, or superior–inferior). Balinese and Thai dance involves a lot of head shifting – side-to-side movement while the eyes stay horizontal. The rib cage likewise can shift to the back or side while still staying relatively vertical relative to the ground (Fig. 11.7A and

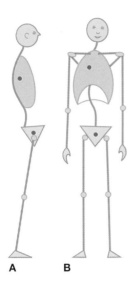

• **Fig. 11.7** In (**A**), there is an anterior tilt of the legs that results in the pelvis being anteriorly shifted relative to the feet, but the pelvis has a posterior tilt relative to the femurs. The rib cage in this diagram is posteriorly shifted relative to the pelvis, and the head is anteriorly shifted relative to the rib cage, in a pattern that is sadly commonplace in the Westernized world. Notice that the ribs are fairly neutral relative to the feet, and the head is fairly neutral relative to the pelvis. Undoing this pattern involves soft-tissue release in nearly every segment of the body. In (**B**), we see the pelvis neutral relative to the feet, but the ribs are right shifted relative to the pelvis, and the head left shifted relative to the ribs. The pelvis and head are thus relatively neutral, but as you begin to shift the rib cage on the pelvis via manipulation or training, the head will generally shift left relative to the pelvis, requiring work between the ribs and head.

B). Such shifts, of course, commonly involve tilts and bends, and often accompany rotations as well. We can use the terminology to specify these particular relationships when called for, but we have found that phrases such as 'left lateral shift of the rib cage' or 'the head is shifted to the right relative to the pelvis' are a useful shorthand when making an initial evaluation.

The mobile scapula is commonly shifted in any of the six modifying directions. The pelvis is commonly described as being anteriorly (as in Fig. 11.7A) or posteriorly shifted relative to the malleoli, with the understanding that some tilts must occur along the way in the upper or lower leg for that to happen. A protracted shoulder involves a lateral shift of the scapula on the ribs, adding in a medial rotation as it slides around the rib cage. A wide stance could be described as a lateral shift of the feet relative to the hips. Genu varus involves a lateral shift (and is probably accompanied by a rotation as well) of the knees.

None of these terms are mutually exclusive. A rib cage can have its center of gravity shifted relative to the pelvis, with or without a tilt, and additionally with or without a rotation. Identifying one event does not preclude the others.

Yet More Detail

Use this simple yet comprehensive vocabulary for a quick sketch or to describe a series of relationships in minute detail. What might initially present as the easily seen 'right tilted shoulder girdle' in our quick sketch (as in Fig. 11.5A) could parse out, with more detailed examination, as 'a right tilted shoulder girdle with an anterior tilt and a medial rotation in the right scapula, and a medially shifted left scapula'. This allows the practitioner to be as detailed or as general as necessary. The description can be noted down quickly, and accurately conveyed to another practitioner or mentor in a phone call or email when seeking assistance or describing a successful strategy for others to follow.

In terms of this greater level of detail, it is worth focusing on the spine, shoulders, and feet to clarify how this vocabulary can be consistently applied. As noted, we could give a general description (e.g. 'the spine in the torso is generally right rotated'), or we could fill it in to whatever level of detail is necessary (e.g. 'the spine is left side tilted and right rotated from the sacrum through L3, right side tilted and left rotated from L3 through T10, and then right rotated from T10 through about T6, forward bent through the upper thoracics, and again left rotated in the cervicals to bring the head to face in the same direction as the pelvis'). The general sketch is quite helpful in getting a global handle on which myofascial meridians might be involved. The more detailed description aids in specific strategy for de-rotating vertebrae and getting specific to local muscle or even particular muscle slips in treatment plans.

Shoulders

Though in a general sketch, the shoulder girdle might be described as a whole, e.g. left or right tilt, or superior shift, closely reasoned strategy requires far more detailed description of each clavicle, scapula, and humerus.

Scapulae are particularly interesting because of their great mobility. To simply describe a shoulder as 'protracted' or 'retracted' can easily, even necessarily, miss much of the detail that lies at the heart of soft-tissue specificity. Imagine a scapula described as follows: 'the right scapula is medially rotated, anteriorly tilted, and posteriorly shifted' (Fig. 11.8). The term 'protracted' might be applied to these scapulae, but would not distinguish the degree of medial rotation, or specify the anterior tilt, or how the shoulder was positioned in the A–P axis on the rib cage. All these characteristics, however, have significant implications for how the person's use pattern is understood and thus for our working strategy. A laterally shifted shoulder would lead us directly to the serratus anterior or the subscapularis fascia or the upper slips of pectoralis minor. The anterior tilt element would send us to the outer part of pectoralis minor and the clavi-pectoral fascia. The posterior shift would lead us to strategize about the middle trapezius and to add work in the axilla. With this level of description, we approach our work with greatly increased precision. It also allows a discourse in the bodywork field where logical thinking can displace magical thinking.

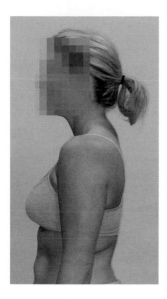

• **Fig. 11.8** Here we see shoulders that are posteriorly shifted – relative to the rib cage – but then medially rotated to bring the glenum anterior to the vertebral border, thus bringing the anterior face of the scapula to face the midline more; hence, a 'medial rotation' of the scapula is an essential part of protraction.

Feet

The human plantigrade foot is complex enough to warrant special attention. When we use 'rotation' in describing the head or spine, we have a good intuitive sense of what is meant. The same is true for tilts of the pelvis and shoulder girdle, and rotations in the humerus and femur. When we get to the feet, however, the long axis of the metatarsals and of the foot itself is horizontal. Therefore, 'lateral rotation' of the foot will designate that the toes are more lateral than the heels – but then we need to say, 'Relative to what?' Does the rotation take place in the foot itself, at the ankle, within the knee, or at the hip?

If the top of the foot is farther lateral than the sole and the weight shifts to the outside (a supinated foot), we would say the foot is 'laterally tilted'. Conversely, falling onto the inside of the foot would be 'medially tilted' (see Fig. 9.49, p. 170). In the extremes of these patterns, one can also have a 'rotation' *within* the foot, meaning that the metatarsals are pointing more lateral or medial than the heel. The person with bunions could be pedantically described as having a 'laterally rotated hallux' or 'laterally rotated big toe' (in other words, use the midline of the body, rather than the midline of the foot, as the reference).

Since the calcaneus is often the key to support of the back body and sacroiliac joint, a few examples of calcaneal description are also offered. For the person who has the top of the calcaneus more toward the body midline than the bottom we would say, 'medially tilted calcaneus'. If a calcaneus has the lateral side farther forward than the medial side, so that the front of the bone faces more medially, it would be termed – consistently but a bit counter-intuitively – a 'medially rotated calcaneus (relative to the tibia or the forefoot)'. Such medial rotation and/or medial

tilt often accompany a so-called pronated foot, fallen arch pattern, but how much of each will guide your strategy. Shifting the Superficial Back Line 'bridle' around the calcaneus is vital to arch restoration, as well as lengthening the *outside* of the foot, along the lateral band of the plantar fascia.

This language requires only a few hours of practice to manage, and only a couple of weeks of regular use of the notation for reasonable facility with the process. Of course, more usual language such as 'low arches' or 'pronated feet' can be used when it meets the needs of the moment, but reversion to this terminology can be used for simplicity and accuracy in the resolution of ambiguity. It also has a pleasing neutrality: 'medially shifted knees with laterally rotated femurs' may be a mouthful, but for the client it is less demeaning than 'knock knees' and less distancing than '*genu valgus*' (see Fig. 11.6C).

Once the skeletal geometry of the client's standing resting posture has been described to the satisfaction of the practitioner, and noted down, either verbally or pictorially on such a form as can be found in Appendix 3 for the reader's use, we proceed to the second stage.

Step 2: an Assessment of the Soft Tissues

The second step is to apply a model to the soft tissues to see how the client's skeletal relationships, as described, might have been created or are maintained. The Anatomy Trains myofascial meridians is one such model, the one we will apply here, but single-muscle strategies or other available models could be employed as well.[14–18]

Step 2 begins with the question: 'What soft tissues could be responsible for pulling or maintaining the skeleton in the position we described in Step 1?' A second question, 'What myofascial meridians do these myofascial units belong to, and how are they involved in the pattern?' follows immediately.

For example, if it is determined that the pelvis has an anterior tilt (as in Fig. 11.4B), then we could look at the hip flexors for the soft-tissue holding – for example, the iliacus, pectineus, psoas, rectus femoris, or tensor fasciae latae (TFL) myofasciae. Limitation in any of the first three would lead us toward the Deep Front Line; the rectus femoris might guide us to look at the Superficial Front Line; the sartorius (unlikely; it is too long and thin for postural maintenance) might lead us to the Ipsilateral Functional Line; and the TFL would suggest Spiral or Lateral Line involvement. Alternatively, the pelvis is being pulled up from behind by the erectors (Superficial Back Line) or the quadratus lumborum (Deep Front Line or Lateral Line).

If the shoulder on the right side lives farther away from the spinous processes than the one on the left, we could look to see whether the serratus anterior is locked short. If treatment of that single muscle results in a stable repositioning of the scapula, all well and good, but if not, we are guided toward assessment of the rest of the left Spiral Line: Are the right ribs closer to the left ASIS than vice versa, as in Fig. 11.5A? Perhaps lengthening of the left internal and right external obliques and their accompanying fascia will allow the work on the serratus to hold and integrate.

Perhaps, however, we find that the scapula is not being pulled into a lateral and inferior shift by a short serratus, but rather that the scapula is medially rotated (which often involves some lateral shift). In this case, we might suspect the pectoralis minor (which pulls down and in on the coracoid process to create a medial rotation or anterior tilt or both). If treatment of the pectoralis minor and associated fascia does not solve the problem, we might be drawn into working on either the Superficial Front Line, the Deep Front Arm Line, or the Front Functional Line to see if 'feeding' the pectoralis minor from its lower trunk connections might help the local work be successfully absorbed.

It is important to keep in mind that portions of lines may be involved without affecting the entire meridian. It is equally important to keep the broad meridian view, since, in our teaching experience, practitioners from almost all schools tend to fall into the mechanist's habit of trying to name the individual muscles responsible for any given position. This is, of course, not wrong, merely unnecessarily limited and ultimately frustrating, since it leaves out the fascial force transmission, progressive hysteresis, and effects over distance.

This 'BodyReading' process of Step 2 is modeled below using client photographs. Although many possible ways of analyzing soft-tissue distribution could be used at this point, we have an understandable prejudice toward employing the Anatomy Trains myofascial meridians schema here. This five-step process, however, can stand independently of any particular method.

By increasing familiarity with the system, it becomes a matter of a minute or two to analyze which lines might be involved in creating the pattern you have observed in Step 1. Trunk and leg rotations generally involve the Deep Front Line or Spiral Line, or both. Arm rotations involve either the Deep Front Arm Line or the Deep Back Arm Line. Side-to-side discrepancies often involve portions of the Lateral Line on the outside and Deep Front Line in the core. The balance between the Superficial Front and Back Line elements is always assessed and noted. If it appears that individual muscles are creating a pattern, we note in which lines this muscle is also involved. The relative positioning among the lines and their fascial planes is also important (e.g. the SFL is inferior relative to the SBL, the DFL has fallen relative to the more superficial lines, etc.).

In summary, analysis of the soft-tissue patterning in Step 2 usually takes note of where tissues seem to be short or fixed, where tissues seem to be overlong or weak, and where the biological fabric of the lines has lost its natural draping, i.e. the common pattern where the Superficial Back Line has migrated upward on the skeleton while the Superficial Front Line has migrated downward, independent of standing muscle tone (see Fig. 4.5). These elements can also be noted on the BodyReading form in practice.

Step 3: the Development of an Integrating Story

In the third stage we bring these skeletal and soft-tissue threads together to weave a story – an inclusive view of the musculoskeletal and movement pattern, based on the client's history and all the factors we can see or ask about taken together.[19] A simple (and single-pointed) version of this process might sound like this:

A client presents with shoulder pain in his dominant right side. In looking at the client's pattern, we observe shortness in the left Spiral Line, the right Front Functional Line, and the right Lateral Line, not unlike the exaggerated posture in Fig. 11.3C. The client is an avid tennis player, and in watching him mock up how he plays tennis, we see all three of these lines are shortened to pull the shoulder down and forward off the rib cage. This short-term attempt to gain more power has long-term negative consequences in straining the trapezius, rhomboids, and/or levator scapulae, and throwing off the head–neck–shoulder balance.

Based on this, you construct a story that aggressive tennis playing has shortened the right side and pulled the shoulder off the torso. The strategy becomes lengthening these lines, while getting the weekend warrior to center his stroke in the middle of his body rather than out at the shoulder. This will both improve his game (after a temporary disruption, of course, which some clients cannot endure) and his longevity with the game.

It could be, of course, that the shoulder being pulled off the axial torso and the shortening of the right side pre-dates the interest in tennis, so hold your story lightly and be ready to abandon it in the face of new information.

Include as much as you can in the story you construct, relating the various elements into a whole. In real life, the story can be much more complex, and may have a strong somato-emotional component. Your story may not account for all of the elements observed; after all, the client has had a long life, and not everything fits in neatly like a jigsaw puzzle. The attempt to relate a tilted pelvis (and accompanying sacroiliac pain) to the medially rotated knee and the medially tilted ankle on the opposite side is an instructive one. The story can help you know where to begin, even though it is some distance away from the site of pain, strain, or injury.

Perhaps you remember those clever Chinese wood puzzle boxes, where, in order to have the drawer open, several little pieces of wood would have to be slid past each other successively. As a child, you struggle to open the drawer, until some adult comes along to show you the sequence. Likewise in manual therapy, we struggle to fix some offending part. What the Anatomy Trains map, and this method of BodyReading in particular, does for us is to show where the other bits are – way on the other side of the 'box' – that need to move beforehand, so that when we return to the offending area, it just slips into place more easily. Tensegrity applied.

Putting the observed skeletal misalignments and the soft-tissue pulls into a comprehensive and self-convincing story is a subjective process, very much subject to revision in light of experience, but a valuable one nonetheless.

Step 4: the Development of a Strategy

Using the story from Step 3, the fourth step is to formulate a strategy for the next move, session, or a series of sessions, based on that global pattern view. Continuing this process for our tennis-playing client (again with the proviso that we are examining only one factor out of the multitude any given client would present), we decide to work up the right Lateral Line from hip to armpit, up the left Spiral Line from left hip to right scapula, and up the Front Functional Line toward the front of the right shoulder – all in an attempt to take away the postural elements that are pulling the shoulder off its supported position on the rib cage. We can then apply trigger point, positional release, cross-fiber friction therapy – whatever is appropriate to the specific injury – to the structure in trouble (perhaps the supraspinatus tendon, or the biceps tendon), secure in the knowledge that it has a far better chance of healing and staying healed if the shoulder is in a position where it can do its job properly without extra strain. Having lengthened the locked-short tissues, we can construct homework for the client to strengthen and tone the locked-long tissues.

In working more complex problems, the strategy may involve more than one session. The general strategy of Structural Integration (as we teach it – see Appendix 3) involves exploring and restoring each line over the full course of about a dozen sessions, resulting in a coherent series of sessions, each with a different strategy. With the role of each line in the story noted down, it is quite possible to stay on a multiple session treatment strategy without addressing the injured part (except for palliation) until it is appropriate and fruitful.

If the strategy is less injury/pain oriented, and the work is being used for performance enhancement or as a 'tonic' for posture and movement, the story and strategy are still important to unwind the details of each person's unique and individual pattern.

Step 5: Evaluation and Revision of the Strategy

Keep reassessing Steps 1 through 4 in light of results and new information. After completing the strategy from Step 4 on our putative client, we find that the shoulder is mostly repositioned, but now immobility or a syncopated scapular rhythm is apparent between the scapula and the humerus in back, so we revise/renew our strategy to include the infraspinatus and teres minor tissues of the Deep Back Arm Line.

After completing any given treatment strategy, an honest assessment is required as to whether the strategy has worked or not, and what, precisely, the results are. We are required to make a fearless re-examination, i.e. go back to Step 1. If our strategy has worked, the skeletal relationships will have altered. We can note these, and go on to Step 2 to see what new set of soft tissues we can address to move the pattern along toward increased balance and support. If there has been no change, then our strategy was wrong, and we go to Step 2 to develop another strategy, addressing a different set of soft tissues in hopes of freeing the skeleton to return to balance. If several successive strategies fail, it is time to consult a mentor, refer the patient to another practitioner, or find some new, as yet untried, strategy.

Virtue

It is very important to note here that there is no virtue involved in having a symmetrical, balanced structure. Everyone has a story, and good stories always involve some imbalance. Without doubt the most interesting and accomplished people with whom we have had the pleasure and challenge to work have had strongly asymmetrical structures, and live far from their optimal posture. In contrast, some people with naturally balanced structures face few internal contradictions, and as a result can be bland and less involved. Assisting someone with a strongly challenged structure out of their pattern toward a more balanced pattern does not make them less interesting, though perhaps it will allow them to be more peaceful or less neurotic or to carry less pain. Just, at this juncture, let us be clear that we are not assigning any ultimate moral advantage to being straight and balanced. Each person's story, with so many factors involved, has to unfold and resolve, unfold and resolve, again and again over the arc of a life. It is our privilege as structural therapists to be present for, and midwives to, the birth of additional meaning within the individual's story.

Postural Analysis of Five 'Clients'

The following analyses of these clients are made solely on the basis of the photographs included herein. They were chosen to demonstrate particular patterns and because the compensations are easily seen in the small photos allowed in a book format. In person, much smaller (but still important) deviations can be observed, noted, and treated. A few other photos are included in the eBook at www.expertconsult.com; and many more photos are included in our BodyReading DVD course (www.anatomytrains.com – video ref: BodyReading, 101).

Except for one set, we have no more history or access to their movement patterns than the reader does. Any photographic process necessarily involves some subjective elements – the happenstance of the clients positioning themselves, principally. Within those limitations, we will run through the steps of this process. In practice of course, the client's history, subjective reports, movement patterning in gait and other activities, and most importantly the repetition of the patterns observed would be part of our assessment. This section is designed simply to give the reader some practice with looking at postural compensation in this way.

Client 1 (Fig. 11.9A–E)

In taking an initial look at a prospective client from the front (**A**), we do well to tot up the advantages and strengths the client brings to the collaborative process before we detail any problems that concern her or ourselves. Here we see a strong young woman who seems securely planted, fairly well aligned, a long core, and with a gentle demeanor and a healthy glow. There is a slight 'down' feeling in the face and chest that goes against this basic vitality, with a deeper tension in what Phillip Latey would call 'the middle fist' or loss of heart energy, seen in the relative lack of depth in the rib cage.[20] The grounding and muscular responsiveness

evident in this client are qualities that will help us in our journey if we call them forth.

Step 1

Having noted these general (and somewhat value-laden, so hold them lightly) considerations, we proceed to Step 1, describing as objectively as possible the relative skeletal position. Looking at lateral deviations from the front, this client presents with a slight left tilt to the pelvis, which causes a slight left shift of the rib cage (note the difference in the waist on the left and right to see this imbalance). This is combined with a right tilt of the ribs that brings the sternal notch back to the midline. The shoulders counterbalance this with a slight right tilt.

The back view (**B**) shows the same picture a little more clearly, and shows that the left leg is the more heavily

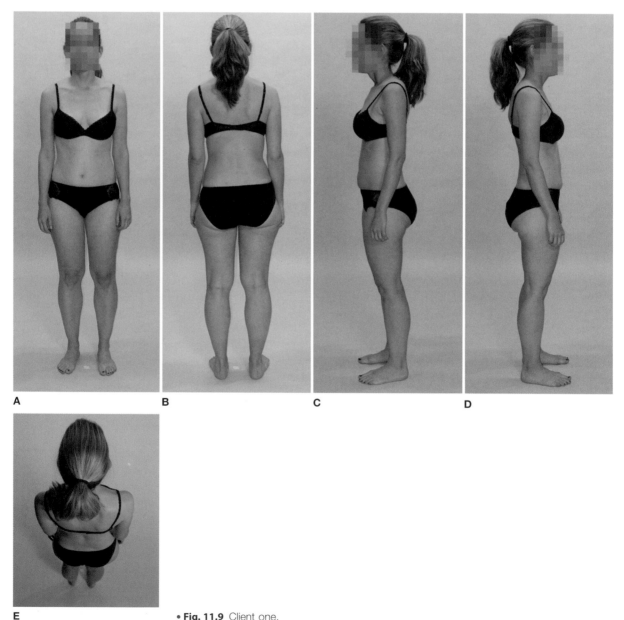

A   B   C   D

E   • **Fig. 11.9** Client one.

weighted one. This makes some sense, because the rotation is in the right leg. As shown by the patella, the right femur seems to be medially rotated compared to the tibia–fibula, which seem laterally rotated. From the back, we can also see that the shoulders look medially shifted (retracted), laterally tilted (downward rotation), and superiorly shifted (lifted).

If we look at the side views (**C** and **D**), we see the head shifted forward (so we can presume an anterior bend in the upper thoracics, and a posterior bend (hyperextension) in the upper cervicals. Old Ida Rolf would have urged her to put her hair on top of her head so that it would not act as a counterweight for her head position. We can see that her shoulders, especially the left one, are superiorly shifted and posteriorly shifted relative to the rib cage. Her right one, though better situated in general on the ribs, has a slight anterior tilt. (Read this from the vertebral border of the scapula: the left is vertical like a cliff; the right is tilted a bit like a roof.)

The lumbars have a long curve, speaking to her long core structure, but what remains for the thoracic spine means a fairly sharp anterior thoracic bend. The long lumbar curve relates to her knees, which are slightly posteriorly shifted (hyperextended). The pelvis, however, looks fairly neutral relative to both the femur in terms of tilt and the feet in terms of shift, though some would feel she has a slight anterior tilt.

Looking down from the top (**E**), and using the feet as a reference, we can see a slight left rotation of the pelvis on the feet and a slight right rotation of the ribs on the pelvis (look at the bra line for this), whereas the shoulders are again left rotated on the ribs.

Step 2

Proceeding to Step 2, we make the following surmises based on our observations in Step 1. Looking from the side, we can see that the Superficial Front Line (SFL) is pulled down along most of its length. The shortness from the mastoid process to the pubic bone is readily visible, and the shortness along the front of the shin accompanies it.

The Superficial Back Line (SBL) is pulled up from the heels to the shoulders, and shortened through the neck and the back of her head.

The right Lateral Line (LL) is shorter than the left from ear to hip, while the left lower LL is shorter than the right on the outside of the leg.

We would expect to find the right upper Spiral Line (SL) shorter than its left complement, as the right ribs are drawn toward the left hip, and the head is tilted slightly to the left. The anterior lower SL (TFL, ITT, and tibialis anterior) is shortened on the right leg, where the left shows a more even-toned balance.

Pectoralis minor is pulling the right shoulder forward over the ribs and there is some adduction going on in both arms, probably due to the coracobrachialis or the myofascia of the back of the axilla. The humeri seem a little laterally

rotated for her body (look at the cubital fossa) but not by much.

Step 3

Bringing all these observations into a coherent story would require weaving them in with a full history, but in general, we can say that most of this woman's pattern is built on:
1. The shortening and downward motion of the fascia in the front of the body, restricting the excursion of the ribs and the placement of the head, requiring compensation (lifting and hiking) in the shoulders and back.
2. She has a slightly longer right leg (probably functional, but we cannot tell without hands-on testing), which accounts for several things: the twist in the right leg is attempting to equalize the leg length, the tilt in the pelvis results from the length discrepancy, and the shift in the ribs away from the high hip is a common compensation. Additionally, the small twists in the torso and legs come from trying to accommodate the differences in what looks like a strong exercise regimen.

Step 4

Based on this assessment, we can move toward Step 4, a general strategy leading to a specific treatment plan. The major elements of the overall plan for this client would include:
1. Lift the tissues of the entire SFL, especially in the areas of the shin, chest and subcostal angle, the neck fascia and sternocleidomastoid.
2. Drop the tissues of the SBL from the shoulder to the heel.
3. Lengthen the tissue of the right LL between the hip and ear, especially in the lower ribs and lateral abdomen. Lengthen the tissues of the left LL along the outside of the left leg.
4. Lengthen the tissues of the upper right SL from the left hip across the belly around the right shoulder and across again to the left occiput.
5. Ease and open the tissues of the right lower SPL and work around the knee to de-rotate the strain in the right knee.
6. Ease out the Deep Front Arm Line, especially the pectoralis minor/coracobrachialis complex on the right. Ease the Superficial and Deep Back Arm Lines to let the scapulae find their proper position farther away from the spine, and balance the rotator cuff.
7. Lift the tissues of the Deep Front Line along the medial side of both legs, and especially in the left groin leading to the left lumbar spine (psoas complex). Lengthen the tissues on the deep anterior of the neck that are anchoring the head into the chest and preventing chest excursion.

This outline covers at least several sessions, and would be sequenced according to the principles of Anatomy Trains treatment and myofascial release work (see Appendix 3). The treatment plan would always be subject to Step 5, reassessing in the light of new observations, the client reports, and palpatory experience.

Client 2 (Fig. 11.10A–E)

Here we see a middle-aged gentleman, clearly active and with his intelligence engaged with the world. He shows basic good balance from front to back, good muscle tone for his years, and solidly planted feet. Core support through the pelvis is fundamentally good, and the structure is basically open. That said we have some significant compensations to usefully read from these photos.

Step 1

Looking from the front, the most prominent feature is the rib cage tilt to the right that helps create a right shift to the head. Bringing some detail into this picture, the right lower leg is laterally rotated and the right leg is shorter than the left (again, we do not know from a photo whether this is anatomical or functional). In either case, this creates a right tilt to the pelvis, and the whole structure of the body seems to 'fall' into the right groin, with the left hip being compressed.

Seeing this from the back, the medially tilting (pronating) right foot and the twist in the tissues of the right leg are prominent, the right tilt of the pelvis is again visible, along with the tilt and shift of the rib cage to the right. Coupled with this is the tilt of the shoulder girdle to the right, a tilt of the neck to the right, and a compensating tilt of the head back toward the left on the neck. We can imagine – but would have to do palpation tests to confirm – a slight left bend in the lumbars, a stronger right bend in the upper thoracics, and a left bend in the upper cervicals.

From the side, the head forward posture predominates, and we note the disparity between the shallower lumbar curve and the deep posterior bend of the mid- to upper

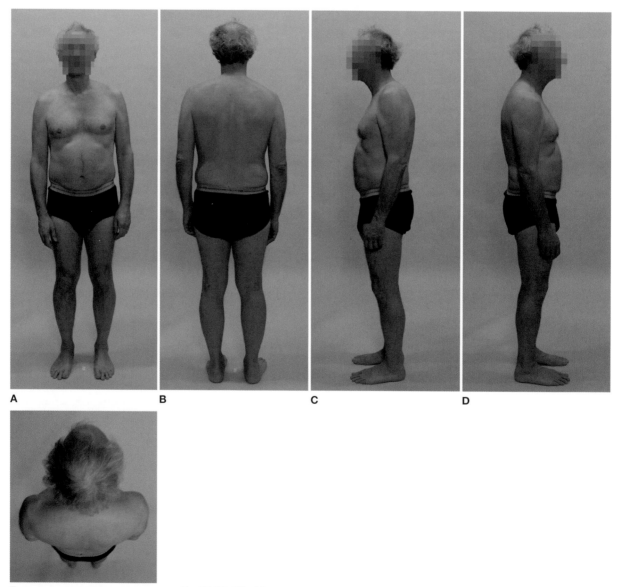

A   B   C   D

E   • **Fig. 11.10** Client two.

cervicals. The shoulders are a bit posteriorly shifted, anteriorly tilted to counterbalance the head. Interestingly, the torso seems posteriorly shifted relative to the femur in the right-hand view, but more aligned over the femur in the left-hand view. This is countered by the view from above (**E**), where a slight left rotation is in evidence from pelvis to shoulders, even though we 'know' that the body cannot have the shifts and bends he shows without accompanying rotations.

Step 2

Based on this sketch of the prominent features, we observe that the SBL has been drawn up along its whole length, but especially from the sacrum up to the shoulders. The suboccipital muscles are also locked up. Correspondingly, the SFL is pulled down all along its length, somewhat similar to Client 1, though with a more male pattern.

On the left, the LL is pulled up from lateral arch to shoulder, and then pulled down from the ear to the shoulder. Work on this side should proceed out in both directions from the shoulder area. On the right, the LL is pulled down to just above the knee, and up from the arch to the knee, so work on this side should proceed out from mid-thigh in both directions.

The left upper SL is clearly the shorter of the two SLs, pulling the head into left lateral tilt, pulling the right shoulder forward, and pulling the right costal arch over toward the left hip. In the legs, the left lower SL is pulled up in its posterior aspect from lateral arch to hip, whereas the right lower SL is shorter in the front, drawing the ASIS down toward the medially tilting inner arch.

The difference in the level of the hands is occasioned by the tilt of the shoulder girdle, which again rests on the tilt of the rib cage. Work with the rib cage position is probably the most effective way of getting the arms to even out, though some supplemental work with the Deep Front Arm Line on the right, and Deep Back Arm Line on the left will be helpful. The right Front Functional Line is clearly shorter than its complement.

In the Deep Front Line, we see a shortness in the right groin which is tied into the inner line of the right leg all the way down to the inner arch. This shortness is clearly pulling on the spine, creating compensatory tension in the opposite quadratus lumborum and other tissue of the left lower back. We can also imagine that the deep tissue on the left side of the neck – the middle and posterior scalenes in particular – is under eccentric strain (locked long).

Step 3

The story here focuses on the shortness in the right groin; much of the other patterning in the torso derives from compensations for this pulling down from the right leg in standing. Whether the fallen medial arch on the right foot pre-dates or post-dates the groin pulling, the arch seems mild in comparison to the hip. The rib and head shift, shoulder tilt, and torso rotation all proceed from this shortening.

This rotational pattern, coupled with the strong head forward posture, accounts for nearly all the compensatory patterning we see in this gentleman.

Step 4

The soft-tissue strategy would begin with lifting the SFL and dropping the SBL, paying particular attention to the tissues of the neck to free the suboccipitals (one suspects years of glasses or computer work). Letting go of the fascial lamina that runs behind the rectus abdominis would be important, and seeing the cervical curve reduce and the head go up on the body should begin with this SFL and SBL work.

The LL work has already been outlined above. On the left side, work the tissues of the LL up from the shoulder to the ear to lengthen the left side of the neck, but work down from the shoulder to the ankle to settle that side down. On the right side, the tissue needs to be lifted from above the knee to ear, and repositioned downward from mid-thigh to the lateral arch. We can surmise with some assurance that the abductors on the left side will be extra short and tight and require some opening work.

The left SL will require lengthening from the left ASIS across the belly to the right ribs, and around the torso to the left side of the neck in back. The left upper SL should require substantially more work and movement than its counterpart on the right. In the legs, the posterior part of both SLs could be dropped toward the outer arch, but in the right leg, the anterior lower SL needs lifting from the arch to the ASIS. The fallen arch and the medial rotation of the knee relative to the tibia and foot are both indicators for this.

The shoulders and arms will require balancing work once the rib cage has taken a more relaxed and centered position.

The key to this overall pattern, however, lies in the Deep Front Line work, which has a chance, if the leg length difference is not anatomical, to open the right groin and allow the upper body to right itself. From the groin, the psoas complex reaches up to the lumbar spine, and freedom from the shortness in the right leg will make all the difference to the lumbars, the rib cage, and the neck.

Client 3 (Fig. 11.11A–E)

In our third model we have a young woman who presents a structure which is superficially like that of Client 2, but with some fundamental differences. Here we see a strong and sturdy structure, well muscled and well founded, with a bright and attentive look from the eyes atop the structure. Nevertheless, this muscular strength is built around some skeletal aberrations that we would want to address before she did any more muscle-building work.

Step 1

The head shows a left tilt and right shift relative to the neck. The shoulder girdle is right tilted, as is the rib cage underneath it. The pelvis is also right tilted, but the alignment of

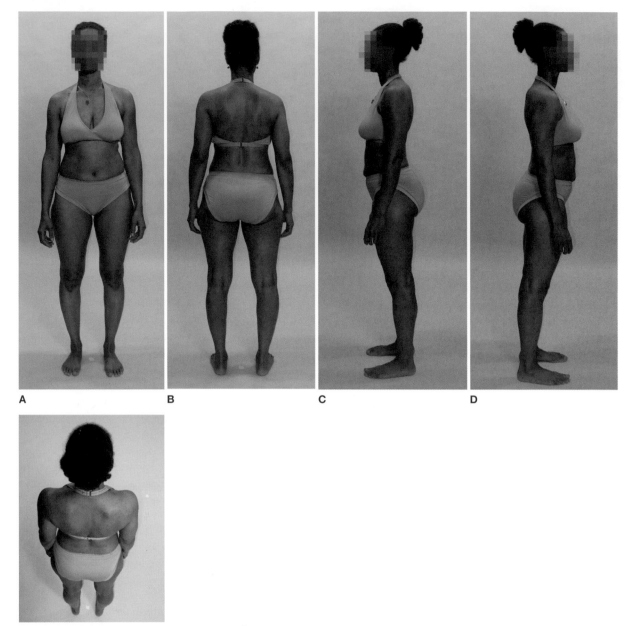

A   B   C   D

E   • **Fig. 11.11** Client three.

the three major torso weight segments – head, ribs, and pelvis – shows that there must be a left bend in both the lumbars and the upper thoracic/lower cervical spine (both visible in the back view).

Although this woman looks somewhat pulled into the right groin – a milder version of what we saw in Client 2 – the cause is not the same. Here, the legs are the same length, and the pattern is almost entirely from a twist in the pelvis on top of the femurs, not a difference in the femurs making itself felt in the pelvis.

Below the pelvis, the knees have a lateral shift (*varus*), sitting on nice, wide, well-grounded feet. The difference in the arm length is once again due to the tilt on the rib cage, not an inherent difference between the arms.

Looking from above, and again remembering to use the feet as a reference, we can see the right rotation and right

tilt of the pelvis relative to the feet, and the left rotation of the ribs relative to the pelvis.

These rotations go some way to explaining the difference we see between the left and right side views. Both show a slight anterior head posture, and both show an anterior shift of the pelvis over the feet, but these shifts on the right side are far more apparent than on the left. Both knees show a posterior shift (hyperextension locking).

Both sides show an anterior tilt of the pelvis relative to the femur, which leads to the long lumbar curve, which we would term a posterior bend of the lumbars. This posterior bend leaves the rib cage with a posterior tilt, which helps keep the head on top of the body. Lift her rib cage in the back and hold it in a vertical position and you would see her head go more out in front. Lengthening work with the anterior scalenes and sternocleidomastoid would be necessary to 'open the calipers' of the angle between the thoracic and cervical spine.

Step 2

We can see some pulling down in the upper SFL, though generally the shortness in the SBL is acting like a bowstring, and pushing the skeleton forward into the SFL. Thus, the SFL would assess as 'tight'; however, this would not be a call for loosening it, but rather to ease the SBL between shoulders and heels. The hamstrings and lumbar erectors and multifidus cry out for work.

In terms of the LLs, both LLs in the thigh are in need of dropping, and the abductors will be short due to the postural abduction of the hip joints. In the upper body, the LL on the right needs lifting from waist to cervicals, and the left side needs dropping from ear to waist, though the deeper structures on that side, like the iliocostalis and quadratus lumborum, need serious lengthening.

As in Client 2, the left SL is shorter than the right in the upper body, with the lower anterior SL shorter on the right, and the lower posterior SL shorter on the left.

The Back Arm Lines, both Deep and Superficial, need release in the proximal tissues to allow the shoulders to sit more comfortably down on the rib cage.

The Deep Front Line, the core, is again the key to opening this structure. The legs form a bow; therefore the inner line of the leg is the bowstring, short from ankle to ischial ramus. The shortening through the psoas complex on the right and the deep lateral rotators on the left will engage our attention to untwist the pelvis. Balancing around the lumbar spine would be our next job, in order to release the right side of the neck from the deep structures of the chest.

Step 3

We do not know whether the pelvis twist might not be occasioned by something internal, such as a rotated cervix, but this is certainly the centerpiece of this structure. It requires a tightening of the Deep Front Line below it, drawing the legs into a bow, and it is pulling down and twisting the torso above, despite her best efforts to stay balanced and symmetrical through her exercise. The key to unlocking this structure will be to free the pelvis from below, from the front, and from the back.

Step 4

This woman will not require so much work in the middle of the SFL, but will require work in the chest and neck to free the head from the ribs, and down in the shins to unlock the knees. The SBL, however, will require substantial work to undo the 'bow', and to loosen the tissue behind the cervical and lumbar curves.

The LLs mostly need spreading in either direction from the waist, but the right needs a lot of lifting in the upper quadrant, and more specific freeing in the lateral abdominals and quadratus lumborum on the left.

As stated, these would be preliminary moves to getting the pelvis to let go of the torque it is putting through the hips below and the spine above. This is primarily Deep Front Line

work, letting go of the adductor fascia and the line of fascia down the inside of the tibia associated with the deep posterior compartment of the leg. The pectineus on both sides will need work to reduce the anterior tilt, but the apparent right rotation of the pelvis on the femur suggests that the right pectineus will engage more of our attention.

Freeing and balancing the pelvis will make for easier breathing. At present, she is tightening the upper abdominals to mediate between the pelvis and ribs, and this is restricting breathing. With the posterior tilt of the ribs, the diaphragm is facing forward rather than facing down toward the pelvic floor, reducing the effectiveness of the posterior portion of the diaphragm.

When the pelvic rotation begins to free (no need to wait until it is perfect), the spinal muscles can be addressed to undo the rotation in the spine and ribs. This would also give us the opportunity to loosen the myofascia in the posterior shoulders, to let them sit down onto the 'new' rib cage and spine.

Clients 4 and 5 (Figs 11.12A–E and 11.13A–E)

If you are intrigued by this type of postural analysis, try your hand by examining these two additional clients in the same way that we have parsed the structures of the previous three. What can you find in terms of shifts, tilts, bends, and rotations? How would you put together their postural 'story'? Test yourself to see what you can detect. You can find our analysis of these two clients in the eBook at www.expertconsult.com.

Summary

We have deliberately presented these photos without recourse to the client histories or symptoms, so that we could see the structure/postural compensations objectively, without the filter of what we 'know' about them. In practice, of course, the two come together in the story-making part of the process. Even so, clients' reports of their own histories can be deceiving, giving added value to more objective analysis of clients or photos prior to getting their history, which can sometimes guide the practitioner down a primrose path.

As a simple example, a young man came for sessions whose lower right leg was clearly jutting laterally out from his knee more than the left. (In our language, his right lower leg was medially tilted, or if he stood with his feet close together and parallel, his right knee would appear medially shifted. In daily practice, we give this pattern the nickname 'kickstand leg', in that it often operates like a bicycle kickstand.) When asked about this, he related that he had skied into a tree at age 22, badly fracturing his right lower leg. Thus reassured as to the source of the pattern, we went to work. Puzzled about the way the area was responding, I asked him to bring in photos of himself, preferably with fewer clothes, before the accident. Next session, he brought in a photo of himself aged 15, on a beach, catching a ball. The right leg was clearly manifesting the same pattern, so it obviously pre-dated the skiing accident. It turned out that

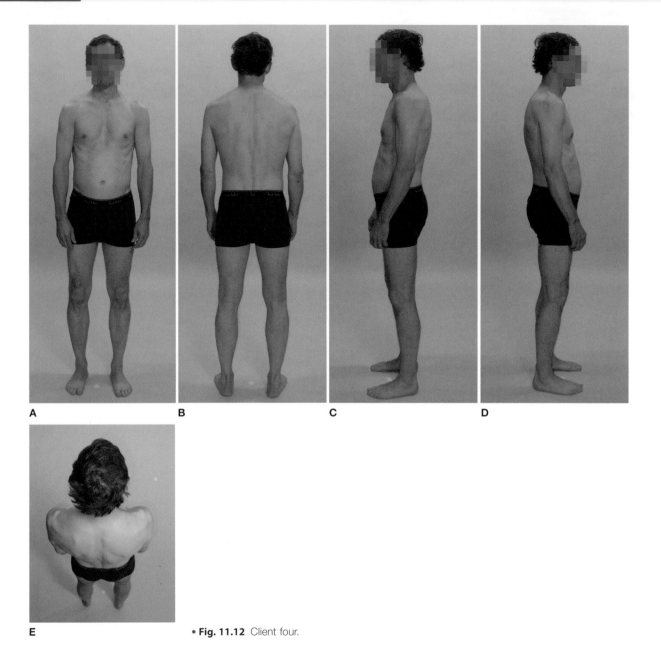

A   B   C   D

E   • **Fig. 11.12** Client four.

the initial pattern began when his tricycle fell on his leg in a spill when he was but three years old. Somebody picked him up, checked him for broken bones, soothed him, and sent him on his way. The soft-tissue strain, however, remained and led to the kickstand compensations up and down the leg. When he ran into the tree, we can surmise, he automatically protected those parts of his body that were clear in his body image, but this lower right leg had been partially out of his kinesthetic picture for a long time – what Hanna calls sensory–motor amnesia.[21] Thus this area of the body may not have received the same amount of attention, or been able to react as quickly, so that, other things being equal, it was more prone to injury. In any case, it illustrates the need to watch the story within the body itself as well as the client's rendition, which must be listened to carefully yet taken with a pinch of salt.

This chapter introduced a method of postural analysis – or, more specifically, habitual patterns of overall compensation – which adds to the efficiency and efficacy of manual/movement therapies. A single chapter is necessarily introductory, and we offer an expanded presentation in DVD form (www.anatomytrains.com – video ref: BodyReading, 101). The great advantages of using the Anatomy Trains myofascial meridians approach in such an analysis are that:

- it encourages the development of a common terminology that could speak across multiple treatment methods
- this description can also be commonly understood by clients and others outside the profession
- the description is objective, internal to each person, and value-free
- it leads to specific treatment plans which are testable hypotheses.

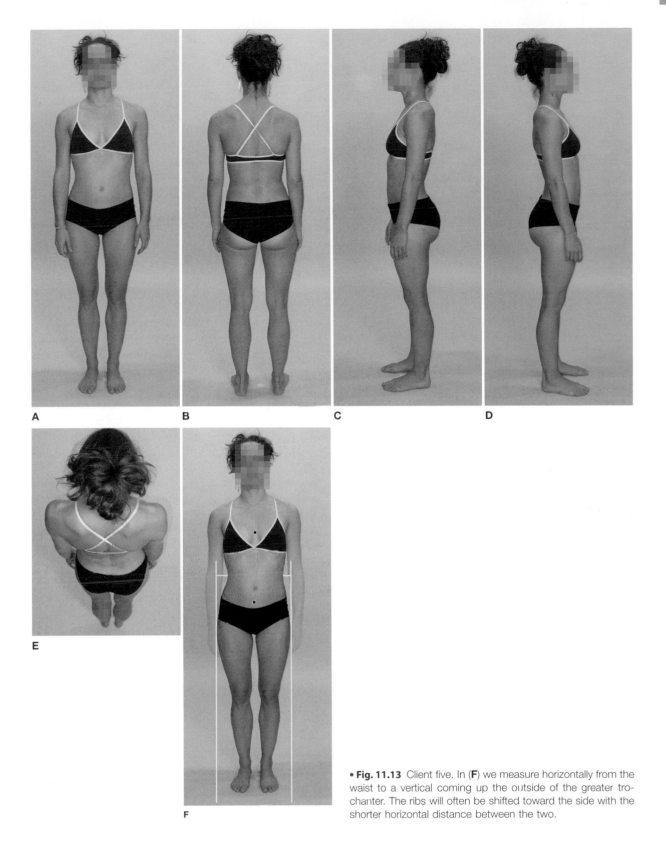

A

B

C

D

E

F

• **Fig. 11.13** Client five. In (**F**) we measure horizontally from the waist to a vertical coming up the outside of the greater trochanter. The ribs will often be shifted toward the side with the shorter horizontal distance between the two.

This is not intended to deny the value of other approaches; we have seen many times that almost any point of entry into viewing the human system can ultimately be followed to a useful description. This Anatomy Trains myofascial meridians approach progresses from the skeletal geometry to a strategy for soft-tissue or movement work without resorting to such value-laden statements as 'She's depressed', or 'He doesn't breathe properly', or 'She is not grounded because she hasn't worked out her "father" issues'. On the other hand, it does allow us to set a personal and inclusive context where the client is viewed not simply as 'a frozen shoulder' or 'an ACL tear' or a pair of flat feet.

It is the fond hope of the author, and of the many people who have contributed to the ideas herein, that this scheme or something like it can begin to bridge the gaps not only among modalities but also between the artist and the scientist who lives within each of us. The same two tendencies, of course, stretch within every one of the manual and movement therapy communities, as well as across 'spatial medicine' as a whole. This book is dedicated to the tireless work of these diverse people who, together, created the renaissance of hands-on and movement healing.

Subjective Elements

In order to round out the 'artistic' side of BodyReading, we include some more subjective suggestions for using these ideas in practice.

While the method above is useful in finding work strategies, the less objectifiable assessments nevertheless have significant value. The following four elements can be included, depending on the predilection of the practitioner or the client, into the process of visual assessment:

1. Do the Assessment in Front of a Full-Length Mirror, With Both You and the Client Looking at the Image

Especially for those clients who are new to this, being looked at in your underwear while being assessed (and perhaps found wanting) can be too reminiscent of bad dating or medical experiences for many people. A lot of these feelings can be circumvented by standing your client in front of the mirror, standing behind and a little to the side (so that you can see both their back directly and their front in the mirror), and asking them what they see. Most people in the Western world have a long and detailed list about what is wrong with their body, and a short and vague list about what is right. Putting both of you in front of a mirror image puts you both on the same team, standing in front of them and ticking off the problems can make you adversaries.

2. Notice Your First Impression

Your first impression carries a wealth of information, only some of which may rise to your awareness.[22] Learn to catch the fleeting perceptions you have on first glance, as they so often contain insights which will only become clear to you later. Do not speak it to the client, but note it for yourself. It is surprising to us how often an initial and uneducated assessment turns out to be insight down the road.

3. Note a Minimum of Three Positive Aspects First

We noted some positive aspects in each of the analyses above. It is surprising how many practitioners only talk about the client's problems and shortcomings. Patients come to us with problems they want solved, so it is natural for both of us to tend to focus on the problems. At any given moment, however, far more is going right in the person in front of you than is going wrong. Be very careful not to reduce your client to a set of faults. Doing so can be damaging for the client – it is no boost to the self-esteem to be given a long list of areas where your carriage or movement falls short of the ideal.

Focusing only on the problems can also be bad for the practitioner – you can miss the strengths that will help carry you and your client over the rough patches to whatever new territory you stake out. Clear skin speaks to a responsive nervous system; stolidity can indicate good grounding; an eager smile denotes an enthusiasm of which you can make use – noting these things to yourself, or, better yet, aloud to the client, can ease the way toward a discussion of real goals, as well as showing you where the client's current physiology may be of real help.

4. Describe the Issues You See in the Objective Language Outlined Above

The tilt–bend–shift–rotate language is less value-laden, and therefore less judgmental, than many other ways of stating the client's problems. These descriptions will lead you into Step 1 of the five-step process outlined above. The discipline of reducing each thing you see to an objective finding makes it much easier to approach the whole client innocently and with humility. Jumping to conclusions can land you in the drink.

Additionally, you may find value in considering an assessment of some of the following more subjective parameters. (These are offered as extra, practically useful, and quick assessments, with references for further study when helpful. None of the following are essential to the Anatomy Trains process *per se*.)

A. Whole Systems Communicators

In Appendix 1, we note that there are three whole-body networks, all of which communicate within themselves and with each other. It is a subjective but worthwhile exercise to call each of these to mind when looking at the client for the first time. What is the state of the neural network? (Are the eyes and skin clear? Are the client's responses timely and appropriate, or awkward and heavy-handed?) What is the state of the fluid network? (How is the skin color, and is it consistent across the body?) What is the state of the fibrous network? (Are they lax or tight? Toned or collapsed?) (See Fig. A1.60, p. 295 for more detail.)

B. Tissue Dominance

Although it is less in vogue these days, noting where your client lies in the endo-, meso-, and ectomorphy scale is definitely worthwhile, as ectomorphs will respond quite differently to manual therapy than will endomorphs. You cannot approach Cassius (who has a 'lean and hungry look') in the same way you would approach Falstaff (who was born with 'something of a round belly', and whose voice was 'lost with hollering and the singing of anthems').[8]

Students of Ayurveda will note the similarity with the *doshas*.

C. Somato-Emotional Orientations

Since many of the patterns people present unconsciously express emotion (especially the unacknowledged ones), it is worth looking to see some of the more obvious telltale signs.

- An anterior pelvic tilt most often indicates a sympathetic, or ergotropic, orientation (a sanguine or choleric character), whereas the posterior pelvis more often accompanies a parasympathetically oriented, trophotropic character (phlegmatic or melancholic).[23]
- Breathing patterns often hover around one end or the other of the respiratory cycle. Those stuck on the exhale side of the pattern tend toward depression and introspection, relying too heavily on their own internal world, while those stuck around the inhale end of the cycle tend toward a false heartiness, relying too heavily on the impressions and responses of others for their sense of self (Fig. 11.14A and B).

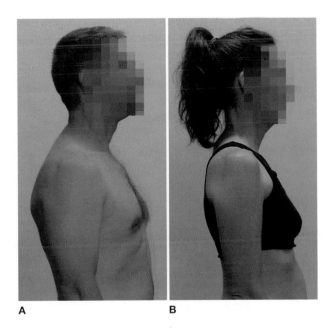

A   **B**

• **Fig. 11.14** Although we are of course looking at still photos, the man on the left shows signs of being 'stuck on the inhale' – with his breath pattern moving around the inhale end, whereas the woman on the right shows signs of being 'stuck on the exhale' – with her breath pattern oscillating around the exhale end of the spectrum.

- Various somatically oriented psychotherapists have coupled particular structural patterns with corresponding psychological tendencies and common behavioral responses.[5–7,15,16] Any of these typological systems can be helpful, though this author's experience has been that they are not totally reliable and can be tempting pigeon-holing traps.

D. Perceptual Orientation

According to Godard, there are two primary orientations – one either grounds to reach out, or reaches out in order to find grounding.[19] Here is a simple test for determining which is dominant: stand behind the client and have them jump lightly on the balls of their feet. It does not matter how high or well they do this. Make two tests, repeating each of these movements on successive jumps for a few seconds: (1) lift them slightly (less than a kilogram) from the sides of their rib cage as they go up, or (2) press them lightly into the earth on their shoulders as they come down. Which movement produces the more organized result in the client jump – pressing down or lifting up?

The ones for whom a slight pressing down results in a more organized spring up are oriented to the ground; those for whom even a few ounces of lift on your part produce a large result in terms of height and delight achieved, are oriented out into the environment around them.

E. Internal and External Orientation/Cylinders

Sultan, building on the flexion–extension preference models in Upledger's version of Craniosacral Therapy, has posited an Internal and External type, which has enjoyed currency at the Rolf Institute of Structural Integration (www.rolf.org).[14,24]

A similar assessment can be made of each segment: it is easy to see that a human being is two cylinders side-by-side when looking at the legs, for that is essentially what we are, and each cylinder can medially or laterally (internally or externally) rotate. Imagine that these two cylinders extend into the trunk. In the pelvis, these two rotational preferences have a name – inflare and outflare – but the phenomenon extends to the belly, ribs, and shoulders. If the cylinders are rotated medially, that segment of the body looks wide in the back and narrow in the front. If the cylinders are rotated laterally, the segment looks wider in the front and narrower in the back.

These patterns can sometimes alternate, with the lower back/belly segment in external rotation, counterbalanced by a chest segment in internal rotation (Fig. 11.15). In these cases, the narrow part of the segments need repeated widening, and the segments where the rotation shifts from internal to external will often be troubled.

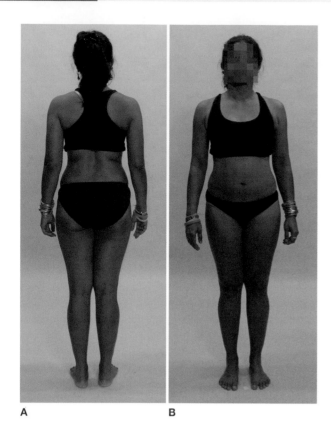

A   B

• **Fig. 11.15** In this model, we see a mild form of the alternation of 'cylinders'. In the torso area, the cylinders are turned outward, so that the front looks wider than the back. In the pelvis and legs, the 'cylinders' appear to be turned in, making the back appear wider than the corresponding area in front.

F. Primary Rotation

Everyone I have worked on or observed over 35 years of practice has had a primary rotation to the spine. (Galaxies and DNA grow in spirals, why not us? Observe the photos of fetuses by Lennart Nilsson and others[25] – each one can be seen to have a nascent spiral in the spine. Could this be a natural part of development, or should it be considered an aberration?) Observing the direction of that rotation, its degree, and the specific areas of counter-rotation that always accompany it are essential data for the most efficient unwinding of the entire pattern.

To observe spinal rotation quickly without benefit of an X-ray, stand behind the client. Place your thumbs on the two posterior superior iliac spines (PSISs), with your fingers resting on the hip. If necessary, de-rotate the client's pelvis so that the PSISs are equally lined up with the heels (thus temporarily and artificially eliminating any rotation in the legs). Now peer down the client's back from above, as we have in all the 'E' pictures above (the short practitioner may need a stool to assess the tall client).

By noting the tissues about an inch (2 cm) on either side of the spinous processes, one can see which side is more anterior or posterior (closer to you or further away). These differences are only rarely due to differential erector development on either side of the spine. At any given level of the

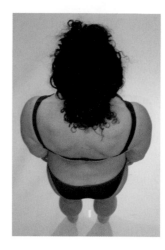

• **Fig. 11.16** A primary thoraco-lumbar rotation to the right.

spine, the side closest to you indicates the direction of rotation of the spine as the transverse processes push the overlying myofascial tissue posteriorly.

In our experience, most clients will show a dominant rotation in the thoracolumbar area, which we term the 'primary' rotation (Fig. 11.16). Counter-rotations frequently occur in the legs or in the neck, but sometimes also within the thoracolumbar area itself. Infrequently, it can be difficult to tell which is the primary and which is the secondary rotation; in which case, further therapy may clear the picture, or the two rotations may indeed be nearly equal, and therefore the designation 'primary' has less meaning. With practice, one can gather quite detailed and specific information about the inherent spinal rotations using this method.

Another simple movement assessment can yield yet more information: kneel behind the client, again with the hands steadying the pelvis and the thumbs on the PSISs. Give the client the instruction to 'look over your shoulder'. By not saying which shoulder, you allow them to choose, and they will almost always choose their preferential side – the side with the primary rotation. As they turn, encourage them to use the whole torso to turn, while you hold the pelvis steady relative to the feet with your hands. Observe where the spine rotates. Have them turn the opposite way, and observe the difference. Anyone with a significant primary rotation will have palpable or observable differences in where in the spine the rotation occurs on the two sides.

G. Pelvic Position

The attention given to pelvic tilt and shift in our system yields four basic types based on pelvic position:

- Anterior tilt, anterior shift – this produces a familiar swayback pattern
- Anterior tilt, posterior shift – favored by toddlers just learning to stand
- Posterior tilt, anterior shift – favored by suppressed neurotics everywhere

- Posterior tilt, posterior shift – favored by plumbers and woodsmen (this posture tends to produce the 'vertical smile' at the top of the back of the jeans).

Soft-tissue strategies peculiar to each of these pelvic positional types can be found elsewhere.[26] In our experience, it is necessary to make liberal allowances for individual patterns in any of these typologies.

H. Weight Distribution in the Feet

It is useful to assess where the weight comes down through the feet. By dropping a real or imaginary plumb line through the ankles in a side view, one can see if the weight is predominantly on the toes or heels, essentially a check on the balance between the Superficial Front and Back Line (Fig. 11.17).

A front view can be used to assess how much of the weight is being taken by the inner arch, and how much by the lateral arch. Wear on shoes can also be indicative in this regard. Generally, the more weight being taken by the lateral arch, the more the Deep Front Line needs to be lengthened and lowered toward the medial arch. The more weight taken by the medial arch, the more the Lateral Line needs to be released and lowered, while the Deep Front Line and the anterior–inferior part of the Spiral Line need to be energized, toned, and lifted.

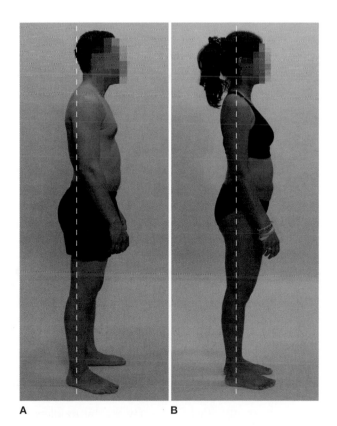

A   **B**

• **Fig. 11.17** Even if we put the vertical line just in front of the ankle, notice how much of the body rests into the front of the foot in these common postures.

The front or back view will also show whether one leg is carrying significantly more weight than the other. (We all have some discrepancy in carrying weight, and we all have a relaxed 'waiting for the bus' posture where we transfer most of the weight to one leg.) The only way to measure this accurately, however, is to have the client step onto two scales, with one foot on each scale, and without looking at the readouts, attempt to stand evenly on both feet. The total of the two scale readouts, of course, will equal the total weight of the person, but the two scales will not necessarily be supporting equal weight. This test will often show that the client's reporting of 'balanced' is actually significantly more weighted on one foot or another. If you adjust the client so that the scales are reporting equal burdens, the client will insist that they are heavily weighted onto the leg that was taking less weight in the initial assessment. This is yet another example of how the client's reports are not always reliable and need to be leavened with the practitioner's acute observation.

I. Balancing Halves

Although the following interpretations need to be taken with some salt, since the realities are quite complex, these simplifications, however subjective, are still quite useful. A quick look at standing posture at the beginning can divide the body into three sets of 'halves': which set has the largest discrepancies between one and the other? It is good to keep the answer in mind in terms of treatment emphasis as therapy proceeds.

- A mid-sagittal line divides the body into right and left. Significant right and left differences often point to internal conflicts between the animus and anima (masculine and feminine tendencies). It is not as simple as right = male and left = female. But those with significant, complex, and intractable differences between the two sides, often involving the eyes and head shape as well as structural differences in the torso and legs, will reveal a significant battle, expressed in uniquely individual ways in work, relationships, artistic endeavor or sexuality, between their inner masculine and feminine aspects (Fig. 11.18).
- A mid-coronal line divides the body, front from back. Of course these two 'halves' are not symmetrical to begin with, but we can still observe the balance between the two. Strong imbalances in this dimension are often expressed as differences in how the person presents in public versus how they act or feel in private (Fig. 11.19).
- A line through the waist divides top from bottom (the exact line can vary individually from an 'empire' waist to just above the iliac crests). Obesity or muscle development can sometimes obscure the underlying bony structure, but what one is looking for here is an evenness of proportion between the shoulder and pelvic girdle, and between the torso and the legs, or the upper and lower body. Those with more weight and substance in the legs and pelvis versus the ribs and shoulders tend toward the

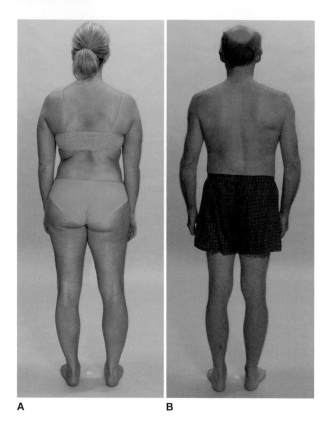

A   **B**

• **Fig. 11.18** The back view is often the easiest – because we tend to make the front look good – to see strong right–left discrepancies, as in these two structures.

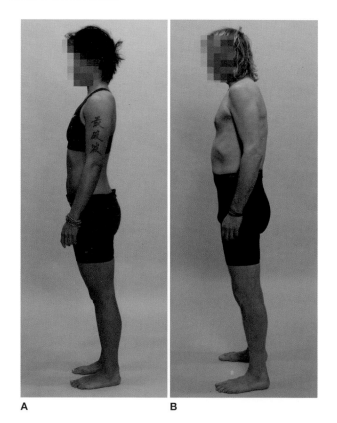

A   **B**

• **Fig. 11.19** The side view is the place to see front–back differences, where what you see in the front is not necessarily what you get in the back.

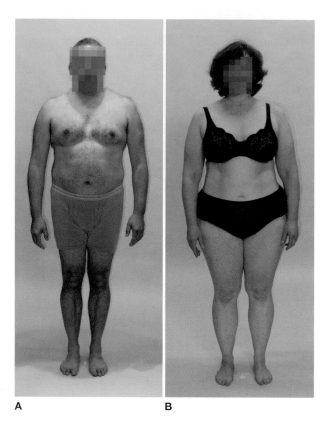

A   **B**

• **Fig. 11.20** Although a large shoulder girdle on top of a cinched-in pelvic girdle is a quintessentially male pattern, and its opposite more often found in the female (as here), you will find the complementary patterns as well.

introverted; those with a large torso and shoulders on top of smaller-built pelves and legs will tend toward the extroverted (Fig. 11.20).

J. Somatic Maturity

Grasping the kind of patterning in the skeletal geometry and myofascial meridians of tension can lead to a different level of seeing, and thus a deeper level of work. One of the most interesting contributions that can be made by quality manual and movement work is related to maturational development (Video 6.26). As an example of what can be accomplished, look at Reginald from the side, (**A**) before Structural Integration, (**B**) just after the completion of a series of sessions (under the direction of Dr Ida Rolf) and (**C**) one year later, with no further work (Fig. 11.21). The pictures have been adjusted only to make them approximately the same size, since Reginald presumably grew over the year.

Before the work, Reginald shows a common randomized postural response: hyperextended knees, an anteriorly tilted pelvis, a posteriorly tilted rib cage, and an anteriorly tilted neck, among other things. His shoulders are integrated neither with the neck nor the rib cage, essentially hanging off the back of the body, putting strain into the upper

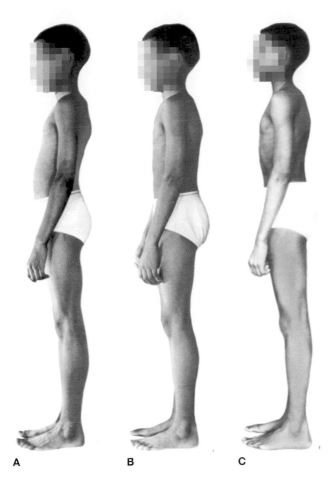

A   **B**   **C**

• **Fig. 11.21** Reginald before intervention (**A**), after (**B**), and one year later with no further work (**C**). (From Toporek (1981), reproduced by kind permission of Robert Toporek (www.handsonparenting.org).)[27]

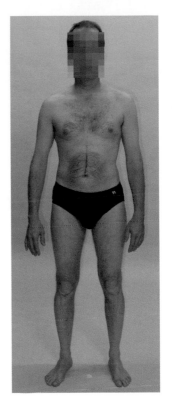

• **Fig. 11.22** Even though this is a full-fledged adult male, can you see the childish remnants in his body structure? The head is the head of an adult; the body is that of a child aged three to six years. What does this mean? Can it be developed and matured at this point?

thoracics and both the superficial and deep pectoral muscles. In (**B**), the post-bodywork picture, he is demonstrably straighter, but not demonstrably better off. (One person, viewing only the first two pictures, accused us of 'somatic colonialism', saying, 'You took away his naturalness and gave him a weedy little white-boy posture! What good is that?')

Picture (**C**), with a year in between to let the work settle, tells a different story. With the knees resting more comfortably forward (although notice that Reginald has 'slipped back' somewhat in this regard over the year), the pelvis has assumed a more horizontal position relative to its former anterior tilt. (And notice that this parameter has improved since the end of the work.) With the pelvis horizontal, the rib cage can orient itself vertically, with a reduced lumbar curvature (see the section in Ch. 3 on primary and secondary curves, pp. 48–50). With the yoke of the shoulder girdle now draped comfortably over the rib cage instead of hanging off behind it, the chest and chest muscles are more free to develop, so Reginald fills out, deepens, and looks a different boy. Our contention is that, left to himself, the boy on the

left would not have developed into the boy on the right in a year, but the boy in the middle could (and did). After the initial work, 'compound essence of time' in gravity is the only medicine necessary to do the job.

Notice that the improvement is not unalloyed. The Reginald of (**C**) has reinstated the tension in the knees and ankles that was present in (**A**) but not in (**B**). Not every element in a pattern responds to any given treatment.

Can you see the underlying very small boy within the postural pattern of the middle-aged man in Fig. 11.22? Can you see that the pelvis of the young woman in Fig. 11.23 looks 'younger' than the rest of her structure? Are such observations clinically useful? In the latter part of this chapter we have stepped over the line from remediation of biomechanical inefficiency toward the realm of the somatic psychologist. In our opinion, being able to recognize such restrictions, parse out the underlying patterns, and realize such potentialities is one of the more important jobs for the manual therapists of the coming century. The Anatomy Trains map, though not specifically developmental, is one way into seeing such underlying patterns.

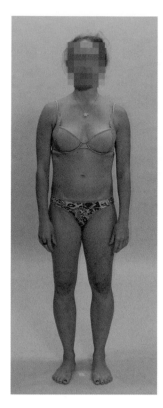

• **Fig. 11.23** While the rest of the structure has grown up, and everything has grown in size, the pelvis of this otherwise strong and balanced young woman nevertheless remains 'young' and immature relative to the rest of her. We see this happen sometimes with sexual trauma, but an early career in gymnastics, hormonal or genetic anomalies, or other factors as yet unmeasured may be in play as well.

References

1. Comeaux Z, Eland DO, Chila A, et al. Measurement challenges in physical diagnosis: refining inter-rater palpation, perception. *J Bodyw Mov Ther.* 2001;5(4):245–253.
2. Sutton C, Nono L, Johnston RG, et al. The effects of experience on the inter-reliability of osteopaths to detect changes in posterior superior iliac spine levels using a hidden heel wedge. *J Bodyw Mov Ther.* 2012;3:1–8.
3. Kendall F, McCreary E. *Muscles, Testing and Function.* 3rd ed. Baltimore: Williams and Wilkins; 1983.
4. Janda V. Muscles and cervicogenic pain syndromes. In: Grand R, ed. *Physical Therapy of the Cervical and Thoracic Spine.* New York: Churchill Livingstone; 1988.
5. Reich W. *Character Analysis.* New York: Simon and Schuster; 1949.
6. Kurtz R. *Body Centred Psychotherapy.* San Francisco: Liferhythms; 1990.
7. Lowen A. *The Language of the Body.* New York: Hungry Minds; 1971.
8. Sheldon WH. *The Varieties of Human Physique.* New York: Harper; 1940.
9. McGill S. *Back Mechanic.* Ontario: Backfitpro Inc; 2015.
10. Aston J. *Aston Postural Assessment Workbook.* San Antonio, TX: Therapy Skill Builders; 1998.
11. Keleman S. *Emotional Anatomy.* Berkeley: Center Press; 1985.
12. Alexander RM. *The Human Machine.* New York: Columbia University Press; 1992.
13. Morrison M. *A Structural Vocabulary.* Boulder, CO: Rolf Institute; Rolf Lines; 2001.
14. Sultan J. Toward a structural logic: the internal–external model. *Notes on Structural Integration* 1992;86:12–18. *Available from Dr Hans Flury, Badenerstr 21, 8004 Zurich, Switzerland.*
15. Keleman S. *Emotional Anatomy.* Berkeley: Center Press; 1985.
16. Pierrakos J. *Core Energetics.* San Francisco: Liferhythms; 1990.
17. Aston J. *Aston Postural Assessment Workbook.* San Antonio, TX: Therapy Skill Builders; 1998.
18. Busquet L. *Les Chaînes Musculaires.* Vol. 1–4. Frères, Mairlot: Maîtres et Cles de la Posture; 1992.
19. McHose C, Frank K. *How Life Moves.* Berkeley: North Atlantic Books; 2006. *Hubert Godard's work is most accessible in English via this book.*
20. Latey P. Themes for therapists (series). *J Bodyw Mov Ther.* 1997;1:44–52, 107–116, 163–172, 222–230, 270–279.
21. Hanna T. *Somatics.* Novato, CA: Somatics Press; 1968.
22. Gladwell M. *Blink.* New York: Little, Brown & Co; 2005.
23. Gellhorn E. The emotions and the ergotropic and trophotropic systems. *Psychol Forsch.* 1970;34:48–94.
24. Smith J. *Structural Bodywork.* Edinburgh: Churchill Livingstone; 2005.
25. Nilsson L. *The miracle of life.* Boston: WGBH Educational Foundation; 1982. Available: www.lennartnilsson.com. Online. Accessed January 14, 2013.
26. Gaggini L. *The Biomechanics of Alignment.* 6th ed. Boulder, CO: Connective Tissue Seminars; 2005. www.connectivetissue.com.
27. Toporek R. *The promise of Rolfing children.* Transformation News Network; 1981.

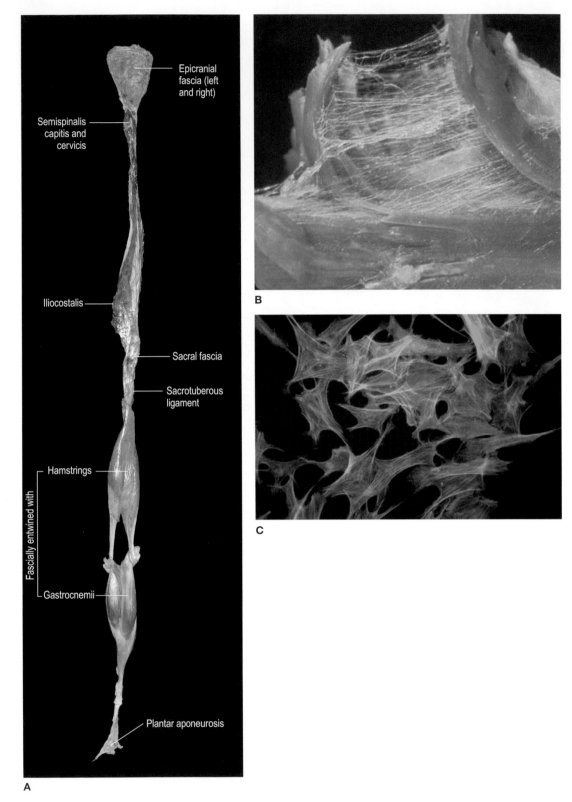

• **Fig. A1.1** (**A**) A fresh-tissue specimen of the myofascial meridian termed the Superficial Back Line, dissected intact by Todd Garcia from the Laboratories of Anatomical Enlightenment. (**B**) A dissection of teased muscle fibers, showing surrounding and investing endomysial and perimysial fascia. (**C**) The ancients and Renaissance artists sought a geometrical ideal for the human form, but the modern equivalent is arising from a consideration of the spatial needs of the individual cells, which could determine a geometric 'ideal' for each body. (A, Photo courtesy of the author; this specimen is explained on video on the accompanying website. B, Reproduced with kind permission from Ronald Thompson; this and other graphics are available and explained in Fascial Tensegrity, available from www.anatomytrains.com. C, photo courtesy of Donald Ingber.)

Appendix 1

A Fascial Reader

Biomechanical Auto-Regulation

Introduction

The following pages are designed to set the current widespread use of the word 'fascia' into context. The entire story of how our body self-regulates its structure and movement extends well beyond the medical (as well as the popular) definition of fascia, running seamlessly through multiple levels of scale from the genetic expression within each cell at a molecular level to the actions and interactions of the entire organism (Fig A1.1; Video B1). It is a complicated story, but it can now be grasped at the level of actionable implications for rehabilitation, training, and all forms of therapy – and physical education as well: how will the next generation of children learn to inhabit their bodies?

The following essays chart how fascia helps living matter self-regulate its growth and form, sustain its physiological processes, and motivate toward its goals. Each of the following sections can be tackled separately, though they are interdependent. Taken in order, it provides a basic narrative of this new story – from definitions to components to properties to applications in training and rehabilitation, and finally into the larger emerging conceptual shift. These forays focus on architecture and structural balance, avoiding discussions of chemistry or connective tissue pathologies.

Besides anatomy, the study of fascia in context leads one into embryology, anthropology, geometry, engineering, hydro- and thermodynamics, neurology, medicine and several other fields where an advanced degree would undoubtedly be helpful. While every attempt has been made to deliver accurate information, research may well replace some of our point of view within the life of this edition, and some of its suppositions may eventually prove to be wrong. The author assumes all responsibility for any inaccuracies with apologies, and is grateful for all the contributions from others in the fast-moving fields of research and therapeutic application.

To look at what everyone has looked at, and see what no one else has seen – this is the essence of all the surprising discoveries detailed in this compendium. In Chapter 1, we showed that Anatomy Trains is part of the historical unfolding of this new understanding, building on previous ideas of kinetic chains, fascial continuities, the neurology of sensing and moving, and systems theory in general (see Fig. A1.4). Here we continue dismantling the 'musculo-skeletal'

structural concept to build a new 'world according to fascia'.

At the very basic level, what do we miss if we follow the standard model implied by the fascia-dissing term 'musculo-skeletal'? In the current model muscles are seen to attach only at their proximal and distal ends and only to bones (origin and insertion). This notional 'single muscle' Newton/Borelli leverage biomechanics we have used for the last 400 years ignores three attachments that all muscles have with a strong effect on *in vivo* biomechanics:

- The longitudinal connections explored in this book, as well as in the 'fascial slings' work of Vleeming and Lee,[1–3] or the lines of Hoepke or Meziére – see Figs. 1.26–28.[4]
- The latitudinal connections of areolar tissue ('fuzz') and intermuscular septa from one muscle to its neighbors,[5] as well as to the ligaments of the joint the muscle crosses,[6] and to the outer unitard layer of the fascia profundis (see Fig A1.6).
- Fascial connections to the neurovascular bundles in their sheaths, which, if shortened, adhered, traumatized, or twisted, may restrict the movement of the area (see Fig A1.10).

We address these specifics as we come to them, but first comes the larger context for the fascial system. The arguments made in this chapter are summarized in less detail on the Fascial Tensegrity program, How Fascia Moves, and other webinars available from www.anatomytrains.com.

Metamembrane – Why Did We Need Fascia?

'Blessed be the ties that bind' goes the old hymn, and fascia is the fabric that binds our cells together into our characteristic shape. Our fascial system evolved as a simple but elegant response to the challenge of becoming a multi-cellular organism. Although we can easily imagine great globs of undifferentiated but still highly organized protoplasm in a fluid continuum ('flow' as envisioned by Aristotle), life on planet Earth committed itself early to building itself around a basic, multiply-repeated unit – the cell (akin to the 'atom' vision of Democritus) (Fig. A1.2).

Modern science posits that for about one-half of the 3.6 billion years or so that life has flourished, all organisms were single-celled – first as simple prokaryotic Protista, which later combined symbiotically to produce the familiar eukaryotic cell.[7] The so-called 'higher' animals – including

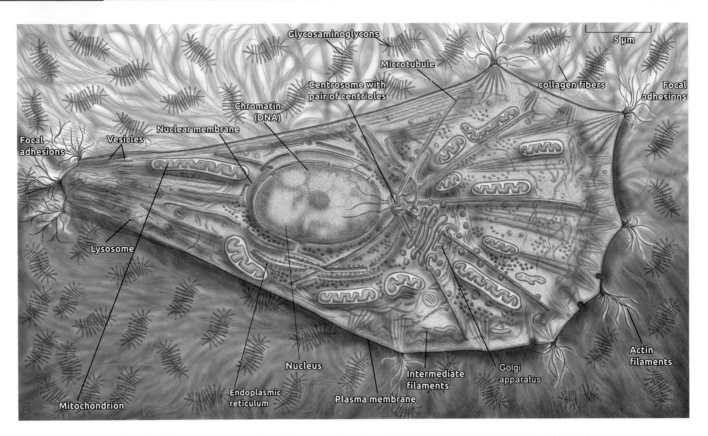

• **Fig. A1.2** The typical eukaryotic cell is a complicated and semi-independent subunit of life, with semi-independent units inside it such as mitochondria. All the large animals, including us, are made up of trillions of these integrated droplets of oily ionised gel.

the humans who are the focus of this book – are not made of bigger cells but are instead coordinated aggregates of ever-higher numbers of these tiny droplet complexes of integrated biochemistry.

In our case, on the order of 10^8 or 10^9 (40–70 trillion is the best recent estimate) of these buzzing little units somehow work together (coupled with a similarly numerous ecology of enteric bacteria in your gut) to produce the event we experience as ourselves. We can recognize bundles of these cells even after years of not seeing them or from several blocks away by observing their characteristic manner of movement. What holds our ever-changing soup of cells in such a consistent physical shape?

While small groups of cells can hook their membranes to each other with adhesive proteins (Fig. A1.3), large groups of cells need a sturdier framework to avoid being smushed out of shape by gravity and the rest of the forces we encounter on Earth's surface. The fascial system, secreted into the intercellular space by connective tissues, is what life invented to keep organized populations of cells working together.

As in human society, cells within a multicellular organism combine individual autonomy with social interaction. In our own tissues, we can identify four basic classes of cells: neural, muscular, epithelial, and connective tissue cells (each with multiple subtypes) (Fig. A1.4). We could oversimplify the situation a bit by saying that each of these emphasizes one of the functions shared by all cells in general (and the fertilized ovum and stem cells in particular). For instance,

all cells conduct along their membranes, but nerve cells have become excellent at it (at a cost, incidentally, to their ability to contract or reproduce well). All cells contain at least some actin, and are thus capable of internal contraction, but muscle cells have become masters of the art. Epithelial cells also contract, but very feebly. Instead, they specialize in lining the surfaces where rapid chemical exchange is necessary, where they absorb nutrition and secrete hormones, enzymes, messenger molecules and other cytokines into the fluid mix of our bodies.

The fourth type, connective tissue cells, are generally less effective at contraction (with one major exception explained later) and fairly good as ionic conductors, but their specialty is to secrete prodigious amounts of an amazing variety of collagenous goo into the intercellular space. This 'slime' sorts itself and undergoes changes to form our bones, cartilage, ligaments, tendons, joints, and fascial sheets (Fig. A1.5). In other words, it is these cells that create the structural substrate to surround and hold all the others, building the strong, pliable 'stuff' that keeps us together. This material in turn becomes the shared and communicative environment for all our cells – Varela[10] termed this 'exo-symbiosis' – shaping us and allowing our 70 trillion cells to coordinate movement toward an organismic intent. If a membrane contains a single cell, the fascia's 'metamembrane' contains our whole organism.

The body-wide net of fascia is the cells' organizing environment, the alembic for all our physiology. And we cannot

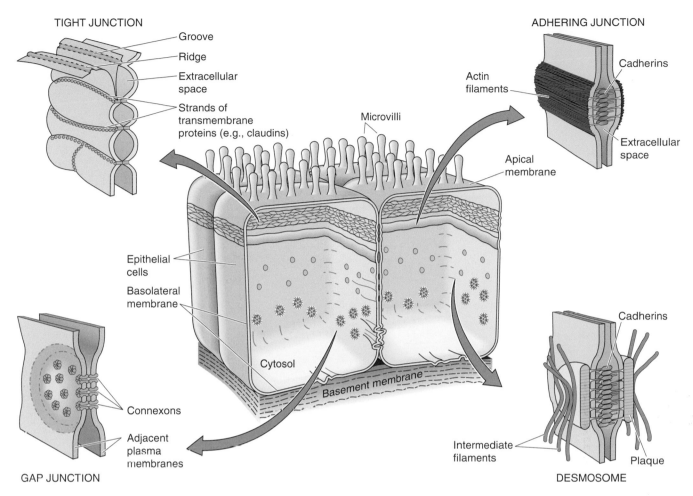

TIGHT JUNCTION

- Groove
- Ridge
- Extracellular space
- Strands of transmembrane proteins (e.g., claudins)

Microvilli

ADHERING JUNCTION

- Cadherins

Actin filaments

- Extracellular space

Apical membrane

Epithelial cells

Basolateral membrane

Cadherins

Cytosol

Connexons

Adjacent plasma membranes

GAP JUNCTION

Basement membrane

Intermediate filaments

Plaque

DESMOSOME

• **Fig. A1.3** Small numbers of cells can hold themselves together – and thus create tissue structure, through cell-to-cell adhesions. Large numbers of cells require an 'exoskeleton' or 'metamembrane' to hold them in relationship to each other. The fascial system is that metamembrane.

let the word 'environment' enter our discussion without quoting from the master of the term, Marshall McLuhan[11]: 'Environments are not passive wrappings, but are, rather, active processes which are invisible. The ground-rules, pervasive structure, and overall patterns of environments elude easy perception.' This may go some way toward explaining why the cellular environment of the extracellular matrix has remained essentially 'unseen' for some centuries of study.

No more. Research on the role and function of fascia, while still nascent, is well underway.[12] It appears we are on the verge of a radically new understanding of how we shape ourselves in space. Accordingly, parts of the following pages reach out beyond current research to some of the promising directions study of our fascial system might take us.

We have noted that the connective tissue matrix is the environment for all our physiology, and of course the fascial system is fully biological – created and maintained internally by our cells on the micro scale (Fig. A1.6). It is thus dependent on functioning genetics, our diet, and our daily breath. It is, however, also fully mechanical, to the point of being increasingly replaceable on the macro scale with manufactured prostheses. A full understanding of our biomechanical auto-regulatory system must span seamlessly from the epigenetic switches in the cell's nucleus to the

entire biopsychosocial organism. This is our ambitious goal; read on.

Definitions

'Fascia' – in a similar manner to 'stress' – is a medical term that has escaped into the wider culture with a more general meaning. Throughout this book, we have used 'fascia' in its wider sense, to discuss its implications. But as with any medical term, 'fascia' has a precise definition, important to maintain for research and applications to pathology. Accompanying terms such as extracellular matrix, connective tissue net, collagenous network, myofascia, and interstitium also need to be differentiated. We start our descent into the geekiness of fascia with a more precise set of definitions (Fig. A1.7).

Fascia

We have referred to this body-wide complex throughout as 'the fascia', or the fascial net. In physiotherapy, the word 'fascia' is usually applied more narrowly to the large sheets of woven fabric that invest, surround, and contain muscular tissues particularly. Medically, according to the Fascial

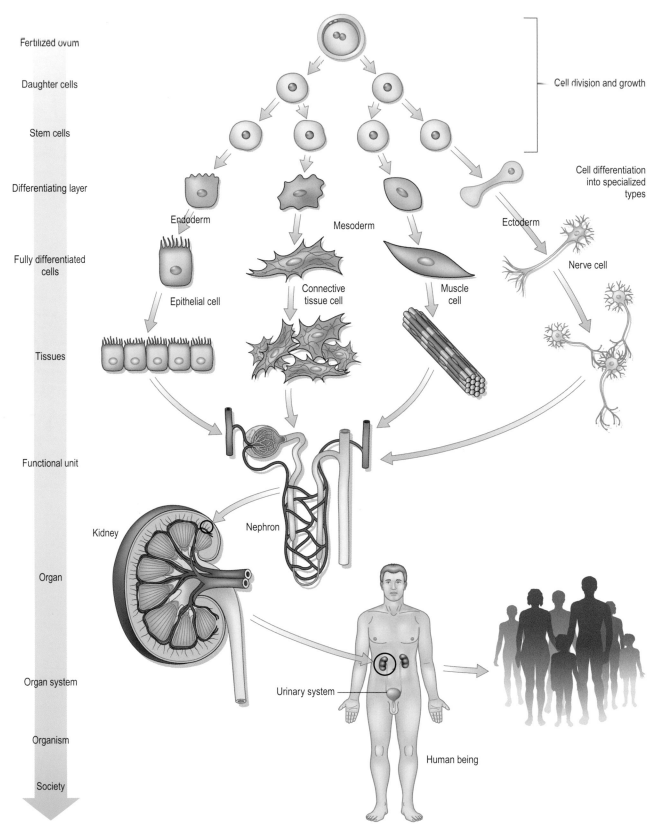

• **Fig. A1.4** Each of the body's major cell types specializes in one of the functions shared by the original ovum and the stem cells, e.g. secretion, conduction, contraction, or support. The specialized cells combine into tissues, organs, organisms, and societies.

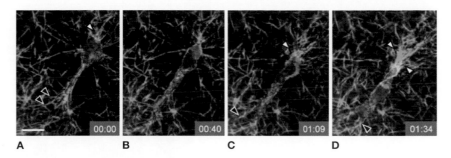

• **Fig. A1.5** Stills from a video of a melanoma cell migrating through a 3-D collagen latticework over an hour's time. Notice how the (green) collagen is remodeled by the passage of the cell, through an interaction with the integrins on the cell's surface. (From Friedl 2004, with kind permission of Springer-Science+Business Media.)

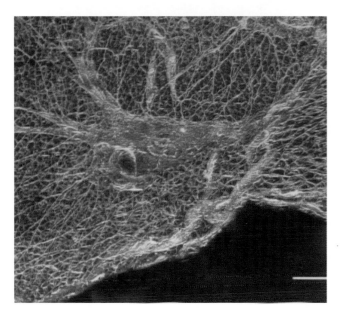

• **Fig. A1.6** The fascial matrix of the lower leg (of a rat), showing the histological continuity among synergistic and even antagonistic muscles. This 3-D reconstruction, using three frozen sections of the anterior and lateral crural compartments, enhances the connective tissue structures within each section. The smallest divisions are the endomysial fibers which surround each muscle fiber. The 'divisions' between these muscles – so sharp in our anatomy texts – are only barely discernible. (Used with kind permission from Prof. Peter Huijing, PhD, Faculteit Bewegingswetenschappen, Vrije Universiteit Amsterdam.)

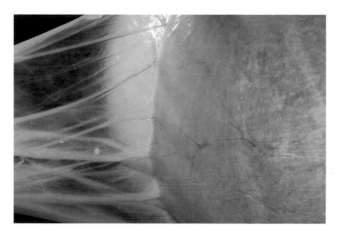

• **Fig. A1.7** The fascial net, considered as a whole, blends a mesh of stronger fibers with a mush of spongy colloids. By shifting proportions, orientation, and chemistry of these sub units, fascia responds within itself to shifting forces – immediately, and over time. (© Fascia Research Society.org/Plastination.)

Research Congress, 'a fascia' is 'a sheath, a sheet, or any other dissectible aggregations of connective tissue that forms beneath the skin to attach, enclose, and separate muscles and other internal organs'.[13]

This is a vague definition – it depends on your dissection skills and how sharp your eyes are as to what constitutes 'a fascia'. Gray's Anatomy complains that 'The practice of attaching a name to any aggregation that is large enough to dissect is of dubious value.'[14] The problem is one of the limitations of human labeling on God's creation. As we argued in Chapter 1, the fascia starts as a whole, lives as a whole, and finishes life as a whole, so what properties must a part have to get a distinct name? What part of this system merits its own label? The debate on anatomical nomenclature continues and likely will not be settled soon. Fortunately, our goal here is not to decide the naming of the details.

Additionally, fascia is so malleable and therefore so variable from person to person and within one person from one time to another, or one spot to another. It is a system defined not by anatomical consistency but by individualized adaptability.

Importantly, experience in the dissection lab shows us that any subset of fascia, from the smallest dissectible piece to any large structure you wish to name, loses its form when removed from the body. This is **not** true in the chemically 'fixed' cadavers used in most medical schools that provide the source material for most modern textbooks and anatomy atlases. Remove a bit of fascia from a standard cadaver, and it stays put in the shape it had when it was part of the body – because the fascia got 'fixed' in place with formaldehyde.

This author has had the privilege of dissecting untreated tissue cadavers for the last decade, without any formaldehyde or other fixative, in a state much closer to living tissue. Remove any bit of untreated tissue, deprive it of its mechanical context, and it reverts to a shapeless blob. Pull on its

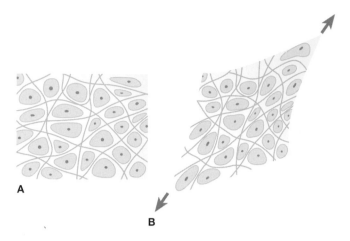

A

B

• **Fig. A1.8** (**A**) The ECM (Extra Cellular Matrix) is designed to allow the relatively free flow of metabolites from blood to cell and back again in the flow of interstitial fluid and lymph. (**B**) Chronic mechanical stress through an area results in increased laying down of collagen fiber and decreased hydration of the ECM's ground substance, both of which result in decreased nourishment to certain cells in the 'back-eddies' caused by the increased matrix.

ends, as would happen in the context of the body, and it takes organized shape again (Fig. A1.8). This property is not evident to those who have worked with embalmed cadavers – and the atlases that proceed from them.

N.B.: Fascial structure is contextual, and it reverts to the formless when deprived of that context. The set of relations to the whole is what matters – and that is what was missed in separating fascia with a blade for these past centuries (see Fascia and tensegrity, in this Appendix). It also demonstrates the fascia's constant ability to adjust by creating structure according to the forces of the moment.[8]

What if we imagine that instead of using a sharp edge, we immersed an animal or a human in some form of detergent or solvent which washed away all the cellular material and left only the fascial system's fabric of collagen. We would see the entire continuum, from the elastic basal layer of the skin, through the subcutaneous fatty/areolar 'neoprene' suit, to the thin fibrous tunic surrounding the muscular body (fascia profundis), down through the cotton investing the muscles and organs, continuous with the leathery scaffolding for cartilage and bones (Fig. A1.9).

Language fails us – even this description of layers suggests a separation that is not present in your body *in vivo*. It would be all one network, connected from top to toe, skin to bone, dense in some spots and gossamer in others, but showing both the external and internal shape of the entire body minus the hair.

If we could fix such a preparation in space so that it would not just collapse like a burst balloon, it would be very valuable in showing us this fascial organ as a continuum. (Early attempts at just such an image are underway, but are fraught with technical difficulties.) This image would emphasize its uniting, shaping nature, rather than simply seeing it as the walls where separations are made. It is the scientific truth that we start whole and end whole; we

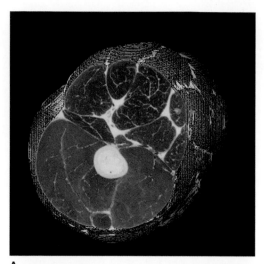

A

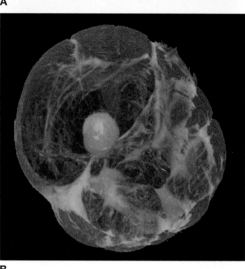

B

• **Fig. A1.9** A section of the thigh, derived from the National Library of Medicine's Visible Human Project by Rolf practitioner Jeffrey Linn. The more familiar view in (**A**) includes muscle and epimysial fascia (but not the fat and areolar layers shown in Fig. A1.24). The view in (**B**) gives us the first glimpse into what the fascial system would look like if that system alone could be abstracted from the body as a whole. (Reproduced with kind permission from Jeffrey Linn.)

are not put together in parts, however convenient and useful these mechanical images are to us.

All naming of parts of the body imposes an artificial, human-perceived distinction on an event that is unitary. Since we are at pains in this book to keep our vision on the whole, undivided, ubiquitous nature of this net, we choose to point to its singularity by calling the whole thing 'fascia'. What we mean, though, is perhaps better described as 'the fascial system'.

The Fascial System

The Fascial Research Congress defines the fascial system as a 'three-dimensional continuum of soft, collagen containing, loose and dense fibrous connective tissues that permeate the body. It incorporates elements such as adipose tissue, adventitiae and neurovascular sheaths, aponeuroses, deep and superficial fasciae, epineurium, joint capsules, ligaments, membranes, meninges, myofascial expansions, periostea, retinacula, septa, tendons, visceral fasciae, and all the intramuscular and intermuscular connective tissues including endo-/peri-/epimysium. The fascial system surrounds, interweaves between, and interpenetrates all organs, muscles, bones and nerve fibers, endowing the body with a functional structure, and providing an environment that enables all body systems to operate in an integrated manner.'

That is more like it, and that is what we see when we open the untreated cadaver. Much of this fascial system must be cut away to produce the pictures we commonly see in anatomy atlases. Arteries or nerves that appear to float freely and separately in Netter's or Sobotta's artwork are in actuality hidden under the adventitial tunics, protected, surrounded, and firmly tied to all the other local fascial structures listed above (Fig. A1.10). A realistic picture would show only fat and fascia, which would not be very useful. But the 'useful' pictures created for these atlases obscure the missing picture of the fascial system as a whole – the surrounding context for all our other structures.

Much of what follows is an expanded definition of the fascial system, so we will let the definition above stand for now. We note, however, that defining the edges of such a system can be difficult. For instance, bones and cartilage are routinely excluded from consideration; the fascial system is only the soft tissues. But the collagenous net extends seamlessly from the soft tissues – the periosteum and perichondrium – into and through the bones and cartilage. We will see, in the section on embryology, how the hard tissues are fashioned from the same processes that form the soft tissues, and there is no discontinuity between the soft and hard

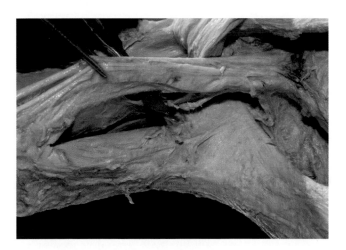

• **Fig. A1.10** The brachial plexus of nerves, artery, and vein protectively wrapped within the medial intermuscular septum of fascia that is part of the Superficial Front Arm Line and divides the Deep Front from the Deep Back Arm Line. Vessels and nerves are often pictured apparently floating within the body, but the reality is that they are wrapped, often together like this, in tunics that are attached to nearby myofascial structures and often anchored to the periosteum. (Photo courtesy of the author.)

tissue network. Out away from the hard tissues, the fascial system is so pervasive, so 'environmental', that it is hard to confine and delineate in the reductive way we humans like to analyze things. Perhaps we should step up one level and get a wider view.

Connective Tissue

The fascial system family of cells is substantial, but only a part of the more expansive connective tissue phylum (Fig. A1.11). According to *Gray's Anatomy*[9]:

> *Connective tissues play several essential roles in the body, both structural, since many of the extracellular elements possess special mechanical properties, and defensive, a role which has a cellular basis. They also often possess important trophic and morphogenetic roles in organizing and influencing the growth and differentiation of the surrounding tissues.*

We will leave the discussion of the defensive support offered by the connective tissue cells to the immunologists. We will touch on the trophic and morphogenetic role of connective tissues when we take up embryology and tensegrity later in these discussions.[15–17] But our main subject here is the mechanical support role the connective tissue cells and their products offer the body in general and the locomotor system in particular.

So when we say 'connective tissues', we are including fat cells, the red and white cells in blood, the glial cells in the brain, and our entire immune system. Intriguing new information is linking these two systems[18] – the immune and the structurally supportive. For our purposes 'connective tissues' is a wide brush that takes in tissues in the same derivation as fascia, but without a mechanical function. That said, 'connective tissues' is quite commonly used to mean the sinewy fibrous portion of the fascial net.

Connective tissue is very aptly named. Although its walls of fabric do act to direct fluids, and create discrete pockets, sacs, and tubes, its uniting functions far outweigh its separating ones. It binds every cell in the body to its neighbors and even connects, as we shall see, the inner network of each cell to the mechanical state of the entire body. Physiologically, according to Snyder,[19] it also 'connects the numerous branches of medicine'.

If the 'connective tissue' is too large a set, and 'a fascia' is too small a target, and 'fascial system' is just right, let us now turn our attention to the manufactured products of this system. If you wish, you can substitute 'collagenous network' or 'connective tissue webbing'; we will use 'extracellular matrix' as described in *Gray's Anatomy*. In public, we will go with the simple 'fascia' or 'fascial system'.[20]

The Extracellular Matrix (ECM)

Connective tissue cells introduce a wide variety of structurally active substances into the intercellular space, including the many types of collagen, along with elastin and reticulin

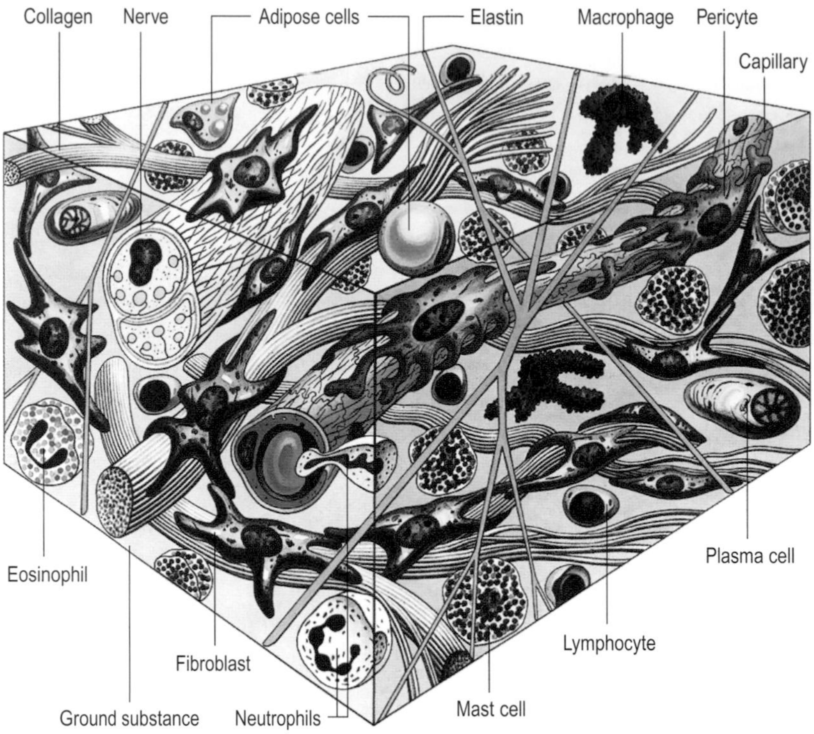

Collagen Nerve Adipose cells Elastin Macrophage Pericyte Capillary

Eosinophil Fibroblast Ground substance Neutrophils Mast cell Lymphocyte Plasma cell

• **Fig. A1.11** All the connective tissues involve varying concentrations of cells, fibers, and interfibrillar ground substance (proteoaminoglycans). (Reproduced with kind permission from Williams 1995.)

fibers, as well as the gluey interfibrillar proteins commonly known as 'ground substance' or more recently as glycosaminoglycans (GAGs) and proteoglycans.

Gray's Anatomy calls this proteinous mucopolysaccharide complex the extracellular matrix:

> *The term extracellular matrix (ECM) is applied to the sum total of extracellular substance within the connective tissue. Essentially it consists of a system of insoluble protein fibrils and soluble complexes composed of carbohydrate polymers linked to protein molecules (i.e. they are proteoglycans) which bind water. Mechanically, the ECM has evolved to distribute the stresses of movement and gravity while at the same time maintaining the shape of the different components of the body. It also provides the physico-chemical environment of the cells imbedded in it, forming a framework to which they adhere and on which they can move, maintaining an appropriate porous, hydrated, ionic milieu, through which metabolites and nutrients can diffuse freely.*[21]

This statement is rich, if a little dense; the rest of this discussion is an expansion on these few sentences, pictured in Figure A1.11.

Dr. James Oschman, PhD, refers to the ECM as the 'living matrix', pointing out that 'the living matrix is a continuous and dynamic "supermolecular" webwork extending into every nook and cranny of the body: a nuclear matrix within a cellular matrix within a connective tissue matrix. In essence, when you touch a human body, you are touching an intimately connected system composed of virtually all the molecules within the body linked together' (Fig. A1.12).[22]

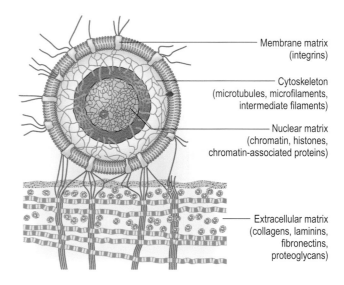

Membrane matrix (integrins)

Cytoskeleton (microtubules, microfilaments, intermediate filaments)

Nuclear matrix (chromatin, histones, chromatin-associated proteins)

Extracellular matrix (collagens, laminins, fibronectins, proteoglycans)

• **Fig. A1.12** The more current view, in which the nuclear material, nuclear membrane, and cytoskeleton are all mechanically linked via the integrins and laminar proteins to the surrounding ECM. (Adapted from Oschman 2000.[41])

Often the fascial webbing is considered to be 'dead' or inert, and certainly characterized as passive. In fact, we will see how very actively it is accommodating and adjusting to momentary and sustained change at various levels. We will examine the responsiveness of the components of the ECM below, but taken together, the connective tissue cells and their products act as a continuum, as our 'organ of form'.[10]

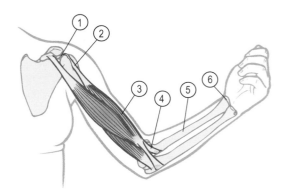

• **Fig. A1.14** The tensile part of mechanical forces is transmitted by the connective tissues, which are all connected to each other. The joint capsule (1) is continuous with the muscle attachment (2) is continuous with the epimysial fascia (3) is continuous with the tendon (4) is continuous with the periosteum (5) is continuous with the joint capsule (6), etc. For dissections of such continuities in the arm, see Figs. 7.4 and 7.29.

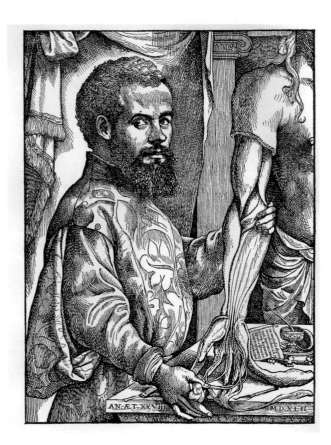

• **Fig. A1.13** Vesalius, like other early anatomists given the opportunity to study the human body, exposed the structures with a knife. This legacy of thinking into the body with a blade is with us still, affecting our thinking about what happens inside ourselves. 'A muscle' is a concept that proceeds not from recorded physiology but directly from the scalpel approach to the body. (Reproduced with permission from Saunders JB, O'Malley C. Dover Publications; 1973.)

Our science has spent more time on the molecular interactions that comprise our function while being less thorough on how we shape ourselves, move through environments, and absorb and distribute impact in all its forms – endogenous and exogenous. Our shape is said to be adequately described by our current understanding of anatomy, but how we think about shape results partly from the tools available to us. For the early anatomists, this was principally the knife. 'Anatomy' is, after all, separating the parts with a blade. From Galen through Vesalius and into our era, it was the tools of hunting and butchery which were applied to the body, and presented to us the fundamental distinctions we now take for granted (Fig. A1.13). These knives (later scalpels, and then lasers) quite naturally cut along the often bi- or multi-laminar connective tissue barriers between different areas, emphasizing the logical distinctions within the ECM, but obscuring the role of the connective tissue web as a whole (Fig. A1.14; Video 6.20). Again we see the need for an image of the fascial system as a single entity – undivided and tuned to all the forces at play across our trillions of working cells – not as our common industrial imagery would have it, as a set of individual parts.

The components of the ECM will be further unpacked in the pages that follow, but for clarity, the ECM includes all the 'stuff' between our cells – fibrous, aqueous, and ground substance.

Collagenous Network

The fibrous network is the hydrophobic part of the fascia – it can be wet but it does not absorb water. It is constructed primarily out of collagen, but includes elastin and reticulin, as detailed below. It is this collagenous network we would see if we dipped the body in solvent and dissolved away all the cells, gels, and fluid.

In the author's mind as he started out in 1975 on this quest, this collagenous spider-web was the fascia in its entirety. Upon further study, we see that the white fibers of collagen are the strongest and most easily seen part of the fascia, but arrayed among the fibers is the clear gel of the ground substance, which has marvelous properties when mixed with this collagenous net, and the interstitial or lymphatic fluid that is the essential third leg of this stool.

The collagenous network is pictured in Figure A1.9 – just the collagen web, abstracted from all it surrounds.

Ground Substance

The ground substance part of the ECM is a nearly amorphous watery gel composed of mucopolysaccharides or glycosaminoglycans such as hyaluronan, chondroitin, keratin, laminin, fibronectin, and heparin. These fern-like colloids are part of the immediate environment of nearly every living cell (Fig. A1.15). Just outside the membrane of most cells is the glycocalyx ('sugary cup'). Similar colloidal gels, at lesser concentrations, fill the interstitial space.

These mucoids bind water in such a way as to allow the easy distribution of metabolites (at least, when these colloids are sufficiently hydrated), and at the same time form

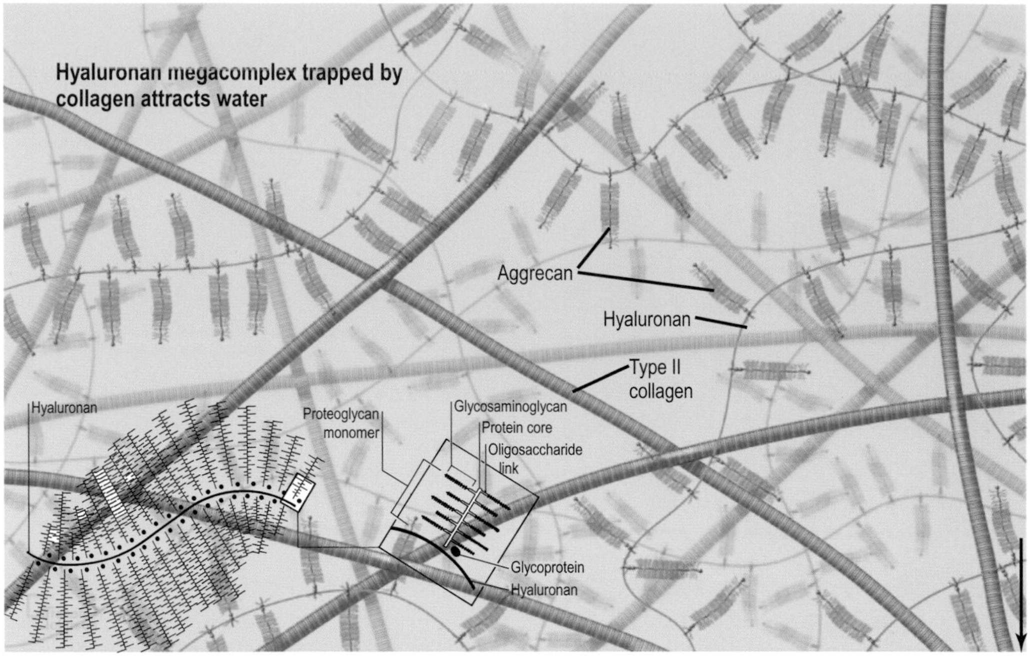

Hyaluronan megacomplex trapped by collagen attracts water

Aggrecan

Hyaluronan

Type II collagen

Hyaluronan

Proteoglycan monomer

Glycosaminoglycan
Protein core
Oligosaccharide link

Glycoprotein
Hyaluronan

• **Fig. A1.15** The sponge-like mucous of the fascial system is a gel of fern-like molecules that spread out through the intercellular and interfibrillar space, soaking up water and binding it into dynamic tissue that at once stabilizes, lubricates, and absorbs shock. This aqueous gel is the background of A1.2.

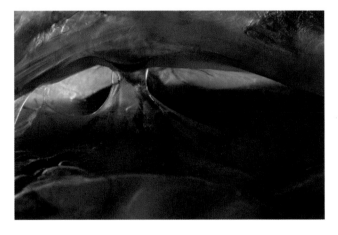

• **Fig. A1.16** The mucopolysaccharide gels and stronger fibers are able to combine to make a full spectrum of building materials from the softest and most pliable to the rigid and reliable. (© FasciaResearch-Society.org/Plastination.)

part of the immune system barrier, being very resistant to the spread of bacteria.

Proteoglycan gel forms a continuous but highly variable 'glue' to help cells both hold together and yet be free to exchange the myriad substances necessary for living. In an active area of the body, the ground substance changes its state constantly to meet local needs (Fig. A1.16). In 'held' or 'still' areas of the body, it tends to dehydrate to become more viscous, more gel-like, and to become a repository for metabolites and toxins. The synovial fluid in the joints and the aqueous humor of the eye are examples where ground substance can be seen in large quantities, but smaller amounts of it are distributed through every soft tissue.

Interstitium

This 'new' word describes something very similar to ECM, but from a more fluid-based point of view. As noted, the connective tissue system is the source for both our immune system and the structural chassis that is the basis for our discussion. The question arises: how are the two related? It turns out cancer researchers were climbing this mountain from the other side, and now they are meeting the structural climbers at the top.

'Through what channels does cancer metastasize?' is a burning question in the quest to cure cancer. In taking histological slices of tissue to examine this question, researchers were confronted with a dense wall of collagen in the slides, with no channels large enough to allow offending cells to slip through. This has been received gospel for a generation or more.

This changed when an imaging system was developed that could examine connective tissue *in vivo* where a regularly irregular network of channels could be clearly seen running between the capillaries and lymph channels and the cells they served. This was a total surprise – they had never seen the openings of these channels in any of their histologically prepared slides.

It was only when they went back to the slide prep that they realized their 'mistake'. In the process of taking the thin slice from the tissue to the slide, it lost the hydration that held the pores open, so they were consistently closed. In the body, they were open for business. They were, in fact, central to the running of the body's water and sewer system. We know now that there is a fluid layer between every fascial plane.

The researchers rushed to publish on the 'new organ system' they had discovered (Fig A1.17A,B).[23] Of course, the 'new' organ system was 'old hat' to the structural fascial researchers: the interstitium was the ground substance, which has been catalogued for years on the structural side, especially via the pioneering videos and writings from Dr Jean-Claude Guimberteau (Fig. A1.17C).[24]

Both sides of the research were interested in 'perfusion' – how the flow of fluids in the body is either effective or disturbed in serving the local cell population. The fundamental insight here is to see how there are channels or conduits within the ground substance (that neither side knew about) where fluid flows faster and more easily from capillary to cell and back again.[25] Other parts of the ground substance were more gel-like and resistant to fluid flow and

cellular migration, while the less resistant 'streams' within the complex allowed greater fluid flow. These canals were generally consistent and regular when left alone, and sometimes lined with undifferentiated fasciacytes. (Guimberteau and Thiese met recently. The author, seeing the work of both, surmises that that the conduits that Thiese describes are the dewy strings that Guimberteau has filmed *in vivo*, as below. Time will tell.)

These canals, however, were not lined with epithelia, and therefore they were not vessels, like the capillaries or lymph canals. They were more akin to unpaved paths through the woods that animals take. If a branch happens to fall on the path, the animals will soon find and beat another path through the underbrush. Similarly, these conduits in the ground substance, or fluid matrix if you will, were not vessels in the formal sense, but the interstitium is still an essential (and adjustably adaptable) 'last mile' of service between the blood system and the more fixed cell populations in need of having nutrition delivered and waste taken away.

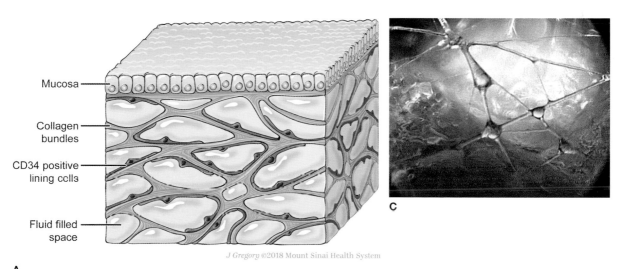

Mucosa

Collagen bundles

CD34 positive lining cells

Fluid filled space

J Gregory ©2018 Mount Sinai Health System

A

C

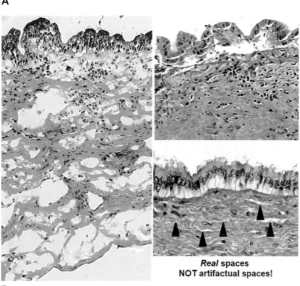

Real spaces
NOT artifactual spaces!

B

• **Fig. A1.17** Long hidden from view due to our histological methods, the newly discovered 'interstitium' expands our knowledge of how substances diffuse through the space between the cells. The dewy, elastic, hollow conduits of the collagenic absorbing system interplay with the vacuoles to create an array of rigging and sails that change with every shift of forces from inside or outside. This gluey areolar network can be said to form a body-wide adaptive system, allowing the myriad small movements which underlie our larger voluntary efforts. (A, Illustration by Jill Gregory. Printed with permission from Mount Sinai Health System, licensed under CC BY-ND. B, Courtesy Dr Neil Thiese. C, Courtesy Dr J-C Guimberteau.)

So, to summarize the preceding terms and make them clear when the reader encounters them in other contexts:

- Connective tissue is a huge kingdom of cells, including all the blood and immune cells, as well as the structural cells that will be our focus in the next section.
- Fascial system is the structural duchy of the connective tissue kingdom, covering all the cells and their products – the collagen-based tissues.
- A fascia is a single dissectible part of the fascial system, often assigned to specific structures such as 'thoracolumbar fascia', 'iliotibial tract', or 'plantar fascia'. (And often named in error – the plantar fascia and superficial thoracolumbar fascia are both actually 'aponeuroses' – a broad sheet for muscles to attach – and the iliotibial tract is simply a dense section of the larger fascia lata.) In this book, and in popular culture, 'fascia' is often an inexact moniker for the fascial system.
- Extracellular matrix (ECM) consists of the cell products (but without the cells themselves) that are interspersed among our cells, including the fibrous nets, the mucous-y ground substance, and the water bound into it.
- Interstitium is about the same as the ground substance, but specifically describes the pathways of least resistance for fluid flow through the ECM.

Given that Anatomy Trains focuses specifically on the muscle fascia, known as myofascia, it is worth noting, while we are in a defining mood, the divisions within the fascia surrounding and investing the muscle.

Myofascia

Myofascia, as noted in Chapter 1, denotes the marriage of muscle and fascial tissue wherever muscle is present. Although fascia appears many places in the body where muscle is absent, wherever muscle is present, fascia must be there to give it shape, direct its contractile strength, and attach it to a bone, cartilage, or some other fascial structure for stability or movement. Muscle without fascia is hamburger, incapable of exerting directed force.

The fascia within the muscle, like the fascia all over the body, is part of a single system, so all three divisions we are about to make are actually one – one net, one system that responds as a whole (Fig. A1.18). But the distinctions are worthwhile.

Around each long, multinucleated muscle cell is the endomysium, the smallest division of fascia within the muscle (Fig. A1.19). It is, in fact, so small that it is not visible to the naked eye or dissectible, so technically it is not 'a fascia' – but it is indivisibly part of the myofascia, and therefore for us, it is fascia, whatever the formal definition.

The endomysial fibers do not run in the same direction as the muscle, but in a double lattice arrangement, like a common mesh onion bag around the cell. The angle of the fibers is 63° to the direction of the muscle fibers, to allow the muscle to contract or be stretched without being limited by the surrounding fascia. This regular arrangement – the double lattice, the consistent angle – is lost if the muscle is not exercised, loaded, or stretched. Without organizing forces, the inner fascia becomes randomly directed, like the fibers in felt, and loses some of its efficiency for transmitting forces faithfully.

Perimysium also lies within the muscle, between fascicles (bundles of 10–100 muscle fibers – Fig. A1.20). The perimysium allows gliding within the muscle, a phenomenon that was only recently recognized on the basis of ultrasound. When fascicles contract, they often must slide on nearby fascicles that are not contracting at that moment. When the perimysium gets 'sticky' from lack of hydration or movement, this sliding within the muscle is lost, and movement efficiency is compromised.

Epimysium is what everybody calls 'fascia' – the cling wrap coating surrounding the muscle, which shapes the muscle and accommodates to its contraction and stretch (Fig. A1.21). It is obvious in observation that the epimysium is continuous with the tendinous attachments at either end of the muscle. Not so obvious is that the endomysium is connected through to the tendon as well. The perimysium, being softer and more lubricating, has less effect on the tendons at either end of the muscle.

To create an accurate picture, we can see the tendon arising from the periosteum of a bone, spreading out when it meets muscle tissue to surround it with epimysium, then invest it down to the single cell level with endomysium, leaving the soft and more liquid perimysium to allow sliding within the muscle. As the muscle tissue attenuates, these fascial layers once more wind themselves tightly into a tendon which is continuous with the periosteum of the target bone (see Fig. A1.18).

Intermuscular Fascia – 'Fuzz'

The discussion of fascia in the muscle would be incomplete without including the fascia between the muscles (Fig. A1.22). Long ignored as the scalpel divides it between one muscle and the other, this intermuscular fascia (dubbed 'fuzz' by anatomist Gil Hedley, and memorialized in several hilarious and informative videos – https://www.gilhedley.com/clips) has been studied extensively by Huijing and his group in Amsterdam.[5] They have shown conclusively that this ignored fascia is a strong carrier of myofascial force sideways from one muscle to its neighbors.

Anatomy Trains focuses on the longitudinal connections that run up and down the body like a chain of sausages. The intermuscular fascia, by contrast, transmits force along the lines of latitude, distributing the shock of landing after a jump, for instance, from only the plantar flexors to **all** the tissues of the lower leg, which is, of course, far more efficient than focusing the force into only the muscles receiving it (see A1.6).

Soft, areolar (loose) fascia such as the perimysium, the fuzz between muscles, and the fascia surrounding the fat beneath the skin does not seem at first like much of a force transmitter, but it is. If a blade is your tool, it is understandable why this phenomenon was ignored, but it is no longer

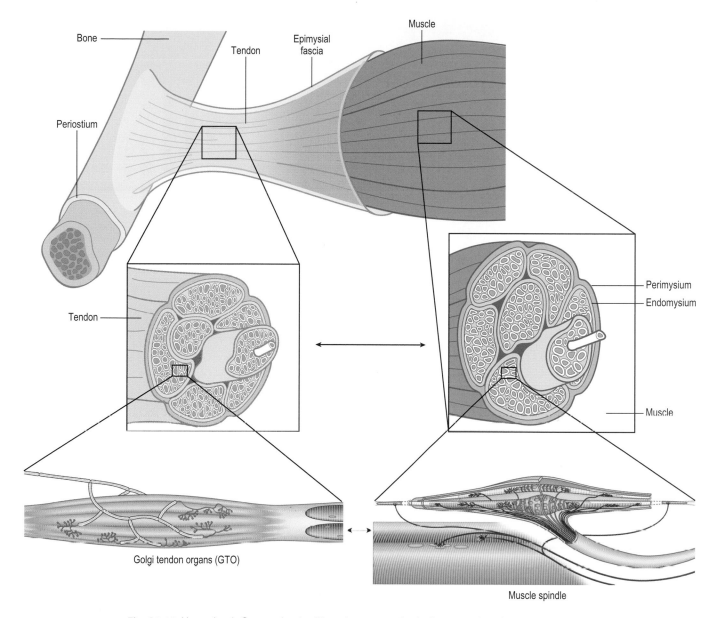

Bone

Periostium

Tendon

Tendon

Epimysial fascia

Muscle

Perimysium

Endomysium

Muscle

Golgi tendon organs (GTO)

Muscle spindle

• **Fig. A1.18** Upper level: Our naming traditions in anatomy imply that a tendon, ligament, periosteum, and a muscle are separate identifiable units. While these are useful terms, it should not obscure the fact that all these named structures blend into each other seamlessly. It might be more useful to start with the idea that the fascial net opens sacs and sleeves in its whole body net for each and every organ – 600 muscles, 200 bones, a dozen visceral organs and one central nervous system with a lot of thin extensions. Middle level: The inner structure of the 'myofascial unit' we name as 'a muscle' is in fact organised into sub-units – fascicles separated by lubricating perimysium as shown here. Lower level: Further, specific muscle spindles link through the fascial web to specific Golgi tendon organs, which both report to the same spot in the spinal cord. The muscle may be the main unit of anatomy, but the brain organizes movement in terms of individual sub-units flickering on and off to meet the challenges presented to the overall myofascial net.

acceptable to slip the scalpel between muscles to isolate them, and then consider their function in this isolated state. The intermuscular fascia is another attachment, an attachment not listed in the books, but nevertheless an important factor in efficient force transmission.

To feel this for yourself, put your finger on your skin of the opposite forearm. You can move the skin with your finger for a centimeter or two in any direction; you can even pinch it and pull it away from your body. 'So that's very soft and loose tissue,' you say, 'incapable of transmitting much force.' Fair enough, but now move your skin up your arm as far as you can, away from your watch. At about 3–5 cm (depends on your native skin elasticity), the soft tissue will 'lock' and begin to transmit serious force, enough to move your watch face a dozen centimeters away. It locks tightly enough that your finger can no longer pull the skin; you will slide over the surface no matter how hard you pull (see Fig A1.8).

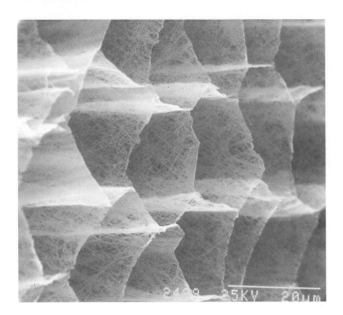

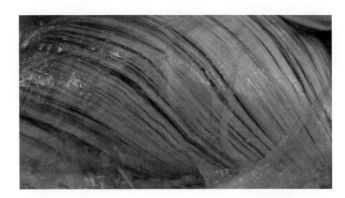

• **Fig. A1.21** The epimysium is the cling-wrap coating around the muscle – here the highly directional surface of the vastus lateralis muscle. Like the endomysium, it is continuous with the tendon. (Photo courtesy of the author.)

• **Fig. A1.19** The endomysium is too small to be called 'a fascia' by anatomical definition, but it is an essential part of the myofascial net and thus the fascial system. One long multi-nucleated muscle cell fits into each one of the honeycomb openings. Notice that the endomysial fibers are not running in the same direction as the muscle, but at an angle that allows for both stretching and concentric contraction. (Reprinted from Purslow PP. Muscle fascia and force transmission. J Bodyw Mov Ther 2010;14:411–17, Copyright 2010, with permission from Elsevier.)

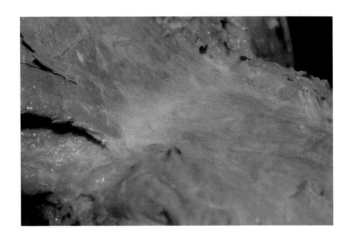

• **Fig. A1.22** The intermuscular areolar fascia, termed 'fuzz' by Gil Hedley, is designed to transfer force at the extremes of load, speed, and dehydration, but permit gliding (low- to no-load transfer) in slow, low-range movement. In regions of inflammation or immobility, as is common here between the subscapularis on the left and the serratus anterior on the right, the intermuscular tissue has a dragging effect on movement. (Photo courtesy of the author.)

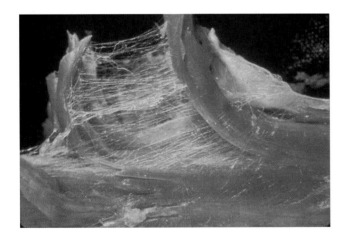

• **Fig. A1.20** The perimysium is a looser, areolar, cotton-like layer which surrounds fascicles of 10–100 muscle fibers and allows glide within the muscles, between the fascicles. (Reprinted with kind permission from Ronald Thompson.)

What is happening under your skin is exactly what is happening between muscles: the intermuscular loose connective tissue allows easy movement between muscles until it locks and transfers force. This is characteristic of loose areolar networks – very easy movement within a short range, until the limit is reached and it 'locks' to transmit force as faithfully as a tendon. The perimysial tissue within the muscle is also like this, but rarely as far as we know is there sufficient movement within the muscle to reach the locking point of the perimysium. But between muscles and in the fat under your skin, this 'loose until it locks' arrangement gives us maximum local adaptability, while providing maximal strain distribution in high load situations.

Fascial 'Layering'

Although the fascial system is one net, the concept of layers is widely used and useful (Fig. A1.23). It is important to say from the outset that while all of these layers show different histology, there are always transition zones and fibers holding each layer to the next. Only in the open spaces of the joints do we see a lack of collagen fibers joining across the surfaces; only synovial fluid – pure ground substance, largely hyaluronan – joins the two bones. Everywhere else collagen fibers run between the layers and must be divided with a scalpel to create these distinct layers.

The outermost layer of fascia is very thin; the dermis is the highly elastic and strong 'carpet-backing' for the skin. Skin is of course very tough to enter with anything other

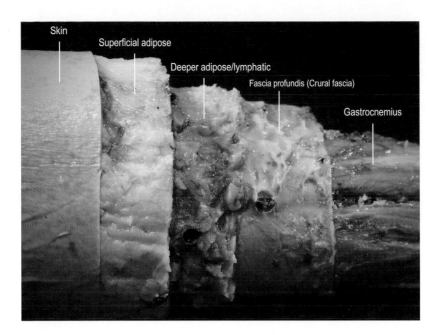

Skin
Superficial adipose
Deeper adipose/lymphatic
Fascia profundis (Crural fascia)
Gastrocnemius

• **Fig. A1.23** Layers in fascia are a widely recognized and useful metaphor, as long as the reader will remember that only in the open spaces of synovial joints is the collagenous web absent. In other words, all these layers are fixed to each other and require a scalpel to be separated. (© FasciaResearchSociety. org/Plastination.)

than a sharp point or blade; the felt-like arrangement and a higher proportion of elastin fibers resist all blunt objects until they come at us with the speed of projectiles.

The next level under the skin is the fat layer, which varies widely in thickness. A loose (areolar) fascial 'loofah' surrounds the fat, and this layer has been termed the subcutaneous layer, hypodermis, or the superficial fascia. Whatever name you give it, this suit of fat, lymph, nerve, and fascia is an outer expression of the inner organs (Fig. A1.24).

Below this mesh of fat and fascia comes the thin but very strong fabric of the tunic around the whole muscular system known as the *fascia profundis*. This fascia forms a unitard around the whole body, providing something steady for the fat to hold on to, but principally to hold the muscles in, wrapping them tightly to the bones. When this layer is removed in an untreated cadaver, the muscles get all floppy, like the triceps on a couch potato. The fascia profundis is called the crural fascia in the leg, the fascia lata in the thigh, the abdominal fascia over the belly, the pectoral fascia over the chest, the fascia colli superficialis around the neck, and the galea aponeurotica under the scalp – but it is all one unitard to hold us in.

Deep to the unitard, we have the epimysium of the muscles described above, and in the muscle tissue we would have the perimysium and endomysium described above as well, though it is too small to see here.

What one can see is the white line of the fascial intermuscular septum ('wall') here between the superficial and deep part of the quadriceps (see Ch. 4 or Fig. A1.9). This wall disappears when the body is dissected in the usual way – half of the wall goes with the rectus femoris, half of it

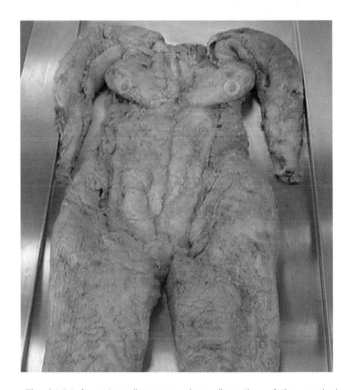

• **Fig. A1.24** An extraordinary one-piece dissection of the areolar/ adipose layer of superficial fascia fills in the picture not covered by Fig. A1.9. This picture does not include the dermis layer of the skin, but does include the fat, the collagen matrix around the fat, and of course the many leucocytes at the histological level. (© Gil Hedley 2005. www.gilhedley.com. Used with kind permission.)

with the intermedius below. If we could make the muscle tissue invisible, this fascia would remain as a wall, as in Fig. A1.9. If glide has been limited by dehydration or adhesion, this septum will act as a drag, not a lubricant.

The periosteal layer, where the muscles really attach, can be found on the outer edge of the bone. The periosteum is highly innervated, and physiologically very active. It is the periosteum that hurts, more than the bone, when you bark your shin. We will have more to say about periosteum and bone development in the section on embryology.

Fascial Components

How to Build a Body

If we take on the thought experiment of building a human body out of materials that could be bought in a local hardware store or builder's supply, what would we need to get? We will imagine that we already have the computer to run it, and that we have already obtained little servo-motors for the muscles, but what would we need to buy to build an actual working model of the body's structure? In other words, what kind of structural materials can connective tissue cells fashion?

You might suggest wood or plastic pipe for the bones, silicon or plastic of some sort for the joint cartilage, spinal discs, and heart valves. We would fill our cart with string, rope, and wire of all kinds, hinges, rubber tubing, cotton wool to pack the empty places, cling-wrap and plastic bags of all sizes to seal things off, oil and grease to lubricate moving surfaces, glass for the lens of the eye, ceramic for the teeth, with lots of cloth, plastic sacks, filters and sponges of various kinds. And where would we be without Velcro® and duct tape?

The list could go on, but the point is made: connective tissue cells make biological correlates of all these materials and more, by playing creatively with cell function and the three elements of the ECM – the available fluid, the tough fiber matrix and the viscous ground substance (Video 6.19). The fibers and ground substance, as we shall see, actually form a continuous spectrum of building materials, but the distinction between the two (non-water-soluble collagen fiber and hydrophilic proteoglycans) is commonly used. The ECM, as we will learn in the section on biotensegrity, is actually continuous with the intracellular matrix as well, but for now, the distinction between what is outside the cell and what is inside is useful.[26]

Fascial Elements

The list of connective tissue elements is short, given that we are not going to explore the chemistry of its many minor variations:

- cells that secrete the intercellular materials, namely:
- tough fibers of collagen and elastin, and
- gluey ground substance, into
- the body's interstitial fluid milieu.

Cells

Fibroblasts

Connective tissue as a whole has the widest variety of cell types, but many of these are the body's wanderers: blood cells, red and white (erythrocytes and leucocytes). Connective tissues also include mast cells, pigment cells, glial cells, fat cells, lymphatic cells, and blood-making (hemopoietic) cells in the bone marrow. We are specifically interested in the cells which create and maintain the ECM, and they are more limited in category, consisting primarily of fibroblasts (fiber-makers – Fig. A1.25).

The fibroblast family is nevertheless diverse, and cells can convert from one type to another, though the limits of that interconversion are not yet fully delineated. Osteocytes (bone cells) and chondrocytes (cartilage cells), fat cells, and even smooth muscle cells can derive from fibroblasts, which are pluripotential like the mesenchymal stem cells from which they themselves derive. The cell type and function can be converted by both chemical agents (such as trophic growth factors) and – because the cells are 'Velcro®-ed' with ligands to the ECM – mechanical changes in the local ECM.[27]

Fibroblasts are thus highly generalized and versatile cells, which crawl through the matrix – laying down new matrix where loads create more piezoelectric charge, and cleaning up old and molecularly 'frayed' collagen with proteolytic enzymes. The fibroblasts are both the planters and the pruners of our fascial garden.

An interesting attribute of fibroblasts is that when the matrix surrounding them is loose and lax, the cells extend processes into the matrix, making the cell bodies small, and using the processes to monitor local tissues and contact other fibroblasts. As the surrounding matrix is loaded, pulled on, subjected to tension, then the fibroblasts pull in these processes, the cytoplasm gathers in the body, and the gears start whirring to produce more matrix to meet the new load (see Fig. A1.25, A–D).

These proteogenic gears grind slowly, so that a momentary new load on the matrix will not produce more fascia, but a sustained or repetitive load will.

This interconvertibility makes the precise classification of this large family of cells problematic. As we can see from Table A1.1, bone has three types of cell – one to build new bone (osteoblast), one to 'eat' old bone (osteoclast), and one to maintain it (osteocyte). Cartilage has only one kind of cell, the chondrocyte. In the fascia itself, we have the fibroblasts, which can convert to myofibroblasts, which are halfway between fibroblasts and smooth muscle cells.

Myofibroblasts

One of the conversions fibroblasts can make is to organize more actin fibers within the cell to become a myofibroblast (MFB – Fig. A1.26). This allows large sheets of fascia to be contractile – the only instance we know of active contraction within the fascia. Let us hasten to add that this mechanism works only under limited and interesting circumstances.

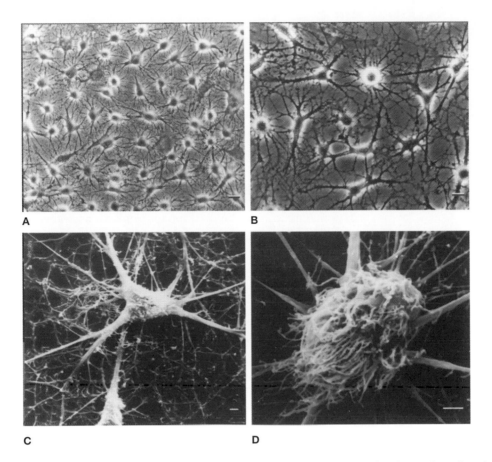

• **Fig. A1.25** (**A**) Cells in relaxed tissue – upper left – extend pseudopods to monitor the nearby web and be in touch with other nearby cells. (**B, C, D**) As the tissue load tightens, the cytoplasm is pulled pack toward the cell body, as it prepares to build more structure. The fibroblasts have intimate connection with the network of fibers they create and maintain (see Fig. A1.12). (A–D from Valentich JD, Popov V, Saada JI, Powell DW. Phenotypic characterization of an intestinal subepithelial myofibroblast cell line. Am J Physiol 1997;272(5 Pt 1):C1513–24.)

TABLE A1.1	**Building Materials**		
Tissue Type	**Cell**	**Fiber Types (Insoluble Fiber Proteins)**	**Interfibrillar Elements, Ground Substance, Water-Binding Proteins**
Bone	Osteocyte, osteoblast, osteoclast	Collagen	Replaced by mineral salts, calcium carbonate, calcium phosphate
Cartilage	Chondrocyte	Collagen and elastin	Chondroitin sulfate
Ligament	Fibroblast	Collagen (with elastin)	Minimal proteoglycans between fibers
Tendon	Fibroblast	Collagen	Minimal proteoglycans between fibers
Aponeurosis	Fibroblast	Collagen mat	Some proteoglycans
Fat	Adipose	Collagen	More proteoglycans
Loose areolar	Fibroblasts, white blood cells, adipose, mast	Collagen and elastin	Significant proteoglycans
Blood	Red and white blood cells	Fibrinogen	Plasma

Connective tissue cells create a stunning variety of building materials by altering a limited variety of fibers and interfibrillar elements. The table shows only the major types of structural connective tissues, from the most solid to the most fluid.

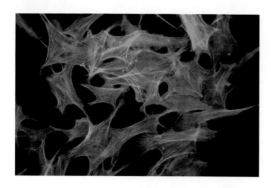

• **Fig. A1.26** Consideration of the spatial needs of the individual cells could determine a geometric 'ideal' for each body. Actin filaments in myofibroblast cells strained green. (Photo courtesy of Donald Ingber.)

Given that all cells contain at least some actin and are therefore able to exert some pull, and given that all the cells are 'Velcro®-ed' into the ECM with adhesive molecules like the integrins, <u>all</u> cells pull on the matrix. MFBs, however, are capable of exerting clinically significant contractile force – enough, for instance, to influence low-back stability.[28] MFBs represent a middle ground between a smooth muscle cell (commonly found in viscera at the end of an autonomic motor nerve) and the traditional fibroblast (the cell that primarily builds and maintains the collagenous matrix). Since both smooth muscle cells and fibroblasts develop from the same mesodermal primordium, it comes as little surprise (in retrospect, as usual) that the body might find some use for the transitional cell between the two, but some surprising characteristics of these cells kept them from being recognized earlier. Apparently, evolution found variable uses for such a cell, as MFBs have several major phenotypes from slightly modified fibroblasts to nearly typical smooth muscle cells.[29,30]

Chronic contraction of MFBs plays a role in chronic contractures such as Dupuytren's contracture of the palmar fascia, fibromatosis of the plantar surface, or adhesive capsulitis in the shoulder.[29] MFBs are clearly very active during wound healing and scar formation, helping to draw together the gap in the metamembrane and build new tissue.[31] To be brief, we will let the reader follow the references for these possibly intriguing roles in body pathology so that we can hew closely to our stated goal of describing how fascia works normally.

It is now clear that MFBs occur in healthy fascia, and in fascial sheets in particular, such as the lumbar fascia, fascia lata, crural fascia, and plantar fascia. They have also been found in ligaments, the menisci, tendons, and organ capsules. The density of these cells may vary positively with physical activity and exercise, but in any case, the density is highly variable in different parts of the body and among people.

Myofibroblasts contract in a spiral motion like smooth muscle cells, not the linear motion of the skeletal muscle fibers. Therefore they pull in on the whole sheet of fascia – say, the crural fascia of your leg when you are on a long plane trip, squeezing the fluid away from your feet back into the venous system. This also pre-stresses the fascial sheet, which allows it to take a larger load and retain its stiffness. MFBs tighten up the system, turning it from a nerf ball to a super ball.

One very surprising aspect of these cells is that – unlike every other muscle cell in the body, smooth or striated – they are *not* stimulated to contract via the usual neural end plate. Therefore, they are beyond the reach of conscious control, or even unconscious control as we would normally understand it. The factors that induce the long-duration, low-energy contraction of these cells are: (1) sustained mechanical tension going through the tissues in question, and (2) specific cytokines and other pharmacological agents such as nitric oxide (which relaxes MFBs) and histamine, mepyramine, and oxytocin (which stimulate contraction). Unexpectedly, neither norepinephrine nor acetylcholine (neurotransmitters commonly used to contract muscle), nor angiotensin or caffeine (calcium channel blockers) have any effect on these MFBs. Many MFBs are located near capillary vessels, the better to be in contact with these chemical agents.[29]

The contraction, when it occurs, comes on very slowly compared to any muscle contraction, building over 20–30 minutes and sustaining for more than an hour before slowly subsiding. Based on the *in vitro* studies to date, this is not a quick-reaction system, but rather one built for more sustained loads, acting as slowly as it does under fluid chemical stimulation rather than neural. One aspect of the fluid environment is of course its pH, and a lower, acidic pH in the matrix tends to increase the contractility of these MFBs.[32] Therefore, activities that produce pH changes in the internal milieu, such as breathing pattern disorder, emotional distress, or acid-producing foods, could induce a general stiffening in the fascial body. Here ends this brief foray into chemistry, which is so well-covered elsewhere.[33]

MFBs also induce contraction through the matrix in response to mechanical loading, as would be expected. With the slow response of these cells, it takes 15–30 minutes or more before the fascia in question gets more tense and stiff. This stiffness is a result of the MFBs pulling on the collagen matrix and 'crimping' it (Fig. A1.27).

Regular fibroblast cells are incapable of mounting the degree of tension or forming the kinds of intracellular and extracellular bonds necessary to pull significantly on the ECM (Fig. A1.28). Under mechanical stress, however, certain fibroblasts will differentiate into a proto-MFB, which builds more actin fibers and connects them to the focal adhesion molecules near the cell surface (Fig. A1.28B). Further mechanical and chemical stimulation can result in full differentiation of the MFB, characterized by a complete set of connections among the fibers and glycoproteins of the ECM through the MFB membrane into the actin fibers connected with the cytoskeleton (Fig. A1.28C).

The contraction produced by these cells – which often arrange themselves in linear syncytia as muscle cells also do, like boxcars on a train – can generate stiffening or shortening of large areas in the sheets of fascia where they often reside, as well as laying down additional reinforcing fascia (see Fig. A1.5).

This discovery, though still in its early stages in terms of research, has implications concerning the body's ability to adjust the fascial webbing. This form of 'pre-stress' – a middle ground between the immediate contraction of voluntary muscle and the fiber-creating remodeling shown by the pure fibroblast – can prepare the body for greater loads or facilitate transfer of loads from one fascia to another. In terms of the responsiveness of myofascial system, we see a spectrum of contractile ability:

- the near instant adjustment of the skeletal muscle
- the more generalized spiral contraction of the smooth muscle cell
- the MFB sustained pre-stress on the larger sheets
- the more passive but still attentive fibroblast.

Given how these MFBs can be stimulated by mechanical loading or by fluid chemical agents, we can also discern in this system the dance among the neural, vascular, and fibrous web that goes into making what we have here termed 'spatial medicine': how the body senses and adapts to changes of shape caused by internal or external forces (see Fascia as a system, p. 282 and ff.

Other Cells

Dr Carla Stecco has recently proposed a new cell type, dubbed the 'fasciacyte', which lines the edges of fascial planes, ensuring that apposite surfaces are able to glide on each other by producing lubricating hyaluronan (hyaluronic acid; see Glycosaminoglycans, below).[35]

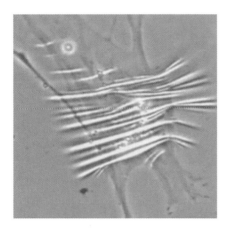

• **Fig. A1.27** A contracting myofibroblast (MFB) can produce visible 'crimping' on the *in vitro* substrate, demonstrating the ability of the motive power of the MFB to affect the surrounding matrix. (From Hinz, et al.[34] Provided by Dr Boris Hinz, Laboratory of Tissue Repair and Regeneration, Faculty of Dentistry, University of Toronto.)

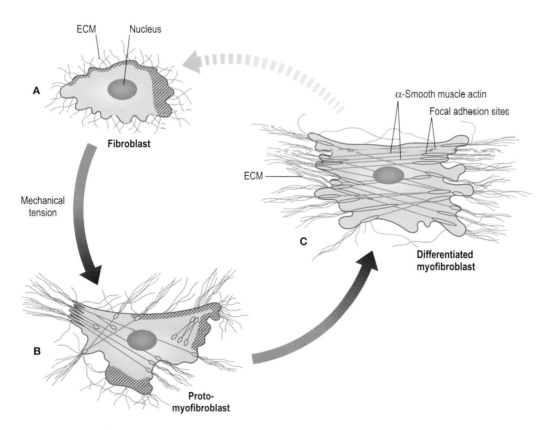

• **Fig. A1.28** MFBs are thought to differentiate in two stages. Though normal fibroblasts have actin in their cytoplasm and integrins connecting them to the matrix, they do not form adhesion complexes or show stress fibers (**A**). In the proto-MFB stage, they do form stress fibers and adhesion complexes through the cell's membrane (**B**). Mature MFBs show more permanent stress fibers formed by the α-smooth muscle actin, as well as extensive focal adhesions that allow the pull from the actin through the membrane into the ECM (**C**). (Redrawn from Tomasek J, et al. Nature Reviews. Molecular Cell Biology; 2002.[28])

A final cell type, telocytes, have been recently identified, and their properties are currently being assessed.[36] Telocytes seem to be the monitors and street sweepers at the end of the connective tissue chain. These cells have long and sinuous telopods – the longest cell processes in the body outside of the neural axons – that reach into the tissue to contact all kinds of local cells, 'listening' for damage or changes in the system.

'The consensus is that telocytes could form an extensive inter-cellular information transmission and executive system …. utilizing electric currents, small molecules, exosomes—and possibly electrical events within the cytoskeleton—to modulate homeostasis, stem cell activity, tissue repair, peristalsis, anticancer activity and other complex functions in many organs.'[37]

Fibroblasts and all their relations, including bone and cartilage cells, fasciacytes and myofibroblasts, and the mysterious telocyte are all at play in the fascia to build, maintain, and repair the ECM for the good of all our cells who live in it.

Fibers

Let us now turn our attention to the elements that lie between these cells – first the strong hydrophobic fibers, then the interfibrillar elements. There are three basic types of fibers: reticulin, elastin, and the ubiquitous collagen (Fig. A1.29).

- Reticulin is a very fine fiber, a kind of immature collagen (now listed as type III collagen) that predominates in the embryo but is largely replaced by collagen in the adult. It does not bundle itself into large fibers, but as a mesh that is used for support in loose connective tissues.

- Elastin, as its name implies, is employed in areas such as the ear, skin, or particular ligaments where large deformation elasticity is required. (These elastic fibers may be better classified as another form of collagen.[38])
- Collagen is by far the most common protein in the body. Collagen is found in the dermis of the skin, bone, tendon, fasciae, organ capsules and many other areas and is readily seen – indeed, unavoidable – in any dissection or even any cut of meat. These fibrils aggregate to form thick bundles of 2–10 μm in diameter and give the connective tissue high tensile strength (500–1000 kg/cm²).

There are currently around two dozen identified types of collagen fiber (Table A1.2), but the distinctions need not concern us here. Type I constitutes about 90% of body collagen. These fibers are composed of amino acids that are assembled like LEGO® in the endoplasmic reticulum and wound around sugars in the Golgi complex of the fibroblast and then extruded into the intercellular space. Here they spontaneously (under conditions described below) form into a variety of arrays. It speaks to the versatility of collagen as a building material that the transparent cornea of the eye, the valves of the heart, the strong tendons of the foot, the spongy lung, and the delicate membranes surrounding the brain are all made from it.

All these fibers ionically repel water – they can get wet, but they will not absorb water, or change their molecular structure in its presence. In every tissue, these fibers interact with the ground substance, which consists of various types of glycoproteins and mucopolysaccharides.

The collagen molecule consists of three chains of amino acid proteins, wound into a triple helix, and kept in that configuration by a glycine chain running down the center of the helix (Fig. A1.30).

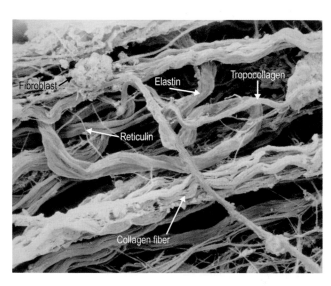

• **Fig. A1.29** This photomicrograph shows very clearly the (purple) fibroblasts in the top third extruding tropocollagen, which combines into the three-strand collagen molecule, apparent in the lower third. There are also bendy yellow elastin fibers, and the much smaller reticulin fibers in the middle third. (© Prof. P. Motta/Dept. of Anatomy/University "La Sapienza", Rome/Science Photo Library. Reproduced with kind permission.)

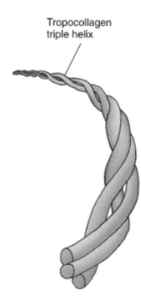

• **Fig. A1.30** Type I collagen is composed of two identical α1(I) chains (blue) and one α2(I) chain (pink). (From Gartner LP. Textbook of Histology, 4e. Elsevier, 2017)

TABLE A1.2   **Types of Collagen**

Type	Characteristic Features	Function	Location in Body
I	Most abundant collagen	Resists tension	Dermis, tendon, ligaments, capsules of organs, bone, dentin, cementum
II	Provides heterofibrils with colix	Resists tension	Hyaline cartilage, elastic cartilage
III	Abundant in elastic tissue	Forms structural framework of spleen, liver, lymph nodes, smooth muscle, adipose tissue	Lymphatic system, spleen, liver, cardiovascular system, lung, skin
IV	Interaction with type IV, laminin, nidogen, integrin	Forms meshwork of the lamina densa of the basal lamina to provide support and filtration	Basal laminae
V	Forms the core of type I fibrils; binds to DNA heparin sulfate, thrombospondin, heparin and insulin	Associated with type I collagen, also with placental ground substance	Dermis, tendon, ligaments, capsules of organs, bone, cementum, placenta
VI	Highly disulphide cross-linked	Ligaments, skin, placenta, cartilage	Bridging between cells and matrix
VII	Forms bundles made of dimmers anchored in anchoring plaques and basal laminae	Forms anchoring fibrils that fasten lamina densa to underlying lamina reticularis	Junction of epidermis and dermis
VIII		Cornea, endothelium	Tissue support, porous network
IX	Interacts with glycosaminoglycans In cartilage	Associates with type II collagen fibers	Cartilage
X		Hypertrophic zone of cartilage growth plate	Calcium binding
XI	Forms core of type II fibrils	Associated with type I collagen as well as type II collagen fibers	Collagenous connective tissue; cartilage
XII	Single transmembrane domain	Associates with type I collagen fibers	Tendons, ligaments, and aponeuroses
XIII			
XIV	Associated with type I	Widespread in many connective tissues	Modulates fibril interactions
XV	Contains antiangiogenic factor	Epithelial and endothelial basement membranes	Stabilizes skeletal muscle cells and microvessels
XVI – XVII			
XVIII		?	Lamina reticularis of the basement membrane
XVIV – XXIII			
XXIV	Displays structural features unique to invertebrate fibrillar collagen	Bone, cornea	Regulation of type I fibrinogenesis
XXV	Extracellular domain deposited in β amyloid plaques	Neurons	Neuron adhesion
XXVI	Disulphide bonds are made into N-terminal noncollagenous domain	Developing and adult testis and ovary	Unknown
XXVII	Presence of triple helix imperfection	Cartilage, eye, ear, lungs	Association of type II fibrils
XXIII–XXIX			

Adapted from: Deshmukh SN, Dive AM, Moharil R, et al. Enigmatic insight into collagen. Journal of Oral and Maxillofacial Pathology 2016; 20 (2): 276–83; and Gartner LP, Textbook of Histology 4e, Elsevier, 2017.

Glycosaminoglycans (GAGs)

Mixed into the fluid with the collagen fibers are the ground substance mucopolysaccharides (Fig. A1.31). All the mucopolysaccharides are hydrophilic, meaning they absorb and bind with water like sponges, and will change their structure and properties in the presence (or absence) of interstitial fluid. Like mucous in your nose, these GAGs can vary in their water content, running from the most serous clear fluid that drips off your nose on a winter day to the middling consistency of egg white to the most viscous, almost solid mucous that accompanies a visit to a dry climate.

The 'strongest' of the GAGs is hyaluronan (HA), which forms a stem structure on which the proteoglycan 'ferns' attach. Indications are the long chains of HA make the tissue 'sticky' and unable to glide, while very short chains of HA are indicative of inflammatory processes. In between is the 'just right' length that allows glide but keeps the tissue from the 'deep freeze' of reduced movement, but away from the fire of inflammation. When the inflammation ferment dies down, the HA can form longer chains again to keep stability and a normal water content. When the chains get too long, movement or manual therapy can help break them up and bring the size to the healthy middle range.

The proteoglycans, or 'fern' part, has a protein core off which the GAGs are suspended. Each GAG complex has multiple sites for water molecules to attach, and water thus bonded to the GAGs is called 'bound' water (as opposed to the 'free' water moving through the interstitium). These bound water molecules are thus arrayed in rows like soldiers, which in turn organizes (binds) nearby water molecules into a liquid crystal array. This ionic array simultaneously allows the free flow of fluids through the conduits of the interstitium while, as we have noted, discouraging the spread of bacteria in our system.

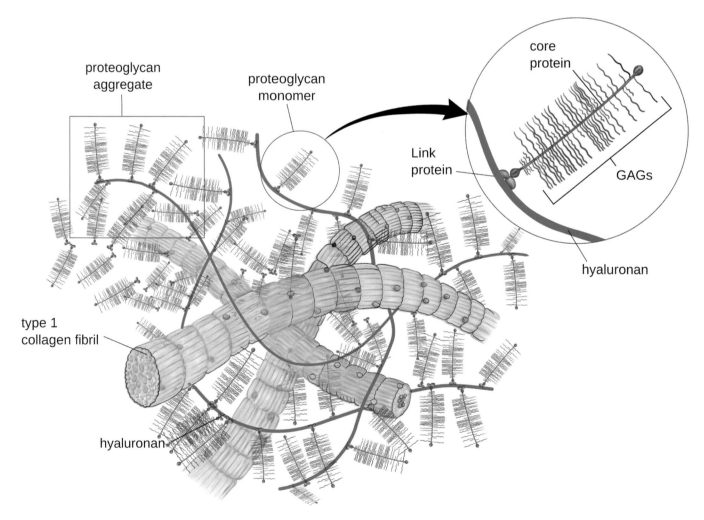

• **Fig. A1.31** The working components of the fascia are few in number but versatile in nature. The tightly ordered array of collagen molecules in the larger collagen fibers (pink) excludes most water and provides a slightly elastic but fundamentally unstretchable component. Hyaluronan chains (green) determine the viscosity – they get longer (and 'sticky') in turgid tissue, but short and hyperreactive in inflamed tissue. The third component are the GAG gels that open like ferns to bind water – the fourth and universal element of the interstitial space – into a loose liquid crystal.

This hydrophilic quality means they are very versatile in handling forces within the body, and come up for more discussion under Fascial properties and Fascial responses to intervention, below. GAGs include chondroitin sulfate, the most prevalent GAG in the body, widely used in cartilage, heparin, an anti-coagulant, and of course HA, the lynchpin of tissues' ability to glide.

The GAGs, taken together with other mucopolysaccharides like fibronectin and laminin, form the basis of what we could call the 'adhesome' – the body's glue. The fibers weave the cells together; mucous glues them together. This is easy to see with the chondroitin sulfate, which is the silicon-like part of cartilage, but it is also true of the hyaluronan, which, like egg white, can both lubricate and 'grip', depending on its water content and the speed with which it is moved.

Discussion

Table A1.1 summarizes the way in which the cells alter the fibers and the interfibrillar elements of connective tissue to form all the building materials necessary to our structure and movement.

Let us take a common example: the bones you have found in the woods or seen in your biology classroom (presuming you are old enough to have handled real as opposed to plastic skeletons) are really only half a bone. The hard, brittle object we commonly call a bone is in fact only part of the material of the original bone – the calcium salts part, the interfibrillar part in the table. The fibrillar part, the collagen, had been dried or baked out of the bone at the time of its preparation; otherwise it would decay and stink.

Perhaps your science teacher helped you understand this by taking a fresh chicken bone and soaking it in vinegar instead of baking it dry. By doing this for a couple of days (and changing the vinegar once or twice), you can feel a different kind of bone. The acid vinegar dissolves the calcium salts and you are left with the fibrillar element of the bone, a gray collagen network with the exact shape of the original bone, but it acts and feels like leather. You can tie a knot in this bone. Living bone, of course, includes both elements, and thus combines the collagen's resistance to tensile and shearing forces with the mineral's reluctance to succumb to compressive forces.

To make the situation more complex (as it always is), the ratio between the fibrous element and the calcium salts changes over the course of your life. In a child, the proportion of collagen is higher, so that long bones will break less frequently, having more tensile resilience.[38] When they do break, they will often break like a green twig in spring (Fig. A1.32A), fracturing on the side that is put into tension, and rucking up like a carpet on the side that goes into compression. For this reason, young bones are difficult to break, but also hard to set back together properly, though they often mend quickly enough due to the responsiveness of the young system and the prevalence of collagen to reknit.

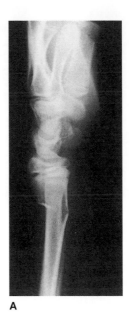
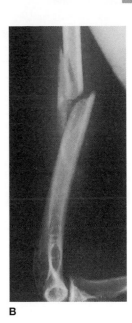

A   B

• **Fig. A1.32** (**A**) Young bone, with a higher fiber content, breaks like green wood, compressing on one side, splintering on the other. (**B**) Old bone, with a proportionally higher calcium apatite content, breaks cleanly like dry wood. (Reproduced with kind permission from Dandy 1998.)

In an older person, by contrast, where the collagen is somewhat frayed and deteriorated, and thus the proportion of mineral salts is higher, the bone is likely to break like an old twig at the bottom of a pine tree (Fig. A1.32B): straight through the bone in a clean fracture. Easily put back in place but hard to heal – precisely because it is the network of collagen that must cross the break and reknit to itself first, to provide a fibrous scaffolding for the hard calcium salts to bridge the gap and recreate solid compressional support. For this reason, bone breaks in older people are often pinned to provide solid contact between the surfaces for the extra time required for the remaining collagenous net to link up across the fracture.

Likewise, the various types of cartilage merely reflect different proportions of the elements within it. Hyaline cartilage – as in your nose – represents the standard distribution between collagen and the silicon-like chondroitin sulfate. Elastic cartilage – as in your ear – contains more of the yellowish elastin fibers within the chondroitin. Fibrocartilage – as in the pubic symphysis or intervertebral discs – has a higher proportion of tough fibrous collagen compared to the amount of chondroitin.[39] In this way, we can see that bone and cartilage are really dense forms of fascial tissue – such that the distinction between 'soft' and 'hard' tissues is a difference in degree, rather than a true difference in type.

In regard to fat, the experienced hands-on practitioner will recognize that some fat allows the intervening hand to enter easily, enabling the therapist to reach deep to the fat layer, while other fat is less malleable, seeming to repel the practitioner's hand and to resist attempts to feel through it. (No prejudice implied here, but certain former rugby

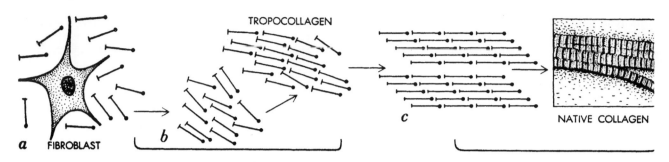

• **Fig. A1.33** The collagen molecules, manufactured in the fibroblast and secreted into the intercellular space, are polarized so that they orient themselves along the line of tension and create a strap to resist that tension. In a tendon, almost all fibers line up in rows like soldiers. (Reproduced with kind permission from Juhan 1987.[40])

players of the author's acquaintance come to mind.) The difference here is not so much in the chemistry of the fat itself, but in the proportion and density of the collagenous honeycomb of fascia that surrounds and holds the fat cells in the subcutaneous layer.

In summary, the connective tissue cells meet the combined need of flexibility and stability in animal structures by mixing a small variety of primarily collagen fibers – dense or loose, regularly or irregularly arranged – within a ground substance matrix that varies from quite fluid, to egg white, to gluey, to plastic, and finally – when the plastic is replaced by minerals – to a crystalline solid. Playing with these two variables, the cells construct the wide variety of mechanically active materials necessary to maintain our structure while having the adaptability to ever-changing movement.

On the more speculative side, the fibrillar and interfibrillar elements together have enough of a regular molecular lattice (Fig. A1.33), especially when loaded evenly, to form a 'liquid crystal'. To what frequencies is this biological 'antenna' sensitive? How can it be tuned to a wider spectrum of frequencies? Can it be made more coherent or harmonized within itself? What movement or other practice supports this coherence in which types of people? This is a challenge of spatial medicine – to find out what works for whom in terms of using movement as both medicine and food for building order in the body and resisting the forces of ageing.

Although this idea may seem farfetched, the electrical properties of fascia have been noted but little studied to date, and we are now glimpsing some of the mechanisms of such 'tuning' (pre-stress – see the section on tensegrity, below).[41–44] The surmise is that beneficial movement practice or manual therapy could increase the coherence of the fiber – GAG – water complex, and lead to better health.

Fascial Properties

A nuanced understanding of fascial properties is vital if we intend to intervene in human structure and movement – and we will explore applications in our next section. What are the properties of this fibrous gel? While our 'building materials' metaphor went some distance towards showing the variety of materials connective tissue has at its disposal, it falls short of the mark in portraying the versatility and responsiveness of the matrix, even after it has been made and extruded from the fibroblasts into the intercellular space. Not only do connective tissue cells make all these materials, these elements also rearrange and remodel themselves and their properties – within limits, of course – in response to the various demands placed on them by individual activity and injury, even after they have been deposited and incorporated into the fascial net. How could supposedly 'inert' intercellular elements change in response to demand?

To continue the metaphor for a moment, the human body is a talented 'building' that is readily movable, self-repairs if it is damaged, and actually reconstructs itself over both the short and long term to respond to different prevailing conditions. Training and rehabilitation can collaborate with these properties to enhance performance, reduce injury, and speed healing.

Genetic Differences in Fascia

We all know the immune system (which is largely connective tissue in origin) has genetic differences in blood types, allergies, and immune reactions, so it is unsurprising that our fascial net shows genetic variation. While this author knows little about genetic variations in fascia, one variable is very relevant to the manual therapist and trainer – the stiffness of the fascial net.

The tightness of the fascial net varies along a spectrum from 'Viking' (probably developed in more Arctic climates: dense and stable, creating a lot of friction and thus heat in movement, and quick to repair) vs 'Temple dancer' (probably developed in more tropical climates, highly elastic and bendy, less stable, low friction sliding, and slower to repair) (Fig. A1.34).[45,46]

The Vikings, well-suited to heavy tasks, tend to be over in the weight room clanking metal while the naturally limber Temple dancers are across the hall in the studio doing yoga – reinforcing the tendencies they already have naturally. It might be better for both groups if they switched places a couple of times per week.

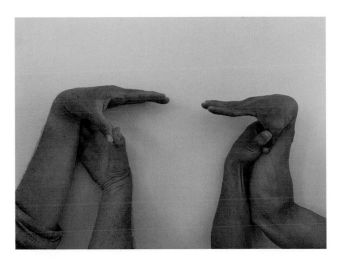

• **Fig. A1.34** 'Ligamentous laxity' as measured by Beighton's or similar tests seems to be a matter of genetic expression, and is generally a condition of the net as a whole, not just ligaments. Some tend toward a more 'Viking' style of fascia, characterized by less range of motion, stable joints, fast wound healing, and high friction (heat production) in movement (left) vs those who tend toward the 'Temple dancer' side, with a wider range of movement, less stable joints, slow injury repair, and reduced friction in movement (right). What diets, treatments, or therapy can do to change one's place on this scale is not clear. Those on either extreme approach pathological conditions.

Vikings appear to have more fibroblasts, and therefore more fascia is laid down in the body, so retaining flexibility is a challenge for the Viking. The same fibroblasts will take charge of a wound and knit it together quickly. Temple dancers, on the other hand, have fewer fibroblasts, and therefore more flexibility, less joint stability, and they take longer for wounds to heal.

To check where you are in this spectrum of tightness or laxity, perform this assessment from the Beighton score: flex your wrist to 90°, and using your other hand, bend your thumb down toward the flexor side of your forearm. The more lax you are, the closer the thumb will get to the arm. If you have 'Viking' fascia, you will not be able to get anywhere close. If you get a 'positive' on this assessment, see whether your elbow goes past 180°, another sign of 'lax ligaments' (so-called in physiotherapy, but this indicates a general laxness in the net as a whole, not just the ligaments).

These statements need two qualifiers: (1) We are all along a spectrum between the two, and (2) other factors – diet, history, training – can be at play here.

We explore the applications of this property at the end of this section.

Fluidity

Fascia is all wet. Although we speak of tissue being 'dehydrated', any cells that are truly dehydrated are busy dying. 'Hydrating your cells' is thus a relative term; cells that are truly dry necrose, while cells in an area of reduced flow simply do not function as well as they could. The only living cells on the surface of your body are your eyeballs, and you wet them regularly to keep them that way. The rest of your skin is covered by hundreds of layers of dead cells until you get to anything living. When you 'exfoliate', you scrub off a few layers of those dead cells. When you scrape your skin enough so it 'weeps', then you are down to the living cells – but not for long, for if they are left exposed to the outside world they will die and crust over. Dry cells are dead cells.

None of the collagen or elastin fibers soak up water, but they are always in a wet environment. The mucousy gel, the ground substance, however, soaks up water like a sponge. The fluid of the interstitium is rich with the flavors of hormones, neuropeptides, stress cytokines, and vesicles of bundled messenger RNA. Heavily ionic, the liquid gel presents a thicket against the expansion of bacterial growth, while allowing conduits through the gel for nutrition.

Water in general, and the two-thirds of the body that is water in particular, is still a mysterious element, as it has been since Thales and the Greeks. The peculiar spread of fern-like proteins (GAGs) through the water lends it toward what Gerald Pollack calls 'the fourth phase of water'.[47] This arrangement is ideal for building viscosity, which allows glide in low-load and slow movements, but provides stability and maximum force transmission in fast, high-load situations. Our gel-rich water is a quick-change artist.

Viscosity

The GAGs impart a viscosity to all our tissues, not just the myofascia. Water has a viscosity of its own (jump off the Golden Gate bridge to have an impactful experience with water's viscosity). The spread of glycoproteins further connects the water molecules in an array that leaves them reluctant to move. Any fast moving wave of force is dampened in this mini-but-continuous shock absorber. The GAGs' huge macromolecules are arranged like Jell-O® (UK: jelly). It only takes a small packet of Jell-O to bind a large bowl of water. In your body the GAGs bind your interstitial water into a thin but connected jelly that is viscous – and this viscosity is a vital element. We are not just bags of water, we are bags of Jell-O.

Clap your hands together, hard. Did you break any bones? Now press your hands palms together slowly but strongly, wiggle them on each other, and feel how close to the surface the edges of your phalanges are. Why are they not damaged when you clap? Or when you catch a 90-mile-an-hour burner over home plate? The gel in your tissues absorbs and distributes the force at the speed of sound through water, long before any neural response can take place.

This is the first example of biomechanical auto-regulation – how our fascial system has evolved to respond, police, and repair itself outside of the neuroregulatory apparatus.

When you land hard on your feet, the same thing happens in your sole with its columns of fat cells wrapped tightly in fascia – forces that would otherwise be concentrated toward the calcaneus are distributed more widely into the tarsum and lower leg.

The viscosity changes almost instantaneously – the very nanosecond you catch a fast ball, your synovial fluid is effectively 'solid', transferring the fast moving force from phalanges to metacarpals to carpals, but a fraction of a second later it turns back to fluid so you can manipulate the ball to throw it to first base.

We do not know how diet, practice, or genetics might affect tissue viscosity, but it is a vital and useful property of the fascial system.

Glide

High densities of hyaluronan and lower densities of collagen in the fluid allow fascial structures more glide on one another, whereas densified intermuscular or surface fascia can act as 'adhesion' to reduce glide locally.[48] Immobility is a prime cause of loss of glide, but inflammation, trauma, bad chemistry, or overloading can also reduce the available glide in the myofascial tissues.

There is an argument that what we call 'stretching' the myofascia, as is commonly taught in yoga and movement warm-ups, is actually best described as 'increasing glide' within and between the muscles. There is a more general argument that many of the manual therapy and movement techniques are simply decreasing the density and increasing the hydration of whichever local area draws the attention of the therapist or trainer. This in turn suggests the primacy of the pattern recognition in movement or the BodyReading outlined in Chapter 11 – to identify key areas which have lost the ability to glide.

Elasticity

The short statement, in the author's every lecture until well into this century, was 'muscle is elastic, fascia is plastic'.[49,50] While this is a clinically useful generalization for the manual therapist, it is definitely not true. The subject of 'stretch' is a fraught one we have attempted to deal with elsewhere and will not repeat here.[51] Elasticity, however, is definitely a property of fascia.

It is curious just how elastic fascia can be. This was clear in the variable elasticity of the ear and the skin, but this is due to the elastin fiber in those tissues. Now we know that even arrangements of pure collagen such as tendons, ligaments, and aponeuroses have elastic properties that allow for the brief storage of significant energy in short ranges of extension and a recoil where the stored energy is 'given back' in shortening. The Achilles tendon/aponeurosis, for instance, is quite compliant, and it has been shown that in human forefoot running the triceps surae (soleus and gastrocnemii) basically contract isometrically while the tendon cycles through stretching and shortening (Fig. A1.35).[52–55]

This storage and return is used in every step (see Ch. 10, James Earls' gait analysis), and certainly in every runner's stride. The recent trend for barefoot running has launched research on how tendons can be trained to reduce their

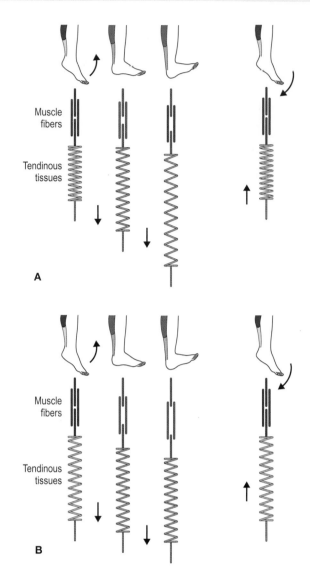

• **Fig. A1.35** It was a surprise to most when research revealed that in running, walking, and most jumps, elastic forces were being stored temporarily in the fascial parts of the myotendinous structure. The muscle operates in near isometric efficiency, tensing just enough to maintain its length. The stored energy is returned in recoil a fraction of a second later, which can be used to advantage by a runner, jumper, or dancer. (With permission from Kawakami Y, Muraoka T, Ito S, et al. *In vivo* muscle fibre behaviour during counter-movement exercise in humans reveals a significant role for tendon elasticity. J Physiol 2002;540:635–46. John Wiley and Sons.)

hysteresis, becoming less like Tempur-Pedic® mattresses and more like steel springs.[56]

The ECM has a combination of viscous and elastic properties, and the important news is that elastic properties can increase in response to specific training (Fig. A1.36).[56,58] Since elastic bounce in rhythmic motion is an observable characteristic of healthy young people and the storage and recoil of fascial elasticity is implicated in efficient running and fast exercise,[59] the suggestion is that cultivating fascial elasticity may contribute to maintaining such capacities into our older years. This is an important finding, in our

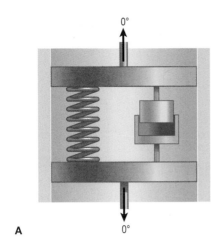

A   0°

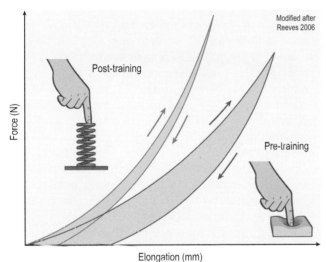

Modified after
Reeves 2006

Post-training

Pre-training

Force (N)

Elongation (mm)

- **Increased elastic storage capacity** (and decreased hysteresis) was found in tendons of an exercise group, using Technogym resistance training which implied stronger tendon loads. *(Reeves 2006)*
- **In contrast:** a controlled exercise study using slow velocity contractions and low resistance demonstrated an increase in muscular strength and volume. However, it failed to yield any change in the elastic storage capacity of the collagenous structures. *(Kubo 2003)*

B

• **Fig. A1.36** (**A**) Fascia combines both elastic (spring) and visco-elastic (damper, plastic, or shock absorber) properties. (**B**) These properties can be trained. (Illustration modified after Reeves et al., 2006.[56] Redrawn from Schleip and Müller[57] with kind permission of Dr Robert Schleip and fascialnet.com.)

sedentary era: we need to encourage the retention of tissue elasticity.

A common use of fascial elasticity is seen in the ubiquitous stretch–shortening cycle, where fascia (and muscle) is 'pre-stressed' by a preparatory counter-movement.[60] Squatting down before a jump, bringing a racquet back before a stroke, or swinging a kettlebell back before lifting it forward would all be examples of this common strategy. Use of this preparatory counter movement makes the subsequent effort smoother and less prone to injury.

A barefoot runner taking maximum advantage of elastic recoil will hold the tibialis posterior, for a prime example, in isometric contraction. During weight acceptance, the musculo-tendinous unit is stretched, but the muscle does not lengthen appreciably, maintaining an efficient limit on the eccentric strain in the muscle. This transfers the deformation to the tendon, which lengthens, and then recoils back, propelling the runner forward at less cost than actually lengthening and concentrically shortening the muscle. Elasticity is efficient, especially in any endurance effort.[61]

Sometimes – a basketball player landing after a jump and wanting to pivot – the need is not to harvest the elastic recoil but to dampen it. By coordinating the muscle to relax and lengthen at that moment, the elastic energy is absorbed back from the tendon without movement. The elasticity of the hip ligaments and spinal ligaments, especially the large nuchal ligament between the sides of the neck, join the ligaments of the feet in being prime areas where the elastic property is of value.

Force Transmission

In spite of its gel like nature, its viscous tendency to deform under slow pressure, and elastically bounce with rapid short pressure, the collagenous net is a highly efficient transmitter of tensional force.[38,62–66] Exerting little force until the fiber net lengthens out to the 'lock' position, any fascia is capable of handling considerable force, as you felt in our finger-on-the-forearm experiment above.[67]

Force transmission and distribution is the principal job of the myofascia and the surrounding fascia profundis holding it in. Anatomy Trains charts common lines of force transmission along the fabric of the body (Fig. A1.37).

Plasticity

Combine the viscosity with the elasticity, and we get fascial plasticity, another unique characteristic of the mammalian fascial system. This characteristic is employed by the yogis, the heirs of Ida Rolf, and increasingly in the athletic arena to create sustained change in the avenues of myofascial force transmission.

Stretched, a muscle's myotatic reflex will attempt to contract it back to its resting length before giving up, eventually adding more cells and sarcomeres to bridge the gap.[68] Stretch fascia quickly and it will tear (the most frequent form of connective tissue injury; Video 4.2). If the stretch is applied slowly enough, and the fascia addressed is thin and healthy enough to be compliant, it will deform plastically: it will change its length and retain that change. Slowly stretch a common plastic carrier bag to see this kind of plasticity modeled: the bag will stretch, and when you let go, the stretched area will remain, and will not recoil like a spring or a TheraBand®.

The mechanism of fascial plastic deformation (viscoelasticity as opposed to elasticity) is incompletely understood, but once it is truly deformed, fascia does not 'snap back'.

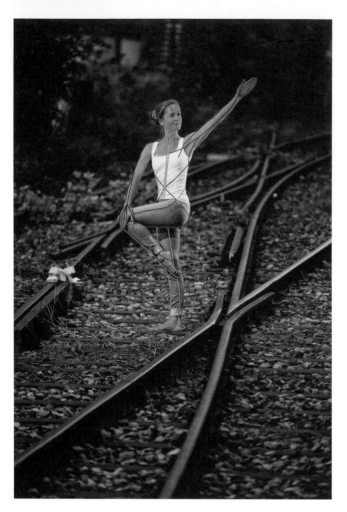

• **Fig. A1.37** Anatomy Trains is a chart of common pathways of myofascial force transmission in humans. A fundamental tenet – only partially proven as of this writing – of this book is that myofascial force transmission occurs beyond muscle attachments.

The mindset – and therefore the pattern of muscle tension – definitely can snap back into place. Fascia, once stretched plastically, will not. We return to this below in the section on fascial responses to intervention.

Fibroblasts can build new fascia, though, to replace the old. If you bring the two surfaces into apposition again and keep them there – as in going back into a familiar slump – your fascial system will lay down new fibers that will rebind the area.[69] But this will take some time (on the order of a couple of months), and is not the same as elastic recoil in the tissue itself. A full understanding of this concept is fundamental to the successful application of sequential fascial manipulation. Practicing therapists, in our experience, make frequent statements that betray an underlying belief that the fascia is either elastic or voluntarily contractile, even though they 'know' it is not. The plasticity of fascia is its essential nature – its gift to the body and the key to unraveling its long-term patterns. We will return to fascial contractility and elasticity at the cellular level in the section on tensegrity, below.

Remodeling – Systemic Plasticity

Cells – the fibroblasts and their cousins – are constantly remodeling your ECM. How does fascia 'know' how to remodel? The fibroblast secretes the matrix into the intercellular space, but does not order it into the various available matrix states – tendon, areolar, cartilage, etc. Stress passing through a material deforms the material, even if only slightly, thereby 'stretching' the bonds between the molecules. In biological materials, this creates a slight electric flow through the material known as a piezo- (pressure) electric charge (Fig. A1.38A,B).[71] This charge, representative of strain through the tissue, can be 'read' by the cells in the vicinity of the charge, and the fibroblasts are capable of responding by augmenting, reducing, or changing the intercellular elements in the area.

The collagen molecules themselves are polarized, with a positive and negative end, so that, once extruded from the cell, they will orient, like a compass needle, along the lines of stress. Do this a million times over and a strap is created in response to the stress, as in Fig. A1.39.

As an example, the head of most everyone's femur is made of cancellous, spongy bone. An analysis of the trabeculae within the bone shows that they are brilliantly constructed, to an engineer's eye, to resist the forces being transmitted from the pelvis to the shaft of the femur. Such an arrangement provides us with the lightest bones possible within the parameters of safety, and could easily be explained by the action of natural selection.

But the situation is more complex than that; the internal bone is shaped to reflect not only species' needs but also individual form and activity. If we were to section the femur from someone with one posture and someone else with a quite different posture and usage, we would see that each femoral head has slightly different trabeculae, precisely designed to best resist the forces which that particular person characteristically creates (Fig. A1.38C). In this way, the connective tissue responds to demand.

Whatever demand you put on the body – continuous exertion or dedicated couch potato, running 50 miles a week or squatting 50 hours a week in the rice paddies – the extracellular elements are altered along the path of the stress to meet the demand within the limits imposed by nutrition, age, and protein synthesis (genetics).

In bone the currents of stress perform this seeming miracle of preferential remodeling within the intercellular elements via a sparse but active community of two types of osteocytes: the osteoblasts and the osteoclasts. Each are sent forth with simple commandments: osteoblasts lay down new bone; osteoclasts clean up old bone. Osteoblasts are allowed to lay down new bone anywhere they like – as long as it is within the periosteum. The osteoclasts may eat of any bone, except those parts that are piezo-electrically charged (mechanically stressed).[72] Allow the cells to operate freely under these rules over time, and a femoral head is produced that is both specifically designed to resist individual forces coming through it, but also capable of

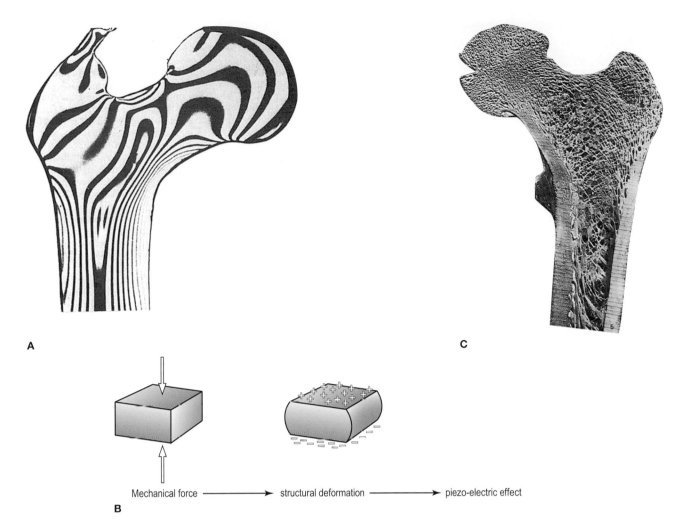

A

B

C

Mechanical force ⟶ structural deformation ⟶ piezo-electric effect

• **Fig. A1.38** 'Virtually all the tissues of the body generate electrical fields when they are compressed or stretched [which are] representative of the forces acting on the tissues involved … containing information on the precise nature of the movements taking place … One of the roles of this information is in the control of form' (Oschman 2000,[41] p. 52). **(A)** Stress lines in a loaded plastic model of the femur. **(B)** Any mechanical force which creates structural deformation creates such a piezo-electric effect, which then distributes itself around the connective tissue system. **(C)** The trabeculae of bone which form in response to individualized stresses. (A, From von Knieff 1977.[70] Reproduced with kind permission from Williams 1995. B, Reproduced with kind permission from Oschman 2000.[41] C, Reproduced with kind permission from Williams 1995.)

changing (given some reaction time) to meet new forces when they are consistently applied.

This mechanism explains how dancers' feet get tougher bones during a summer dance camp: the increased dancing creates increased forces which create increased stresses which reduce the ability of the osteoclasts to remove bone while the osteoblasts carry on laying it down – and the result is denser bone. This is also part of the explanation for why exercise is helpful to those with incipient osteoporosis: the forces created by the increased stress on the tissues serve to discourage the osteoclastic uptake. The reverse process operates in the astronauts and cosmonauts deprived of the force of gravity to create the pressure charge through the bones: the osteoclasts have a field day and the returning heroes must be helped off their ship in wheelchairs until their bones, back in gravity, become less porous.

This extraordinary ability to respond to demand accounts for the wide variety in joint shapes across the human spectrum, despite the consistent pictures averaged into most anatomy textbooks. A recent study detailed distinct differences in the structure of the subtalar joint.[73] Smaller differences can be observed over the entire body. In Figure A1.40A we see a 'normal' thoracic vertebra. However, in Figure A1.40B, we can see the body distorted as pressure creates a demand for remodeling under Wolff's law,[74] and hypertrophic spurs forming as the periosteum is pulled away by excess strains from the surrounding connective tissues and muscles (see also Ch. 3 on heel spurs). A non-union fracture can often be reversed by creating a current

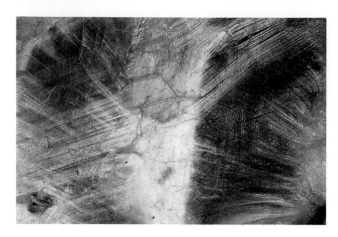

• **Fig. A1.39** A dissection of the superficial pectoral fascia in the sternal area. Notice how one leg of the evident 'X' across the sternum, from upper right to lower left in the picture, is more prevalent than the other, almost certainly as a result of use patterns. (Reproduced with kind permission from Ronald Thompson.)

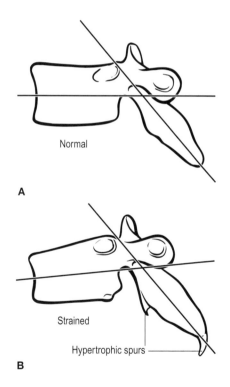

Normal

A

Strained

Hypertrophic spurs

B

• **Fig. A1.40** (**A,B**) Even bones will alter their shape within certain limits, adding and subtracting bone mass, in response to the mechanical forces around them. (Reproduced with kind permission from Oschman 2000.[41])

flow across the break, reproducing the normal piezo-electric flow, through which the collagen orients itself and begins the process of bridging the gap, to be followed by the calcium salts and full healing.[15,75]

This same process of response occurs across the entire extracellular fibrous network, not just inside the bones. We can imagine a person who develops for whatever reason (e.g. shortsightedness, depression, imitation, or injury) a common 'slump': the head goes forward, the chest falls,

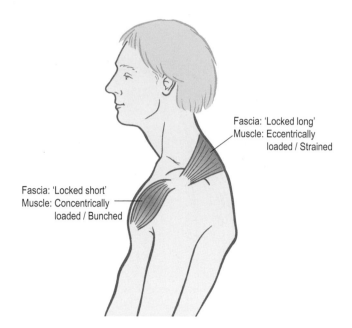

Fascia: 'Locked long'
Muscle: Eccentrically loaded / Strained

Fascia: 'Locked short'
Muscle: Concentrically loaded / Bunched

• **Fig. A1.41** When body segments are pulled out of place and muscles are required to maintain static positions – either stretched/contracted ('locked long') or shortened/contracted ('locked short') – then we see increased fascial bonding in the surrounding intercellular matrix (ECM), as well as an increase in trigger points and 'knots'.

the back rounds (Fig. A1.41). The head, a minimum of one-seventh of the body weight in most adults, must be restrained from falling further forward by some muscles in the back. These muscles must remain in isometric contraction (eccentric loading) for every one of this person's waking hours.

Muscles are designed to contract and relax in succession, but these particular muscles are now under a constant eccentric strain, robbing them of their full ability, and facilitating the development of trigger points. The strain transmits through the fascia within and around the muscle (and often beyond in both directions along the myofascial meridians). Essentially, these muscles or parts of muscles are being asked to act like straps (see Fig. A1.8).

More serious deformations of the fascial net may require more time, remedial exercise, peri-articular manipulation (such as is found in osteopathy and chiropractic), outside support such as orthotics or braces, or even surgical intervention, but the process described above is continual and ubiquitous. Much restoration of postural balance, whether via the Anatomy Trains scheme or any other model, is attainable using non-invasive techniques.

Fascial Responses to Intervention

Can we translate the findings on the properties into practical steps for the working professional? There are pointers, certainly, but few certainties yet. We divide the following into a section for movement practitioners and another for manual therapists, though they cross-pollinate.

Training Fascia

It is important to emphasize from the outset that training fascia is not new, for all the recent attention paid to fascia in training circles.[76] Our connective tissue web has always been with us; we cannot avoid training it, stretching it, and allowing (or hindering) its job of repairing itself. Fascia provides a substrate for the muscle tissue to work on the skeletal and articular framework. Of course trainers and physiotherapists have considered it all along – as individual tendons, ligaments, and attachments considered as separate parts. The fascia as an interactive system – the thesis of this book – is now being given more consideration by the athletic and performance fields.

All methods – dance, martial arts, yoga, Alexander Technique, strength conditioning, or any of their modern offshoots – train our fascia one way or another. (In fact, the ubiquitous sitting we do in the Western world is also a form of 'fascial training' or 'stretching' that can occupy many hours of an office-worker's week, with some deleterious effects – see the section on Sitting in Chapter 10.) The emerging picture from the research suggests that we can do a better job if we are conscious of fascial properties and responses in addition to nutritional support, neurological coordination, and muscle strength and balance.

The other side of this coin is that 'fascia' is not a miracle or the answer to all training problems; it is a down-to-earth event, a versatile and variable tissue that handles a variety of movement demands within the generous but not unlimited capabilities of a biological fabric.

As always with a newly minted concept, the less informed enthusiast may make exaggerated claims. Nevertheless, the developing research picture, referenced for the rest of this section, suggests a fairly radical re-thinking of our basic concepts of anatomy is in the offing, worthy of the overused 'paradigm shift'. Fascial study is ushering Einstein's relativity – only a century late – into the world of movement training and rehabilitative medicine. Especially exciting is the established link between movement training, brain science, and epigenetics, a field which promises to yield objective data as to which program of movement would most suit any given person.

Here our focus is once again on the function of healthy fascia. Fascial dysfunction, pathology, and the intricacies of body pain are beyond the scope of this volume. The following is only a partial and truncated set of bullet points; a more complete picture of the relevant research can be gathered elsewhere.[57,76–81]

Healthy Loading Positively Remodels Fascial Architecture

Perhaps the most significant finding for trainers is that regular loading (read: exercise) within the healthy limits of the tissue induces a regular spiral double lattice pattern through the myofascia, while a lack of regular loading produces a felt-like irregular architecture (Fig. A1.42).[82–84] This

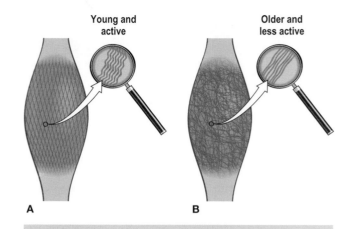

Young and active   **Older and less active**

- Staubesand 1996 found a 2-directional **lattice** orientation in fasciae of young women compared with older women
- Jarvinen 2002: **immobilization** induces multidirectional collagen arrangement and crimp-reduction
- Wood 1998 reported an increased collagen **crimp** formation in daily running rats

• **Fig. A1.42** Healthy loading induces a regular spiral lattice in the myofascia (**A**). A sedentary life leaves the fascia without directing forces, and it orients randomly, like felt (**B**). (Redrawn from Schleip and Müller[57]; reproduced courtesy of Robert Schleip and fascialnet.com.)

lattice pattern is the most efficient for myofascial force transmission, as well as for fluid perfusion.

Lack of fascial loading also reduces the molecular 'crimp' in the fascia over time, which not only provides a healthy first 'bounce' of elasticity to the tissue, but also is the method by which the Golgi tendon organs (GTOs) read the load on the tissue.[84,85] Reduce the crimp through inactivity and the perception of load will be less accurate (Fig. A1.43).[86] Thus the sedentary person leaving the couch or the hospital bed to return to exercise faces two fascial challenges in addition to his muscle weakness: remodeling the spiral double lattice and building the crimp (and thus the sensitivity) back in.

Both of these require longer time scales than building muscle, as collagen turnover in the less-vascular fascia is far slower than protein turnover in the well-irrigated muscle, so that early in any new training program is a more likely time for injury, when the muscles are outdistancing their supporting fascia.[87] After some months the fascia has 'caught up', and the probability of injury lowers.

Part of the training process is a forced remodeling of the fascia as the muscle cells grow in volume or number, bursting their limits. This so-called 'tear and repair' is a normal process that does involve soreness from the released Substance P, but this remodeling of small tears is accomplished within a day or days, depending on their physiology – their sleep, diet, and the rest.

Take Advantage of Elasticity

Elasticity, as we saw above, can be trained. Water is squeezed slowly out of tendons as they build the elastic infrastructure. Whether you are using running, skipping rope, or swinging

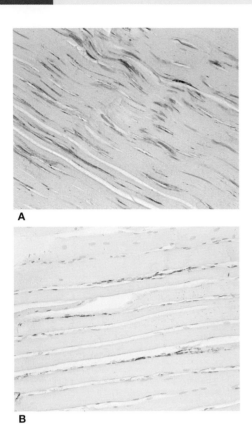

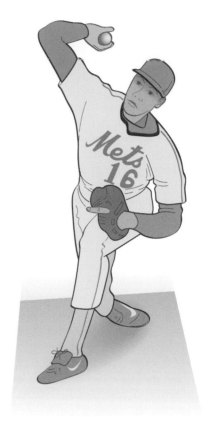

• **Fig. A1.43** Healthy crimp (A) provides a first response of elasticity, and also is the means whereby the Golgi tendon organs can assess load. Reduced crimp (B) means less bounce and less load sensitivity. (Reproduced with kind permission of Dr Robert Schleip and fascialnet. com.)

• **Fig. A1.44** Training long myofascial chains makes maximum use of long lever arms, coordination, fascial elasticity, and the whip-like motion of proximal initiation with distal delay.

weights – always a yield–bounce–recoil stimulus – you are building youth into your body as you keep yourself elastic.

To take advantage of the elastic recoil, there is only a one-second window (actually 0.8–1.2 seconds[88]) between the weight acceptance and the recoil. You do not build elasticity into the body at yoga or Tai Chi speeds. (These arts have many benefits, but fascial elasticity is not one of them.) Even bicycling is too slow to build much elasticity. Look at a bicyclist's calves – that is muscle power, and the fascia around those gastrocnemii is strong, but not necessarily elastic.

To feel the power of elasticity, first put your hand on your thigh, lift your index finger and, using your muscles, slam it into your leg. Use all the muscle power you have. To check out the power of elasticity, lift up that index finger to its full hyperextension with your other hand, then let it go to feel the elastic power in the tendon. Coordinate them both together for the greatest power.

Take Advantage of Plasticity

Making the fascia 'longer' (increasing glide and thus effective range-of-motion) depends on moving slowly or 'hanging out' at or near the end range, where the fascia in the target area 'locks out', keeping the stretch going long enough for the stretch reflex to fade and the muscles relax. Only then

does increased plastic glide in the fascia begin, so stay in the stretch for at least 30–90 seconds **after** the muscles relax.[89]

If elasticity does not happen at yoga and Tai Chi speeds, plasticity does not happen at athletic speeds. For fibers and ground substance to interact in a lengthening way, sustained tension at the stretching edge, not fleeting tension in mid-range, is called for to regain the ability to shear between the fascial planes.

Train the Fascial System More Globally by Using Variable Vectors Over Long Kinetic Chains

Training isolated to individual muscle groups with linear motion may sculpt that muscle well, but may not extend to neighboring fascial tissues necessary to the body's health in functional movement.[90] For instance, training the quadriceps in a seated position by weighting the ankle and extending the knee – as is common in many gyms – may strengthen the quads, but will not build the necessary concomitant strength in the contralateral SI joint ligaments and piriformis (for force closure), leading to the likelihood of pelvic dysfunction and pain.[1]

Training the myofascial meridians as open or closed kinetic chains builds the fascial strength between and around the muscles, and allows for the greater coordination of proximal initiation and distal delay (Fig. A1.44; Video 1.2).[90]

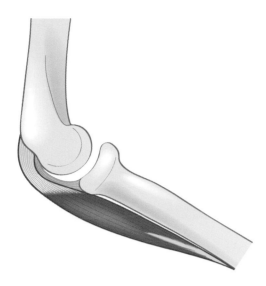

• **Fig. A1.45** Most ligaments run in series with nearby muscles and are not the parallel system depicted in most texts. (After van der Waal 2009.)

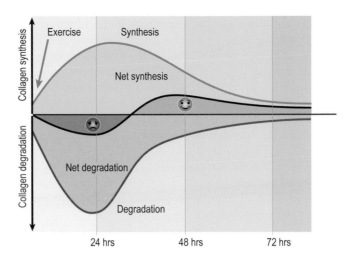

• **Fig. A1.46** Heavy workouts perturb the fibroblasts, which in turn both dissolve old collagen and create new fibers. This process results in a net degradation after 24 hours, but a net synthesis after 72 hours. (Illustration modified after Magnusson et al., 2010.[93] Redrawn from Schleip and Müller[57] with kind permission of Dr Robert Schleip and fascialnet.com.)

Varying the load, the rhythm, and the vectors of pull or stretch while training – as in club or rope work, kettlebells or parkour; machines and weights in gravity tend to be more linear – insures an even development of the supporting fascia in and around the muscles. Conversely, logic suggests that repeating the same exercises, katas, or yoga asanas in the same way day after day will train only the certain pathways of fascia that are loaded, leaving nearby fascia unloaded and untrained and unbalanced – and thus subject to injury when life comes at you from a different angle. Not that repetition is bad in itself – routines are invaluable in absorbing a complex dance or martial art, but exclusively repeated routines without variation has questionable value as preparation for real life.

Ligaments Dynamically Stabilize Joints at All Angles

We have assumed that ligaments are passive structures until we reach the end-range of motion, at which point they come into play to save the joints.[91] Van der Waal's careful dissections show that ligaments are not the parallel system we thought them to be: most ligaments are in dynamic series with the surrounding muscles.[6] Our common dissection method only made them appear separate by sliding the scalpel between muscle and ligament to break their natural connection (Fig. A1.45).

The implications for joint strengthening of this simple but radical finding are vast and will take time to assess and apply. Just the realization that ligaments are being trained at every angle of movement is revelatory. Again, multivector exercise and sufficient time investment to build or lengthen ligaments recommends itself.

Fascial Training Takes Gentle Perseverance

Most common body injuries involve fascia.[92] Gentle perseverance works on three time scales. Firstly, muscles develop

faster than fascia, due to slow collagen turnover, so a program to build fascial resilience should be undertaken with a long-term view, such as that promoted by yoga and the martial arts. Since the half-life of collagen is about one year, a period of 6–24 months (depending on age, exercise, and nutrition) is required to make a thorough change in the fascial system.[87] The 'gotta get back in shape fast for summer' attitude of pushing the muscles to 'pop' in a few-weeks is a recipe for myotendinous junction injury (based on over 40 years of anecdotal experience).

Secondly, research confirms the fascia in your body likes the idea of staggering heavy workouts as it needs recovery time. After a heavy stimulus (stretching or muscle work) fibroblasts are stimulated to produce more fascia (in Vikings especially) and the fascia busting enzymes like the collagenases and other proteinases begin breaking down older, frayed fascia.[93] By 24 hours after the workout, there is a net loss of collagen, implying that the system might be a bit weaker, and thus not ready for another heavy stimulus, but by 48 hours there is a net gain, and by 72 hours the system has settled for most of us and is ready for another strong stimulus (Fig. A1.46).

Thirdly, most injuries occur when local fascia tissue is loaded and then required to move too quickly. A rough parallel lies in the common plastic carrier bag: stretch it slowly and it will plastically deform for quite a distance; stretch it quickly and it will tear. In our experience, a movement or exercise that can be performed slowly is ready to be done quickly in a safer manner than starting out trying to learn it quickly first – a strategy that can lead to local tissue failure and the necessity for long-term recovery.

All Clients Are Different

We detailed the differences between a 'Viking' and a 'Temple dancer' – they will not respond in the same way to training.

As this and other genetic differences in fascia are understood, training programs will need to accommodate these differences, instead of 'one-size fits all'. Those with ligamentous laxity may gravitate toward stretching classes, given their natural affinity for it, but they are better advised to go against their tendency to build a more resilient balance. Vikings should balance out their heavy tasks with sustained stretches and non-directed undulating movement to stay limber.

Getting it right for each client is a lifetime's work in the art of training. A good trainer or movement teacher can work with all types of people, not just the folks with a similar body type to them.

Manual Therapy and Fascia

No manual therapy can target only fascia. Every hands-on intervention, like every training session, will involve all four types of tissue. That said, targeting short or adhered fascia requires patience. Neuromuscular responses are quick; fascial responses are slow. How slow? You can see the speed we recommend in the accompanying videos, but the watchword is to listen to the tissue, as everyone is different.

We often engage, for example, with the fascia over the sternum, pictured in Figure A1.39, a spot where the fascia is frequently tied down to the sternal periosteum and sternochondral joint tissues. What will determine our speed? First, we go deep enough to engage the fascial layers between the back of the skin and the front of the bone. As you lift the tissue cephalad (toward the head), you can feel a wave, not right under your fingers but about a centimeter in front of them. Pay attention to that wave and adjust your speed so you neither fall behind it nor get in front of it. That wave is the tissue opening and hydrating in front of your applicator – fingers, knuckles, elbow, whatever you are using (see video Opening the Breath, 1:17:05–1:20:42, available from www.anatomytrains.com).

Then comes the question: where to work? First, stop chasing pain. In the slump pictured in Figure A1.41 (reminiscent of Vladimir Janda's upper crossed syndrome[94]), the muscles in the back of the neck and top of the shoulders will have become tense, fibrotic, and strained, and will require some work. But the concentric pull in the front, be it from the chest, belly, hips, or elsewhere, will need lengthening first, and the structures beneath it rearranged to support the body in its 'new' (or more often 'original', natural) position.

In other words, manual therapists must look globally, act locally, and then act globally to integrate our local remedies into the person's entire structure. In strategizing our therapy in this global–local–global way, we are acting exactly as the ECM itself does (Video 6.23), as we explore below in the section on tensegrity. Connective tissue cells produce ECM in response to local conditions, which in turn affect global conditions that re-impinge on local conditions in an unending recursive process.[10] Understanding of the myofascial meridians assists in organizing the search for both the silent culprit and the necessary global decompensations – reversing the downward spiral of increasing immobility.

Back to our slump: eventually, fibroblasts in the area (and additional mesenchymal stem cells or fibroblasts that may migrate there) secrete more collagen in and around the muscle to create a better strap. The long collagen molecules, secreted into the intercellular space by the fibroblasts, are polarized and orient themselves like compass needles along the line of mechanical tension (see Fig. A1.33). They bind to each other with numerous hydrogen bonds via the interfibrillar glue (proteoglycans or ground substance proteins like decorin), forming a strap-like matrix of fibrils around the muscle.

Figure A1.39 illustrates this phenomenon very well. It shows a dissection of some of the fascial fibers running over the sternum between the two pectoral muscles. If we compare the fibers running from upper right to lower left, we can see that they are denser and stronger than those running from the upper left to the lower right. This means that more strain was habitually present in that one direction, perhaps from being left-handed, or (entirely speculatively) from being a big city bus driver who used his left hand predominantly to swing his horizontal steering wheel. This strain caused lines of piezo-electricity, and the fibroblasts responded by laying down new collagen, which oriented along the lines of strain to create more resistance.

Meanwhile, the muscle, overworked and undernourished, may show up with reduced function, trigger-point pain, and weakness, along with decreased hydration in the surrounding ground substance, and increased metabolite toxicity. Fortunately – and this is the tune sung by Structural Integration, yoga, and other myofascial therapies – this process works pretty well in reverse: strain can be reduced through manipulation or training, the fascia enzymatically reabsorbed, and the muscle restored to full function. Two elements, however, are necessary for successful resolution of these situations, whether achieved through movement or manipulation:

1. a reopening of the tissue in question, to help restore fluid flow, muscle function, and connection with the sensory–motor system, *and*
2. an easing of the biomechanical pull that caused the increased stress on that tissue in the first place.

Either of these alone produces temporary or unsatisfactory results. The second point urges us to look beyond 'chasing the pain' and calls to mind the prominent physiotherapist Diane Lee's admonition: 'It is the victims who cry out, not the criminals.' Taking care of the victims and collaring the local thugs is addressed by point 1; going after the 'big shots' is the job of point 2.

The 'big shots' in human structure are rarely felt by the client as painful. The secondary areas can be painful to the client, or sore to the touch or when stretched. The important primary areas are usually 'numb' for the client, and it is the job of the manual therapist to be able to spot the cause, rather than getting caught messing around with the effects. To build this insight, develop the BodyReading skills outlined in Chapter 11 (and see BodyReading webinar at www.anatomytrains.com/product/bodyreading-visual-assessment-of-the-anatomy-trains-webinar-series/)

Manual therapy has very limited tools for building elasticity into fascial tissue – that is a matter for rhythmic loaded exercise. On the other hand, manual therapy is well-placed to create plastic change by working slowly and specifically on short and densified tissues to restore the ability to glide.

The client can also do self-help with their myofascia by undertaking any of the Self-Myofascial Release (SMR) systems out there, with balls, sticks, or other tools that get more sophisticated by the year.[95–98] They vibrate, they have knobs or other unique selling points – but the essence of these practices is awareness, the mindful part. Just rolling yourself up and down on a tool is not necessarily beneficial in and of itself, and less likely if your mind and attention are elsewhere. How much progress is being made by the jogger on the treadmill who is lost to her earbuds?

A preventive program of structural awareness (call it 'kinesthetic literacy') could also be productively incorporated into public education.[99 102]

The entry of the word 'awareness' draws us to the relationship between the nervous system and the fascial system.

Fascial Kinesthesia

Kinesthesia – our sense of body in space and in motion – is unique among the senses in that it is hard to imagine a life without it. We can imagine being blind or deaf, or living without taste or smell, but our 'sense of self' is so tied up with what we feel in our bodies, could we live without it?[103–105]

Often called the sixth sense, but really integrating several 'senses', our appreciation of our inner selves has evolved from a very simple sense of stretch in the tissues to the complex and sophisticated coordination required to play the flute, take out the appendix, climb a rock face, or deal with a rebellious teenager. But we can isolate kinesthesia easily: close your eyes and touch the ring finger of your non-dominant hand to your nose. Only your kinesthetic sense can help you do this.

The summary version of the neuromyofascial story to keep in mind is this: the brain listens to the fascia and talks to the muscles. Mechano-sensitive nerve endings abound in the fascia and the interstitial space. But no motor nerves have been discovered going to fascia, and the one instance of active contraction in fascia, caused by the myofibroblasts (see fascial components above), is not modulated by nerves.

Fascia happens to be the most wired organs in the body, with more sensory nerves in it than you have even in your eye or your tongue.[106] But we only get information from each ending if it moves. If it is held 'still' in the tissue and not stimulated, it eventually 'falls out' of the body image.

Part of the goal of manual therapy or movement training is to create as complete as possible a body image in the client, with no gaps or lacunae of 'forgotten' areas of the body. 'Self-remembering' is an important – nay, vital – part of any restorative therapeutic process.

We will divide the kinesthesia of the fascial system into proprioception, interoception, and nociception. The first is more objective – 'Where am I in space?' The second is more subjective: 'How do I feel about what I'm sensing?' The third is pain perception. All are important, and all rely heavily on the fascial system reporting in.

Proprioception in Fascia

Your sense of yourself in space is assembled from a variety of sources – the inner ear, the eyes if they are open, the temporomandibular joint, the hip joint, and the skin sensors on the bottom of the feet figure largely in our inner orientation – but so do the nerve endings deployed throughout the myofascial and fascial tissues.

These nerve endings need to learn to work, it does not come automatically. A lot of this comes in our first year on the planet, when, after a few fally-down months, we get pretty good at matching our inner sense of our body with the world outside.

(Although you only have to step into a room whose floor is 2 inches/5 cm lower than you thought it was going to be to understand how precisely your system 'guesses'/calculates what it is about to encounter, how it can be fooled, and how much of a shock goes through the system when it prepares for the wrong set of forces.)

Proprioception is the word given specifically to our sense of position in space and how it is moving. We often talk about 'feeling the stretch in our muscles', but we have perhaps six times the number of receptors in the fascia around any given muscle than we do in the muscle itself.[107] Muscle tissue in general is comparatively numb compared to the fascia around it. (The neurally rich muscles such as the suboccipitals, eye muscles, tongue, and plantaris are exceptions.)

The brain is clearly vitally interested in what's going on interstitially in the fascia. Along with the vestibular system and the many skin sensors, we absolutely need all the fascial sensors to know what is going on with our body in space.[108] The suggestion here is that bulldozing through our sense data ('no pain, no gain') paves the way toward short-term or long-term fascial injury, and that cultivation of a refined sense of proprioception, interoception, and kinesthesia will serve us well in refining our skills and extending them into older age.

So the first surprise is that muscle provides less feeling, and the surrounding collagenous tissues provide more feeling, more information. In terms of response, the fascia is limited to the slow physiology we detailed above in the section on fascial plasticity while the neuromuscular system can respond in a fraction of a second to adjust the tension in the myofascial web.

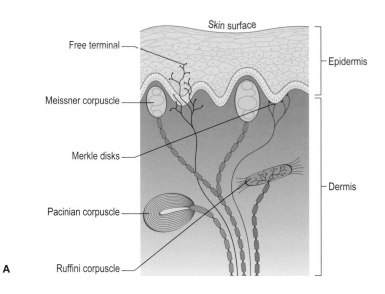

A

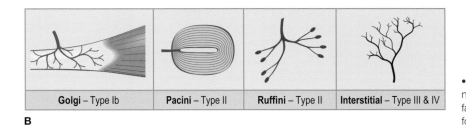

| Golgi – Type Ib | Pacini – Type II | Ruffini – Type II | Interstitial – Type III & IV |

B

• **Fig. A1.47** The nervous system has a large number of generalized receptors in the interstitial fascia, and has also developed specialized endings for stretch, load, pressure, and shear.

Proprioception makes use of five basic receptor endings in the myofascial body, each with sub-types that we will not detail: muscle spindles, Golgi tendon organs (GTOs), Paciniform corpuscles, Ruffini endings, and free nerve terminals (Fig. A1.47).

Without rehearsing all the well-known data about these endings, we note muscle spindles are the only type of receptor inside a muscle – the rest are in the interstitium or in the fascia itself. The spindle is a tiny fascial capsule surrounding a few elastin fibers, with the annulospiral ending wrapping around them. As the muscle is stretched or contracted, the ending reports the change in length, which also gives the brain a readout over time of the rate of change of length. We can note that even the muscle spindles inside the muscles are reading the change in length of the connective tissue to infer the change of length in the muscle, but even so let us give these sensors to the muscle.

These spindles offer us the chance to 'fool' the spinal cord into thinking the muscle has been stretched by tweaking the spindle at its ends – the so-called Gamma motor system. The spindle, thinking the muscle is elongating, sends a message to the spinal cord and that portion of the muscle governed by that spindle is contracted through reflex. This allows for much smoother movement, but only in the movements where we 'know' what is going to happen and can thus prepare. The Gamma system does not help us in new movements – compare the concentration of the toddler

learning to tie his shoes to the reflexive movements of the regular runner (see Fig. A1.18).

Muscle spindles thus offer us a reading of the length of the muscle, and give us the opportunity to pre-program known movements, but they tell us nothing about load. This is the job of the GTO, a fundamental stretch receptor that is located all over the fascial system. Its mechanism is simple: a sensory ending winds itself among the fibers of a tendon (or other fascia). Those fibers are crimped and wavy, and get straighter as the fascia takes on more load. The nerve ending simply measures the degree that the crimp has straightened to get a readout on the amount of load on that tissue (see Fig. A1.43).

If the crimp is no longer present, due to age or inactivity, then the GTOs cannot read the load properly, and thus the perception of the old or out-of-shape client may not be as refined as it could be.

To visualize all this: if you close your eyes and hold your hand out with the elbow bent, and someone drops a book onto your hand, your hand will go down and then come right back up again as the spindle senses the sudden shift in length, and alerts the spinal cord to correct the muscle back to its previous resting length. As far as the spindle is concerned, what is the difference between the initial reading and the resultant reading? None, it is the same as before, because the muscle is the same length as before. But you will have the distinct sense that things are different, you can feel the weight of the book, even though the spindle says we are back to normal.

The weight of the book – the load – is measured by the straightening of the crimp in the tendon, and the crimp is still slightly straightened at the end, so we feel it and register it as weight on the hand. Keep adding books, and eventually the GTO reflex will encourage the muscle to relax and let go to avoid damaging the tendon. But these two simple machines – one for length and one for load – do the majority of the work of telling us what is happening in our body.

One more fact about the spindles and GTOs is important to our thesis here. Years ago, we thought the spindles and GTOs were distributed randomly through the muscle and tendon. Now we know that the muscle is bundled into sections (called fascicles) by the fascia, and that these persevere into the tendons as identifiable bundles within the tendon. Further, we know that the muscle spindle and GTO associated with a particular fascicle bundle are linked at the spinal cord (see Fig. A1.18).

This is a very important concept to understand, as it underlines that the brain does not think in terms of whole muscles. We conceive the body that way because of our method of dissection, but the nervous system does not organize movement in terms of named muscles, rather in terms of these distinct neuromotor units within the muscle, each with their own supply of linked spindles and GTOs.

Outside the muscle tissue proper are other well-distributed and clever specialized sensory endings in the fascial net, including:

- GTOs outside the tendon measuring load in the surrounding tissues
- Paciniform corpuscles for measuring pressure
- Ruffini endings for measuring shear between adjacent fascial planes
- The most prolific ending of them all, the free nerve terminals which report a little bit of everything, and also connect to the nociceptic (pain) tracts (Fig. A1.47).[109]

We will return to nociception in fascia, but first we need to understand the new information about interoception.

Interoception

To pay attention. This is our endless and proper work.
MARY OLIVER

Whatever is happening to the tissue under our hands, we are also communicating with the client's nervous system. The nervous system is the 'meaning maker', and our construction of meaning has a number of layers to it. Interoception is part of that process of gleaning the relevant data out of the myriad and endless signals we are getting from our body. Therapists deal in perception and therefore must study how the brain perceives the body and the body–mind interface. There is plenty that science has yet to learn about how we sense the body in motion, and how our clients 'make sense' of our work in themselves.

In studying how the brain monitors the body in kinesthesia, scientists have distinguished proprioception and interoception. Traditionally, proprioception has been applied, as we did, to our sense of position in space, including all the receptors we listed in the parietal myofasciae. Interoception was originally assigned to the signals coming from our organs. Interoceptors are also, like proprioceptors, mostly modifications of stretch receptors, but also include thermoceptors and other regulatory parameters. Perception of stretch in the bladder or rectum tells us we need to find a bathroom. Lack of stretch in our stomach tells us it's time to find lunch. Stretch receptors in our lungs modulate breathing, and similar receptors in our arteries help regulate blood pressure.

In other words, interoception can be described as *a sense of the physiological position of the body* (as opposed to the literal positional sense of the proprioceptors), and thus a connection to '*how* we feel about *what* we feel'.[110] We represent our body from within with interoception. By contrast, we represent how our body is relating to the outside world – what we are touching, what is its weight, and what we are moving through – through the skin sense (somesthetic) and proprioception.

This affords a neat distinction, but like many of our presumptions about the machinery of our body – never as simple as we would like it to be – not true. We have recently discovered that interoception extends into our musculoskeletal body as well as our organs. 'How you feel about what you feel' is present in our movement self as well as our physiological self (Box A1.1).

• BOX A1.1   Tools to Appreciate Your Own 'Felt Sense'

Slower Movements: In bodywork, speed is the enemy of sensitivity – the slower you go, the more you feel. When we do slow movement practices like yoga or Tai Chi, when we allow the mind to move beyond the actual sequence (the proprioceptive aspect), we can shift our attention to how movements feel in the body (the interoceptive aspect). Try slowing your techniques down to be able to be able to listen deeply – to someone else with your hands if you are doing manual therapy, or in movement to yourself or your client.

Simple Breath Meditation: This slowing down is especially effective for the autonomic system when you apply it to the breath. Focus on the coolness of the air as you inhale, and the warmth of the air as you exhale – and watch the feelings inside yourself as a result of the slower breath.

Change your routine: Take your autopilot experiences and turn them into something new. Doing a particular sequence of yoga or training repetitively will develop mastery of the skill, but introducing novelty by changing your routine may give you access to a deeper listening. Even changing the position of your massage table in your room or the music you play during sessions may provide a finer tuning of your interoceptive awareness.

Self-massage: When using any SMR (Self Myofascial Release) tool – a foam roller or balls – slow down and feel. You will invite a deep parasympathetic response and an overall deeper listening to both proprioceptive and interoceptive cues.

To feel this, simply hold one arm out to the side, level with your shoulder – in other words, shoulder abducted, elbow extended. Keep it there as you read on. Right from the beginning, you can appreciate the proprioception – the contraction in the deltoid and trapezius, the joint receptors telling you where your arm is and how much it weighs without you having to look at it.

As time passes, though, you will begin to notice other feelings. You will begin to look for excuses to take your arm down. It is not painful, exactly, and there is no tissue damage from holding your arm out there for a few minutes, but now we know it is the interoceptors that are letting you know 'how you feel about what you feel' even in the fascia, muscles, and joints.

You can take your arm down anytime now, but it is an interesting test to leave your arm out there as long as possible to watch the process of interoception – how annoyed and agitated you can get as the sensations increase. Proprioception is emotionally neutral; interoception – from your organs or your musculoskeletal body – has a motivating force in it. Followers of Wim Hoff test themselves against these kinds of interoceptive feelings by taking ice baths and such, and there may well be value in expanding the limits of sensation tolerance in this way.

The feeling difference is because interoceptive endings tickle a different part of the brain than proprioceptive ones. According to fascial researcher Dr Robert Schleip, 'These sensations are triggered by stimulation of unmyelinated sensory nerve endings (free nerve endings) that project to the insular cortex rather than to the primary somatosensory cortex which is usually considered as the main target of proprioceptive sensations.'

Though interoceptive endings are important to help us maintain homoeostasis in the body, these sensations not only have a sensory aspect, but also come with an affective, motivational, or emotional aspects. The relief you felt when your mom rubbed your 'boo-boo' had been ascribed to the 'gate control' theory of pain, but the mechanism now appears to be through your interoceptors – you may still have the pain, but you feel better about it because the interoceptors have been calmed by Dr Mom.

Distressed interoception and altered insular processing is associated with conditions such as irritable bowel syndrome, eating disorders, anxiety, depression, alexithymia (emotional blindness), schizophrenic disorders, post-traumatic stress disorder (PTSD), and possibly fibromyalgia.[110] It has been proposed that the neural pathways associated with interoception may be considered as an essential component for consciousness, a fundamental part of 'presence'.

The interoceptors can be seen as an extension of the organic self out into the neuromotor self. These responses integrate seamlessly with the autonomic nervous system's sympathetic alarm and parasympathetic restorative calm. These issues are beyond our scope here, and are competently dealt with elsewhere[111–113] (see also the Stress webinar at www.anatomytrains.com/product/physiology-emotional -release-webinar/).

Nociception – Fascia and Pain

The problem of body pain is still a mystery, and this book will not solve it. Although pain and tissue damage are associated strongly, we have incidents of pain without damage (as in holding your arm out in the experiment above, or the traditional laboratory test of putting your fingers in ice water. There is no damage, but given time you will take your fingers out as a certainty.) On the other hand, many people have significant fibroids or other tumors, or accidents where there has been damage but the subject feels no pain. Freud's first intimation of the jaw cancer that would eventually lead to his death was a drop of blood dripping out of his beard onto the paper he was reading – no pain, but certainly tissue damage underway.[114]

Only the free nerve terminals convey pain signals, and only up the nociceptive tracts.[109,115] The recent biopsychosocial model of pain locates the perception of pain in the central nervous system (CNS), a higher processing level event.[116] This contrasts with the bodyworker's common talk of 'pain stored in the body' – a phrase this author has used with frequency. Such talk is metaphoric – all perception, as far as we know, happens in the CNS.

But the CNS is also a metaphor. Think of it this way: itch is also carried by the nociceptive tracts. That does not mean we have to scratch the CNS to relieve the itch. The perception of the itch is in the CNS, but we do not therefore scratch our brains – scratching the bug bite out in the arm relieves the sensation in the CNS. Likewise with body pain, touching an area that 'carries pain' can help change the CNS interpretation of the sensation. Is the pain in the body? Certainly something that links to the pain is.

Future research will sort this out for us, and in the process, so this author believes, we will revolutionize our understanding of how the nervous system works, as our understanding of the brain's control of movement – a subject we do not even attempt in this book – is at this point very rudimentary. Meanwhile, for those who wish to pursue the issue of fascial and myofascial pain, we recommend these references.[117,118]

Fascia as a System

With these prefatory concepts in place, we now build out this new picture of the fascial system acting as a whole in terms of three specific but interconnected ideas:
- physiologically by looking at it as one of the 'holistic communicating systems'
- embryologically through seeing its 'double bag' arrangement
- geometrically through comparing it to a 'tensegrity' structure.

These metaphors are presented in brief and general terms as we attend to our primary purpose of laying out the Anatomy Trains myofascial meridians. While certain aspects of these metaphors run ahead of the supporting research, nevertheless, some speculative exploration seems useful at this point.

Anatomy has been thoroughly explored in the previous 450 years. New discoveries and new therapeutic strategies will not come from finding new structures, but from looking at the known structures in new ways.

Taken together, the following sections expand the notion of the role of the fascial net as a whole, and form a supporting framework for the Anatomy Trains concept. This appendix concludes with a new image of how the fascial system may put all these concepts to work together *in vivo* – to function as our biomechanical regulatory system.

The Three Holistic Networks

Let us begin with a thought experiment, fueled by this question: which physiologic systems of the body, if we could magically extract them intact, would show us the precise shape of the body, inside and out? In other words, which are the truly holistic systems?

Imagine that we could magically make every part of the body invisible except for one single anatomic system, so that we could see that system standing in space and moving as in life. Which systems would show us the exact and complete shape of the body in question?

There are three positive answers to our question in palpable, anatomical terms: the nervous system, the circulatory system, and the fibrous (fascial) system – an idea, we must admit, so unoriginal that Vesalius, publishing in 1548, rendered versions of each of them. We will examine each of these in turn (in full knowledge that they are all fluid systems that are incompletely separate, all interwoven, and have never functioned without each other), before going on to look at their similarities and specialties, and speculate on their place in the somatic experience of consciousness.

The Neural Net

If we could make everything invisible around it and leave the nervous system standing as if in life (a tall order even for magic, considering the nervous system's fragility), we would see the exact shape of the body, entirely and with all the individual variations (Fig. A1.48). We would see the brain, of course, which Vesalius unaccountably omitted, and the spinal cord, which he left encased in the vertebrae. All the main trunks of the spinal and cranial nerves would branch out into smaller and smaller twigs until we reached the tiny tendrils which insinuate themselves into every part of the skin, locomotor system, and organs. Vesalius presents only the major trunks of nerves, the smaller ones being too delicate for his methods. A more modern and detailed version, albeit still with only the major nerve trunks represented, can be seen in the Sacred Mirrors artwork at www.alexgrey.com.

We would clearly see each organ of the ventral cavity in the filmy autonomic system reaching out from the sympathetic and parasympathetic trunks. The digestive system is surrounded by the submucosal plexus, which has as many neurons spread along the nine yards of the digestive system

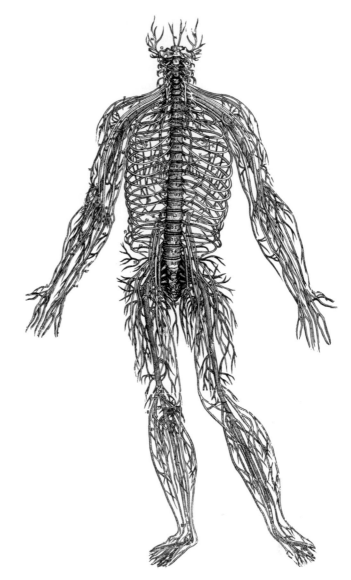

• **Fig. A1.48** It is amazing, given the methods available at the time, that Vesalius could make such an accurate version of the delicate nervous system. A modern and strictly accurate version of just this system would not include the spine, as Vesalius did, and would, of course, additionally include the brain, the autonomic nerves, and the many finer fibers he was unable to dissect out. (Reproduced with permission from Saunders JB, O'Malley C. Dover Publications; 1973.)

as are in the brain.[119] The heart would be particularly vivid with the bundles and nodes of nerves that keep it tuned.

Of course, this system is not equally distributed throughout; the tongue and lips are more densely innervated than the back of the leg by a factor of 10 or more. The more sensitive parts (e.g. the hands, the face, the genitals, the eye and neck muscles) would show up with greater density in our filmy 'neural person', while the otherwise dense tissues of bones and cartilage would be more sparsely represented. No part of the body, however, save the open lumens of the circulatory, respiratory, and digestive tubes, would be left out.

If your nervous system is working properly, there is no part of you that you cannot feel (consciously or subconsciously), so the whole body is represented in this network. And no ganglion of nerves operates on its own, separately from the rest of the nervous system.

If we are going to coordinate the actions of trillions of quasi-independent cells, we need this informational system that 'listens' to what is taking place all over the organism, weighs the totality of the many separate impressions, and produces speedy coordinated chemical and mechanical responses to both external and internal conditions. Therefore, every part of the body needs to be in close contact with the rapid-fire tentacles of the nervous system.

The functional unit of this system is the single neuron, and its physiological center is clearly the largest and densest plexus of neurons within it – the brain.

The Fluid Net

Similarly, if we made everything invisible but the vascular system, we would once again have a filmy representation that would show us the exact shape of the body in question (Fig. A1.49). Centered around the heart's incessant pump, its major arteries and veins go to and from the lungs, and out through the aorta and arteries to the organs and every part of the body via the wide network of capillaries.

Although the concept can clearly be seen in the early attempt by Vesalius, notice that in his conception the veins and arteries do not join with each other – it would take another two centuries for William Harvey to discover capillaries and the closed nature of the circulatory net. A full accounting would show tens of thousands of miles (about 100,000 km) of capillary nets, giving us another filmy 'vascular body' that would be complete down to the finest detail (Figs A1.50–A1.52; or see the complete system modeled at www.bodyworlds.com). If we included the lymphatic and the cerebrospinal fluid circulation in our consideration of the vascular system, our 'fluid human' would be even more complete, down to the finest nuances of everything except hair and some gaps created by the avascular parts of cartilage and dense bone.

In any multicellular organism – and especially true for those who have crawled out onto dry land – the inner cells, which are not in direct communication with the outside world, depend on the vascular system to bring nourishing chemistry from the outer edges of the organism to the middle, and to take otherwise toxic chemistry from the middle to the edge where it can be dispersed. The organs of the ventral cavity – the lungs, the heart, the digestive system, and the kidneys – are designed to provide this service for the inner cells of the body. To provide a comprehensive 'inner sea' complete with nourishing and cleansing currents, the network of capillaries must penetrate into the immediate neighborhood of most individual cells, of whatever type, to be able to deliver the goods via diffusion from the capillary walls. Cartilage and ligament injuries take longer to heal because their cells are so far from the shores of this inner sea that they must rely on seepage from farther away.

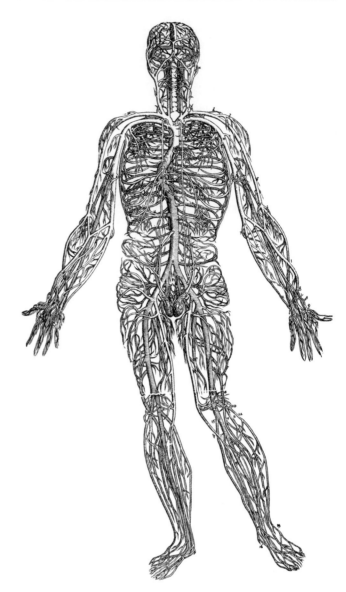

• **Fig. A1.49** Vesalius, in 1548, also created a picture of our second whole-body system, the circulatory system. Again, working in the mid-16th century, only the larger vessels were included. William Harvey and the discovery of the closed circulatory net of capillaries was still in the future. (Reproduced with permission from Saunders JB, O'Malley C. Dover Publications; 1973.)

The Fibrous Net

It can be no surprise, given our subject, that the fascial system is our third whole-body communicating network; the only surprise is how little the importance of this network has been recognized and studied as a whole until recently (Fig. A1.53).

If we were to render all tissues invisible in the human body except the collagenous elements of the connective tissue, we would see the entire body, inside and out, in a fashion similar to the neural and vascular nets. The areas of density would once again differ: the bones, cartilage, tendons, and ligaments would be thick with leathery fiber, so that the area around each joint would be especially well represented. Each muscle would be sheathed with it, and

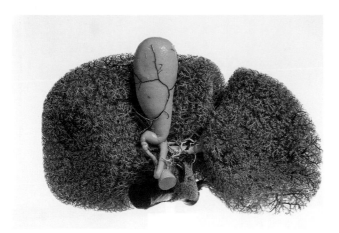

• **Fig. A1.50** A cast of the venous system inside the liver from below. The sac in the center is the gall bladder. (© Ralph T. Hutchings. Reproduced from Abrahams, et al. 1998.)

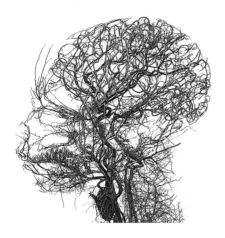

• **Fig. A1.51** Even with just these few large arteries represented, we can see something about this person. You might guess a Nilo-Hamitic person, for instance, from the shape of the head but it is, in fact, a full-term infant. (© Ralph T. Hutchings. Reproduced from Abrahams, et al. 1998.)

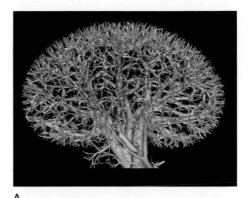

A

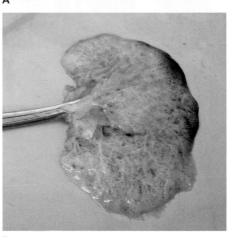

B

• **Fig. A1.52** (A) BriteVu® is a novel contrast agent used to evaluate organ vasculature, in this case a rat kidney. This kidney was CT scanned at 21 µm, which clearly shows the major and minor vasculature within. Image courtesy of Dr Scott Echols and www.ScarletImaging.com. (B) A largely decellularized kidney (some purple epithelia remain at the outer edge) using a combination of detergents and salts to reveal the fascial structure within – the non-hyrdophilic fibers of its ECM (extracellular matrix). Notice the similarity between the internal vascular structure in A) and the loose internal fascial structure here that allows the rapid fluid exchange necessary to the kidney's complex sorting process. With thanks to Anatomy Trains faculty and dissector Prof. Laurice D. Nemetz for creating the process (following Dr Doris Taylor) and the resulting image at the Laboratories of Anatomical Enlightenment.

infused with a cotton-candy net surrounding each muscle cell and bundle of cells (see Fig. A1.1B). The face would be less dense, as would the more spongy organs like the breast or pancreas, though even these are encased by denser, tough bags. Although it arranges itself in multiple folded planes, we emphasize once again that no part of this net would be distinct or separated from the net as a whole; each of these bags, strings, sheets, and leathery networks is linked to each other, top to toe. The center of this network would be our mechanical center of gravity, located in the middle of the lower belly in the standing body, known in martial arts as the 'hara'.

The bald statement is that the fascial web so permeates the body as to be part of the immediate environment of every cell. Without its support, the brain would be runny custard, the liver would spread through the abdominal cavity, and we would end up as a puddle at our own feet. Only in the open lumens of the respiratory and digestive tracts is the binding, strengthening, connecting, and separating web of fascia absent. Even in the circulatory tubes, filled with flowing blood, itself a connective tissue, the potential exists for fiber to form a leak-stopping clot (and in some places where we do not need one, as when plaque builds in an artery).

We could not extract a cubic centimeter, let alone Shylock's pound of flesh, without taking with us some of this meshwork of collagen. With any touch we contact the tone of this web, registering it whether we are conscious of it or not, and affecting it, whatever our intention.

This ubiquitous network has enough of a regular molecular lattice (see Fig. A1.33A) to qualify as a liquid crystal, which begs us to question: to what frequencies this biological 'antenna' is tuned, and how it can be tuned to a wider spectrum of frequencies or harmonized within itself?

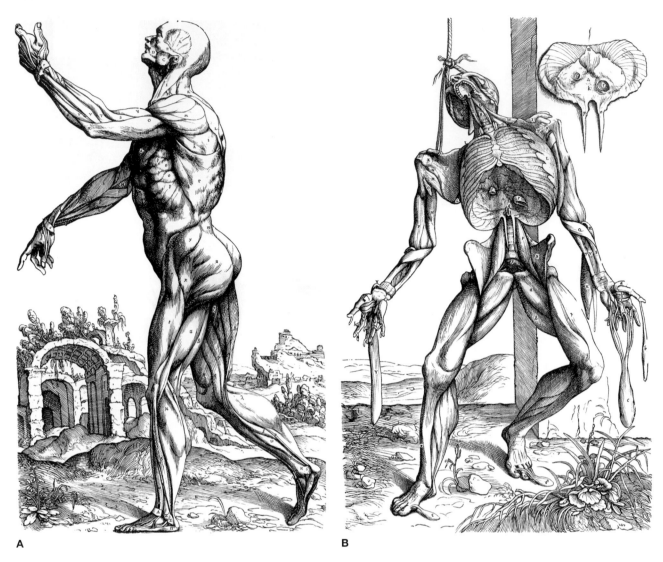

A   B

• **Fig. A1.53** (**A**) Vesalius shows the fibrous net in the familiar way – as a layer of muscles – but the overlying layers of fascial fabric have been removed. (**B**) The second view shows a deeper layer of musculature; fascial septa would fill in all the gaps and lines among the muscles. In (**B**), notice the black line extending from the bottom of the diaphragm to the inside arch of the foot, and compare it to the Deep Front Line (see Ch. 9). (Reproduced with permission from Saunders JB, O'Malley C. Dover Publications; 1973.)

Although this idea may seem farfetched, the electrical properties of fascia have been noted but little studied to date, and we are now glimpsing some of the mechanisms of such 'tuning' (pre-stress – see the section on tensegrity, below).[41–44]

In contrast to the neural and vascular net, the fascial net has yet to be depicted on its own by any artist we have seen to date. Vesalius's closest rendering is the familiar écorché view of the body (Fig. A1.53), which certainly gives us some idea of the grain of the fabric of the fibrous body, but really renders the myofascia – muscle and fascia together, with a heavy emphasis on the muscle. This is a prejudgment that has been continued in many anatomies, including those in wide use today: the fascia is largely removed and discarded to give visual access to the muscles and other underlying tissues.[120–122]

These common depictions have also removed and discarded two important superficial fascial layers: the dermis that provides a carpet backing for the skin, and the fatty areolar layer with its well-funded store of white blood cells (see Fig. A1.24). If we left these hefty layers in the full picture, we would see the animal equivalent of a citrus 'rind' beneath the very thin skin. Removing these layers and the rest of the 'packing material' helps contribute to a view of the fascial net as a 'dead' scaffolding around the cells, to be parted and discarded on the way to the 'good stuff'. Now, however, we are at pains to reverse this trend to create a picture of the fascial net with *everything else*, including the muscle fibers, removed.

New methods of depicting anatomy have brought us very close to this picture. Structural Integration practitioner Jeffrey Linn,[123] using the Visible Human Project data set, created Figure A1.9 by mathematically eliminating everything that was not fascia in a section of the thigh; he gives us the closest approximation of a 'fascial human' we yet have – though this view also omits the two superficial fascial layers.

If we can imagine extending this method to the entire body, we would see an entirely new anatomical view. We would see the fascial sheets organizing the body's fluids into areas of flow. We would recognize the intermuscular septa for the supporting guy-wires and sail-like membranes they really are (Video 6.21). The densely represented joints would be revealed as the connective tissue's organ system of movement.

It will be some time before such methods can be used to show the entire fascial system, for it would include (as Fig. A1.9 does not, but Fig. A1.1B does) the cotton wool infusing each and every muscle, as well as the perineural system of oligodendrocytes, Schwann cells, and glial cells and attendant fats which cuddle the nervous system, as well as the complex of bags, ligaments, and spiders webs that contain, fix, and organize the ventral organ systems.

If we could then take such a rendition into motion, we would see the forces of tension and compression shifting across these sheets and planes, being met and accommodated in all normal movements.

A grapefruit provides a good metaphor for what we are trying to envision (Fig. A1.54). Imagine that you could somehow magically extract all the juice out of a grapefruit without disturbing the structure within. You would still have the shape of the grapefruit intact with the rind of the dermis and areolar layers. You would see all the supporting walls of the sections (which, if pulled apart would turn out to be double-walled membranes, one half going with each section – just like our intermuscular septa in standard dissection). Plus we would see all the little filmy walls that separated the single cells of juice within each section. The fascial net provides the same service in us, except it is constructed out of pliable collagen instead of the more rigid cellulose. The fascial bags organize our 'juice' into discrete bundles, resisting the call of gravity to pool at the bottom. This role of directing and organizing fluids within the body is primary to an understanding of how manual or kinetic therapy of this matrix can affect health.

When you roll the grapefruit under your hand prior to juicing it, you are breaking up these walls and making it easier to juice. Fascial work (more judiciously applied of course) does much the same in a human, leaving our 'juices' more free to flow to otherwise 'drier' areas of our anatomy.

If we were to add the interfibrillar or ground-substance elements to our fascial human, that picture would fill in substantially, making the bones opaque with calcium salts, the cartilage translucent with chondroitin, and the entire 'sea' of intercellular space gummy with acidic glycosaminoglycans (GAGs; Video 6.12).

It is worth our while to focus our microscope in for a moment, to see this sugary glue in action. For the layman, the closest correlate to GAGs is mucous.

In Figure A1.8, we imagine ourselves at the cellular level (similar to Fig. A1.11). The cells are deliberately left blank and undefined; they could be any cells – liver cells, brain cells, muscle cells. Nearby is a capillary; when the blood is pushed into the capillary by systole of the heart, its walls expand and some of the blood is forced – the plasma part, as the red blood cells are too stiff to make it through – into the interstitial space. This fluid carries with it the oxygen, nutrients, and chemical messengers carried by the blood, all intended for these cells.

In between lies the stuff that occupies the intercellular realm: the fibers of the connective tissue, the interfibrillar mucousy ground substance, and the interstitial fluid itself, which is very similar (indeed, readily interchangeable) to the blood's plasma and lymph. The plasma, termed interstitial fluid when it is pushed through the capillary walls, must run the gauntlet of the connective tissue matrix – both fibrous and gluey – to get the nourishment and other messenger molecules into the target cells. It does so through the conduits – unlined pathways in we described in the section above on the interstitium. The denser the mesh of fiber and the less hydrated the ground substance, the more difficult that job becomes. Cells lost in the 'back-eddies' of fluid circulation will not function optimally. (See Fig. A1.8.)

How easily the nutrients make it to the target cells is determined by:
1. the density of the fibrous matrix (Video 6.20)
2. the viscosity of the ground substance in the interstitium.

If the fibers are too dense, or the ground substance too dehydrated and viscous, then these cells will be less thoroughly fed and watered. It is one basic intention of manual and movement interventions – quite aside from the educational value they may have – to open both of these elements to allow free flow of nutrients to, and waste products from, these cells. The condition of the fibers and ground substance is of course partially determined by genetic and nutritional

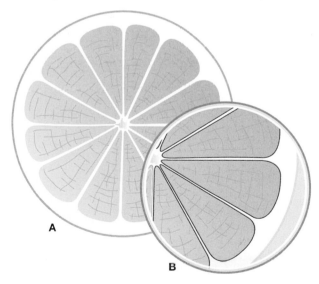

A

B

• **Fig. A1.54** A person is not unlike a grapefruit in construction. The skin is much like our own skin – designed to deal with the outside world. The rind is akin to the 'fat suit' we all wear, seen in Figure A1.24. Each segment is separated from the next by a wall we see when we cut the grapefruit through the equator for breakfast (**A**). But if we peel it and separate the sections as we might with an orange, we realize that the seeming one wall is actually two walls – one half goes with each section (**B**). The intermuscular septa are the same way. We often separate them with a knife, so we think of them as simply the epimysium of each muscle. But just as the walls are left after we eat a grapefruit, the walls are what is left in Figure A1.9, and we can see what strong structures they are, worthy of separate consideration.

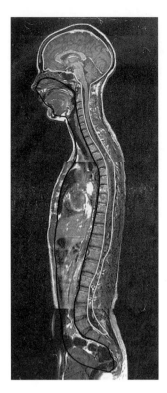

• **Fig. A1.55** The subject of this book is the myofascia in the body's locomotor chassis. But the connective tissue net extends into the dorsal (yellow) and ventral (red) cavities as well, to surround and invest the organs. (Image provided by Dr N. Roberts, Magnetic Resonance Centre, University of Liverpool. Reproduced with kind permission from Williams 1995.)

factors, as well as exercise, but local areas can be subject to 'clogging' from either fiber or glue when excess strain, trauma, inflammation, or insufficient movement has allowed such clogging to occur. Once the clog is dispersed, by whatever means, the free flow of chemistry to and from the cells allows the cell to stop functioning on metabolism-only, 'survival' mode to resume its specialized 'social' function, be that contraction, secretion, or conduction. 'There is but one disease,' says Paracelsus,[124] 'and its name is congestion.'

Back at the macro level, we need one final note on the distribution of the net in general: it is worthwhile making a separation, for clinical analysis only, among the fibrous elements inhabiting the two major body cavities – dorsal and ventral (Fig. A1.55).

The dura mater, arachnoid layer, and pia mater are connective tissue sacs that surround and protect the brain, and are in turn surrounded by and awash in the cerebrospinal fluid (CSF) (see Fig. A1.16). These membranes arise from the neural crest, a special area at the junction between the mesoderm and ectoderm in the developing embryo.[125] They interact with the central nervous system and the CSF to produce a series of palpable pulses within the dorsal cavity, and by extension, to the fascial net as a whole.[126–128] These pulses are well known to the cranial osteopaths and others who use them therapeutically, though the mechanism is not yet well understood, and even the existence of these wave motions is still denied by some.[129,130]

Besides the billions of neurons that make up the brain and spinal cord, within the dorsal cavity there are additional connective tissue cells that surround and infuse the entire nervous system, called the perineural network. These astrocytes, oligodendrocytes, Schwann cells, and other neuroglia are 'greater in number [than the neurons] but have received less attention because they were not thought to be directly involved in neural transmission', according to Charles Leonard.[131] In fact, the neuroglia outnumber the neurons about 10:1. Now they are 'beginning to cast a shadow over the performing brilliance of the neurons'.

During development, support cells guide the neurons to their final destination, provide nutrients to neurons, create protective barriers, secrete neuroprotective chemicals, and literally provide the glue and skeleton to hold the nervous system together. Recent research has pointed to the participation of the neuroglia in brain function, particularly in the area of emotional feelings.[132] Neuroglia also apparently act as 'gatekeepers' to the synapse, sorting which of the neuropeptides are allowed into the synaptic space to affect neural transmission, as well as helping to sweep up excess neurotransmitter in the synaptic cleft.[133]

If we could lift the perineural system intact from the body, it would show the exact outline of the nervous system, as every nerve, both central and peripheral, is covered or surrounded by this system. These coatings speed neural signal transmission (myelinated fibers transmit faster than unmyelinated fibers). Many so-called 'neurological' diseases such as Parkinsonism, polio, diabetic neuropathy, or multiple sclerosis are in fact problems of the neuroglia, which then interrupt the easy working of the nerves themselves.

The perineural cells also have a signal transmission system of their own, perhaps a more ancient precursor to the highly specific digital capabilities of neuronal transmission. In normal functioning and in wound healing, the slow waves of DC current that run along the perineural network help to organize generation and regeneration, and may act as a kind of integrating 'pacemaker' for the organism.[15,134,135]

In embryological development, the perineural cells take on a morphogenetic role. For example, the cells of the neocortex are born deep in the brain on the shores of the ventricles. Yet they must locate themselves incredibly precisely in the neocortex layer exactly six cells thick, on the very surface of the brain. These developing neurons use long extensions of neighboring neuroglia, gliding up the extension like a diver using a guide rope, ushered to their precise final position on the brain's surface by this supporting connective tissue network.[136]

The temptation to jump the gun and give this perineural network a role in consciousness is barely resistable.[137,138]

In the ventral cavity, the fibrous net organizes organic tissues, providing some of the trophic and morphogenetic support referred to in the beginning of this appendix in the quote from *Gray's Anatomy*, and to which we will return shortly. The bags that envelop the heart, lungs, and abdominal organs develop from the linings of the coelom during embryonic development (Video 4.10). The result is a series of differently thickened organ 'puddings' in cloth bags, tied loosely or tightly to the spine and each other, and moved about within a limited range by the continual waves of the muscular diaphragm in the middle, and to a lesser degree by other bodily movements as well as exogenous forces such as gravity.

The French physiotherapist and osteopath Jean-Pierre Barral has made an interesting observation that these inter-facing surfaces of serous membranes moving on each other could be thought of as a series of inter-organ 'joints'.[139] He has made a fascinating study of the normal excursion of the organs within their fascial bags during breathing, as well as their inherent motility (a motion similar to the craniosacral pulse). According to Barral, the ligaments that attach these organs to surrounding structures determine their normal axes of movement. Any additional minor adhesions that restrict or skew these motions (which are, after all, repeated close to 17,000 times each day) can not only adversely affect organ function over time, but also expand into the sur-rounding myofascial superstructure.

If the dorsal cavity contains one section of the fibrous net, and the ventral cavity another, the domain of the book in your hand is the third segment of the fascial net: the myofascia of the locomotor system that surrounds both of these cavities. It is interesting that a therapeutic approach has been derived for each of these sections of the fascial net. Practitioners of both visceral and cranial manipulation posit that effects from twists and restrictions in their respec-tive systems are reflected in the musculoskeletal structure. That is an assertion we have no desire to refute, though we assume that such effects are carried both ways. To be clear, however, our domain for the rest of this book is (arbitrarily) confined to that portion of the entire fascial net that com-prises the 'voluntary' myofascial system around the skeleton.

Spatial Medicine

This suggests that a complete approach to the 'fibrous body' – a 'spatial medicine' approach, if you will – would best be obtained by a practitioner having skill in four ultimately and intimately connected, but still distinguishable, areas:

- The meninges and perineurium that surround and pervade the predominantly ectodermal tissues of the dorsal cavity, currently dealt with by the methods similar to cranial osteopathy, craniosacral therapy, sacro-occipital technique, and methods of dealing with adverse neural tension in the cranial and peripheral nerve sheaths;
- The peritoneal, pleural, and pericardial sacs and their ligamentous attachments that surround and pervade the predominantly endodermal tissues of the ventral cavity, addressed by the techniques and insights of visceral manipulation and Asian organ releases;
- The 'outer bag' (see the following section on embryology for an explanation of this term) of myofascia, which contains all of the myofascial meridians described herein, and yields to the many forms of soft-tissue

bodywork such as strain–counterstrain, trigger-point therapy, myofascial release, and structural integration;
- The 'inner bag' of periostea, joint capsules, thickened ligaments, cartilage, and bones that comprise the skeletal system, are responsive to the joint mobilization and thrust techniques common to chiropracty and osteopathy, as well as deep soft-tissue release techniques found in structural integration.

A fifth skill set that encompasses all four of these areas is to set them all in motion, implying the host of skills in movement addressed by physiatry, rehabilitation medicine, physiotherapy, yoga, Pilates, Feldenkrais, the Alexander Technique, and a host of personal and postural training programs, including our own Anatomy Trains in Train-ing and Anatomy Trains in Motion programs featured in Chapter 10.

When can we create an educational program where prac-titioners would be conversant with all these five sets of skills? Many schools pay lip service to inclusion, but vanish-ingly few practitioners can navigate the entire fibrous body with ease and set it into balanced motion as well.[140,141]

Three Holistic Networks: a Summary

Before going on to the embryological origin of this fascial net, it is useful to compare these three holistic networks for similarities and differences.

All Three Are Networks

At the outset, we note that they are all complex networks, with a fundamental genetically-determined core form, but distributed chaotically (in its mathematical sense) in their outer reaches. This fractal nature suggests that they would be fairly labile in their smaller scale structures, but quite stable in their larger structures. As an example, the aorta in each of us is determined largely genetically, and is quite regular in its form. If we were to take a postage stamp sized square of skin from each of our hands and examine the blood vessels under a microscope, the general structure would be similar from person to person. The detailed map of the capillaries, however, would completely differ from one person to another.

In vivo, these three nets are also, of course, utterly inter-meshed with each other both anatomically and functionally, and this entire separation exercise is simply a useful fantasy (Table A1.3 and see Fig. A1.58).

All Three Are Made From Tubes

We can also note that the units for these networks are all tubular. The cylindrical tube is a fundamental biological shape – all the early multi-celled organisms had a basically tubular shape, an extended toroid which still lies at the very core of all the higher animals.[142] Each of these communicat-ing systems is also built around tubular units (Fig. A1.56). (These tubes do not exhaust the use of the tubes in the body, of course: the digestive system is a tube, the spinal cord is a tube, as well as the bronchioles, the nephrons of the kidney, the common bile duct and other glandular ducts – tubes are literally everywhere.)

The neuron is a one-celled tube, holding an imbalance of sodium ions on the outside of the tube and potassium ions inside until a pore in the membrane opens via an action potential. The capillary is a multicellular tube containing blood with walls of epithelial cells, confining the flow path of red blood cells while allowing the diffusion of plasma and the escape of white blood cells. The basic unit of the fascial web is a collagen fibril, which is not cellular like the other two, but rather a cell product. The molecular shape, however, is also tubular, a triple helix (like three-stranded rope). Some have suggested that this tube also has a hollow center, though whether this is true or whether anything flows through this tiny tube is still open to investigation.[143] So, while all the networks are tubular, the construction of the tubes is not the same.

Neither is the scale. The axons of the nerve 'tubes' range from about 1 μm to 20 μm in diameter,[144] while capillaries vary from 2 μm to 7 μm.[145] The collagen 'tube' is much smaller, each fiber being only 0.5–1.0 μm in diameter, but very long and cable-like.[146] If a three-strand rope – a triple helix like the collagen fiber – were 1 cm thick, it would have to be more than a meter long to match the proportions of a collagen molecule.

All Three Convey Information

Although each of these networks communicates, the information carried by these networks differs. The neural net carries encoded information, usually in a binary form: on or off. Starling's law dictates that either the stimuli to a nerve achieve a threshold allowing the nerve to fire, or they do not and it remains quiet.[147] The nervous system, in other words, works on frequency modulation (FM) not amplitude modulation (AM). A loud noise does not make bigger spikes up cranial nerve VIII, it simply makes more of them – interpreted by the temporal lobe as a louder noise. But whatever information is sent, it is encoded as 'dots and dashes' and must be decoded properly.

As an example of the limitation of such coding, press the heel of your hand on the orb of your closed eye until you 'see' light. Was there any light? No, the pressure merely stimulated the optic nerve. The optic nerve goes to a part of

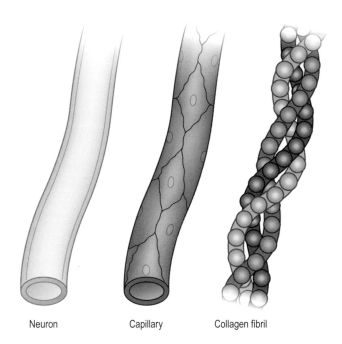

Neuron   Capillary   Collagen fibril

• **Fig. A1.56** Each of the major body communicating networks is made up of tubular subunits. The nerves are unicellular tubes, the capillaries are multicellular tubes, and the tubes of the collagen fibers are cell products, woven by the fibroblasts.

TABLE A1.3   Summary of the Holistic Communicating Nets

Variable	Neural	Fluid	Fibrous
		All Networks	
		All Tubular	
Tube type	Unicellular (neuron)	Multicellular (capillary)	Cell products (fibril)
Information	Digitally coded/binary	Chemical	Mechanical (tension/compression)
Function	Environment simulator	Milieu (inner sea) balance	Spatial organization
Cell metaphor	Meta-nucleus	Meta-cytoplasm	Meta-membrane
Speed of transmission	Seconds	Minutes–hours	1. Speed of sound (force transmission) 2. Days–years (adjustment/compensation)
Element	Time	Matter	Space
Consciousness	Temporal memory	Emotional memory	Belief systems

The table summarizes the information carried on the three holistic communicating nets. Exceptions and caveats can be found to these generalizations, but the overall idea stands. The bottom line (what kind of consciousness is held in each system) is pure speculation on the part of the author, based on empirical observation and experience. It represents a plea to expand consciousness from being solely the domain of the brain to include the accumulated wisdom of the rest of the nervous system, the chemical wisdom of the fluid system, and the spatial wisdom found in the semiconducting fluid crystal of the connective tissue web.

the brain that can only interpret incoming signals as light. Therefore, the signal 'pressure' was erroneously decoded as 'light'. The late famed neurologist Oliver Sacks has produced a compendium of books detailing many stories of conditions where the neurological system 'fools' its owner into seeing, feeling, or believing that the world is something other than it appears to the rest of us. One of his less celebrated books recounts his personal experience of sensorimotor amnesia so relevant to the manual or movement therapist, *A Leg to Stand On*.[148]

The circulatory net carries chemical information around the body in a fluid medium. The myriad exchanges of actual physical substance (as opposed to the encoded information carried by the nervous system) take place through this most ancient of conduits.

Though we must be clear that these two systems work seamlessly in the living body, the difference between these two types of information conveyed is easily explained. If I wish to lift a glass to my mouth, I can conceive of this idea in my brain (perhaps stimulated by thirst, perhaps by my discomfort on a first date, it matters not), turn it into a code of dots and dashes, send this code down through the spine, out through the brachial plexus, and down to my arm. If some security agency intercepted this message halfway in between the two, the actual signal would be meaningless – just a series of on–off switches, as in Morse code. At the neuromuscular junction, the message is decoded into meaning – and the relevant muscles contract according to the coded sequence.

Suppose, however, that in order to carry out the nervous system's command, that muscle's mitochondria require more oxygen. It is simply not possible for me, even if I could conceive that idea in my brain, to encode some signal that could be decoded somewhere down the nervous system as an oxygen molecule. It is instead necessary that the actual oxygen molecule be captured from the air by the surfactant bordering the epithelium of the alveolus, cross through this surface layer, over the interstitial space and connective tissue layer, pass through the alveolar capillary wall, 'swim' through the plasma until it finds a red blood cell, pass through the membrane of the red blood cell and hook itself on to a bushy hemoglobin molecule, ride with the red blood cell out to the arm, detach itself from the hemoglobin, escape from the red blood cell, pass with the plasma through the capillary wall, pass between the fibers and the ground substance in the interstitial space and squiggle through the membrane of the cell in question, finally to enter the Krebs cycle in the service of raising my arm. As complex as this series of events may seem, it is happening millions and millions of times every minute in your body.

These systems have social correlates, which may also serve to illustrate the differing functions of the neural and circulatory nets. It is increasingly common for us as a society to encode data into an unrecognizable form and have it decoded at the other end. Although this book would be a primitive form of such encoding, phone calls, webinars, and the internet provide a better example. My daughter lives far

from me; when I write 'I love you' on email, it is turned into a pattern of electrons that bears no resemblance to the message itself, and would carry no meaning for anyone else who might intercept it along the way. At the other end, though, is a machine that decodes the electrons and turns it back into a message with meaning that I hope brings a smile. This is quite similar to how the neural net coordinates both sensory perception and motor reaction.

If, on the other hand, an email or phone call will simply not do, and she needs a genuine hug, I must get into my little 'blood cell' of an automobile, and travel the 'capillaries' of the roadways and 'arteries' of the airways until I reach the physical proximity that allows a genuine, non-virtual hug. That is the way the circulatory fluid net works to provide direct chemical exchange.

The third system, the fascial system, conveys mechanical information – the interplay of tension and compression – along the fibrous net, the gluey proteoglycans, and even through the cells themselves (Video 4.9). Please note that we are *not* talking here of the muscle spindles, Golgi tendon organs, and other stretch receptors we covered earlier. These proprioceptive sense organs are how the nervous system informs itself, in its usual encoded way, about what is going on in the myofascial net. The fibrous system has a far more ancient way of 'talking' to itself: simple pulls and pushes, communicating along the grain of the fascia and ground substance, from fiber to fiber and cell to cell, directly (Fig. A1.57).[149]

Biomechanical transmission of mechanical information has been studied less than the neural or circulatory communication, but it is clearly important.[150] We will return to its particulars below in the section on tensegrity. For now, we note that the Anatomy Trains myofascial meridians are simply some common pathways for this kind of tensile communication.

A tug in the fascial net is communicated across the entire system like a snag in a sweater, or a pull in the corner of an empty woven hammock. This communication happens

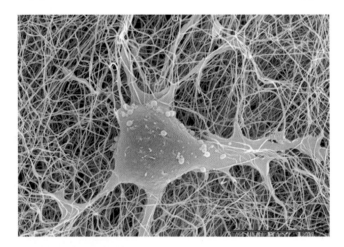

• **Fig. A1.57** The connective tissue forms a syncytium – a continuity of cells and the intercellular fibers – in which the cells can exert tension through the entire network of the ECM (see also A1.25). (Reproduced with permission from Jiang H, Grinnell F. American Society for Cell Biology; 2005.)

below our level of awareness for the most part, but through it we create a shape for ourselves, registered in the liquid crystal of the connective tissue, a recognizable pattern of posture and 'acture' (defined as 'posture in action' – our characteristic patterns of doing – by Feldenkrais[40]), which we tend to keep unless altered for better or worse.

As well as the type of information carried, the timing of the communication within these systems differs as well. The nervous system is widely regarded as the fastest, working in milliseconds to seconds at speeds of 7–170 miles per hour (10–270 km per hour) – not like electricity at the speed of light.[147] The slowest neural message, throbbing pain, runs along tiny nerves at about one meter per second, and thus might take about two seconds to get from the stubbed toe of a tall man to his brain. Other messages pass more quickly but still on the same order – the reaction time of a trained martial artist is $\frac{1}{30}$ of a second from the reception of a stimulus to the beginning of a response in movement. This approaches the reaction time for a simple reflex arc like the knee-jerk response.

The circulatory system works on a slower time scale. The standard is that most red blood cells return through the heart every 1.5 minutes.[147] Despite the recurring movie motif of the instant drug knockout, even injected drugs will take a few minutes to make it to the brain. Many chemical levels in the blood (e.g., salt and sugar levels) fluctuate on several-hour cycles, so we can set this system's average responsive rhythm as minutes to hours. Of course, many fluid rhythms work at slower scales – from the slow pulse of the 'long tide' (around 90 seconds) in the cranial system through the 28-day cycle of the menstrual system.

The nervous system and fluid systems developed in tandem, both in the individual and in our species, so the division between them is purely an analytical exercise. Still, the distinction is useful.

The timing of the fascial system is interesting in that it has two rhythms; at least, two that have interest to us. On the one hand, the play of tension and compression communicates around the body as a mechanical 'vibration', so it travels at the speed of sound. This is roughly equivalent to 720 mph (1100 kph), which is more than three times faster than the nervous system. So, contrary to conventional wisdom, the fibrous net communicates more quickly than the nervous system. One can feel this communication if one steps from one room to another in which there is an unexpected drop or rise. The nervous system, setting the springs of responsive muscles to the expected level of floor, is unprepared for the sharp shock that does come, which is thus absorbed instead almost entirely by the fascial system over a fraction of a second. We will take up the mechanism of this immediate communication in the tensegrity section below; for now we note that every nuance of changing mechanical forces is 'noticed' and communicated along the fabric of the fibrous net.

On the other hand, the speed at which this system responds with compensation around the structural body is much slower. Structural bodyworkers commonly find that this year's neck pain was built on last year's mid-back pain, which derived in turn from a sacroiliac problem three years earlier, which in fact rests on a lifelong tendency to sprain that left ankle. A careful history-taking is always necessary in working with the fibrous system because even small incidents can have repercussions, removed at some space and time from the initial incident.

These patterns of compensation, often with a fixation in the myofascia well away from the site of pain, are daily bread for Structural Integration practitioners. 'Where you think it is, it ain't' was one of Ida Rolf's aphorisms. Another: 'If your symptoms get better, that's your tough luck.' Her interest was in resolving patterns of compensation, not merely eradicating symptoms, which would then tend to pop up some months or even years later in another form.

For example, a middle-aged woman came to my practice a while ago, complaining of pains in the right side of her neck. An office worker, she was sure that the pain was related to her computer workstation and 'repetitive strain' from keyboard entry and mouse use. She had run the gamut of healing, having seen a chiropractor, physiotherapist, and a massage therapist. Each of these methods offered temporary relief, but 'as soon as I start working again, it comes back.'

When presented with a situation like this, there are two possible 'causes': the one offered, that work really is producing the problem, or, conversely, that some other area of the client's pattern is not supporting the new position demanded by her workstation. By examining this woman (using the method of seeing outlined in Ch. 11), we found that the rib cage had shifted to the left, dropping the support out from under the right shoulder (a similar pattern can be seen in Fig. 1.14). The rib cage had moved to the left to take weight off the right foot. The right foot had not taken its share of the weight since a mild skiing injury to the medial side of the knee three years earlier. The whole pattern was now set into the neuromyofascial webbing.

By working manually with the (by now long-healed but not yet resolved) tissues of the knee and lower leg, then with the quadratus lumborum, iliocostalis, and other determinants of rib cage position, we were able to support the right shoulder from below, so that it no longer 'hung' from the neck. The woman was able to point and click to her heart's content without any recurrence of her 'work-related' problem.

In summary, we may view the connective tissue as a living, responsive, semiconducting crystal lattice matrix, storing and distributing mechanical information. As one of the three anatomic networks that govern and coordinate the entire body, the ECM can be seen as a kind of *metamembrane*, according to Deane Juhan.[151] Just as the membrane is now seen to envelop the inside as well as the surface of a cell, our fibrous metamembrane surrounds and invests all our cells, our tissues, our organs, and ourselves. We develop this idea further in the section on embryology, below.

All Systems Intertwine

Of course, examining these holistic networks apart from each other has been just another reductionist analytical trick

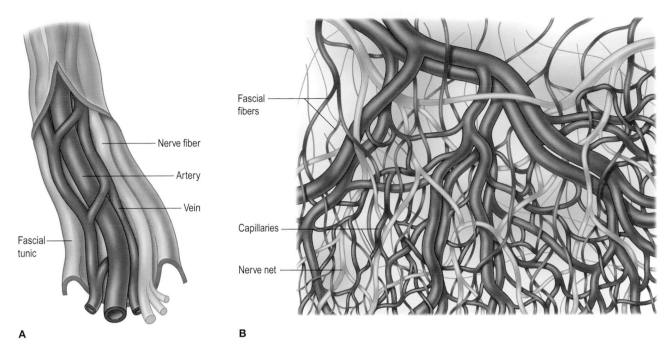

A

B

• **Fig. A1.58** The neural, vascular, and fascial systems run parallel in the neurovascular bundles (**A**) that extend the viscera out into the limbs and farther recesses of the body, with the connective and neural tissues forging the way. When they reach their destination, however, they spread into three enmeshed networks all occupying the same space (**B**).

– they always are interacting, and always have within the individual and the species, time out of mind (Fig. A1.58). We could as easily speak of a single 'neuromyofascial' web that would encompass all three of these networks acting singly to respond to the changes in the environment (Video 4.9).[152] We cannot entirely divorce the mechanical communication of the fibrous net from the neurological communication that would occur nearly simultaneously. Likewise, neither of these networks can be considered separately from the fluid chemistry that brings the nourishment that allows each of them to work in the first place. In fact, each and every biological system is fundamentally a fluid chemical system, and thus dependent on flow.

Persisting in this metaphor for one more image, each system has a set of 'ambassadors' that run in both directions, with the ability to alter the state of the other systems and keep them inter-informed (Fig. A1.59). Hormones and neurotransmitters inform the circulatory net of what the neural net is 'thinking'; neuropeptides and other hormone-like chemicals keep the nervous system up to date in what the circulatory system is 'feeling'. The circulatory net feeds proteins to the fibrous net and maintains turgor within the pressure-system bags in the body; the fibrous net guides the flow of fluids, allowing and restricting for better or worse as we have described above. It also affects the tonus of the myofibroblasts through fluid chemistry, as we noted above.

The nervous system feeds into the fibrous system by means of the motor nerves that change the tonus of muscles. Perhaps the most interesting leg of this three-legged stool for the clinician is the set of mechanoreceptors that feed information from the fascial net back to the nervous system

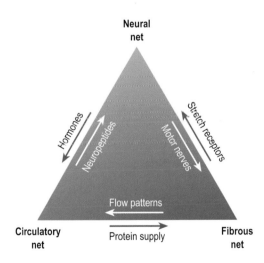

• **Fig. A1.59** Relationships among these holistic nets are complex. Each of the nets has 'ambassadors' to the other nets to alter their state and to keep the systems inter-informed and regulated.

– see the section on proprioception and interoception above. This fascial network is the largest 'sense organ' in the body, dwarfing even the eyes or ears in its rich diversity and proliferation of primarily stretch receptors.[153]

These sensory nerves frequently outnumber their motor compatriots in any given peripheral nerve by nearly 3:1. They pick up and pass along information concerning changes in stretch, load, pressure, vibration, and tangential (shear) force. The free nerve endings are especially interesting, in that they are the most abundant (they are even found within bone), they are connected to interoceptive and autonomic functions such as vasodilation, and they can function as mechanoreceptors or as nociceptors (pain).[154]

Obviously, the nervous system is highly responsive, and can change muscle tone in response to signals. We have previously described how the fascial system has its own (generally slower) responses to mechanical changes. Woven together, as they always are in a living person, they point to a rich diversity of modes of intervention into the fibrous body itself or to the neurological web within it.

Applying Spatial Medicine

We can demonstrate the spatial medicine approach to this interweaving of the three systems with an example: the person who becomes depressed, for whatever reason, will generally express that feeling in somatic form as being stuck on the exhale – they will generally appear to the observer as having a sunken chest, without full excursion upward of the ribs on the inhale. Put the other way around, few people with a high, full chest go around saying, 'I'm so depressed'.

The depressive posture may begin as a perception within the nervous representation of the self-versus-the-world, involving guilt, pain, or anxiety, but that soon is expressed out through the motor system as a recurrent pattern of contraction. This chronic contraction pattern is accommodated after a time by the fascial system, often reaching out over the whole body – the pattern in the chest requires compensation in the legs, neck, and shoulders as well as the ribs, and the ventral cavity's pressure systems. The diminution of the breathing in turn creates a different balance of chemistry in the blood and body fluids, lowering oxygen and raising cortisol levels. Simply changing the rate of serotonin re-uptake with antidepressant drugs (the material medicine/drug approach) or even changing the internal perception of self-worth (the temporal medicine/psychiatric approach) may not be fully effective in changing this whole pattern, because the pattern is also written into a habit of movement, a 'set' of fascial net.

In modern medicine, the neural and chemical aspects of such patterns are often considered, while the 'spatial medicine' aspect of these patterns is too often ignored. Effective treatment considers all three, but individual treatment methods tend to favor one over any other. The old saying goes: 'If your hand is a hammer, everything looks like a nail.' Whatever tool we are using to intervene, we do well to remember all three of these holistic communicating systems, and their relative dominance within each person.

The consideration of the fibrous system as an 'equal branch of (physiological) government' to find which conditions have a spatial medicine/fibrous body component will fill in a gap that has existed for the last 400 years of anatomy and physiology.

Embryology/Fascial Morphology/the Double-Bag Theory

When the BBC asked the great British naturalist J. B. S. Haldane if his lifelong study had taught him anything about the mind of the Creator, he replied, 'Why, yes, He shows an inordinate fondness for beetles.' (Haldane was so fond of this answer that he arranged to be asked the same question a number of times, so that he could delight himself and others with minor variations of the same reply.)

The modern anatomist, given the same question, can only answer, 'an inordinate fondness for double-bagging'. Two-layered sacs show up so often in connective tissue anatomy, often derived from embryology, that it is worth a brief separate exploration, before returning to its relevance to the Anatomy Trains theory *per se*. We also take the opportunity, while rummaging around in embryology, to point out a few of the larger mileposts in the development of the fascial net in general.

Each cell is double-bagged (Fig. A1.60); the heart and lungs are both double-bagged; the abdomen is double-bagged; and the brain is at least double-bagged, if not triple-bagged. It is the contention of this section that it is worth looking at the musculoskeletal system as a double-bagged system as well.

If we return to the very beginnings, we find that the ovum, even before it is expelled from the ovarian follicle (Fig. A1.61), is surrounded by the double bag of the internal and external theca.[155] Once released, like most cells, it is bounded with a bilaminar phospholipid membrane, which acts as a double bag around the cell's contents.

The ovum expelled from the follicle at ovulation is further surrounded by another membrane, a translucent coating of mucopolysaccharide gel called the zona pellucida (Fig. A1.62), an especially thick glycocalyx, through which the successful sperm must pass before reaching the actual membrane of the egg. While we commonly retain a Darwinian picture of fertilization, with victory going to the fastest-swimming and most aggressive sperm, the fact is that between 50 and 1000 of the fastest sperm beat their heads uselessly against the zona pellucida, making pockmarks with the hyaluronidase in their heads (and dying) until some lucky slowpoke comes along and comes in contact with the cell membrane itself and is accepted by the ovum for the actual fertilization.

When the fertilized egg divides, it is this zona pellucida that contains the zygote (Fig. A1.62A). The huge size of the original ovum allows it to divide again and again within the zona pellucida, and each successive set of cells takes up nearly the same amount of space as the original large cell. Thus this 'ground substance' shell around the zygote forms the first *metamembrane* for the organism. This is the first of the connective tissue products to do so, later to be joined by the fibrillar elements of reticulin and collagen (Video 1.1). This mucousy exudate is the initial organismic environment, and the original organismic membrane.

With the first division, a small amount of cytoplasm escapes the two daughter cells, forming a thin film of fluid surrounding the two cells, and between the cells and the zona pellucida (Fig. A1.62B).[156] This is the first hint of the fluid matrix, the lymphatic or interstitial fluid that will be the main means of exchange among the community of cells within the organism.

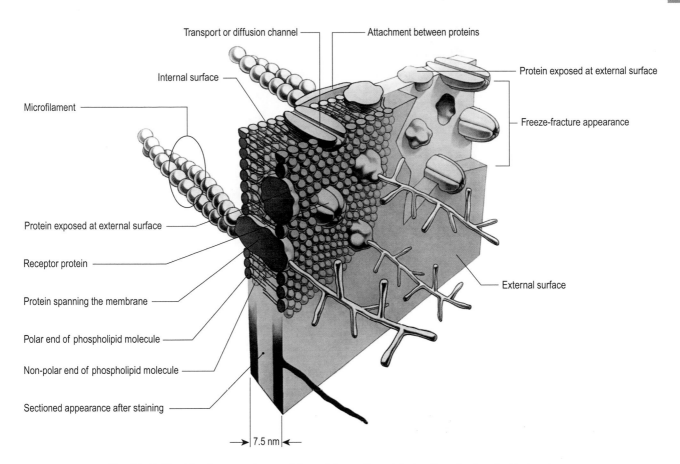

- **Fig. A1.60** The bilaminar membrane of the cell forms the original pattern for the double-bag image, which is repeated over and over again in macro-anatomy. (Reproduced with kind permission from Williams 1995.)

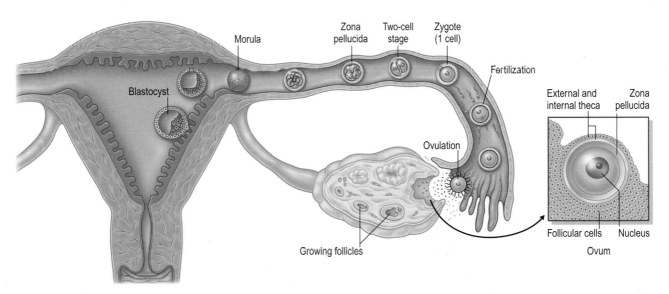

- **Fig. A1.61** The mucousy zona pellucida surrounds the ovum, and continues as an organismic membrane around the morula and blastocyst until it thins and disintegrates at the end of the first week of embryonic development as the blastosphere expands, differentiates, and prepares for implantation.

Note also that while the single cell is organized around a point, the two-celled organism is organized around a line drawn between the two centers of the cells. The early zygote will alternate between these two – organization around a point, then organization around a line. Further, the two-celled organism resembles two balloons (two pressurized systems) pushed together, so that their border is a double-layered diaphragm, another popular shape throughout embryogenesis.

The cells continue to divide, creating a 50–60-cell morula (bunch of berries) still within the confines of the zona (see

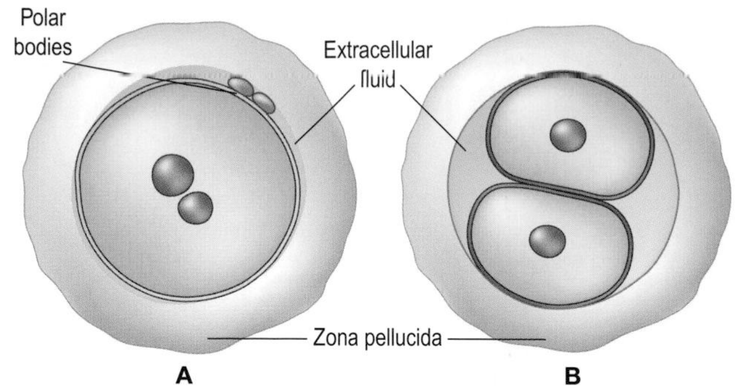

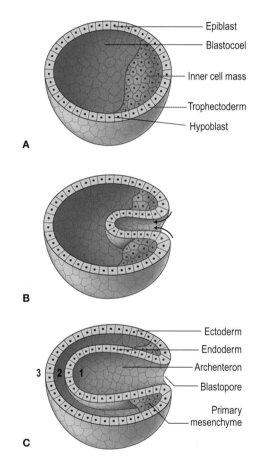

• **Fig. A1.62** When the ovum is fertilized, its membrane and the gummy zona pellucida surround the same space (**A**). With the first cell division, the two-celled organism is held in place by the *metamembrane* of the zona (**B**). The zona persists as the organismic limit right up through the blastocyst stage.

• **Fig. A1.63** The first definitive autonomous motion of the embryo is to fold the blastosphere in upon itself to form a double bag, which connects the epiblast and hypoblast into the bilaminar membrane. This motion forms the first double bag.

Fig. A1.61). After five days, the zona has thinned and disappeared, and the morula expands into a blastosphere (Fig. A1.63A), an open sphere of cells (which thus echoes in shape the original sphere of the ovum).

In the second week of development, this blastosphere invaginates upon itself during gastrulation (Fig. A1.63B). Gastrulation is a fascinating process where certain cells in one 'corner' of the sphere send out pseudopods which attach

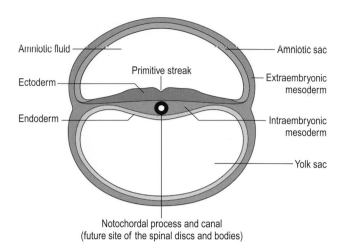

• **Fig. A1.64** Gastrulation, a turning inside-out motion of the embryonic sock, forms the trilaminar disc (ecto-, meso-, and endoderm) between the two large sacs of the amnion and yolk (transverse section). This action turns the double bag into a tube. Notice the similarity in shape to Figure A1.62B.

to other cells, and then, by reeling in the extensions, create first a dimple, then a crater, and finally a tunnel that creates an inner and an outer layer of cells (Fig. A1.63C).[157] This is the basic double-bag shape, a sock turned halfway inside-out or a two-layered cup. Notice that this ancient tunicate-like shape creates three potential spaces:

1. the space within the inner bag
2. the space between the inner and the outer bag
3. the environment beyond the outer bag.

If the 'mouth' of the structure is open, then there can be little difference between space 1 and space 3, but if the sphincter of the mouth is closed, they are three distinct areas separated by the two bags.

This inversion results in the double bags of the amnion and yolk sac, with the familiar trilaminar disc of ectoderm, mesoderm, and endoderm sandwiched between (Fig. A1.64 – note the similarity to the two-celled shape with the 'diaphragm' in between in Fig. A1.62 – now what will be the baby is the diaphragm between 'mother' yolk and 'father' amnion). The ectoderm, in contact with the amniotic sac and fluid, will form the nervous system and skin (and is thus associated with the 'neural net' as described above). The endoderm, in contact with the yolk sac, will form the linings of all our circulatory tubing, as well as the organs of the alimentary canal, along with the glands (and is the primary source of the fluid vascular net). The mesoderm in between the two will form all the muscles and connective tissues (and is thus the precursor of the fibrous net), as well as the blood, lymph, kidneys, most of the genital organs, and the adrenal cortex glands.[157]

The Formation of the Fascial Net

Digressing from double-bagging for a moment to follow the development of the fibrous net within the embryo, this initial cellular specialization within the embryo is a very important moment which occurs at about two weeks into development. Up until this point, most cells have been carbon copies of each other; very little differentiation has taken place. Therefore, spatial arrangement is not crucial – shuffling a deck of cards makes no difference if they are all copies of the same card. During this time, the mucousy 'glue' among the cells and their intermembranous junctions have sufficed to keep the tiny embryo intact (see Fig. A1.62 and A1.3). Now, however, as increasing specialization takes place, it is imperative that concrete spatial arrangements be maintained while still allowing movement, as the embryo begins to increase exponentially in size and fold into unimaginable complexity.

If we look more closely at this middle layer, the mesoderm, we see a thickening in the middle below the primitive streak, called the notochord, which will ultimately form the spinal column, i.e., vertebral bodies and discs. Just lateral to this, in the paraxial mesoderm, is a special section of the mesoderm called the mesenchyme (literally, the mess in the middle).[157] Mesenchymal cells, which are the embryonic stem cells for fibroblasts and other connective tissue cells, migrate among the cells throughout the organism, to inhabit all three layers (Fig. A1.65). There they secrete reticulin (an immature form of collagen with very fine fibers) into the interstitial space.[158] These reticulin fibers mesh with each other, chemically and like Velcro®, to form a body-wide net – even though the entire body is only about 1 mm long at this point.

As an aside, some of these pluripotential mesenchymal cells are retained in the tissues of the body, ready to convert themselves into whatever connective tissue function is most called upon. If we eat too much, they can convert to fat cells to handle the excess; if we are injured, they can become fibroblasts and help heal the wound; or if we are subject to a bacterial infection, they can convert to white blood cells and go forward to fight the infection.[19] They are a perfect example of the supreme adaptability and responsiveness of this fibrous/connective tissue system to our changing needs. This is a type of 'vital capacity' which can be used up over time with illness, continuing traumatic distress, inflammation, continued injury, and binge/purge dieting.

The reticular fibers these mesenchymal cells generate will gradually be replaced, one by one, by collagen fibers, but

the fact remains: this is the source of our singular fibrous net, and the reasoning behind our favoring of the singular 'fascia' over the plural 'fasciae'. While we may, for analytical purposes, speak of the plantar fascia, the falciform ligament, the central tendon of the diaphragm, lumbosacral fascia, or dura mater, each of these is a man-made distinction imposed on a net that is in truth *unitary* from top to toe and from birth to death. Only with a knife can these or any other individual parts be separated from the whole. This fibrous net can fray with age, be torn asunder by injury, or be divided with a scalpel, but the fundamental reality is the unity of the entire collagenous network.[159] The naming of parts has been one of our favorite human activities since Genesis, and indeed a very useful one, as long as we do not lose sight of the fundamental wholeness.

Once the three layers and the binding net of fascia are established, the embryo performs a magnificent feat of auto-origami, folding and refolding itself to form a human being from this simple trilaminar arrangement (Fig. A1.66A). The mesoderm reaches around the front from the middle,

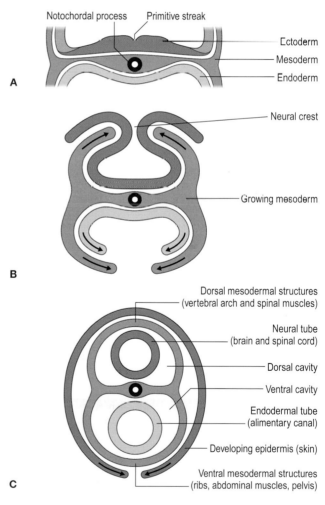

• **Fig. A1.66** The middle layer of the trilaminar disc, here seen (as in Figs A1.64 and A1.65) in transverse section, grows so fast that the cells boil out around the other two layers to form two tubes – digestive and neural – and to surround them in two protective cavities – the dorsal and ventral cavities. Part of the ectoderm 'escapes' to form the skin – another tube outside all the others.

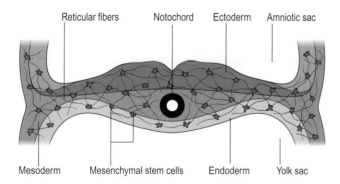

• **Fig. A1.65** Mesenchymal cells from the paraxial mesoderm disperse through all three layers of the embryo to form the reticular net, the precursor and foundation for the fascial net, in order to maintain spatial relationships among the rapidly differentiating cells.

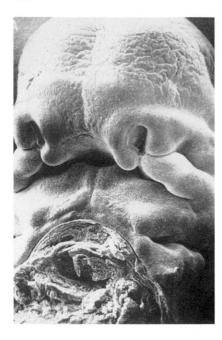

• **Fig. A1.67** In the complex origami of embryological development, the formation of the face, cranial base, and upper neck is especially intricate. One of the last folds, seen here under the developing eye sockets, is to bring the two halves of the palate together. Thus this is a common area for congenital defects. (Reproduced from Larsen 1993, with permission.[159])

forming the ribs, abdominal muscles, and pelvis, creating and supporting the endodermal alimentary canal within (Fig. A1.66B). It also reaches around to the back, forming the neural arch of the spine and the cranial vault of the skull, which surrounds and protects the central nervous system (the fasciae within these cavities were briefly described at the end of the section on the fibrous net earlier in this chapter – Fig. A1.66C). One of the last bits of origami is the fold that brings the two halves of the palate together. Since it is one of the last bricks in the wall of developmental stages, if any brick below it is missing it could result in a cleft palate, which explains why this is such a common birth defect (Fig. A1.67).[161]

Just lateral to the mesenchyme, near the edge of the embryo, lie the tubes of the intraembryonic coelom.[162] This tube (also, interestingly, the first hint of circulation) runs up each side of the embryo, joining in front of the head. These tubes will form the fascial bags of the thorax and abdomen. The very top part of the coelomic tube will, by means of the sagittal fold, pass in front of the face and surround the developing heart with the double bag of the endocardium and pericardium (Fig. A1.68) as well as forming the central part of the diaphragm. The upper part on either side will fold in to surround the lungs with the double bag of the visceral and parietal pleura (Fig. A1.69). The upper and lower parts will be separated by the invasion of the two domes of the diaphragm. The lower outside part of each tube will fold in to form the double bag of the peritoneum and mesentery.

The double- and triple-bagging around the brain and spinal cord is more complex, developing from the neural

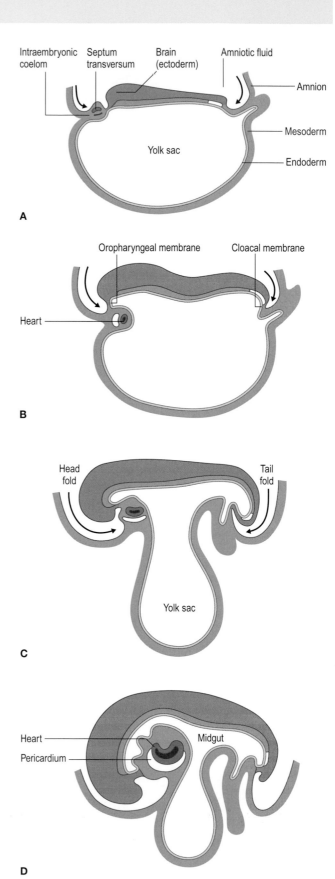

• **Fig. A1.68** A sagittal section of the embryo through the 4th week. The tube of intra-embryonic coelom which runs through the embryo is divided into separate sections which 'double bag' the heart as it folds into the chest from the transverse septum 'above' the head. A similar process happens from the side with the lungs in the thorax and intestines in the abdominopelvic cavity. (Adapted from Moore and Persaud 1999.[125])

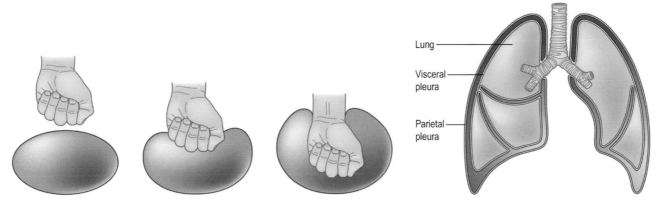

• **Fig. A1.69** Although they differ in form when they reach mature stages, the fundamental structure of the balloon pushed in to form a double bag by the tissue of the organ is found around nearly every organ system, in this case with the double-layered pleura around the lung.

crest, the area where the mesoderm 'pinches' off the ecto-derm (with the skin on the outside and the central nervous system on the inside), so that the meninges (the dura and pia mater) form from a combination of these two germ layers.[163]

Double-Bagging in the Musculoskeletal System

We have given short shrift to this fascinating area of morphogenesis, but we must return to the subject at hand – the myofascial meridians in the musculoskeletal system.

With such an 'inordinate fondness' for double-bagging, might we not look for something similar in the musculo-skeletal system? Yes, in fact: the fibrous bag around the bones and muscles can be viewed as having much the same pattern as we see in the way the fascial bag surrounds the organs (Fig. A1.70; Video 6.21). The inner bag surrounds the bones and the outer bag surrounds the muscles.

To create a simple model for this idea, imagine that we have an ordinary plastic carrier bag lying on the counter with its open end toward us (Fig. A1.71). Now lay some wooden thread spools on top of the bag in a row down the middle. Insert your hands into the bag on either side of the spools, and bring your hands together above the spools. Now we have:

1. spools
2. an inner layer of plastic fabric
3. hands
4. another outer layer of plastic fabric.

Substitute 'bones' for 'spools', 'muscles' for 'hands', and 'fascial' for 'plastic' and we are home free.

The human locomotor system is, like nearly every other fascial structure in the body, constructed in double-bag fashion – although this is speculative (Fig. A1.72). The content of the inner bag includes very hard tissues – bone and cartilage – alternating with almost totally fluid tissue – synovial fluid; the spools and spaces between them in our simple model. The inner fibrous bag that encases these materials is called *periosteum* when it is the cling-wrap sleeve

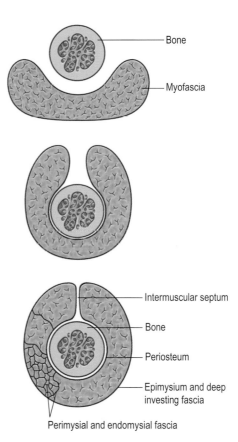

• **Fig. A1.70** We can imagine, whether it is embryologically correct or not, that the bones and muscles share a similar double-bag pattern.

around the bones, and *joint capsule* when it is the ligamen-tous sleeve around the joints.

These connective tissue elements are continuous with each other, and have always been united within the fascial net, but, once separated for analysis, tend to stay separate in our conception. This is strongly reinforced for every student by ubiquitous anatomical drawings in which all the other fabric around a ligament is carefully scraped away to expose the ligament as if it were a separate structure, rather

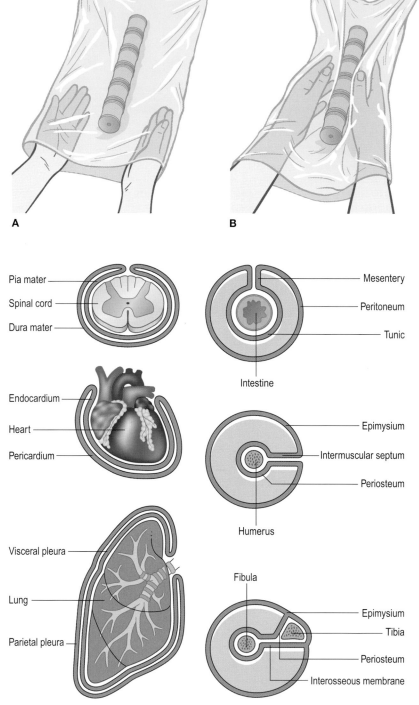

• **Fig. A1.71** Perform this little demonstration yourself with a common carrier bag and some spools or similar cylindrical objects to see how the bones and muscle tissue interact in a continuous 'double bag' of fascial planes.

Pia mater — Spinal cord — Dura mater

Mesentery — Peritoneum — Tunic

Intestine

Endocardium — Heart — Pericardium

Epimysium — Intermuscular septum — Periosteum

Humerus

Visceral pleura — Lung — Parietal pleura

Fibula

Epimysium — Tibia — Periosteum — Interosseous membrane

• **Fig. A1.72** Examining the fascia of the upper arm and lower leg reveals a suspiciously similar 'echo' in the pattern of disposition by other organic 'double-bagged' fascial layers.

than just a thickening within this continuous inner bag of the net (Fig. A1.73). Taken altogether, the ligaments and periostea do not form separate structures, but rather a continuous inner bag around the bone–joint tissues. Even the cruciate ligaments of the knee – often shown as if they were independent structures – are part of the knee capsule and thus this continual inner bag.

The content of the outer bag – where our hands were in the model – is a chemically sensitive fibrous jelly we call

muscle, which is capable of changing its state (and its length) very quickly in response to stimulation from the nervous system. The outer side of the bag we call the deep investing fascia, *fascia profundis*. The double-walled part between our thumbs we call the intermuscular septa (see Fig. 5.7A). Our tendons are our fingers, pulling on the spools within. Within this conception, the individual muscles are simply pockets within the outer bag, which is 'tacked down' to the inner bag in places we call 'muscle

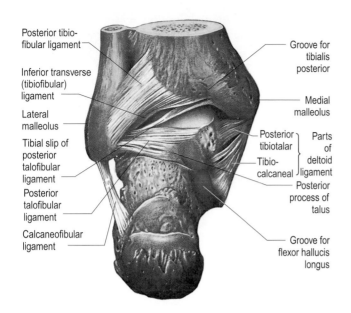

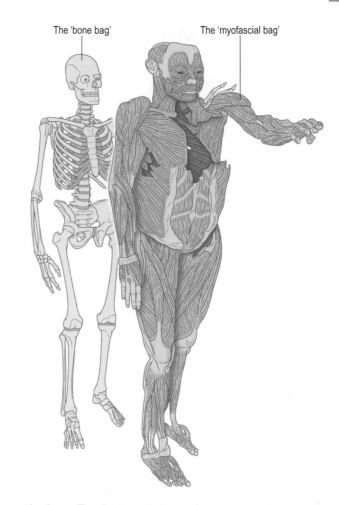

• **Fig. A1.73** The ligaments we see separated and detailed in the anatomy books are really just thickenings in the continuous encircling 'bone bag' part of the musculoskeletal double-bagging system termed by osteopaths as the 'ligamentous bed'. (Drawn from a specimen in the museum of the Royal College of Surgeons of England, with permission from the Council. Reproduced with kind permission from Williams 1995.[147])

attachments' or 'insertions'. The lines of pull created by growth and movement within these bags create a 'grain' – a warp and weft – to both muscle and fascia.

We need to remind ourselves once again at this point that muscle never attaches to bone. Muscle cells are caught within the fascial web like fish within a net. Their movement pulls on the fascia, the fascia is attached to the periosteum, the periosteum pulls on the bone.

There really is only one muscle; it just hangs around in 600 or more fascial pockets (Fig. A1.74). We have to know the pockets and understand the grain and thickenings in the fascia around the muscle – in other words, we still need to know the muscles and their attachments. All too easily, however, we are seduced into the convenient mechanical picture that a muscle 'begins' here and 'ends' there, and therefore its function is to approximate these two points, as if the muscle really operated in such a vacuum. Useful, yes. Definitive, no.

Muscles attach to other muscles by their sides, muscles are in series with ligaments, and muscles attach to nearby neurovascular bundles – these 'attachments' get little consideration in modern anatomy, but the research referenced here shows the importance of each and all of them in our assessment of efficient biomechanics.[5,6,164]

Muscles and ligaments are almost universally studied as isolated units, as in Figure A1.75. Such study ignores the longitudinal effects through this outer bag that are the focus of this book, as well as latitudinal (regional) effects now being exposed by research.[165] It is now clear that fascia

• **Fig. A1.74** The Anatomy Trains tracks are some of the common continuous lines of pull within this 'muscle bag', and the 'stations' are where the outer bag tacks down onto the inner bag of joint and periosteal tissue around the bones. This image, redrawn after a photo of the plastinated bodies in the Korperwelten project of Dr Gunter van Hagens, shows more clearly than any other the connected nature of the myofascia and the fallacy (or limitation, at least) of the 'individual muscle connecting two bones' image we have all learned. To connect this image to this chapter, the 'inner bag' would be the ligamentous bed surrounding the skeleton on the left, as if we wrapped the entire skeleton with cling wrap. The 'outer bag' would be the fascia surrounding (and investing) the tissue of the figure on the right. To prepare this specimen, Dr van Hagens removed the entire myofascial bag in large pieces and reassembled them into one whole. The actual effect is quite poignant; the skeleton is reaching out to touch the 'muscle man' on the shoulder, as if to say, 'Don't leave me, I can't move without you.' (The original plastinated anatomical preparation is part of the artistic/scientific exhibition and collection entitled Korperwelten (BodyWorlds). The author recommends this exhibition without reservation for its sheer wonder as well as the potency of its many ideas. Some taste of it can be obtained through visiting the website (www.bodyworlds.com) and purchasing the catalog or the video.)

distributes strain laterally to neighboring myofascial structures; so that the pull on the tendon at one end is not necessarily entirely taken by the insertion at the other end of the muscle (see Fig. A1.6).[166] The focus on isolating muscles has blinded us to this phenomenon. In retrospect stringing individual muscles is a definitively inefficient way to design a system subject to varying stresses. It is far more efficient

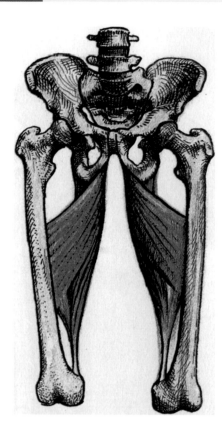

• **Fig. A1.75** Contrast the living reality of the myofascial continuity in Figures 9.18 and A1.86 with the isolated single muscle pictured here. No matter how much we can learn from this excellent and unique depiction of the strange adductor magnus, the common practice of isolating muscles in anatomies results in 'particulate' thinking that leads us away from the synthetic integration that characterizes animal movement. (Reproduced with kind permission from Grundy 1982.)

to distribute the force as widely as possible – using the visco-elastic properties of the medium we discussed above. Likewise, we have focused on individual muscles to the detriment of seeing the synergistic effects along these fascial meridians and slings.

Applying the Anatomy Trains scheme within this vision, the myofascial meridians can now be seen as the long lines of pull through the outer bag – the myofascial bag – which both form, deform, reform, stabilize, and move the joints and skeleton – the inner bag. The lines of continuous myofascia within the outer bag we have called the 'tracks', and the places where the outer bag tacks down onto the inner bag we have called 'stations' – not end points, but merely stops along the way – points of transmission or 'braking'. Some of the intermuscular septa – the ones that run superficial to profound like the walls of the grapefruit sections – join the outer to the inner bag into the single fascial balloon (compare the lower figure of A1.70 to the reality of Fig. A1.9).

Anatomy Trains maps the layout of lines of pull in the outer bag, and begins the discussion of how to work with them. Work with the inner bag – manipulation of peri-articular tissues as practiced by chiropractors, osteopaths,

and others with joint mobilization – as well as the inner double-bags of the meninges and coelomic peritonea and pleura, are likewise very useful, but are not within the scope of this book. Given the unified nature of the fascial net, we may assume that work in any given arena within the net might propagate signaling waves or lines of pull that would affect one or more of the others. As every researcher writes at the end of her paper: more research is necessary.

After the nine months of *in utero* gestation, we emerge from the womb for about 9 months' *ex utero* gestation, a potent time for developmental movement learning, as outlined in the developmental movement section of Chapter 10. The 'gestational' time allows us to double the size of our brains, as well as to solidify the bones and cartilage, strengthen the muscles, and pull the fascial sheets like the iliotibial band and plantar aponeurosis into being.

The unity of the fascial net is easier to understand if we see its unified beginnings. The connections among the meninges, visceral attachments, and the outer and inner bags of fascia around the musculoskeletal system – each has its own rhythm within the larger net. Each responds to its own manual or movement approaches, such that developing unified principles and application will be the job of spatial medicine for some decades to come.

Fascia and Tensegrity – the Musculoskeletal System as a Tensegrity Structure

To summarize our arguments so far, we have posed the fibrous system as a body-wide responsive physiological network on a par (in terms of importance and scope) with the circulatory and nervous systems. The myofascial meridians are useful patterns discernible within the locomotor part of that system.

Secondly, we have noted the frequent application of the double bag (a sphere turned in on itself) in the body's fasciae. The myofascial meridians describe patterns of the 'fabric' within the parietal myofascial bag connected down onto (and thus able to move) the inner bone–joint bag.

In order to complete our particular picture of the fascial system in action and its relation to the Anatomy Trains, we beg our persistent reader's patience while we place one final piece of the puzzle: to view the body's architecture in the light of 'tensegrity' geometry (Video 1.2).

Taking on 'geometry' first, we quote cell biologist Donald Ingber quoting everybody else: 'As suggested by the early 20th century Scottish zoologist D'Arcy W. Thompson, who quoted Galileo, who in turn cited Plato: the book of Nature may indeed be written in the characters of geometry.'[167]

While we have successfully applied geometry to galaxies and atoms, the geometry we have applied to ourselves has been generally limited to levers, vectors, and inclined planes, on the Newtonian-based, Borelli-applied 'isolated muscle' theory outlined in Chapter 1. Though we have learned much from the standard view of mechanics that underlie our current understanding of kinesiology, this line of inquiry has still not produced convincing models of movements as fundamental as human walking (see some new thinking in this regard in James Earls' contribution in Ch. 10). Getting a robot to play chess is relatively easy, compared to getting a robot to walk.

A new understanding of the mechanics of cell biology, however, is about to expand the current kinesiological thinking, as well as give new relevance to the search of the ancients and Renaissance artists for the divine geometry and ideal proportion in the human body. Though still in its infancy, the recent research summarized in this section promises a fruitful new way to apply this ancient science of geometry in the service of modern healing. This section shows how spatial medicine works without interruption across several levels of scale from the molecular to the organismic (see A1.4).

In this section we examine the macroscopic level of the body architecture as a whole, and then at the microscopic level of the connection between cell structure and the extracellular matrix. As with the hydrophilic and hydrophobic fibrous building blocks of connective tissue discussed earlier (see section above on fascial components), these two levels actually form part of a seamless whole, but for discussion the macro-/micro-distinction is useful.[168] While the macro-level

argument is directly relevant to Anatomy Trains, both levels contain implications for the entire spectrum of manual and movement work in medicine. Following the argument is worth your attention.

'Tensegrity' was coined from the phrase 'tension integrity' by the designer R. Buckminster Fuller (working from original structures developed by artist Kenneth Snelson – Fig. A1.76A,B). It refers to structures that maintain their integrity due primarily to a balance of woven tensile forces continual through the structure as opposed to relying on continuous compressive forces like any common wall or column. 'Tensegrity describes a structural relationship principle in which structural shape is guaranteed by the finitely closed, comprehensively continuous, tensional behaviors of the system and not by the discontinuous and exclusively local compressional member behaviors.'[169]

Notice that spiderwebs, trampolines, and cranes, as wonderful as they are, are anchored to the outside and are thus not 'finitely closed'. Every moving animal structure, including our own, must be 'finitely closed', i.e. independent, and able to hang together whether standing on your feet, standing on your head, or flying through the air in a swan dive. Also, although every structure is ultimately held together by a balance between tension and compression, tensegrity structures, according to Fuller, are characterized

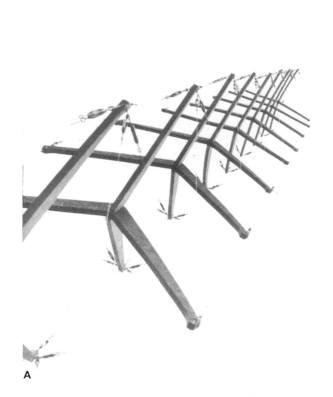

A

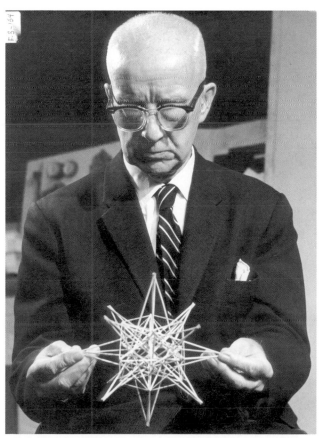

B

• **Fig. A1.76** (**A**) More complex tensegrity structures like this mast begin to echo the spine or rib cage. (**B**) Designer R. Buckminster Fuller with a geometric model. (Reproduced with kind permission from the Buckminster Fuller Institute.)

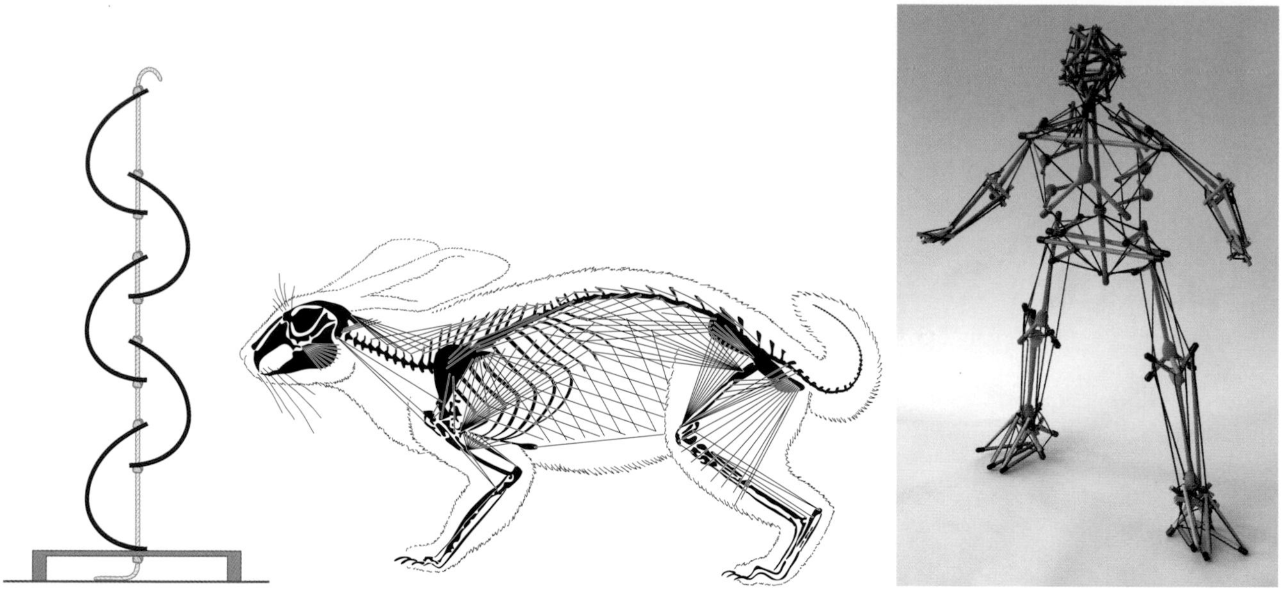

• **Fig. A1.77** (**A**) A tensegrity-like structure where the tensional 'core' is held aloft by rib-like structures. (**B**) A tensegrity-like rendition of a rabbit. This was created by drawing a straight line from origins to insertions for the rabbit's muscles. (Compare to Fig. 1.4A.) (**C**) An attempt to 'reverse engineer' a human in tensegrity form, a fascinating line of inquiry by inventor Tom Flemons. (B, From Young 1957. Reproduced by permission of Oxford University Press.[170] C, © 2008 T. E. Flemons, www.intensiondesigns.com.)

by *continuous tension around localized compression*. Does this sound like any 'body' you know?

'An astonishingly wide variety of natural systems, including carbon atoms, water molecules, proteins, viruses, cells, tissues, and even humans and other living creatures, are constructed using … tensegrity.'[167] All structures are compromises between stability and mobility, with savings banks and forts strongly at the stability end while kites and octopi occupy the mobility end (Video 6.11). Biological structures lie in the middle of this spectrum, strung between widely varying needs for rigidity and mobility, needs which can change from second to second (Fig. A1.77). The efficiency, adaptability, ease of hierarchical assembly, elastic energy storage, and sheer beauty of tensegrity structures would recommend them to anyone wanting to construct a biological system.[171]

Explaining the motion, interconnection, responsiveness and strain patterning of the body without tensegrity is simply incomplete and therefore frustrating. With tensegrity included as part of our thinking and modeling, its compelling architectural logic is leading us to re-examine our entire approach to how bodies initiate movement, develop, grow, move, stabilize, respond to stress, and repair damage.[150]

Macrotensegrity – How the Body Manages the Balance Between Tension and Compression

There are but two ways to offer support in this physical universe – via tension or compression; brace it or hang it. No structure is utterly based on one or the other; all structures mix and match these two forces in varying ways at different times. Tension varies with compression always at 90°: tense a rope, and its girth goes into compression; load a column and its girth tries to spread in tension. Blend these two fundamental centripetal and centrifugal forces to create complex bending, shearing, and torsion patterns. A brick wall or a table on the floor provides an example of those structures that lean to the compressional side of support (Fig. A1.78A). Only if you push the wall sideways will the underlying tensional forces be evident. Tensional support can be seen in a hanging lamp, a bicycle wheel, or in the moon's suspended orbit (Fig. A1.78B). Only in the tides on earth can the 90° compressional side of that invisible tensional gravity wire between the earth and the moon be observed.

Our own case is simultaneously a little simpler and more complex: our myofasciae and the collagenous webbing provide a continuous network of restricting but adjustable tension around the individual bones and cartilage as well as the incompressible fluid balloons of organs and muscles, which push out against this restricting tensile membrane (Video 6.16). Ultimately, the harder tissues and pressurized bags can be seen to 'float' within this tensile network, leading us to the strategy of adjusting the tensional members in order to reliably change any malalignment of, or even intraosseous strain within, the bones (Fig. A1.79).

Tensegrity Structures Are Maximally Efficient

The brick wall in Figure A1.78 (or almost any city building) provides a good example of the contrasting common class

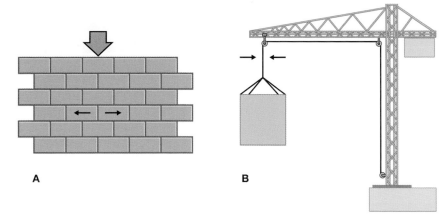

A   **B**

• **Fig. A1.78** There are two ways to support objects in our universe: tension or compression, hanging or bracing. Walls brace up one brick on top of another to create a continuous compression structure (**A**). A crane suspends objects via the tension in the cable (**B**). Notice that tension and compression are always at 90° to each other: the wall goes into tension horizontally as the pressure falls vertically, while the cable goes into compression horizontally as the tension pulls vertically.

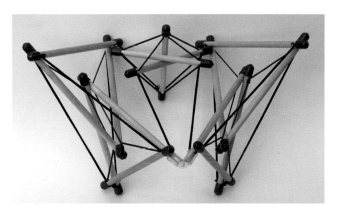

• **Fig. A1.79** A complex model shows how the pelvis, for instance, could be made up of smaller pre-stressed tensegrity units. (Photo and concept courtesy of Tom Flemons, www.intensiondesigns.com.)

of structures based on continuous compression. The top brick rests on the second brick, the first and second brick rest on the third, the top three rest on the fourth, etc., all the way down to the bottom brick, which must support the weight of all the bricks above it and transmit that weight to the earth. A tall building, like the wall above, can also be subject to tensile forces – as when the wind tries to blow it sideways – so that most compressive-resistant 'bricks' are reinforced with tensile-resistant steel rods. These forces are minimal, though, compared to the compressive forces offered by gravity operating on the heavy building. Buildings, however, are seldom measured in terms of design efficiencies such as performance-per-pound. Who among us knows how much our home weighs?

Biological structures, on the other hand, have been subjected to the rigorous design parameters of natural selection.[167] That mandate for material and energetic efficiency has led to the widespread employment of tensegrity principles:

All matter is subject to the same spatial constraints, regardless of scale or position ... It is possible that fully triangulated

tensegrity structures may have been selected through evolution because of their structural efficiency – their high mechanical strength using a minimum of materials.[172]

Tensional forces naturally transmit themselves over the shortest distance between two points, so the elastic members of tensegrity structures are precisely positioned to best withstand applied stress. For this reason tensegrity structures offer a maximum amount of strength for any given amount of material.[169] Additionally, either the compression units or the tensile members in tensegrity structures can themselves be constructed in a tensegrity manner, further increasing the efficiency and 'performance/kilo' ratio (Fig. A1.80). These nested hierarchies can be seen from the smallest to the largest structures in our universe.[173,174]

Now, our commonly held (and widely taught) impression is that the skeleton is a continuous compression structure, like the brick wall: that the weight of the head rests on the 7th cervical, the head and thorax rest on the 5th lumbar, and so on down to the feet, which must bear the whole weight of the body and transmit that weight to the earth (Fig. A1.81). This concept is reinforced in the classroom skeleton, even though such a representation must be reinforced with rigid hardware and hung from an accompanying stand. According to the common concept, the muscles (read: myofascia) hang from this structurally stable skeleton and move it around, the way the cables move a crane (Fig. A1.82). This mechanical model lends itself to the traditional picture of the actions of individual muscles on the bones: the muscle draws the two insertions closer to each other and thus affects the skeletal superstructure, depending on the physics.

In this traditional mechanical model, forces are localized. If a tree falls on one corner of your average rectangular building, that corner will collapse, perhaps without damaging the rest of the structure. Most modern manipulative therapy works out from this idea: if a part is injured, it is because localized forces have overcome local tissues, and local relief and repair are necessary.

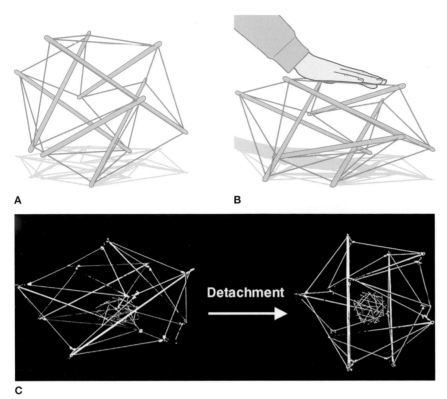

A

B

Detachment

C

• **Fig. A1.80** (**A**) In the class of structures known as 'tensegrity', the compression members (dowels) 'float' without touching each other in a continuous 'sea' of balanced tension members (elastics). When deformed by attachments to an outside medium or via outside forces, the strain is distributed over the whole structure, not localized in the area being deformed. (**B**) That strain can be transferred to structures on a higher or lower level of a tensegrity hierarchy. (**C**) Here we see a model within a model, roughly representing the nucleus within a cell structure, and we can see how both can be de- or reformed by applying or releasing forces from outside the 'cell'. (C, Photo courtesy of Donald Ingber.)

Tensegrity Structures Are Strain Distributors

A tensegrity model of the body paints an altogether different picture – forces are distributed, rather than localized (Fig. A1.83; Video 1.2). An actual tensegrity structure is difficult to describe – we offer several pictures here, though building and handling one gives an immediate felt sense of the properties and differences from traditional views of structure – but the principles are simple. (Kits with directions to build the structure pictured in Fig. A1.80 as well as more complex models are available from www.anatomytrains.com.)

A tensegrity structure, like any other, combines tension and compression, but here the compression members are islands floating in a sea of continuous tension. The compression members push outwards against the tension members that pull inwards. As long as the two sets of forces are balanced, the structure is stable. Of course, in a body, these tensile members often express themselves as fascial membranes, such as the fascia lata or thoracolumbar fascia, not just as tendinous or ligamentous strings (Fig. A1.84).

The stability of a tensegrity structure is, however, generally less stiff but more resilient than the continuous compression structure. Load one 'corner' of a tensegrity structure and the whole structure – the strings and the dowels both – will give a little to accommodate (see Fig. A1.80A,B). Load it too much and the structure will ultimately break – but not necessarily anywhere near where the load was placed. Because tensegrities distribute strain throughout the structure along the lines of tension, the tensegrity structure may 'give' at some weak point far removed from the area of applied strain, or it may simply break down or collapse.

In a similar analysis, a bodily injury at any given site can be set in motion by long-term strains in other parts of the body. The injury happens where it does because of inherent weakness or previous injury, not purely and always because of local strain. Discovering these pathways and easing chronic strain at some remove from the painful portion then becomes a natural part of restoring systemic ease and order, as well as preventing future injuries.

Thus we can see the bones as the primary compression members (though the bones can carry tension as well) and the myofascia as the surrounding tension members (though big balloons, such as the abdominopelvic cavity and smaller balloons such as cells and vacuoles can also carry compression forces). The skeleton is only apparently a continuous compression structure: eliminate the soft tissues and watch the bones clatter to the floor, as they are not locked together but perched on slippery cartilage surfaces. It is evident that soft-tissue balance is the essential element that holds our skeleton upright – especially those of us who walk precariously on two small bases of support while lifting the center of gravity high above them (Fig. A1.85).

In this concept, the bones are seen as 'spacers' pushing out into the soft tissue, and the tone of the tensile myofascia becomes the determinant of balanced structure (Fig. A1.86). Compression members keep a structure from collapsing in on itself; tensional members keep the compression struts

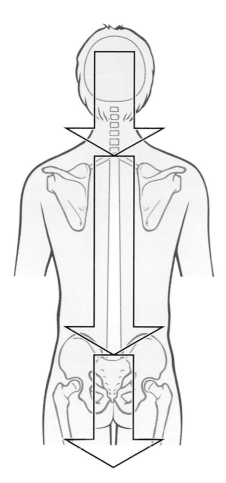

• **Fig. A1.81** Given the ease of building and simplicity of continuous compression structures, and given how many of them we make to live and work in, it is not surprising that the principles of tensegrity remained obscured for so long. This figure shows a familiar continuous compression model of the body – the head resting on C7, the upper body resting on L5, and the entire body resting like a stack of bricks on the feet.

relating to each other in specific ways. In other words, if you wish to change the relationships among the bones, change the tensional balance through the soft tissue, and the bones will rearrange themselves. This metaphor speaks to the strength of sequentially applied soft-tissue manipulation, and implies an inherent weakness of short-term repetitive high-velocity thrust manipulations aimed at bones. A tensegrity model of the body – unavailable at the time of their pioneering work – is closer to the original vision of both Dr Andrew Taylor Still and Dr Ida Rolf.[175,176]

Even the most solid-seeming part of the body – the neuro-cranial vault – has been interestingly modeled as a tensegrity structure, bringing the work of Dr William Sutherland into this same domain (Fig. A1.87).[177]

In this tensegrity vision, the Anatomy Trains myofascial meridians described in this book are frequent (though by no means exclusive) continual bands along which this tensile strain runs through the outer myofasciae from bone to bone. Muscle attachments ('stations' in our terminology)

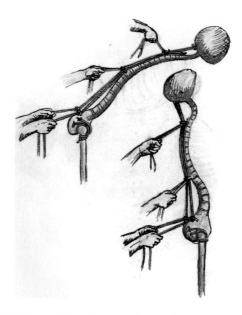

• **Fig. A1.82** The erector spinae muscles can be seen as working like a crane, holding the head aloft and pulling the spine into its primary and secondary curves. The actual biomechanics seem to be more synergistic, less isolated, requiring a more complex model than the traditional kinesiological analysis. (Reproduced with kind permission from Grundy 1982.)

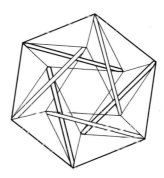

• **Fig. A1.83** A simple tensegrity icosahedron gets not-so-simple when you try to make one. (Reproduced with kind permission from Oschman 2000.[41])

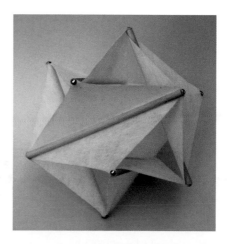

• **Fig. A1.84** While most tensegrity sculptures are made with cable-like tension members, in this model (and in the body) the tension members are more membranous, as in the skin of a balloon. (Photo and concept courtesy of Tom Flemons, www.intensiondesigns.ca.)

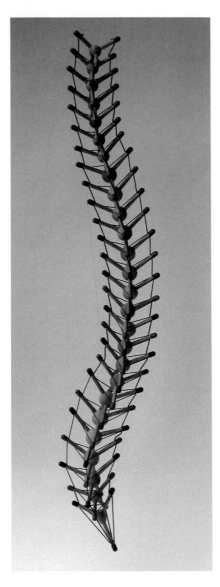

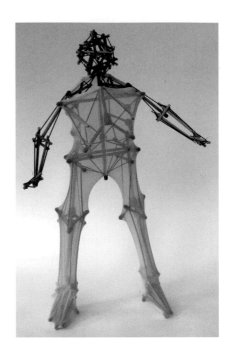

• **Fig. A1.86** The rest of the body in a simple tensegrity rendition. This structure is resilient and responsive, like a real human, but is of course static compared to our coordinated myofascial responses. The position of the wooden struts (bones) is dependent on the balance of the elastics (myofasciae) and the surrounding superficial fascial 'membrane'. The feet, knees, and pelvis of this model have very lifelike responses to pressure. If we could integrate the spine pictured in Figure A1.85 and a more complex cranial structure (as in Figure A1.88 or see www.tensegrityinbiology.co.uk), we would have a closer working model. (Photo and concept courtesy of Tom Flemons, www.intension-designs.ca.)

A Spectrum of Tension-Dependent Structures

Some writers do not agree with this macrotensegrity idea at all, seeing it as a spurious modeling of human structure and movement.[178] Others, notably orthopedist Stephen Levin, MD, who has pioneered the idea of 'biotensegrity' for over 30 years (www.biotensegrity.com), see the body as entirely constructed via different scale levels of tensegrity systems hierarchically nested within each other.[172,179,180] Levin asserts that bony surfaces within a joint cannot be completely pushed together, even with active pushing during arthroscopic surgery, though others cite research to show that the weight is indeed passed through the knee via the harder tissues of bone and cartilage.[181,182]

Further research is required to quantify the constituent tensional and compressional forces around a joint or around the system as a whole, to see if it can be analyzed in a manner consistent with tensegrity engineering. Clearly, though, the traditional notions of inclined planes and levers needs, at minimum, an update – if not a total overhaul – in light of the increasing evidence for 'floating compression' as a universal construction principle in our biomechanics.

Allowances must be made in this vision of tensegrity for the reality of the body in motion. In this author's opinion, the body runs the gamut, in different individuals, in

• **Fig. A1.85** The spine is modeled in wooden vertebrae with processes supported by elastic 'ligaments' in such a way that the wooden compression segments do not touch each other. Such a structure responds to even small changes in tension through the elastics with a deformation through the entire structure. It is arguable whether this simple model really reproduces the mechanics of the spine, but can the spine be said to operate in a tensegrity-like manner? (Photo and concept courtesy of Tom Flemons, www.intensiondesigns.ca.)

are where the continuous tensile net attaches to the relatively isolated, outwardly pushing compressive struts. The continuous meridians one sees in dissection photos throughout this book result, essentially, from turning the scalpel on its side to separate these stations from the bone underneath, while retaining the connection through the fabric from one 'muscle' to another (Fig. A1.88). Our work seeks balanced tone along these tensile lines and sheets so that the bones and muscles will float within the fascia in resilient equipoise, such as is seen at nearly all times in the incomparable Fred Astaire (Fig. A1.89).

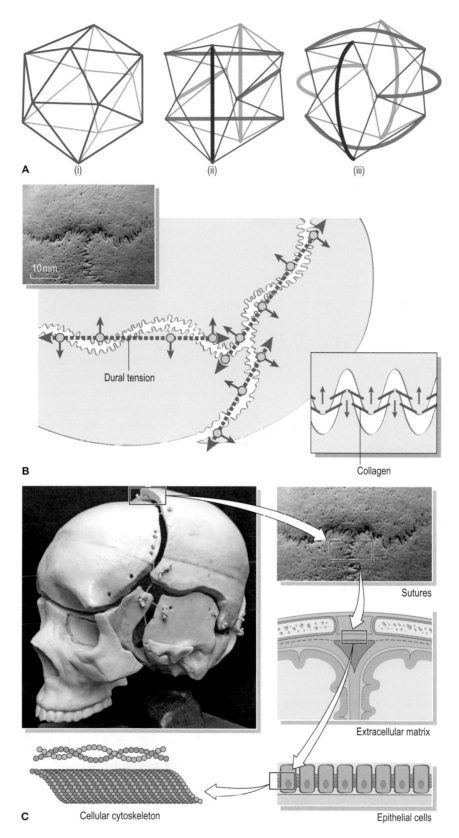

• **Fig. A1.87** The work of Dr Graham Scarr models the cranium as a tensegrity structure. (**A**) In our simple icosahedronal unit, straight dowels can be replaced with curved ones. (**B**) Because of the squiggly sutures, the dural and periosteal membranes act to keep the sutures apart, ensuring sutural patency. (**C**) This process is a tensegrity from overall down to the cellular level. (A–B, Adapted with permission from Scarr G. A model of the cranial vault as a tensegrity structure and its significance to normal and abnormal cranial development. Int J Osteopath Med 2008;11:80–89. C, Adapted with permission from Scarr (2008) and Scarr G. Simple geometry in complex organisms. J Bodyw Mov Ther 2012;14:424–44.)

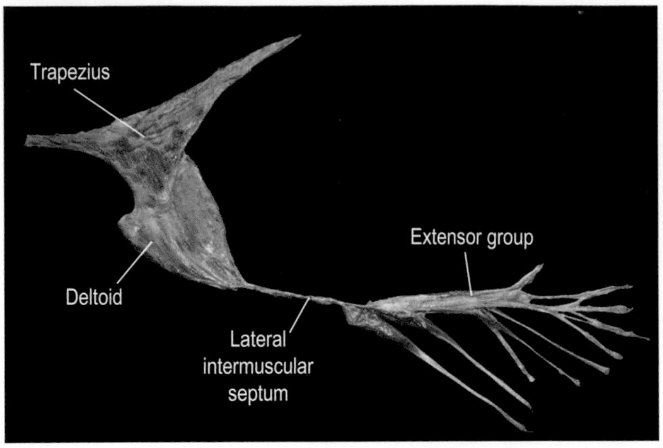

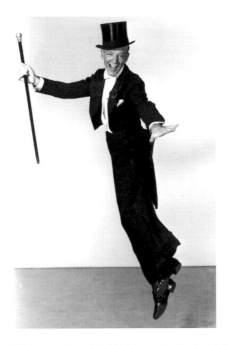

• **Fig. A1.88** This dissection clearly shows how, by changing the angle of the scalpel by 90°, it is possible to demonstrate a fascial continuity over the distal attachments of one muscle (or soft-tissue structure) to the next, forming a continuous fascial line of tension from the skull and spine to the back of the fingers – the Superficial Back Arm Line (see Ch. 7).

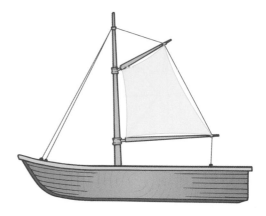

• **Fig. A1.90** A sailboat is not strictly a tensegrity structure, but its structural integrity still depends somewhat on the tension members – the shrouds, stays, halyards, and sheets that take some of the excess strain so that the mast can be smaller and lighter than it otherwise would have to be.

• **Fig. A1.89** Who more than Fred Astaire embodies the lightness and easy response suggested by the tensegrity model of human functioning? While the rest of us slog around as best we can, trying to keep our spines from compressing like stacks of bricks, his bones eternally float with a poise rarely seen elsewhere.

different parts of the body, and in different movements in various situations, from the security offered by a continuous compression structure to the sensitive poise of pure, self-contained tensegrity. We term this point of view 'tension-dependent spectrum' – the body operating through different mechanical systems dependent on local need.

A herniated disc was thought to be surely the result of trying to use the spine as a continuous compression structure, contrary to its design. Recent evidence, however,

points to microstrains in the annulus from too much grinding in rotation as a cause, more often than direct traumatic compression.[183,184] Common sense dictates that a long jumper landing at the far end of his leap relies momentarily but definitely on the compressive resistance of all the leg bones and cartilages taken together. (Though even in this case, where the bones of the leg could be thought of as a 'stack of bricks', the compressive force is distributed through the collagen network of the bones, and out into the soft tissues of the entire body in 'tensegrity' fashion.) In daily activities, the body employs a spectrum of structural models from tensegrity to more compression-based modeling.[185]

Filling in the range from the pure compression of a stack of blocks to the self-contained tensegrity of Figure A1.86, a sailboat provides one of several 'middle ground' structures (Fig. A1.90). At anchor, the mast will stand on its own, but when you 'see the sails conceive, and grow big-bellied with the wanton wind' – Shakespeare, A Midsummer Night's Dream, the fully loaded mast must be further supported by the tensional shrouds and stays or it will snap (Video 1.2). By means of the tensile wires, forces are distributed around the boat, and the mast can be thinner and lighter than it otherwise would be. Our spine is similarly constructed to depend on the balance of tension member 'stays' (the erector spinae, longissimus specifically) around it to reduce the necessity for extra size and weight in the spinal structure, especially in the lumbars (Fig. A1.91).

The structures of Frei Otto, beautiful membranous biomimetic architecture that relies on tensional principles but is not pure autonomous tensegrity (because it is anchored to and relies on its connections to the ground), can be seen in Denver's airport, or at www.freiotto.com (Fig. A1.92). Here we can see, especially with the cable and membrane structures that characterize the Munich Olympiazentrum, a further exploration of a tension–compression balance which leans strongly toward reliance on the tensional side of the spectrum. The core is flexible, held aloft only by a balance

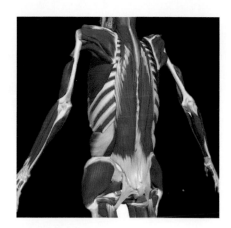

• **Fig. A1.91** In a similar way to A1.90, the erectors, specifically the longissimus, act as our 'stays' in the spine, allowing the spine to be smaller than it would otherwise have to be if it were a continuous compression structure. The iliocostalis is constructed and acts like the mast in A1.92. (Image provided courtesy of Primal Pictures, www. primalpictures.com.)

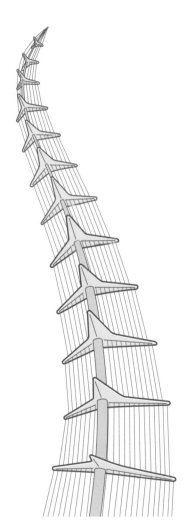

• **Fig. A1.92** This mast of Frei Otto relies even more heavily on tension for its integrity. The core is flexible, and would fall over without the cables to hold it up. By adjusting the cables and then securing them, this mast can be made a solid support in any number of different positions.

of the cords attached to its 'processes'. With the cords in place, pulling on them can put the mast anywhere within the hemisphere defined by its radius. Cut the cords, and the flexible core would fall to the ground, unable to support anything. This arrangement parallels the iliocostalis muscles, seen on the outer edge of the erectors in Figure A1.91.

While we are convinced that the body's overall architecture will ultimately be fully described by tensegrity mathematics, the safer statement at this point is that it potentially can be so employed, but frequently and sadly is used less efficiently, as described above (see Fig. A1.81). While this is a subject for further research and discussion, what is clear is that the body's tensile fascial network is continuous and pulls in toward the bones, which push out against the netting. Our body distributes strain – especially sustained long-term strain – within itself in an attempt to equalize forces on the tissues. It is clinically clear that release in one part of the body can produce changes at some distance from the intervention, though the mechanism is not always evident. This all points toward tensegrity as an idea at least worthy of consideration, if not the primary geometry for constructing a human. The models of the late inventor Tom Flemons (www.intensiondesigns.com and Figs A1.79, A1.84–A1.86) are wonderfully evocative. These early 'force diagrams' of human plantigrade posture approach, but do not yet replicate in their resilience and behavior, a human architectural model. They are brilliantly suspended in homeostasis, but are of course not self-motivating (tropic) as with a biological creature.

Pre-Stress and Elastic Energy Storage

(Fascial elasticity as a property is further discussed earlier in this appendix.) Every tensegrity system contains stored energy – it is inherent to the system: compression members have a constant compressive force pushing out, as the elastic tensional network pulls in toward the center. The resting tensegrity structure is a balance of opposing forces, not equilibrium. Deform the tensegrity, as in Figure A1.80, and additional energy is stored, to be 'given back' when the deforming force is taken away and the structure returns to its original form and balance of forces.

If any element of a tensegrity breaks – a compression strut, an elastic, or a junction – this dynamic balance is disturbed, and the structure will change shape until it either collapses completely or another balance point is reached. In our bodies, we can see this in action: in a wound that cuts the dermis, we see the sides of the wound move apart from each other, and edema rush in to the area, passively 'sucked' there by the spongy GAGs, once the restraining tensional 'squeeze' of the dermal and profundis layer has been relieved by the opening of the cut. The myofibroblasts (see section on cells, above) must pull the sides together and new fascia knit to repair the damage and restore dynamic balance again between the ground substance's desire to expand via soaking up water vs the circumferential tension of the surrounding collagen mesh. The relative hydration of our tissues, and especially the interstitial ground substance, is determined by the balance between these centripetal and centrifugal forces.

Once we take these tensegrity models into motion and differing load situations, we need more adjustability. Loose tensegrity structures are 'viscous' – they exhibit easy deformation and fluid shape change, but they will collapse under any significant load. Tighten the tensile membranes or strings – especially if this is done evenly across the board – and the structure becomes increasingly resilient, approaching rigid, columnar-like resistance. In other words, increasing the pre-stress increases the capacity of the structure to accept load without deformation.

As Ingber[167] puts it: 'An increase in tension of one of the members results in increased tension in members throughout the structure, even ones on the opposite side.' All the interconnected structural elements of a tensegrity model rearrange themselves in response to a local stress. And as the applied stress increases, more of the members come to lie in the direction of the tensional part of the applied stress, resulting in a linear stiffening of the material (though distributed in a non-linear manner) (Fig. A1.93).

This is certainly reminiscent of the reaction of the fibrous system's response to pull stresses that we described earlier in this appendix. Take a wad of loose cotton wool and gently pull on the ends to see the multidirectional fibers accommodate your stretch until suddenly the stretching comes to a stop as the lined up fibers bind. Our fibrous body reacts similarly when confronted with extra strain, just like a tensegrity structure or a Chinese finger puzzle. We can continue to pull, overcome these binding forces, and tear the cotton ball or finger-puzzle in two. When that happens in the body, it is a fascial injury.

In other words, tensegrity structures show resilience, getting stiffer as they are loaded up to the point of breakage or collapse. As stated above, if a tensegrity structure is loaded beforehand, especially by tightening the tension members ('pre-stress'), the structure is able to bear more of a load without deforming. Being adjustable in terms of 'pre-stress' allows the biological tensegrity-based structure to quickly and easily stiffen (with muscle contraction) in order to take greater loads of stress or impact without deforming, and just as quickly unload the stress so that the structure as a whole is immediately far more mobile and responsive to smaller loads (Fig. A1.94).

This leads to a more 'fascial stiffness strategy' in high-load predictable situations (weight-lifting, moving a piano) and toward a 'neuromuscular control strategy' in conditions of low-load unpredictable situations (jumping over a stream, playing ping-pong).[187] (High load and unpredictability is a recipe for injury.)

We have described two ways in which the myofascial system can remodel in response to stress or the anticipation of stress: (1) the obvious speedy one – muscle tissue can contract very quickly at the nervous system's whim within the fascial webbing to pre-stress an area or line of fascia; and (2) long-term stresses can be accommodated by the remodeling of the ECM around the stress patterns, adding matrix where more is demanded (see Fig. A1.94). Myofibroblast (MFB) contraction is a middle-ground way to add small levels of pre-stress to the fascial sheets.[154,188]

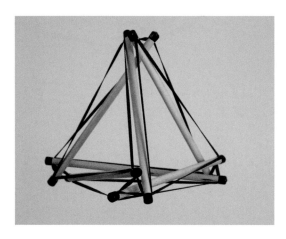

• **Fig. A1.93** A slight modification of the icosahedron in Figures A1.80 and A1.83 – simply sliding the dowel ends along the rubber bands results in a slightly truncated tetrahedron and a closer approximation of the actual human situation. In this form, the 'myofascial' elastics run in closer parallel to the 'bone' dowels (as most muscles do, especially in our limbs). The short bits of elastic near the vertices act as a kind of 'ligament' holding the dowel/bones close but not touching, in the close approximation Fuller called a 'locked kiss'. Human bones (except the hyoid and some sesamoids) do not float in isolated splendor; they are tied closely together at joints, which direct and limit movement between the bones in a definitive way compared to the total freedom offered by the idealized tensegrity of Figures A1.80 and A1.83. Apply sudden external pressure to this model to see why so many impact injuries result in ligament rather than muscle damage.

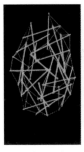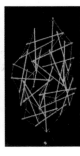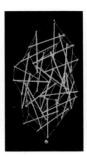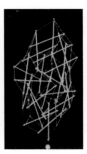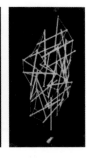

• **Fig. A1.94** By 'pre-stressing' a tensegrity structure, that is, putting a particular strain on it beforehand, we notice that (1) many of the members, both compressional and tensional, tend to align along the lines of the strain, and (2) the structure gets 'firmer' – prepared to handle more loading without changing shape as much. (Reproduced with permission from Wang, et al. 1993.[186])

The unique role of the myofibroblasts, already discussed, provides a perfect transition between the tissue-and-bone world of macrotensegrity to the cytoskeletal world of microtensegrity which is the subject of our next and last dive into the esoterica of fascia.

Biomechanical Auto-Regulation – Microtensegrity: How the Cells Balance Tension and Compression

Up to this point, we have been discussing tensegrity on the macroscopic level, as it relates to our Anatomy Trains model. In discussing the MFBs, we saw how the internal cell structure could hook to the macrostructure of the ECM. This end of the tensegrity geometry argument has recently been boosted with extensive research, now more familiar under the name mechanobiology, with relevance to movement training and manual intervention of all types. Before we leave tensegrity, we repair once again to the microscope. Here we find a new set of connections with an unexpected glimpse into the effect of movement and repositioning on cellular function, including epigenetic expression.

On the basis of this book, one could be forgiven, saving our few paragraphs about MFBs, for thinking that the cells 'float' independently within the ECM we have been describing, and indeed that is how I myself taught it for years. 'Medicine has done great things', I would pontificate, 'by concentrating on the biochemistry within the cells, while manual and movement therapists concentrate on what goes on between the cells'. The cell has been viewed as 'a water-filled balloon', in which the organelles float, in the same way the cell floats in the medium of the ECM.

This new research – and here we rely heavily on the work of Dr Donald Ingber and his faculty at the Children's Hospital in Boston – has knocked any such separation into a cocked hat. It has been definitively shown that there is a very structured and active 'musculo-skeletal system' within the cell, called the cytoskeleton, to which each organelle is attached, and along which they move.[189] The cytoskeleton is slightly misnamed in that it also contains actomyosin molecules that can contract to exert force within the cell, on the cell membrane, or – as we saw with the MFBs – through the membrane to the matrix beyond, so it is really the cell's parallel to the musculoskeletal or myofascial system. These mechanically active connections – compression-resisting microtubules, tensile microfilaments, and interfibrillar elements – run from the inner workings of nearly every cell and the ECM, a mutually active relationship that forever puts to rest the idea that independent cells float within a sea of 'dead' connective tissue products.

It has been known for some time that the 'double bag' of the phospholipid cell membrane is studded with globular proteins that offer receptor sites and ion channels both within and without the cell, to which many but highly particular chemicals could bind, changing the activity of the cell in various ways (see Fig. A1.60). Candace Pert's research

summarized in the *Molecules of Emotion*, making endorphins a household word, is one example of the kinds of links in which the chemistry beyond the cell, binding to these cross-membrane receptors, affects the physiological workings within the cell.[190]

The 'Adhesome'

The newer discovery, and one even more relevant to our work, is that in addition to these chemoreceptors, some of the membrane-spanning globular proteins (a family of chemicals known as integrins, including selectins, cadherins, and a host of new additions to the adhesome) are mechanoreceptors which communicate tension and compression from the cell's surroundings – the ECM – into the cell's interior, even down into the nucleus (Fig. A1.95). So, in addition to chemoregulation, we may now add the idea of cellular mechanoregulation.

By the early 1980s, it was understood in scientific circles that the ground substance and adhesive matrix proteins were linked into the system of the intracellular cytoskeleton.[189] It is that linkage – from the nucleus to the cytoskeleton to the focal adhesion molecules inside the membrane, through the membrane with the integrins and other transmembranous connectors, and then via the glycocalyx[191] and proteoglycans such as fibronectin to the collagen network itself (Fig. A1.96) – which is extraordinarily strong in the MFBs, working generally from the cell out onto the matrix, but the same kind of mechanoregulatory process extends to every cell, often working from the outside in: movements in the mechanical environment of the ECM can affect, for better or worse, how the cell functions.

While it is obvious that some kind of cell adhesion is necessary to hold the body together, the mechanical signaling within the 'adhesome', now called mechanotransduction, extends importantly into a wide variety of diseases, including asthma, osteoporosis, heart failure, atherosclerosis, and stroke, as well as the more obvious mechanical problems such as low back and joint pain.[192] 'Less obviously, it helps to direct both embryonic development and an array of processes in the fully formed organism, including blood clotting, wound healing, and the eradication of infection'.[167,193]

For instance:

A dramatic example of the importance of adhesion to proper cell function comes from studies of the interaction between matrix components and mammary epithelial cells. Epithelial cells in general form the skin and lining of most body cavities; they are usually arranged in a single layer on a specialized matrix called the basal lamina. The particular epithelial cells that line the mammary glands produce milk in response to hormonal stimulation. If mammary epithelial cells are removed from mice and cultured in laboratory dishes, they quickly lose their regular, cuboidal shape and the ability to make milk proteins. If, however, they are grown in the presence of laminin (the basic adhesive protein in the basal lamina) they regain their usual form, organize

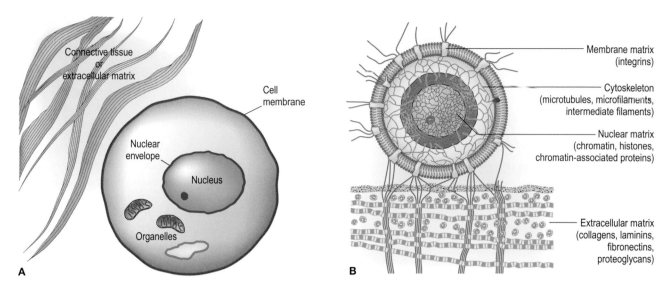

• **Fig. A1.95** Two views of the relationship between the cell and the surrounding ECM. (**A**) The traditional view, in which each element has its autonomy. (**B**) The more current view, in which the nuclear material, nuclear membrane, and cytoskeleton are all mechanically linked via the integrins and laminar proteins to the surrounding ECM. (Adapted from Oschman 2000.[41])

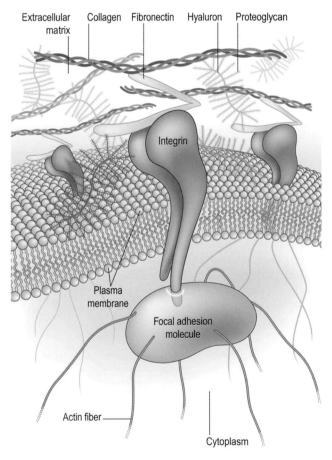

• **Fig. A1.96** The integrins – 'floating' in the phospholipid membrane – make Velcro®-like connections between the cellular elements shown in Figure A1.95 and the extracellular elements of the ECM.

a basal lamina, and assemble into gland-like structures capable once again of producing milk components.[194]

In other words, the mechanical receptors and the proteins of the ECM are linked into the cell in a communicating system via the integrins on the cell's surface. These connections act to alter the shape of the cells and their nuclei (see Fig. A1.80C), and with that, their physiological properties. How do cells respond to changes in the mechanics of their surroundings?

The response of the cells depends on the type of cells involved, their state at the moment, and the specific makeup of the matrix. Sometimes the cells respond by changing shape. Other times they migrate, proliferate, differentiate, or revise their activities more subtly. Often, the various changes issue from the alterations in the activity of genes.[194]

Information conveyed on these spring-like 'mechanical molecules' travels from the matrix into the cell to alter epigenetic or metabolic expression, and, if appropriate, out from the cell back to the matrix:

We found that when we increased the stress applied to the integrins (molecules that go through the cell's membrane and link the extracellular matrix to the internal cytoskeleton), the cells responded by becoming stiffer and stiffer, just as whole tissues do. Furthermore, living cells could be made stiff or flexible by varying the pre-stress in the cytoskeleton by changing, for example, the tension in contractile microfilaments.[167]

The actual mechanics of the connections between the extracellular matrix and the intracellular matrix is generally achieved by numerous weak bonds – a kind of Velcro® effect – rather than a few strong points of attachment. The MFBs, with their very strong connections, would be an exception. These focal adhesion and outside integrin bonds respond to changing conditions, connecting and unconnecting rapidly at the receptor sites when the cell is migrating, for instance.[195] Mechanically stressing the chemoreceptors on the cell's surface – the ones involved in metabolism, as in Pert's work – did not effectively convey force inside the cell. This job of communicating the picture of local tension and compression is left solely to the adhesive molecules, principally integrins, which appear 'on virtually every cell type in the animal kingdom'.[167]

This brings us to a very different picture of the relationship among biomechanics, perception, and health. The cells do not float as independent 'islands' within a 'dead' sea of intercellular matrix. The cells are connected to, and active within, a responsive and actively changing matrix, a matrix that is communicating meaningfully to the cell, via many connections (see Figs A1.95B and A1.96).

The connections are linked through a tensegrity geometry of the entire body, and are constantly changing in response to the cell's activity, the body's activity (as communicated mechanically along the trails of the fiber matrix), and the condition of the matrix itself.[196]

Microtensegrity and Optimal Biomechanical Health

It appears that cells assemble, function, and stabilize themselves much as we as organisms do – as a stretch activated system. Via tensional signaling, they communicate with and move through the local surroundings via adhesive molecules, and that the musculo-fascial-skeletal system as a whole functions largely as a tensegrity. According to Ingber: 'Only tensegrity, for example, can explain how every time that you move your arm, your skin stretches, your extracellular matrix extends, your cells distort, and the interconnected molecules that constitute the internal framework of the cell feel the pull – all without any breakage or discontinuity.'[167]

The sum total of the matrix, the receptors, and the inner structure of the cell constitute our 'spatial' body. Though this research definitively demonstrates its biological responsiveness, a question remains concerning whether this system is 'conscious' in any real sense, as posited earlier in this chapter, or whether we perceive its workings only via the neural stretch receptors and muscle spindles arrayed throughout the muscle and interstitia of the fibrous body.

Structural intervention – of whatever sort – works through this system as a whole, changing the mechanical relations among a countless number of individual tensegrity-linked parts, and linking our perception of our kinesthetic self to the dynamic interaction between cells and matrix.

Research into integrins has just begun to show us the beginnings of 'spatial medicine' – and the importance of spatial health:

To investigate the possibility further [researchers in my group] developed a method to engineer cell shapes and function. They forced living cells to take on different shapes – spherical or flattened, round or square – by placing them on tiny adhesive 'islands' composed of extra-cellular matrix. Each adhesive island was surrounded by a Teflon®-like surface to which cells could not adhere.[194]

By simply modifying the shape of the cell, they could switch cells among different genetic programs. Cells that were stretched and spread flat became more likely to divide, whereas rounded cells that were prevented from spreading activated a suicidal apoptotic gene. When cells are neither too expanded nor too hemmed in, they spend their energy neither in dividing nor in dying. Instead they differentiated themselves in a tissue-specific manner; capillary cells formed hollow capillary tubes, liver cells secreted proteins that the liver normally supplies to the blood, and so on.

Thus, mechanical information apparently combines with chemical signals to tell the cell and cytoskeleton what to do. Very flat cells, with their cytoskeletons overstretched, sense that more cells are needed to cover the surrounding substrate – as in wound repair – and that cell division is necessary. Rounding and pressure from all sides indicates that too many cells are competing for space on the matrix and that cells are proliferating too much; some must die to prevent tumor formation. In between those two extremes, in the 'Goldilocks', 'just right' tensional environment normal tissue function is established and maintained. Understanding how this switching occurs could lead to new approaches in cancer therapy and tissue repair and perhaps even to the creation of artificial-tissue replacements.[196]

The New Proportion

This research points the way toward a holistic role for the mechanical distribution of stress and strain in the body that goes far beyond merely dealing with localized tissue pain.[196] If every cell has an ideal mechanical environment, then there is an ideal 'posture' – likely slightly different for each individual, based on genetic, epigenetic, and personal use factors – in which each cell of the body is in its appropriate mechanical balance for optimal function. This could lead to a new and scientifically based formulation of the old search for the 'ideal' human proportion – an ideal not built on the geometry of proportion or on musical harmonics, but on each cell's ideal mechanical 'home'.

Thus, creating an even tone across the myofascial meridians, and further across the entire collagenous net, could have profound implications for health, both cellular and general. 'Very simply, transmission of tension through a tensegrity array provides a means to distribute forces to all interconnected elements, and, at the same time to couple or 'tune' the whole system mechanically as one.'[196]

For manual and movement therapists, this role of tuning the entire fascial system could have long-term effects in immunological health, improved physiology, and prevention of future breakdown, as well as in the sense of self and personal integrity. It is this greater purpose – along with coordinating movement, augmenting range, and relieving pain – that is undertaken when we seek to even out the tension to produce an equal tonus, like the lyre's string or the sailboat's rigging, across the Anatomy Trains myofascial meridians (see Fig. 1.1).

In fact, however, every cell is involved in what we could term a 'tensile field' (see also the appendix on acupuncture meridians for more in this vein). When the cell's need for space is disturbed, there are a number of compensatory moves, but if the proper spatial arrangement is not restored by the compensations, the cell function is compromised – that is what this research makes clear.[28] The experienced therapist's hand or eye can track disturbances and excesses in the tensile field, although an objective way to measure these fields would be welcome. Once discovered, any variety of treatment methods can be weighed and essayed in order to relieve the mechanical stress.

The Self-Adjusting Mechanosome

The body has to relieve and distribute such stress continually. The mechanism for doing so – a fascinating fractal adapting system in the connective tissues – has recently been uncovered and documented. We cannot leave the world of fascia without sharing some of the insights and beautiful images that have come from the work of the French plastic and hand surgeon Dr Jean-Claude Guimberteau (Video 6.13).[24,197] These images show the interface between microtensegrity and macrotensegrity (an artificial distinction in the first place as tensegrity works seamlessly across levels of scale) in action in the living body (Fig. A1.97).

So many of the images, both verbal and visual, that we present here are taken from *in vitro* laboratory experiments or from cadaverous tissue. The photos in this section were by contrast photographed *in vivo* during surgery, with permission. How well they demonstrate the healthy functioning of normal fascia, revealing a surprising new discovery of how fascial layers 'slide' on each other.

Fascial layers in the hand, specifically tendons in the carpal tunnel, must slide on each other more than any other apposite surfaces, so it is understandable that a hand surgeon like Dr Guimberteau would seek more precision on this question (Video 6.12). Every fascial plane, however, has to slide on every other if movement is not to be unnecessarily restricted. Yet, when doing dissection, one does not see fascial planes sliding freely on each other; one sees instead either a delicate fascial 'fuzz' or stronger cross-linkages that connect more superficial planes to deeper ones, as well as laterally between the epimysia.[198] This fits with the 'all-one fascia' image of continuity that is the motif for this book, but it calls into question what constitutes 'free' movement within the fascial webbing (Fig. A1.98).

Such movement within the carpal tunnel and with the lower leg tendons around the malleoli is usually depicted in the anatomies as having tenosynovial sheaths, or specialized bursae for the tendons to run in – often rendered in blue in anatomy atlases such as Netter's[120] or Gray's.[147] Dr Guimberteau has poked his camera inside these supposed bursae of the 'sliding system' and come up with a startling revelation that applies not only to his specialized area of the hand,

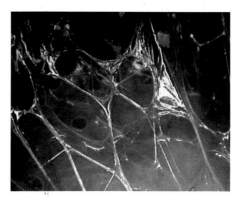

• **Fig. A1.98** 'The fibrils, made of collagen and elastin, delimit the microvacuoles where they cross each other. These microvacuoles are filled with hydrophilic jelly made of proteoaminoglycans.' What a still photo cannot convey is the fractal way these microvacuolar structures roll over each other, elasticize, reform, blend, and separate. Guimberteau synthesizes the predictions made by tensegrity geometry with the pressure system concepts from visceral manipulation proffered by another Frenchman, Jean-Pierre Barral. This system responds to all the forces under the skin – tensegrity and optimal use of space/closest packing, osmotic pressure, surface tension, cellular adhesions, and gravity. The gluey, elastic, hollow fibrils in ever-responsive interplay with the vacuoles create an array of rigging and sails that changes with every traction or movement from the outside. This gluey areolar network could be said to form a body-wide adaptive system (roughly approximated by the new term 'interstitium') allowing the myriad small movements that underlie larger voluntary efforts. (Photos (and quote) from Promenades Sous La Peau. Paris: Elsevier; 2004. With kind permission of Dr J.C. Guimberteau, Plastic and Hand Surgeon and Endovivo Productions.)

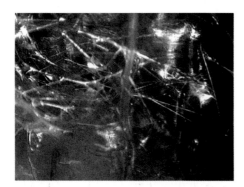

• **Fig. A1.97** Actual *in vivo* photos of the connective tissue network by Dr J.C. Guimberteau show the varying polygonal shapes of the microvacuolar sliding system – in this picture resembling the trabeculae of the bones. One can see here how the capillaries are held within the extensible connective tissue network. (With kind permission of Dr J.C. Guimberteau, Plastic and Hand Surgeon and Endovivo Productions. These illustrations are taken from 'Strolling Under the Skin' and subsequent videos, available at www.anatomytrains.com.)

but to many of the loose interstitial areas of the body: there is no discontinuity between the tendon and its surroundings. The necessary war between the need for movement and the need for maintaining connection is solved by a constantly changing, fractally divided set of polyhedral bubbles which he terms the 'multimicrovacuolar collagenic absorbing system'.[24]

The skin of these bubbles is formed from elastin and collagen types I, II, IV and VI. The bubbles are filled with 80% water, 5% fat, and 15% hydrophilic proteoglycoaminoglycans. The fern-like molecules of the sugar–protein mix (GAGs) spread out through the space, turning the contents of the microvacuole into a slightly viscous jelly. When movement occurs between the two more organized layers on either side (the tendon, say, and the flexor retinaculum), these bubbles roll and slide around each other, joining and dividing as soap bubbles do, in apparently incoherent chaos. 'Chaos', understood mathematically, actually conceals an implicate order. This underlying order allows all the tissues within this complex network to be vascularized (and therefore nourished and repaired), no matter which direction it is stretched, and without the logistical difficulties that present themselves whenever we picture the sliding systems the way we have traditionally done (Fig. A1.99).

This kind of tissue arrangement occurs all over the body, not just in the wrist. Whenever fascial surfaces are required to slide over each other in the absence of an actual serous membrane, the proteoglycans-cum collagen gel bubbles ease the small but necessary movements between the skin and the underlying tissue, between muscles, between vessels and nerves and all adjacent structures, accommodating a wide variety of forces automatically. This arrangement is almost literally everywhere in our bodies; tensegrity at work on a second-by-second basis.

There is little to add to these images; they speak for themselves. To see this system in motion, Dr Guimberteau's videos are available from www.endovivo.com and www .anatomytrains.com. (No still photo can convey how the microvacuoles and microtrabeculae rearrange themselves to accommodate the forces exerted by internal or external movement.) The trabecular 'struts' (actually parts of the borders between vacuoles) shown in Figures A1.97–A1.99, which combine collagen fibers with the gluey mucopolysaccharides, spontaneously change nodal points, break and reform, or elasticize back into the original form. Also not visible in the still pictures is how each of these sticky guy-wires is hollow, with fluid moving through the middle of these bamboo-like struts (which are perhaps the same as the conduits viewed in the interstitium – see the section above on fluid motion in fascia (Fig. A1.100).

Guimberteau's work brings together the tensegrity concepts on both a macroscopic and microscopic level. It shows how the entire organismic system is built around the pressure balloons common to both cranial osteopathy and visceral manipulation. It suggests a mechanism whereby even light touch on the skin could reach deeply into the body's structure. It demonstrates how economical use of materials can result in a dynamically self-adjusting system.

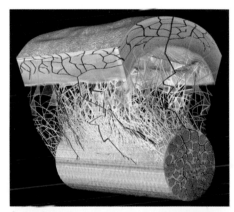

A

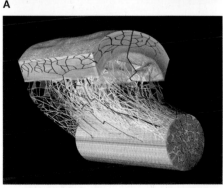

B

• **Fig. A1.99** The 'microvacuolar collagenic absorbing system' diagrammed from skin to tendon, showing how there is no discontinuity among fascial planes, just a frothy relationship of polygons that supports the vascular supply to the tendon while still allowing sliding in multiple directions. (With kind permission of Dr J.C. Guimberteau, Plastic and Hand Surgeon and Endovivo Productions.)

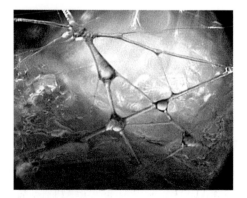

• **Fig. A1.100** The gluey, elastic, hollow fibrils in ever-responsive interplay with the vacuoles create an array of rigging and sails that changes with every traction or movement from the outside. Again, a still photo fails to convey the dynamism and ability to instantly remodel that characterizes this ubiquitous tissue. This gluey areolar network could be said to form a body-wide adaptive system allowing the small adjustments which underlie larger voluntary efforts. (With kind permission of Dr J.C. Guimberteau, Plastic and Hand Surgeon and Endovivo Productions.)

Biomechanical Auto-Regulation

One last personal note, however familiar it is, on the scientific method: it is not simply observing, but observing with understanding that makes the difference. I and many other somanauts have observed these microvacuoles as we dissected tissue. Each year at a class in the Alps we dissected the paschal lamb just after slaughtering and before it became dinner. For years I observed these bubbles between the skin and the fascia profundis and in other areolar tissue, but dismissed them as artifacts of either the dying process or being exposed to the air. Figure A1.101A is a microscopic photo we took at a fresh-tissue dissection 6 months before I was exposed to Dr Guimberteau's work. This photograph is part of a short video (Video 4.2) in which we were watching the behavior of the fascial fibers and ground substance, but completely ignored the role of the microvacuoles in the tissue samples, again dismissing them as an unimportant artifact (Fig. A1.101B).

In summary, we can see that the 70 trillion cells we call 'us' are held in place through this body-wide network of variably elastic fibers in a variably viscous hydrated glycoprotein gel. The cells are guided into place and stretched (or not) into their proper shape, and this shaping can alter their epigenetic function. This tensional environment is constantly changing with the endogenous and exogenous forces from fluid flow to gravity.

This vision – which is not visionary, it is what we can understand right now about physiology – is so beyond what the public knows about 'fascia' ('Oh yes, I know about fascia, I foam roll after my workout.') – that it requires a new term to grasp it comprehensively. Guimberteau, as noted, calls it the 'multimicrovacuolar collagenic absorbing system'. Bordoni calls it RAIN – Rapid Adapability of Internal Network.[199] We choose to call it BARS – our Biomechanical Auto-Regulatory System – since it extends from everything catalogued by the term 'fascial system' down into the very genetic programming of our cells. Whatever it is finally called, which matters little, this new vista of human physiology has the potential to marry physiotherapy, physical education, athletic performance, along with elements from psychology and medicine as we connect the mechanisms within each cell to the organic whole.

The BARS operates with the help of the nervous system, of course, but has many regulatory functions that operate beyond, faster than, and below the notice of the human nervous system. The viscous elements act like a shock absorber, a non-Newtonian fluid that auxetically absorbs and dissipates fast forces, e.g. we have noted that the synovial fluid in your finger joints is effectively 'solid' at the moment of impact from a ball, and effectively fluid a second later as you manipulate it in your hand to throw it back. The gel elements allow for free perfusion to the cells and maintain a hydration level suitable to the tissues within. The fibrous elements maintain the overall shape and the apposition of the anatomical elements.[200] In health it all works together as a supremely well-designed biomechanical regulatory system.

The challenge for the researchers and practitioners of the coming decades is to integrate this thoroughly new vision of how our cells hold together and adjust, running seamlessly from the genetic material within the nucleus all the way out to the level of the whole organism. Our practices in training, rehabilitation, and physical education across the board – what we have called 'spatial medicine' – will rise to match this model, with benefits to all those with a body that moves.

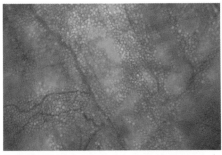

A

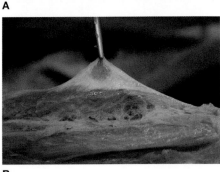

B

• **Fig. A1.101** (**A**) Microvacuoles embedded in the gluey proteoaminoglycans with capillaries running through. This photo was taken of human tissue through a microscope at a dissection conducted by the author some months before his acquaintance with the work of Dr Guimberteau. At the time, we did not know what we were looking at; in retrospect, its importance is obvious. (**B**) Similar bubbles are visible to the unaided eye in fresh animal dissection or occasionally, as here, in embalmed cadavers. Again, before being exposed to the work of Guimberteau, we took this as an artifact of death or tissue exposure during the dissection, and therefore did not realize the significance of what we were seeing. (A, Photo courtesy of Eric Root. B, Photo courtesy of the author.)

References

1. Vleeming A, Stoeckart R. The role of the pelvic girdle in coupling the spine and the legs: a clinical-anatomical perspective on pelvic stability. In: Vleeming A, Mooney V, Stoeckart R, eds. *Movement, Stability, and Lumbopelvic Pain, Integration of Research and Therapy*. Edinburgh: Elsevier; 2007.
2. Vleeming A, Pool-Goudzwaard AL, Stoeckart R, et al. The posterior layer of the thoracolumbar fascia: its function in load transfer from spine to legs. *Spine*. 1995;20:753.
3. Lee DG. *The Pelvic Girdle*. 3rd ed. Edinburgh: Elsevier; 2007.
4. Busquet L. Les chaînes musculaires. In: Frères M, Mairlot MB, eds. *Maîtres Et Clés De La Posture*. Vol. 1–4. Paris: Frison-Roche; 1992.

5. Huijing PA. Intra-, extra-, and intermuscular myofascial force transmission of synergists and antagonists: effects of muscle length as well as relative position. *Int J Mech Med Biol*. 2002;2:1–15.

6. Van der Waal JC. The architecture of connective tissue as parameter for proprioception – an often overlooked functional parameter as to proprioception in the locomotor apparatus. *Int J Ther Massage Bodywork*. 2009;2(4):9–23.

7. Margulis L, Sagan D. *What Is Life?* New York: Simon and Schuster; 1995:90–117.

8. Guimberteau J. *Strolling Under the Skin*. Paris: Elsevier; 2004.

9. Williams P. *Gray's Anatomy*. 38th ed. Edinburgh: Churchill Livingstone; 1995:75.

10. Varela F, Frenk S. The organ of form. *J of Soc Bio Structure*. 1987;10:73–83.

11. McLuhan M, Gordon T. *Understanding Media*. Corte Madera, CA: Gingko Press; 2005.

12. *Fascia Research Society*. Available: https://fasciaresearchsociety.org/.

13. *Fascia Congress. Fascia glossary of terms*. Available: https://fasciacongress.org/congress/fascia-glossary-of-terms/. Accessed April 25, 2019.

14. Williams P. *Gray's Anatomy*. 38th ed. Edinburgh: Churchill Livingstone; 1995:782.

15. Becker RO, Selden G. *The Body Electric*. New York: Quill; 1985.

16. Sheldrake R. *The Presence of the Past*. London: Collins; 1988.

17. Kunzig R. Climbing through the brain. *Discover Magazine*. 1998;(August):61–69.

18. Benias PC, Wells RG, Sackey-Aboagye B, et al. Structure and distribution of an unrecognized interstitium in human tissues. *Sci Rep*. 2018;(March):article 4947.

19. Snyder G. *Fasciae: Applied Anatomy and Physiology*. Kirksville, MO: Kirksville College of Osteopathy; 1975.

20. Langevin HM, Huijing P. Communicating about fascia: history, pitfalls, and recommendations. *Int J Ther Massage Bodywork*. 2009;2(4):3–8. *This gives a fuller discussion of the terminological issues.*

21. Williams P. *Gray's Anatomy*. 38th ed. Edinburgh: Churchill Livingstone; 1995:80.

22. Oschman J. *Energy Medicine*. Edinburgh: Churchill Livingstone; 2000:48.

23. Rettner R. Meet your interstitium, a newfound "organ". *Sci Am*. 2018;(March).

24. Guimberteau J. The subcutaneous and epitendinous tissue behavior of the multimicrovacuolar sliding system. In: Schleip R, Findley TW, Chaitow L, et al, eds. *Fascia: The Tensional Network of the Human Body*. Edinburgh: Churchill Livingstone; 2012:143–146.

25. Friedl P. Intravital microscopy of the tumor microenvironment: escape and relevance for immunotherapy. *J Acquir Immune Defic Syndr*. 2019;81:42.

26. Oschman J. *Energy Medicine*. Edinburgh: Churchill Livingstone; 2000:45–46.

27. Alberts B, Johnson A, Lewis J, et al. *Molecular Biology of the Cell*. 4th ed. New York: Garland Science; 2002.

28. Tomasek J, Gabbiani G, Hinz B, et al. Myofibroblasts and mechanoregulation of connective tissue modeling. *Nat Rev Mol Cell Biol*. 2002;3:349–363.

29. Schleip R, Klinger W, Lehmann-Horn F. Fascia is able to contract in a smooth muscle-like manner and thereby influence musculoskeletal mechanics. In: Leipsch D, ed. *Proceedings of the 5th World Congress of Biomechanics*. Munich: Medimand S.r.l.; 2006:51–54.

30. Langevin H, Cornbrooks CJ, Taatjes DJ. Fibroblasts form a bodywide cellular network. *Histochem Cell Biol*. 2004;122:7–15.

31. Gabbiani G, Hirschel B, Ryan G, et al. Granulation tissue as a contractile organ, a study of structure and function. *J Exp Med*. 1972;135:719–734.

32. Papelzadeh M, Naylor I. The in vitro enhancement of rat myofibroblast contractility by alterations to the pH of the physiological solution. *Eur J Pharmacol*. 1998;357(2–3):257–259.

33. Chaitow L, Bradley D, Gilbert C. *Multidisciplinary Approaches to Breathing Pattern Disorders*. Edinburgh: Elsevier; 2002.

34. Hinz B, Gabbiani G, Chaponnier C. The NH2-terminal peptide of α–smooth muscle actin inhibits force generation by the myofibroblast in vitro and in vivo. *J Cell Biol*. 2002; 157(4):657–663.

35. Stecco C, Fede C, Macchi V, et al. The fasciacytes: a new cell devoted to fascial gliding regulation. *Clin Anat*. 2018;31: 667–676.

36. Chaitow L. Telocytes: connective tissue repair and communication cells. *J Bodyw Mov Ther*. 2017;21(2):231–233.

37. Edelstein L, Smythies J. The role of telocytes in morphogenetic bioelectrical signaling. *Front Mol Neurosci*. 2014;7:41.

38. Van den Berg F. Extracellular matrix. In: Shleip R, Findley TW, Chaitow L, et al, eds. *Fascia: The Tensional Network of the Human Body*. Edinburgh: Churchill Livingstone; 2012:165–170.

39. Williams P. *Gray's Anatomy*. 38th ed. Edinburgh: Churchill Livingstone; 1995:475–477.

40. Feldenkrais M. *The Potent Self*. San Francisco: Harper Collins; 1992.

41. Oschman J. *Energy Medicine*. Edinburgh: Churchill Livingstone; 2000.

42. Ho M. *The Rainbow and the Worm*. 2nd ed. Singapore: World Scientific Publishing; 1998.

43. Sultan J. Lines of transmission. In: *Notes on Structural Integration*. Rolf Institute; 1988.

44. Keleman S. *Emotional Anatomy*. Berkeley: Center Press; 1985.

45. Wall ME, Banes AJ. Early responses to mechanical load in tendon. role for calcium signaling and gap junction intercellular communication. *J Musculoskelet Neuronal Interact*. 2005;5(1):70–84.

46. Banes A, Archambault J, Tsuzaki M, et al. Regulating signaling and gene expression in tendon cells with mechanical load. *Annual International Conference of the IEEE Engineering in Medicine and Biology – Proceedings*. 2002;1:429–433.

47. Pollack G. *The Fourth Phase of Water*. Seattle: Ebner & Sons; 2013.

48. Fede C, Angelini A, Stern R, et al. Quantification of hyaluronan in human fasciae: variations with function and anatomical site. *J Anat*. 2018;233(4):552–556.

49. Rolf I. *The Body Is a Plastic Medium*. Boulder, CO: Rolf Institute; 1959.

50. Currier D, Nelson R, eds. *Dynamics of Human Biologic Tissues*. Philadelphia: FA Davis; 1992.

51. Myers T, Frederick C. Stretching and fascia. In: Schleip R, Findley T, Chaitow L, et al, eds. *Fascia, the Tensional Network of the Human Body*. Edinburgh: Churchill Livingstone; 2012: 433–439. (2nd ed. planned for 2020)

52. Bobbert M, Huijing P, van Ingen Schenau G. A model of the human triceps surae muscle-tendon complex applied to jumping. *J Biomech*. 1986;19:887–898.

53. Muramatsu T, Kawakami Y, Fukunaga T. Mechanical properties of tendon and aponeurosis of human gastrocnemius muscle in vivo. *J Appl Physiol*. 2001;90:1671–1678.

54. Fukunaga T, Kawakami Y, Kubo K, et al. Muscle and tendon interaction during human movements. *Exerc Sport Sci Rev.* 2002;30:106–110.

55. Alexander RM. *Tendon Elasticity and Muscle Function.* School of Biology: University of Leeds, Leeds; 2002.

56. Reeves ND, Narici MV, Manganaris CN. Myotendinous plasticity in aging and resistance exercise in humans. *Exp Physiol.* 2006;91(3):483–498.

57. Schleip R, Müller G. Training principles for fascial connective tissues: scientific foundation and suggested practical applications. *J Bodyw Mov Ther.* 2013;17:103–115.

58. Kubo K, Kanehisa H, Miyatani M, et al. Effect of low-load resistance training on the tendon properties in middle-aged and elderly women. *Acta Physiol Scand.* 2003;178(1):25–32.

59. Kawakami Y, Muraoka T, Ito S, et al. In vivo muscle fiber behavior during countermovement exercise in humans reveals a significant role for tendon elasticity. *J Physiol.* 2002;540(2):635–646.

60. Roberts TJ, Marsh RL, Weyand PG, et al. Muscular force in running turkeys: the economy of minimizing work. *Science.* 1997;75(5303):1113–1115.

61. Daniel E, Lieberman D, Bramble D. The evolution of marathon running capabilities in humans. *Sports Med.* 2007;37(4–5): 288–290.

62. Huijing P. Force transmission and muscle mechanics. In: Schleip R, Findley TW, Chaitow L, et al, eds. *Fascia: The Tensional Network of the Human Body.* Edinburgh: Churchill Livingstone; 2012:113–116.

63. Huijing P. Myofascial force transmission, An introduction. In: Schleip R, Findley TW, Chaitow L, et al, eds. *Fascia: The Tensional Network of the Human Body.* Edinburgh: Churchill Livingstone; 2012:117–122.

64. Richter P. Myofascial Chains, a review of different models. In: Schleip R, Findley TW, Chaitow L, et al, eds. *Fascia: The Tensional Network of the Human Body.* Edinburgh: Churchill Livingstone; 2012:123–130.

65. Levin S, Martin D-C. Biotensegrity, the mechanics of fascia. In: Schleip R, Findley TW, Chaitow L, et al, eds. *Fascia: The Tensional Network of the Human Body.* Edinburgh: Churchill Livingstone; 2012:137–142.

66. Guimberteau J-C. The subcutaneous and epitendinous tissue behavior of the multimicrovacuolar sysetm. In: Schleip R, Findley TW, Chaitow L, et al, eds. *Fascia: The Tensional Network of the Human Body.* Edinburgh: Churchill Livingstone; 2012:143–148.

67. https://www.youtube.com/watch?v=r0uQYBQoBcc. Also see the many pioneering dissection films of Gil Hedley, including the remarkable ability of the subcutaneous fascial network to transmit force, at www.gilhedley.com.

68. Williams P, Goldsmith G. Changes in sarcomere length and physiologic properties in immobilized muscle. *J Anat.* 1978;127:459.

69. Williams P. *Gray's Anatomy.* 38th ed. Edinburgh: Churchill Livingstone; 1995:413.

70. von Knief J-J. Quantitative Untersuchung der Verteilung der Hartsubstanzen in Knochen in ihrer Beziehung zur lokalen mechanischen Beanspruchung. Methodik und biomechanische Problematik dargestellt am Beispiel des coxalen Femurendes. *Z Anat Entwickl-Gesch.* 1967;126:55–80.

71. Williams P. *Gray's Anatomy.* 38th ed. Edinburgh: Churchill Livingstone; 1995:448–452.

72. Williams P. *Gray's Anatomy.* 38th ed. Edinburgh: Churchill Livingstone; 1995:415.

73. Hively W. Bruckner's anatomy. *Discover Magazine.* 1998;11: 111–114.

74. Wolff J, Wessinghage D. *Das Gesetz Der Transformation Der Knochen.* Berlin: Hirschwald; 1892.

75. Bassett CAL, Mitchell SM, Norton L, et al. Repair of non-unions by pulsing electromagnetic fields. *Acta Orthop Belg.* 1978;44:706–724.

76. Lindsey M, Robertson C. *Fascia: Clinical Application for Health and Human Performance.* New York: Delmar; 2008.

77. Schleip R, Findley T, Chaitow L, et al, eds. *Fascia, the Tensional Network of the Human Body.* Edinburgh: Churchill Livingstone; 2012.

78. Schleip R, Bayer J. *Fascial Fitness.* London: Lotus Publishing; 2018.

79. *Anatomy Trains.* Online. Available: www.anatomytrains.com. Accessed September 6, 2019.

80. Myers T. *Fascial fitness: training in the neuromyofascial web.* Online. Available: https://www.anatomytrains.com/wp-content/uploads/2013/06/Fascial_Fitness__Training_in_the_Neuromyofascial_Web1.pdf. Accessed September 6, 2019.

81. Earls J, Myers T. *Fascial Release for Structural Balance.* London: Lotus, Berkeley: North Atlantic; 2010.

82. Staubesand J, Li Y. Zum Feinbau der Fascia cruris mit besonderer, Berücksichtigung epi- und intrafaszialer, Nerven. *Manuelle Medizin.* 1996;34:196–200.

83. Staubesand J, Baumbach KUK, Li Y. La structure fin de l'aponévrose jambiére. *Phlebol.* 1997;50:105–113.

84. Jarvinen TA, Jozsa L, Kannus P, et al. Organization and distribution of intramuscular connective tissue in normal and immobilized skeletal muscles. An immunohisto chemical, polarization and scanning electron microscopic study. *J Muscle Res Cell Motil.* 2002;23:245–254.

85. Wood TO, Cooke PH, Goodship AE. The effect of exercise and anabolic steroids on the mechanical properties and crimp morphology of the rat tendon. *Am J Sports Med.* 1988;16: 153–158.

86. Franchi M, Torricelli P, Giavaresi G, Fini M. Role of moderate exercising on Achilles tendon collagen crimping patterns and proteoglycans. *Connect Tissue Res.* 2013;54(4–5).

87. Neuberger A, Slack H. The metabolism of collagen from liver, bones, skin and tendon in normal rats. *Biochem J.* 1953;53:47–52.

88. Kubo K, Kawakami Y, Fukunaga T. Influence of elastic properties of tendon structures on jump performance in humans. *J Appl Physiol.* 1999;87(6):2090–2096.

89. Schoenau E. From mechanostat theory to development of the 'functional muscle-bone-unit'. *J Musculoskelet Neuronal Interact.* 2005;5(3):232–238.

90. Gracovetsky S. *The Spinal Engine.* New York: Springer Verlag; 1989.

91. Hamilton N, Weimar W, Luttgens K. *Kinesiology: The Scientific Basis of Human Motion.* New York: McGraw Hill; 2011.

92. Renstrom P, Johnson RJ. Overuse injuries in sports. A review. *Sports Med.* 1985;2(5):316–333.

93. Magnusson SP, Langberg H, Kjaer M. The pathogenesis of tendinopathy: balancing the response to loading. *Nat Rev Rheumatol.* 2010;6:262–268.

94. Janda V. Muscles and cervicogenic pain syndromes. In: Grand R, ed. *Physical Therapy of the Cervical and Thoracic Spine.* New York: Churchill Livingstone; 1988.

95. *MELT method.* Online www.meltmethod.com. Accessed September 6, 2019.

96. *Tune Up Fitness*. Online www.tuneupfitness.com. Accessed September 6, 2019.

97. *Yamuna*. Online www.yamunausa.com. Accessed September 6, 2019.

98. *Ellen Saltonstall*. Online www.ellensaltonstall.com. Accessed September 6, 2019.

99. Myers T. Kinesthetic dystonia. *J Bodyw Mov Ther*. 1998;2(2):101–114.

100. Myers T. Kinesthetic dystonia. *J Bodyw Mov Ther*. 1998;2(4):231–247.

101. Myers T. Kinesthetic dystonia. *J Bodyw Mov Ther*. 1999;3(1):36–43.

102. Myers T. Kinesthetic dystonia. *J Bodyw Mov Ther*. 1999;3(2):107–116.

103. Cole J. *Losing Touch: A Man Without His Body*. Oxford: Oxford University Press; 2016.

104. Schleip R, Mechsner F, Zorn A, Klingler W. The bodywide fascial network as a sensory organ for haptic perception. *J Mot Behav*. 2014;46(3):191–193.

105. Mitchell JH, Schmidt RF. Cardiovascular reflex control by afferent fibers of the skeletal muscle receptors. In: Shepherd JT, et al, eds. *Handbook of Physiology 2*. Vol. III. Part 2. Baltimore: Waverly Press, Inc; 1997:623–658.

106. Grunwald M. *Homo Hapticus*. Munchen: Droemer Knauer; 2018.

107. Barker D. The morphology of muscle receptors. In: Barker D, Hunt C, McIntyre A, eds. *Handbook of Sensory Physiology*. Vol. II. Muscle receptors. New York: Springer Verlag; 1974.

108. Schleip R. Fascial plasticity – a new neurobiological explanation. Part 1. *J Bodyw Mov Ther*. 2003;7(1):11–19.

109. Hoheisel U, Taguchi T, Mense S. Nociception: the thoracolumbar fascia as a sensory organ. In: Schleip R, Findley T, Chaitow L, et al, eds. *Fascia, the Tensional Network of the Body*. Edinburgh: Churchill Livingstone; 2012.

110. Craig AD. *How Do You Feel? An Interoceptive Moment With You Neurobiological Self*. Princeton, NJ: Princeton U Press; 2015.

111. Porges S. *The Polyvagal Theory*. New York: WW Norton & Co; 2011.

112. van der Kolk B. *The Body Keeps the Score*. New York: Penguin; 2015.

113. Selye H. *The Stress of Life*. 2nd ed. New York: McGraw Hill; 1978.

114. Gay P. *Freud: A Life for Our Time*. New York: WW Norton & Co; 1988.

115. Bagg M, McCauley J, Mosely GL, Benedict MW. Recent data from radiofrequency denervation trials further emphasise that treating nociception is not the same as treating pain. *Br J Sports Med*. 2019;53(13):841–842.

116. Mosley GL, Gatchel RJ, Peng YB, et al. The biopsychosocial approach to chronic pain: scientific advances and future directions. *Psychol Bull*. 2007;133(4):581–624.

117. Pongratz D, Mense S, Spaeth M. *Soft-Tissue Pain Syndromes*. Bingham, NY: Haworth Press; 2016.

118. Taguchi T, Tesarz J, Mense S. The thoracolumbar fascia as a source of low-back pain. *Pain*. 2009;138:119–129.

119. Gershon M. *The Second Brain*. New York: Harper Collins; 1998.

120. Netter F. *Atlas of Human Anatomy*. 2nd ed. East Hanover, NJ: Novartis; 1997.

121. Clemente C. *Anatomy: A Regional Atlas*. 4th ed. Philadelphia: Lea and Febiger; 1995.

122. Rohen J, Yoguchi C. *Color Atlas of Anatomy*. 3rd ed. Tokyo: Igaku-Shohin; 1983.

123. See www.anatomytrains.com. *Access to a movie version of this image plus many other fascinating views can be obtained at this website. Developed by Jeffrey Linn using the Visible Human Data Project*.

124. Read J. *Through Alchemy to Chemistry*. London: Bell and Sons; 1961.

125. Moore K, Persaud T. *The Developing Human*. 6th ed. London: WB Saunders; 1999.

126. Magoun H. *Osteopathy in the Cranial Field*. 3rd ed. Kirksville, MO: Journal Printing Company; 1976.

127. Upledger J, Vredevoogd J. *Craniosacral Therapy*. Chicago: Eastland Press; 1983.

128. Milne H. *The Heart of Listening*. Berkeley: North Atlantic Books; 1995.

129. Ferguson A, McPartland J, Upledger J, et al. Craniosacral therapy. *J Bodyw Mov Ther*. 1998;2(1):28–37.

130. Chaitow L. *Craniosacral Therapy*. Edinburgh: Churchill Livingstone; 1998.

131. Leonard CT. *The Neuroscience of Human Movement*. St Louis: Mosby; 1998.

132. Fields RD. The other half of the brain. *Sci Am*. 2004;290(4):54–61.

133. Koob A. *The Root of Thought: Unlocking Glia*. NY: FT Science Press; 2009.

134. Becker R. A technique for producing regenerative healing in humans. *Frontier Perspectives*. 1990;1:1–2.

135. Oschman J. *Energy Medicine*. Edinburgh: Churchill Livingstone; 2000:224.

136. Kunzig R. Climbing up the brain. *Discover Magazine*. 1998;8:61–69.

137. Oschman J. *Energy Medicine*. Edinburgh: Churchill Livingstone; 2000:[Ch 15].

138. Becker R. Evidence for a primitive DC analog system controlling brain function. *Subtle Energies*. 1991;2:71–88.

139. Barral J-P, Mercier P. *Visceral Manipulation*. Seattle: Eastland Press; 1988.

140. Schwind P. *Fascial and Membrane Technique*. Edinburgh: Churchill Livingstone Elsevier; 2003. (German), 2006 (English).

141. Paoletti S. *The Fasciae*. Seattle: Eastland Press; 2006. (English).

142. Wainwright S. *Axis and Circumference*. Cambridge, MA: Harvard University Press; 1988.

143. Erlingheuser RF. *The Circulation of Cerebrospinal Fluid Through the Connective Tissue System*. Academy of Applied Osteopathy Yearbook; 1959.

144. Fawcett D. *Textbook of Histology*. 12th ed. New York: Chapman and Hall; 1994:276.

145. Rhodin J. *Histology*. New York: Oxford University Press; 1974:353.

146. Rhodin J. *Histology*. New York: Oxford University Press; 1974:135.

147. Williams P. *Gray's Anatomy*. 38th ed. Edinburgh: Churchill Livingstone; 1995.

148. Sacks O. *A Leg to Stand on*. New York: Summit Books; 1984.

149. Grinnell F. Fibroblast-collagen-matrix contraction: growth-factor signalling and mechanical loading. *Trends Cell Biol*. 2002;10:362–365.

150. Discher D, Dong C, Fredberg JJ, et al. Biomechanics: cell research and applications for the next decade. *Ann Biomed Eng*. 2009;37(5):847–859.

151. Juhan D. *Job's Body*. Barrytown, NY: Station Hill Press; 1987.

152. Schleip R. *Explorations in the Neuromyofascial Web. Rolf Lines*. Boulder, CO: Rolf Institute; 1991.

153. Grunwald M. *Homo Hapticus*. Munchen: Droemer Verlag; 2018.

154. Schleip R. Active fascial contractility. In: Imbery E, ed. *Proceedings of the 1st International Congress of Osteopathic Medicine, Freiburg, Germany*. Munich: Elsevier; 2006:35–36.

155. Moore K, Persaud T. *The Developing Human*. 6th ed. London: WB Saunders; 1999:23.

156. Moore K, Persaud T. *The Developing Human*. 6th ed. London: WB Saunders; 1999:30.

157. Moore K, Persaud T. *The Developing Human*. 6th ed. London: WB Saunders; 1999:53–56.

158. Moore K, Persaud T. *The Developing Human*. 6th ed. London: WB Saunders; 1999:60.

159. Schultz L, Feitis R. *The Endless Web*. Berkeley: North Atlantic Books; 1996:8–10.

160. Larsen WJ. *Human Embryology*. New York: Churchill Livingstone; 1993:328.

161. Moore K, Persaud T. *The Developing Human*. 6th ed. London: WB Saunders; 1999:216–221.

162. Moore K, Persaud T. *The Developing Human*. 6th ed. London: WB Saunders; 1999:60–71.

163. Moore K, Persaud T. *The Developing Human*. 6th ed. London: WB Saunders; 1999:61–63.

164. Wilke Jan, Krause F, Vogt L, Banzer W. What is evidence-based about myofascial chains: a systematic review. *Arch Phys Med Rehabil*. 2016;97(3):454–461.

165. Huijing PA, Baan GC, Rebel GT. Non-myotendinous force transmission in rat extensor digitorum longus muscle. *J Exp Biol*. 1998;201:682–691.

166. Huijing PA, Yaman A, Ozturk C, et al. Effects of knee joint angle on global and local strains with human triceps surae muscle: MRI analysis indicating in vivo myofascial force transmission between synergistic muscles. *Surg Radiol Anat*. 2011;33(10):869–879.

167. Ingber D. The architecture of life. *Sci Am*. 1998;(January):48–57.

168. Ingber D. The origin of cellular life. *Bioessays*. 2000;22:1160–1170.

169. Fuller B. *Synergetics*. New York: Macmillan; 1975:[Ch 7].

170. Young JZ. *The Life of Mammals*. NY: Oxford University Press; 1957.

171. Levin SM. *Space Truss: A Systems Approach to Cervical Spine Mechanics*. San Antonio: IOP publishing; 1988.

172. Levin S. A suspensory system for the sacrum in pelvic mechanics: biotensegrity. In: Vleeming A, ed. *Movement, Stability, and Lumbopelvic Pain*. 2nd ed. Edinburgh: Elsevier; 2007.

173. Lakes R. Materials with structural hierarchy. *Nature*. 1993;361:511–515.

174. Ball P. *The Self-Made Tapestry; Pattern Formation in Nature*. New York: Oxford University Press; 1999.

175. Still AT. *Osteopathy Research and Practice*. Kirksville, MO: Journal Printing Company; 1910.

176. Rolf I. *Rolfing*. Rochester, VT: Healing Arts Press; 1977.

177. Scarr G. A model of the cranial vault as a tensegrity structure, and its significance to normal and abnormal cranial development. *Int J Osteopath Med*. 2008;11:80–89.

178. Simon H. The organization of complex systems. In: Pattee H, ed. *Hierarchy Theory*. New York: Brazilier; 1973.

179. Levin S. The scapula is a sesamoid bone. *J Biomech*. 2005; 38(8):1733–1734.

180. Levin S. *The Importance of Soft Tissues for Structural Support of the Body*. Spine: State of the Art Reviews; 1995:9(2).

181. Tyler T. Online. Available: http://hexdome.com/essays/floating_bones/index.php. Accessed September 6, 2019.

182. Ghosh P. The knee joint meniscus, a fibrocartilage of some distinction. *Clin Orthop Relat Res*. 1987;224:52–63.

183. Hu SS, Tribus C, Tay B, et al. Lumbar disc herniation section of Disorders, diseases, and injuries of the spine. In: Skinner HB, ed. *Current Diagnosis and Treatment in Orthopedics*. 4th ed. New York: McGraw-Hill; 2006:246–249.

184. Werbner B, Spack K, O'Connell GD. Bovine annulus fibrosus hydration affects rate-dependent failure mechanics in tension. *J Biomech*. 2019;89:34–39. doi:10.1016/j.jbiomech.2019.04.008. [Epub 2019 Apr 10].

185. Myers T. Tensegrity continuum. *Massage*. 1999;5/99:92–108. *This provides a more complete discussion of this concept, plus an expansion of the various models between the two extremes.*

186. Wang N, Butler JP, Ingber DE. Mechanotransduction across the cell surface and through the cytoskeleton. *Science*. 1993;260(5111):1124–1127.

187. Brown S, McGill S. How the inherent stiffness of the in vivo human trunk varies with changing magnitudes of muscular activation. *Clin Biomech (Bristol, Avon)*. 2008;23(1):15–22.

188. Shleip R, Findley T, Chaitow L, et al. *Fascia: The Tensional Network of the Human Body*. Edinburgh: Churchill Livingstone; 2012:157–164.

189. Ingber DE. Cellular tensegrity revisited I. Cell structure and hierarchical systems biology. *J Cell Sci*. 2003;116:1157–1173.

190. Pert C. *Molecules of Emotion*. New York: Scribner; 1997.

191. Saladin K. *Anatomy & Physiology: The Unity of Form and Function*. 5th ed. McGraw Hill; 2010:94–95. *Glycocalyx refers to extracellular glycoprotein produced by cells. The slime on the outside of a fish is considered a glycocalyx. External to the plasma membrane, all animal cells have a fuzzy coat called the glycocalyx. Only identical twins have chemically identical glycocalices; everyone else is unique. The glycocalyx is a type of identification that the body uses to distinguish between its own healthy cells and transplanted tissues, diseased cells, and invading organisms. The glycocalyx also includes the cell-adhesion molecules that enable cells to adhere to each other and guide the movement of cells during embryonic development. This definition marries the structural and immunological functions of the ECM and its attendant cells.*

192. Ingber D. Mechanobiology and the diseases of mechanotransduction. *Ann Med*. 2003;35:564–577.

193. Ingber D. Mechanical control of tissue morphogenesis during embryological development. *Int J Dev Biol*. 2006;50:255–266.

194. Horwitz A. Integrins and health. *Sci Am*. 1997;(May):68–75.

195. XVIVO. *Scientific Animation*. Online. Available: http://www.xvivo.net/the-inner-life-of-the-cell. Accessed September 6, 2019. *If a video could be included in a book, this one from XVIVO commissioned by Harvard would be front and center – go here for a visual feast of mechanotransduction.*

196. Ingber DE. Cellular mechanotransduction: putting all the pieces together again. *FASEB J*. 2006;20:811–827.

197. Guimberteau JC. *Promenades Sous La Peau; Strolling Under the Skin: Edition Bilingue*. Paris: Elsevier Masson SAS; 2004.

198. Hedley G. *Fascia and stretching: the fuzz speech*. Online. Available: https://www.youtube.com/watch?v=_FtSP-tkSug. Accessed September 6, 2019. *No mention of fascial fuzz can be complete without reference to Gil Hedley's 'fuzz speech'.*

199. Bordoni B, Marelli F, Morabito B, Castagna R. A new concept of biotensegrity incorporating liquid tissues: blood and lymph. *J Evid Based Integr Med*. 2018;https://doi.org/10.1177/2515690X18792838.

200. Gatt R, Vella Wood M, Gatt A, et al. Negative Poisson's ratios in tendons: an unexpected mechanical response. *Acta Biomater*. 2015;24:201–208. doi:10.1016/j.actbio.2015.06.018. [Epub 2015 Jun 20].

Appendix 2

A Note on the Meridians of Latitude: The Work of Dr Louis Schultz (1927–2007)

This book concerns itself primarily with the myofascial connections that run the full length of the body and limbs, the longitudinal meridians if you will. What we have described, of course, are only a few of the myriad fascial connections within the body. Another set, identified and written about by the late Dr Louis Schultz and Dr Rosemary Feitis, DO,[1] are local horizontal bands or straps within the body's myofascia, which act somewhat like retinacula. Like the retinacula at the ankle or wrist, they are thickenings in the deep investing layer of fascia and in the areolar layer of loose connective tissue (superficial to the myofascial layers we have been discussing; see also the discussion of Guimberteau's exploration of this layer at the end of Appendix 1) which restrain, for better or worse, the movement of the underlying tissues.

The Endless Web discusses these body retinacula in detail. However, I learned these ideas directly from Dr Schultz, to whom I owe a deep debt of gratitude. Ideas in this book about fascial embryology and fascial connectivity were all inspired by his teaching, and the myofascial meridians described are extensions of his original concept.

These straps are not described in traditional anatomy texts, but are readily visible and often palpable in the more superficial layers of tissue. Fig. A2.1 shows seven bands commonly seen in the torso. The bands are variable in their exact positioning and in their degree of tension or binding.

The chest strap – roughly corresponding to the location of a bra strap – is visible on most people in the front, at or just above the level of the xiphoid. It is easy to see how excessive tightness or binding in this strap would restrict breathing, as well as the free movement of the SFL, FFL, and SL in the superficial musculature under the strap. The other straps are more variable, but readily identifiable in many people. Since the bands lie superficially, they tend to restrict fat deposition; bands can often be identified in adipose tissue contours.

These straps can restrict or divert the pull through the superficial myofascial meridians, linking the lines together at a horizontal level, or restricting the free flow of movement through a meridian where it passes under the strap.

In structural or postural misalignment the binding nature of the straps is increased to try to stabilize an unstable structure. Interestingly the straps occur at the level of the spinal junctions (Fig. A2.2; with a similar take from another author in Fig. A2.3):

- the sphenobasilar junction connects with the eye band
- the craniocervical junction connects with the chin band
- the cervicothoracic junction connects with the collar band
- the dorsal hinge (a functional mid-thoracic hinge, usually around the level of T6) connects with the chest band
- the thoracolumbar junction connects with the umbilical band
- the sacrolumbar junction connects with the inguinal band
- the sacrococcygeal junction connects with the groin band.

The temptation to further link these levels with the autonomic plexi or endocrine glands is barely resistible.

Schultz and Feitis offer some intriguing anecdotal correlates to emotional and developmental events in connection with these bands. Since our purpose here is less explanatory and more descriptive, we simply point out the empirical existence of these bands and refer the reader to *The Endless Web* for further development of these and other related ideas.

1. The lowest band in the torso (pubic band) extends from the pubic bone in front across the groin (which is thereby shortened), around the top of the greater trochanter of the femur and across the lower buttocks, including the junction of the sacrum and coccyx.
2. The band across the lower abdomen (inguinal band) is frequently more prominent in men. It connects the two projections of the pelvic bones in front (the anterior superior spines of the ilia). It usually dips slightly downward in front, like an inverted arch. Its lower margin tends to include the inguinal ligament, connecting the band downward to the region of the

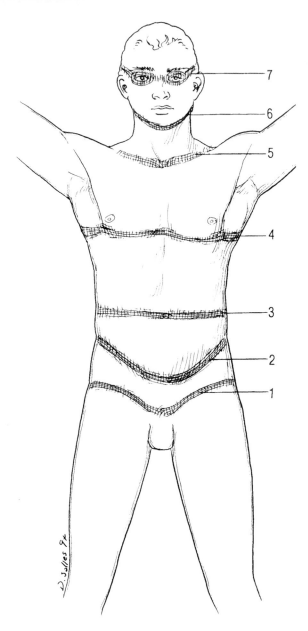

• **Fig. A2.1** Body retinacula: the seven body bands of the torso (see also Fig. A2.2). Dr Schultz has described another useful set of fascial meridians: the meridians of latitude. These bands lie in the more superficial layers of fascia for the most part, but may have connections into underlying layers and can thus affect the working transmission of the myofascial meridians described in this book. (Reproduced with kind permission from Schultz and Feitis 1996.)

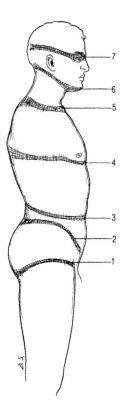

• **Fig. A2.2** Body straps, side view. The meridians of latitude girdle the body at various levels (mostly, please note, at the levels of spinal transitions). (Reproduced with kind permission from Schultz and Feitis 1996.)

pubic bone. This band extends laterally along the upper margin of the large wings of the ilia, ending at the lumbosacral junction.

3. The 3rd band crosses the abdomen (belly/umbilical band) and is perhaps the most variable in location. It may cross at the umbilicus (sometimes creating a crease in the abdominal wall extending out on either side of the umbilicus), or it may lie midway between the umbilicus and the midcostal arch (tying together the two sides of the costal arch). In either case, it will extend laterally to form an arch across the abdomen to

the lower ribs on each side – particularly to the free tip of the 11th rib. It travels backward along the lower ribs, ending at the junction of the thoracic and lumbar vertebrae.

4. The 4th band is in the area just below the nipples (chest band) and is visually the most apparent. It is usually a non-moving depressed area on the chest; the skin seems glued down onto the ribs and muscle. Laterally, it extends along the lower border of the pectoralis major, across the mid-lateral chest, and down the lateral margin of the latissimus dorsi where it begins to run parallel to the scapula toward the arm. The strap appears to tie the lower tip of the scapula to the back ribs and includes the dorsal hinge of the spine. When this strap is pronounced, there is not only a depressed mid-chest, but also an inability to expand the ribs sideways in breathing.

5. The 5th strap at the shoulders (collar band) involves the clavicle and is part of the tissue gluing the clavicle to the 1st and 2nd ribs in front. It can be felt as a pad of tissue just below and deep to the collar bone (clavicle). It extends laterally to the tip of the shoulder, with some fibers fanning down into the armpit. The strap continues toward the back on the inside and outside of the upper border of the shoulder blade (scapula), and ends at the junction of cervical and thoracic vertebrae.

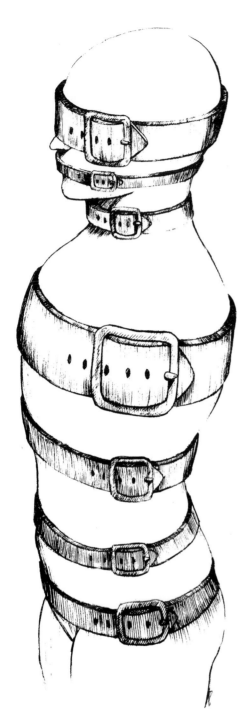

6. The area below the chin (chin band) is an area of concentration of fibers and padding which includes the hyoid bone and the base of the jaw, passing just below the ear, and including the base of the skull where it joins the first cervical vertebra (atlas).

7. The top band (eye band) is the most difficult to visualize. It originates on the bridge of the nose, travels across the eye sockets and above the ears, and includes the back of the skull just above the occipital crest and inion (the bump at the back of the skull).

Reference

1. Schultz L, Feitis R. *The Endless Web*. Berkeley: North Atlantic Books; 1996.
2. Keleman S. *Emotional Anatomy*. Berkeley: Center Press; 1985.

• **Fig. A2.3** This somewhat more pessimistic view of the horizontal body straps, drawn from Keleman's brilliant *Emotional Anatomy*,[2] nevertheless shows how these meridians of latitude act as controls on the pulsation, flow, pressure, and shape of the inner tubes and pouches of the organism. (Reproduced with kind permission from Keleman 1985.[2])

Appendix 3

Structural Integration

Since initial publication, the Anatomy Trains scheme has served a wide field of manual and movement workers, including orthopedists, orthodontists, physiatrists, nurses, midwives, physical therapists, osteopaths, chiropractors, massage therapists, yoga teachers, athletes and their conditioning coaches, martial artists, personal trainers, and body-centered psychologists.

The Anatomy Trains map derived from our own attempt to organize a progressive series of sessions to unravel the postural and functional compensations discussed throughout the book and assessed in Chapter 11 (a sample chart for noting such assessments is shown in Fig. A3.1). This 'recipe' for working the lines in progression follows the same principles the author learned from Dr Ida Rolf (see Fig. 1.15, p. 10), and the resultant approach accordingly retains her term for it – 'structural integration'. Graduates of our Anatomy Trains Structural Integration (ATSI – www.anatomytrains.com/atsi) program are certified in structural integration and eligible to join the International Association of Structural Integrators (IASI – www.theIASI.net) (Fig. A3.2).

The idea in structural integration is to use connective tissue manipulation (myofascial work) and movement reeducation to lengthen the body and organize it around its vertical axis. By 'redraping' the myofascial cape over the skeletal frame (see Fig. A1.74; Video 1.1) or by achieving the 'floating bones' of coordinated fascial tensegrity, if you prefer (see Fig. A1.77), we see generally greater symmetry around the Euclidian planes. This restores the feeling of 'lift' as the person elongates from whatever random pattern they may have had toward the highest potential and kinetic energy of an easy upright alignment. In physical terms, this process seeks to lower the moment of inertia around the vertical axis, readying our bodies for all available movements without initial preparation (Figs A3.3 and A3.4).

The ATSI approach differs somewhat from other Rolf-derived schools in that our series of 12 soft-tissue manipulation sessions is based around reading and treating the cohesive myofascial continuities of the Anatomy Trains, rather than following any set formula. We include this brief guide to how our particular approach to this method unfolds, in hopes that this might be useful for others wishing to put the Anatomy Trains into practice (Video 1.5). Of course, such an overview elides many complexities and the varying application to individual peculiarities. Some of the actual techniques that are employed in the training program are written up in this book, more appear in *Fascial Release for Structural Balance*,[1] others in our video presentations including those on this book's website, and still others (for safety reasons) only in our training programs.

So, with the proviso that this Appendix is not meant to limit experimentation and innovation, we present an outline of how we currently apply the Anatomy Trains map in our training programs. This Appendix will perhaps mean less to movement therapists, but more to manual therapists, especially those who employ 'direct' myofascial techniques.

The general order in myofascial release procedures dictates that we begin with the more superficial lines – the Superficial Front Line, the Superficial Back Line, the Lateral Line, and finally the Spiral Line. This is followed by work with what is popularly called 'core', gathered in the Deep Front Line. The final stage of the process calls for integrating sessions that bring the core and the superficial 'sleeve' together in a coordinated symphony of movement with an 'easy' relaxed posture and 'acture'.

Looking at the overall sequence before we outline each session (Fig. A3.5), we note some elements that differ from other, similar approaches:

1. The Arm Lines, and shoulder myofascia in particular, come in for significant differentiating work for each of the first four sessions, since the myofascia of the arms is even more superficial than the Front, Back, and Lateral Lines. They have a session of their own at the end, when the shoulder and arm assembly must be reintegrated into the new support from the decompensated trunk. The Functional Lines, joining the arms to the contralateral leg across the front and back of the trunk, generally come in for consideration during these integrating sessions.

2. Opening the lower leg, line by line, compartment by compartment, is spread over the first five sessions, giving plenty of time to open, de-adhere, and balance the foundations of our structure. This area comes up again for integration in the 9th and 12th sessions as well.

3. The middle four sessions really explore and reorganize the core in a manner not attempted by other bodywork approaches. These sessions extend the connections of 'core' far beyond the usual meaning of the pelvic floor and inner abdominal muscles to a coherent fascial unity that runs from the bottom of the

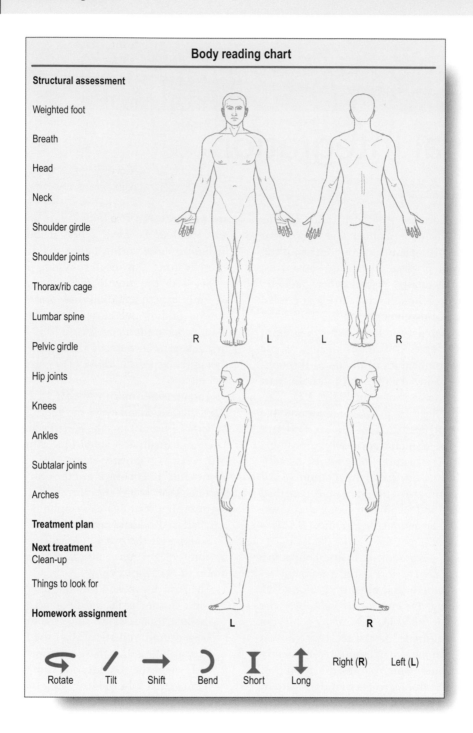

Body reading chart

Structural assessment

Weighted foot

Breath

Head

Neck

Shoulder girdle

Shoulder joints

Thorax/rib cage

Lumbar spine

Pelvic girdle

Hip joints

Knees

Ankles

Subtalar joints

Arches

Treatment plan

Next treatment
Clean-up

Things to look for

Homework assignment

R   L   L   R

L   R

Rotate   Tilt   Shift   Bend   Short   Long   Right (**R**)   Left (**L**)

• **Fig. A3.1** Body reading chart for assessment purposes.

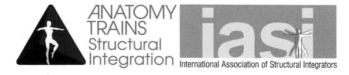

ANATOMY TRAINS Structural Integration   **iasi** International Association of Structural Integrators

• **Fig. A3.2** The logo for Anatomy Trains Structural Integration, a brand of Structural Integration based on the Anatomy Trains, and the logo for the International Association of Structural Integrators, the professional organization for all Structural Integration practitioners worldwide.

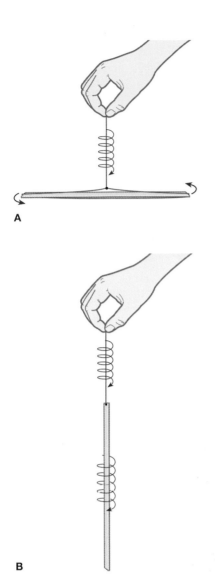

A

B

• **Fig. A3.3** Given that the stick on the top and the stick on the bottom have the same mass, the stick on the bottom has a lower 'moment of inertia'. Imagining that the stick is suspended from its middle, a large number of turns in the string would be necessary to set the stick in motion. On the bottom, we can intuit that only a few turns of the string would set the stick in rapid motion. The mass is the same in both; the difference between the two is the distance from the axis of rotation of the mass. One sees the same effect in figure skating, where the skater starts to spin slowly with her arms out. When she brings her arms into her body, lowering her moment of inertia, the speed increases to a blur. Putting the arms back out allows her to slow again. Slouching, taking a wide stance, or any of the tilts and shifts described in Chapter 11 will increase our moment of inertia and make stabilization of movement just that much harder, necessitating excess muscle tension and fascial binding that forces compression into the joints.

foot to the skull. The last of these, the 8th session (for the neck and head) is a fulcrum between the differentiation and integration – it both completes the first and begins the second.

With the proviso that each session differs in emphasis, method, and order depending on the client's individual pattern, the sessions unfold in the following manner (more detail regarding the details of addressing each line listed can be found in the chapters, as well as on the website – www.anatomytrains.com).

The Anatomy Trains 'Recipe'

Superficial Sessions

Session 1

Open the Superficial Front Line, and differentiate Superficial and Deep Front Arm Lines from axial body (Fig. A3.6).
   Goals:
- Successfully introduce the client to deep, direct fascial work
- Open the breath in the front, disengage patterns of fear
- In general, lift the Superficial Front Line, and open the proximal portions of the Front Arm Lines.
   Key structures (Videos 3.1–3.3):
- Ankle retinacula and crural fascia
- Subcostal arch and sternal fascia
- Sternocleidomastoid and superficial neck fascia.

Session 2

Open the Superficial Back Line, and differentiate the Superficial Back and Deep Back Arm Lines from axial body (Fig. A3.7).
   Goals:
- Deepen the touch into the heavy fascia and endurance fibers of the posterior musculature
- Improve grounding, bringing the client onto their legs and feet
- Bring initial balance to the primary and secondary curves
- In general, drop the Superficial Back Line, and even the tonus of the Back Arm Lines.
   Key structures (Videos 3.4, 3.6):
- Plantar aponeurosis
- Hamstring fascia
- Erector spinae
- Suboccipital muscles.

Session 3

Open the Lateral Line, differentiate all four Arm Lines from above and below, and open lateral aspects of the Deep Front Line at either end of the rib cage (Fig. A3.8).
   Goals:
- Open the body's sides, spread the 'wings' of the breath
- Contact and balance the body's stabilizing system
- Contact the body's 'lateral core'.
   Key structures (Videos 3.8–3.10):
- Peroneal fascia
- Iliotibial tract
- Lateral ribs
- Quadratus lumborum and scalene myofascia.

Session 4

Balance superficial myofasciae in terms of tonal balance of both right and left Spiral Line (Fig. A3.9).

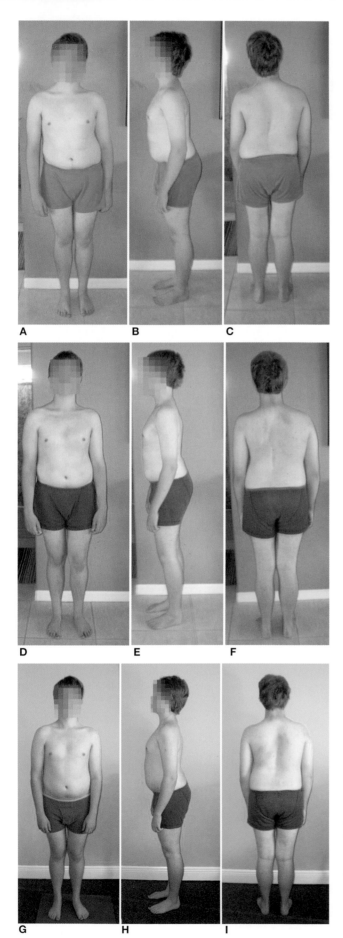

A B C

D E F

G H I

• **Fig. A3.4** Most clients achieve a smaller moment of inertia around the vertical axis during structural integration processing. Here we see a child with considerable imbalance before structural integration (**A–C**), in the midst of the process (**D–F**), at completion (**G–I**). Notice the progressive establishment of alignment around a central axis. After some months of 'absorption' time, this boy would be ready for more intervention to continue the process until no more could be achieved. Assigning specific exercises between rounds of Structural Integration could be very helpful if the child complies, but the results shown were attained through manual intervention only. (Courtesy of Lauree Moretto.)

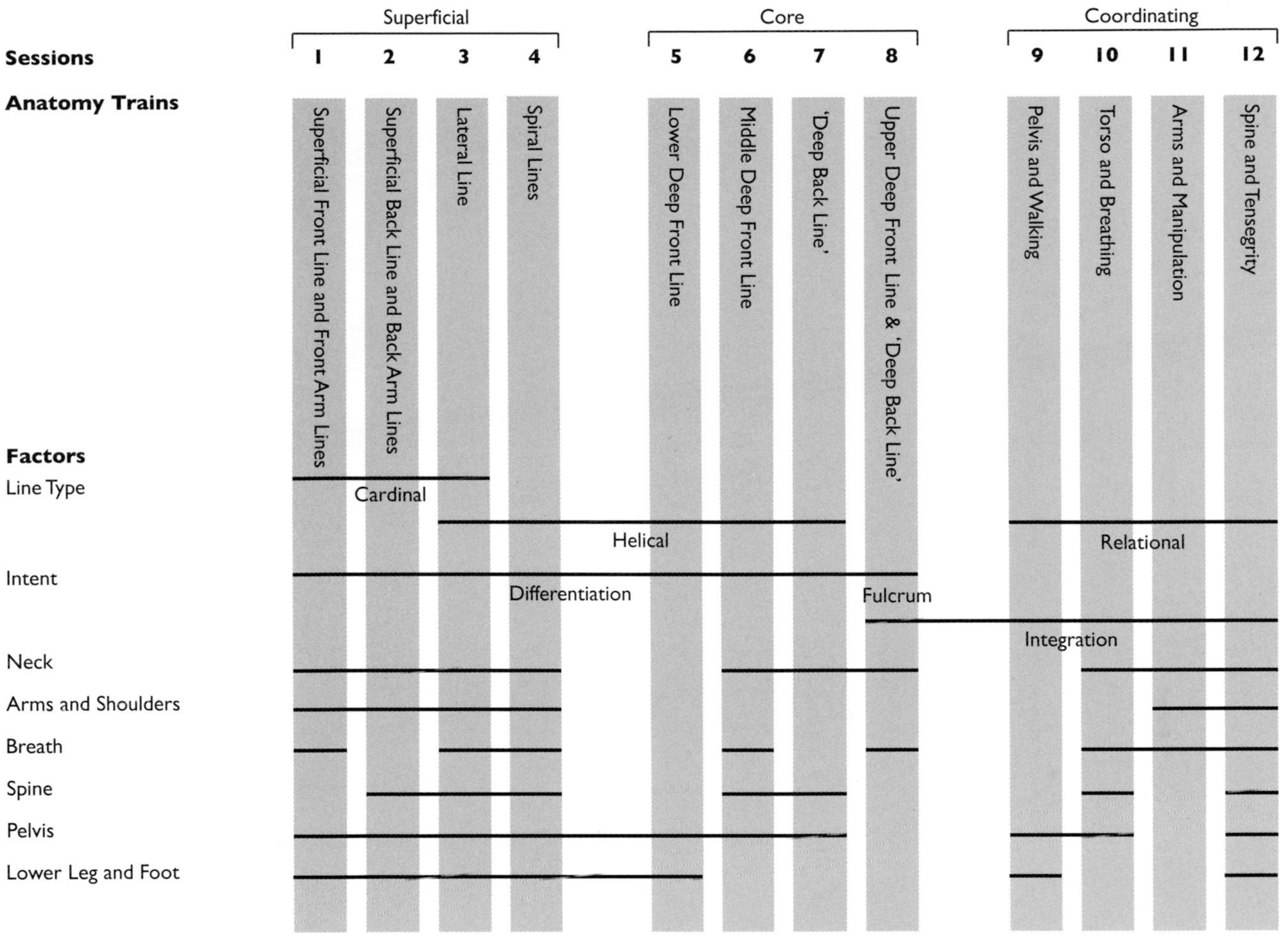

	Superficial				Core				Coordinating			
Sessions	1	2	3	4	5	6	7	8	9	10	11	12
Anatomy Trains	Superficial Front Line and Front Arm Lines	Superficial Back Line and Back Arm Lines	Lateral Line	Spiral Lines	Lower Deep Front Line	Middle Deep Front Line	'Deep Back Line'	Upper Deep Front Line & 'Deep Back Line'	Pelvis and Walking	Torso and Breathing	Arms and Manipulation	Spine and Tensegrity

Factors

Line Type — Cardinal / Helical / Relational

Intent — Differentiation / Fulcrum / Integration

Neck

Arms and Shoulders

Breath

Spine

Pelvis

Lower Leg and Foot

• **Fig. A3.5** The Anatomy Trains recipe in diagrammatic summary.

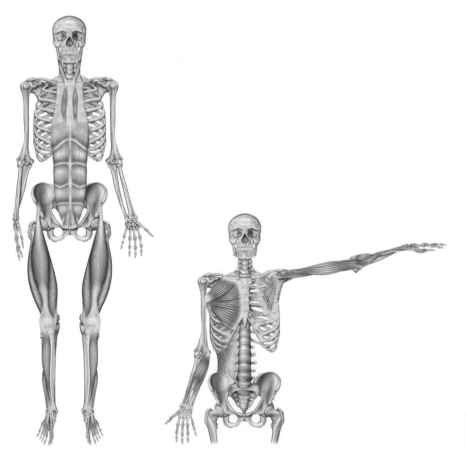

• **Fig. A3.6** The first session concentrates on lifting the Superficial Front Line and opening the two Front Arm Lines.

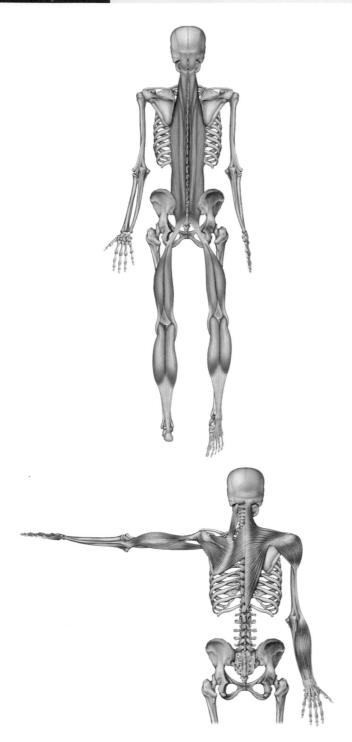

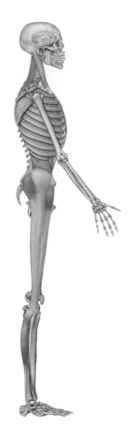

• **Fig. A3.8** The third session focuses on the Lateral Line, and balancing the shoulders onto it.

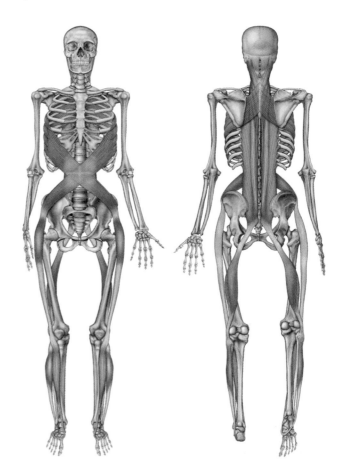

• **Fig. A3.7** The second session grounds the Superficial Back Line and opens the two Back Arm Lines.

• **Fig. A3.9** The fourth session balances the double helix of the Spiral Lines, including the sling under the arch of the foot and the scapular position relative to the head and ribs.

Goals:
- Ease the restrictions in any superficial rotations
- Balance the sling around the scapula
- Balance the sling under the foot arches
- Complete the work on the superficial sleeve lines.
  Key structures (Videos 3.12, 6.9, 6.24):
- Rhombo-serratus complex
- Abdominal obliques
- Tibialis anterior–peroneus longus sling.

Core Sessions

Session 5

Open the lower portion of the Deep Front Line, and balance with Lateral Line (Fig. A3.10).
Goals:
- Build support through the inner leg
- Open and balance the adductor compartment
- Release the pelvis from below.
  Key structures (Videos 3.17, 6.3):
- Deep posterior compartment of leg
- Adductor group
- Pelvic floor/levator ani
- Psoas complex attachments at lesser trochanter.

Session 6

Open the trunk portion of the Deep Front Line, and revisit the Front Arm Lines, especially the Deep Front Arm Line (see Figs A3.6 and A3.10).
Goals:
- Find appropriate support and positioning for the lumbars
- Balance psoas and diaphragm to release the 'deeper breath'
- Find reciprocity between the pelvic floor and respiratory diaphragm.
  Key structures:
- Psoas
- Diaphragm
- Anterior longitudinal ligament, visceral attachments (Fig. A3.11)
- Deep laminae of abdominal myofascia.

Session 7

Open the 'Deep Back Line', relate to the Deep Front Line, with attention to the inner bag issues of support from calcaneus to ischial tuberosities to sacrum to mid-dorsal hinge of spine (Fig. A3.12).
Goals:
- Align the bony support in the back of the body
- Free the intrinsic motions of the sacrum
- Ease spinal bends and rotation.
  Key structures (Video 6.7):
- Piriformis and deep lateral rotators
- Pelvic floor muscles
- Calcanei
- Multifidi and transversospinalis muscles.

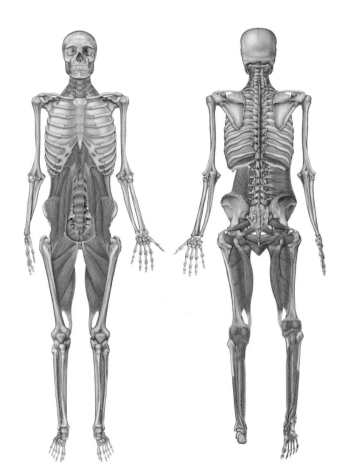

• **Fig. A3.10** The core sessions, beginning with session 5, concentrate on the Deep Front Line, which runs from the inner arch up through and around the pelvis and viscera to the jaw.

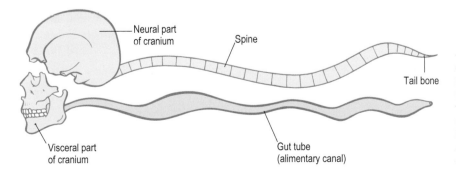

• **Fig. A3.11** The 'core sessions, especially session 6, make much of the separation and proper 'span' between the neuro-muscular body (what Maria Montessori called the 'white man', above) distinct from the visceral body (what she called the 'red man', below). The division is right at the anterior longitudinal ligament, running from the tail bone and anus caudally to the separation between the viscerocranium and neurocranium at the top end.

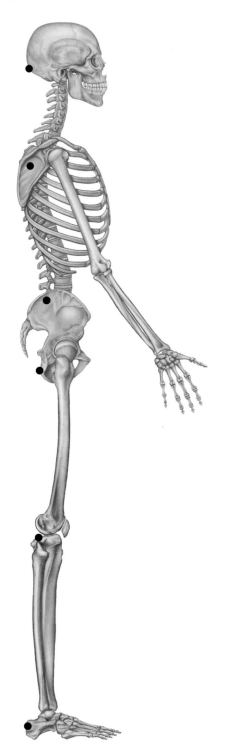

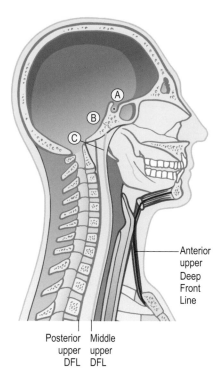

Anterior upper Deep Front Line

Posterior upper DFL

Middle upper DFL

• **Fig. A3.13** Session 8 is an opportunity to 'put the head on'. At a deeper level, it is about bringing together the multiple physiologies of the neck and head, where the ectoderm, mesoderm, and endoderm meet very closely (see p. 296).

- Balance the jaw and 'viscerocranium'
- Begin the integration via the neck.
  Key structures:
- Sphenoid bone
- Temporomandibular joint and jaw muscles
- Hyoid complex
- Cervical vertebrae, deep anterior neck muscles.

Integration Sessions (Fig. A3.14)

Session 9

Promote tonal balance, generous movement, and integration in the seven lines that run through the pelvis and legs, with emphasis on gait and pelvic support.

Session 10

Promote tonal balance, generous movement, and integration in the eleven lines that run through and around the rib cage, with emphasis on breathing and functional integration of the trunk.

Session 11

Promote tonal balance, generous movement, and balanced integration in the four lines of the arms and shoulder girdle, with emphasis on functional integration of client's arm movements (Videos 3.13–3.15).

• **Fig. A3.12** Session 7 works with the deeper tissues on the back of the body to align the major bony landmarks – the heels, ischial tuberosities, sacroiliac joints, mid-dorsal hinge, and the occiput. The deep lateral rotators are key to this session.

Session 8

Open the neck and head portions of the Deep Front and 'Deep Back' Lines, and relate to Arm Lines (Fig. A3.13).
  Goals:
- Align the head atop the body

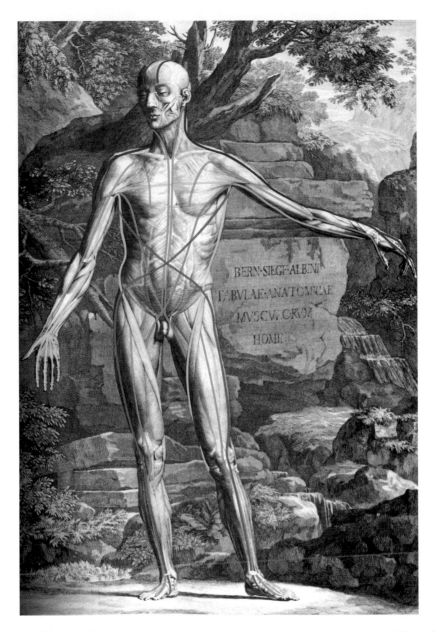

• **Fig. A3.14** The integrating sessions are a chance to bring harmony and coordination to the 12 myofascial meridians, moving progressively up the body. Session 9 deals with the pelvis and legs, session 10 with the torso and breath enhancement, session 11 with the shoulders and arms, and session 12 with the spine and neck relating out to the whole body. (With thanks for use of Albinus's brilliant drawing, courtesy of Dover Publications.)

Session 12

Promote balance of deep muscles of the spine, and tonal balance across the entire body, with emphasis on movement integration of the spine.

Principles of Treatment

The recipe above is derived from these principles:

1. There must be sufficient *energy* available – nutritional, physical, hormonal, etc. – to reach the stated goals for both practitioner and client. If the energy available is insufficient, then one must either find more or persuade the client to lower their sights.
2. Use the available energy to seek increased functional and tissue *adaptability* in any given area.
3. Via the new tissue adaptability, change segmental relationships to gain increased *support*.
4. Once support is improved, seek *release* of underlying strain patterns.
5. When release occurs, *integrate* the new pattern into everyday function and posture.

Guidelines for Strategy

The following offers some general guidance in using the Anatomy Trains myofascial meridians system in manual therapy:

- *In palpatory assessment, start from the affected/restricted/injured/painful area and move out along the trains.* If treatment to a local area is not working, seek other areas along the meridian that may yield results at the affected area (e.g. if the hamstrings are not yielding to direct manipulation or stretching, try elsewhere along the Superficial Back Line – the plantar fascia or suboccipital areas can be fruitful, for example).
- *Work on the meridians can often have distant effects.* By whatever mechanism, work on one area of a meridian can show its effect somewhere quite distant, either up or down the meridian involved. Be sure to reassess the whole structure periodically to see what global effects your work may be having.
- *Work the tissue of the meridian in the direction you want it to go.* If you are simply loosening a muscular element of a meridian, direction is not as crucial. If you are shifting the relation among fascial planes, it is. 'Put it where it belongs and call for movement', was Dr Ida Rolf's terse summary of her method. Frequently, for instance, the tissues of the Superficial Front Line need to move up in relation to the tissues of the Superficial Back Line, which need to move down to more effectively 'drape the toga' of the myofascia over a balanced skeleton (see Fig. 4.5).
- *Work from the outside in, and then inside out.* Sort out the compensations in the more superficial layers first, as far as is practical, before taking on the more deeply embedded patterns. In general, look for a uniform resilience and adaptability in the Superficial Front and Back Lines, and the Lateral and Spiral Lines before attempting to unravel the Deep Front Line. Going for deep patterns too quickly, before loosening the overlying layers, can result in driving patterns deeper or reducing the body's coherence, rather than resolving problems. Once some resilience and balance is established in the Deep Front Line, return to the issues remaining in the more superficial lines, and drape the Arm and Functional Lines over the rebalanced structure.

Principles of Body and Hand Use

General principles for fascial and myofascial manipulation are as follows:

- *Pay attention.* Though we tend to pay attention to how we contact the client or patient, i.e. what is coming out of your hands toward the client, less time is given in training to what the practitioner is feeling, i.e. what is coming up your arm *from* the client. Be sure you are attentive to what the tissue is telling you at all times.

- *Layering.* Go in only as far as the first layer that offers resistance, and then work within and along that layer.
- *Pacing.* Speed is the enemy of sensitivity; move at or below the rate of tissue melting.
- *Body mechanics.* Minimal effort and tension on the part of the practitioner leads to maximum sensitivity and conveyance of intent to the client. Using your weight and 'compound essence of time' is always better than using your strength to force tissue change. Principles of body mechanics are widely taught in training and widely ignored in practice.
- *Movement.* Client movement makes myofascial work more effective. With each move you make, seek a movement direction to give the client. Again, 'put it where it belongs and call for movement.' The client's movement, even a small movement, under your hands serves at minimum two purposes:
  - it allows the practitioner to feel with ease in which level of myofascia he is engaged
  - it involves the client actively in the process, increasing the proprioception and interoception from muscle spindles and fascial stretch receptors.
- *Pain.* Pain is sensation accompanied by the client's 'motor intention to withdraw'. It is a reason to stop, let up, or slow down, or if entering the area is necessary to the therapy, to obtain full and informed consent from the client.
- *Trajectory.* Each move has a trajectory or an arc – a beginning, a middle, and an end, and each move involves depth, direction, and duration. Each session has an arc, each series of sessions has an arc – know where you are in these overlapping arcs.

Goals

The goals of myofascial or movement work include the following:

- *Complete body image.* The client has access to the information coming from, and motor access to, the entire kinesthetic body, with minimal areas of stillness, holding, or 'sensory–motor amnesia'.
- *Skeletal alignment and support.* The bones are aligned in a way that allows minimum effort and maximum poise for standing and action.
- *Tensegrity/palintonicity.* The myofascial tissues are balanced around the skeletal structure such that there is a general evenness of tone, rather than islands of higher tension or slack. The opposite of structural integration is structural isolation.
- *Length.* The body lives its full length in both the trunk and limbs, and in both the muscles and the joints, rather than moving in shortness and compression.
- *Resilience.* The ability to bear stress without breaking, and to resume a balanced existence when the stress is removed. Ultimately, resilience is the ability to learn from stressful situations.

- *Ability to hold and release somato-emotional charge.* The ability to hold an emotional charge without acting it out, and to release it into action or simply into letting go when the time is appropriate.
- *Unity of intent with diffuse awareness.* Structural Integration implies the ability to focus on any given task or perception while maintaining a diffuse peripheral awareness of whatever is going on around this focused activity. Focus without contextual awareness breeds a fanatic; awareness without focus breeds a space cadet.
- *Reduced effort.* Reduced effort in standing and movement – less 'parasitic' tension or unnecessary compensatory movement involved in any given task.

- *Range of motion.* Generosity of movement, less restriction in any given activity, and that – within the limits of health, age, history, and genetic make-up – the full range of human movement is available.
- *Reduced pain.* Standing and activity be as free of structural pain as possible.

Reference

1. Earls J, Myers T. *Fascial Release for Structural Balance*. Berkeley: North Atlantic; London: Lotus Publishers; 2010.

Myofascial Meridians and Asian Medicine

The Anatomy Trains myofascial meridians evolved solely within the Western anatomical tradition. Initially, we deliberately omitted any comparison to the acupuncture and similar meridians used in traditional Asian medicine, in order to emphasize the anatomical basis of these continuities. The close relationship between the two, however, is inescapable, especially in light of recent research detailing the effects of acupuncture on and through the extracellular matrix produced by the connective tissue cells. Here we include a comparison of the acupuncture meridians, the Sen lines of Thai yoga massage, and the Anatomy Trains. Since we are all studying the same human body, it is unsurprising that we find overlap near the summit of two different routes of ascent.

To correct our ignorance of Asian medicine, we enlisted Dr Peter Dorsher,[1] Dr C. Pierce Salguero,[2–6] Dr Helene Langevin,[7–22] and Dr Phillip Beach, DO[23] to help in accurately depicting these meridians and teasing out their details. There is much variation among the many Asian medicine traditions in how the meridians are portrayed, so we have chosen the road more traveled and have not strayed into the underbrush of such variations.

As the accompanying illustrations from Dr Dorsher show, the Superficial Front Line (SFL), Superficial Back Line (SBL), and Lateral Line (LL) myofascial continuities show significant overlap with the energetic continuities of the Stomach meridian, Bladder meridian, and Gallbladder meridian, respectively (Fig. A4.1A–D).

The four Arm Lines, from Superficial Front to Superficial Back, correspond quite closely to the Pericardium, Lung, Small Intestine, and Triple Heater meridians respectively (Fig. A4.2A–D).

The Deep Front Line, which is only occasionally accessible near the surface of the body, corresponds to the Liver meridian, which likewise travels through and around the ventral viscera, but in some areas parallels the Kidney meridian that traverses the inner line of the leg (Fig. A4.3A,B).

When it comes to the so-called helical lines – the Spiral Line and the Functional Lines – we find a problem in that they cross the body's front and back midline to join biomechanically with structures on the other side of the body, whereas no acupuncture meridian crosses the midline. The Stomach meridian most closely approximates the anterior portion of the Spiral Line; when combined with the Bladder meridian, most of the Spiral Line is duplicated, but this correspondence is a bit contrived (Fig. A4.4).

If we switch our attention to the Sen lines used in traditional Thai massage, we find that while no meridians cross in the posterior aspect, many lines seem to meet and cross at the navel or *hara* in the front (Fig. A4.5).

Specifically, the Kalatharee line crosses in the front, joining (and mirroring the Anatomy Trains map) the front of the arm (Superficial Front Arm Line) across the body's midline to the contralateral femur (Front Functional Line), and connecting from the adductor longus down through the inner line of the leg to the inner arch (via the Deep Front Line – Fig. A4.6).

Recent research highlights the link in both form and function between the workings of acupuncture and the fascial network in general. Findings by prominent acupuncture researcher and neuroscientist Dr Helene Langevin and others have shown that connective tissue – specifically the hydrophilic proteoglycans along with collagen fibers and fibroblasts – winds around the end of the acupuncture needle when it is rotated in place, creating detectable mechanical tissue effects (Fig. A4.7). These effects have been noted 4 cm away from the site of needle insertion (as this was the limit of the field of view; new experiments are underway to establish if the effect can be detected at a greater distance).

Additionally, Langevin postulated that Asian acupuncture meridians may follow intermuscular or intramuscular fascial planes. These findings, taken together, link the possible effects of acupuncture stimulation with the mechanical transduction within fascial planes of the extracellular matrix (ECM) detailed in Appendix 1 (although of course other effects may be taking place with acupuncture as well). Langevin found an 80% correspondence in the arm between the sites of traditional acupuncture points and these fascial planes of division in the interstitial connective tissue.

This suggests that the clear 'signaling' and action at a distance which one associates with acupuncture is connected at the cellular and histological level with the new mechanotransduction communication channels being discovered among the connective tissue cells, such as fibroblasts and leucocytes, and the interstitium – the ECM

Text continued on p. 353

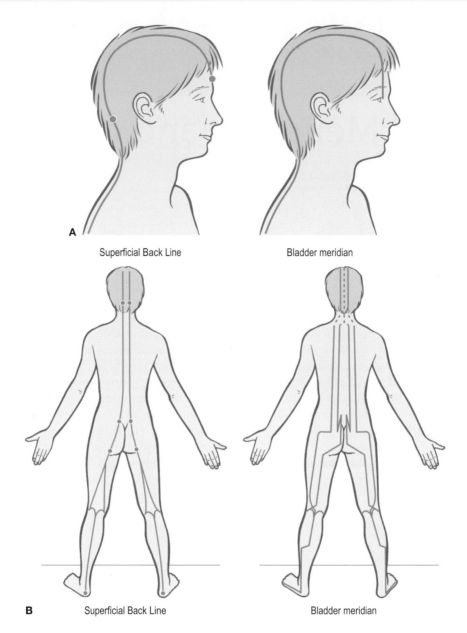

A

Superficial Back Line   Bladder meridian

B   Superficial Back Line   Bladder meridian

• **Fig. A4.1** There is a fairly close correspondence between the path of the Back, Front, and Lateral Lines and the Bladder (**A–B**), Stomach (**C**), and Gallbladder (**D**) meridians, respectively. (Used with the kind permission of Dr Peter Dorsher.)

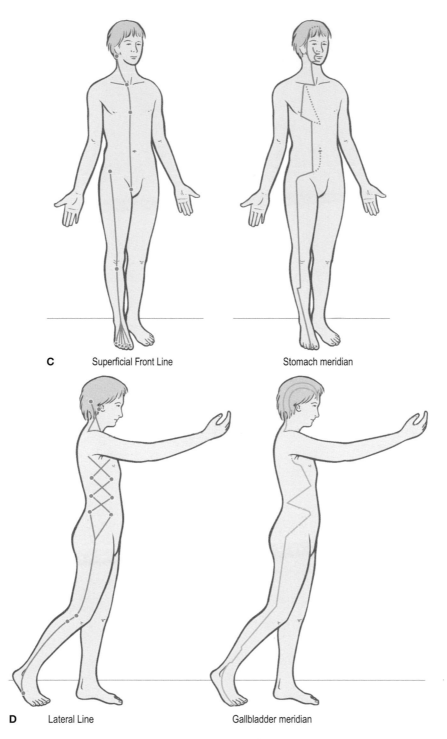

C   Superficial Front Line   Stomach meridian

D   Lateral Line   Gallbladder meridian

• Fig. A4.1, cont'd

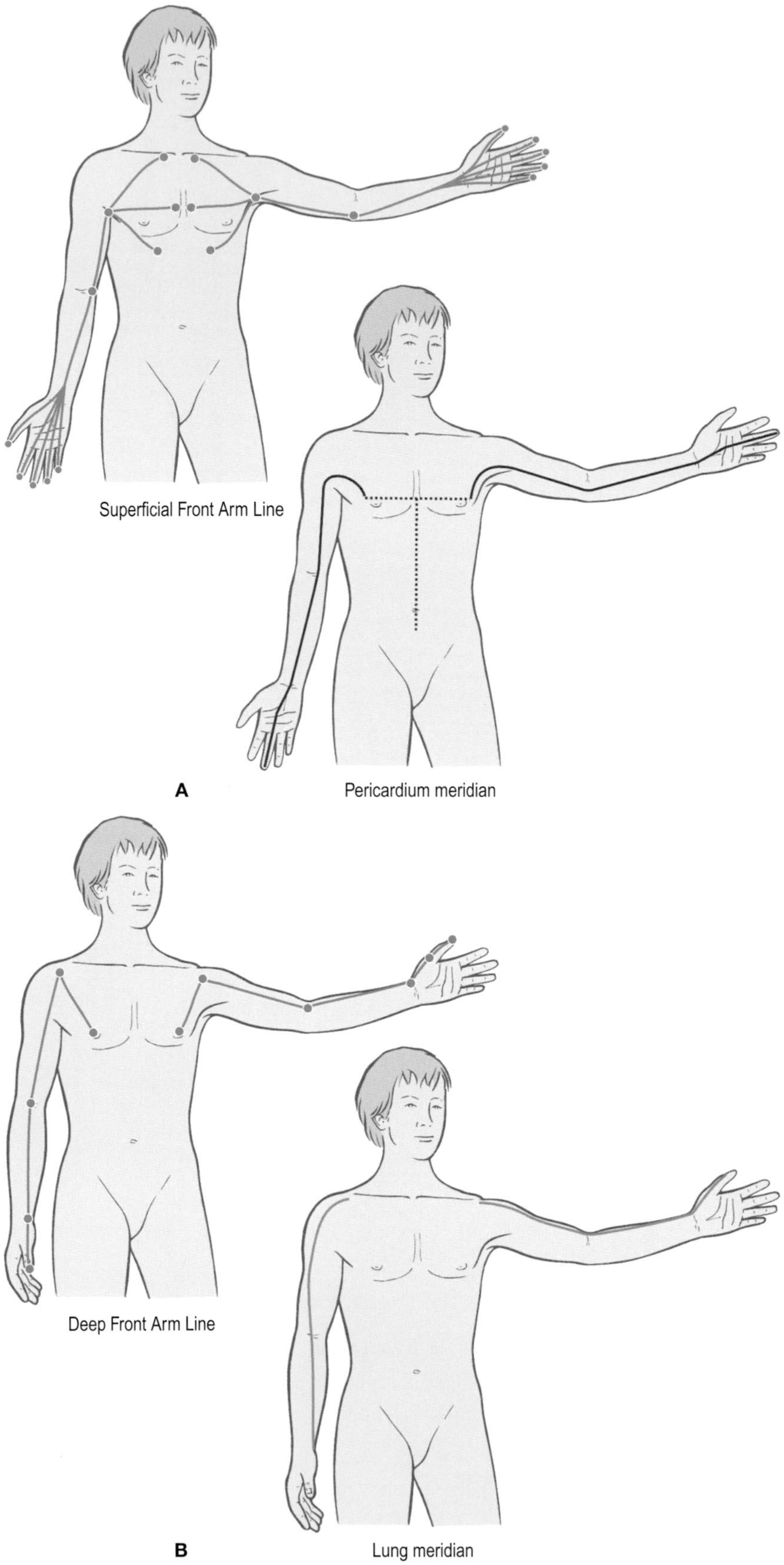

Superficial Front Arm Line

Pericardium meridian

A

Deep Front Arm Line

Lung meridian

B

• **Fig. A4.2** There is a quite close correspondence between the paths of the four Arm Lines and the Pericardium (**A**), Lung (**B**), Triple Heater (**C**), and Small Intestine (**D**) meridians. (Used with the kind permission of Dr Peter Dorsher.)

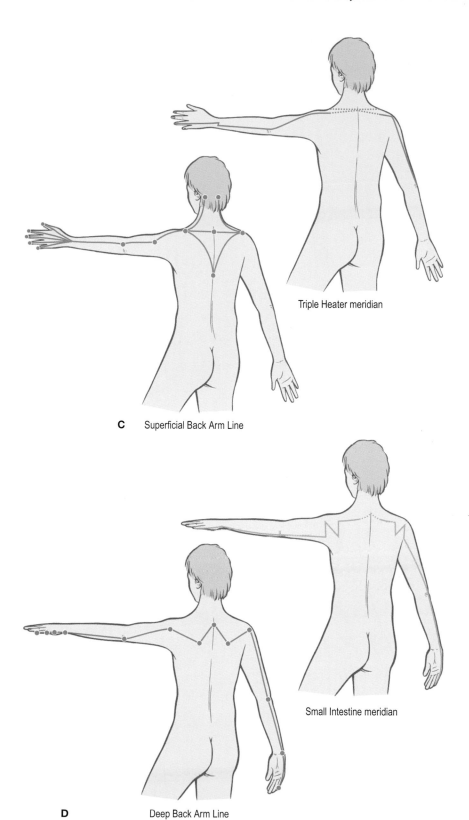

Triple Heater meridian

C   Superficial Back Arm Line

Small Intestine meridian

D   Deep Back Arm Line

• **Fig. A4.2, cont'd**

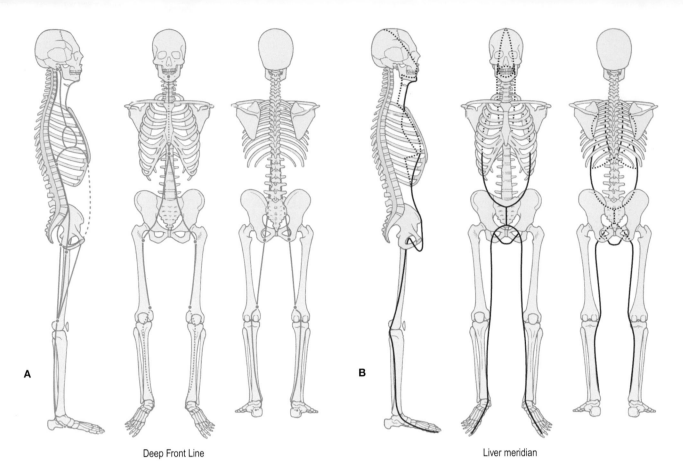

Deep Front Line

Liver meridian

• **Fig. A4.3** The Deep Front Line corresponds with the Liver meridian, though the inner line of the leg seems to have a lot in common with the Kidney meridian as well, which terminates in the inner arch as the Deep Front Line also does. (Used with the kind permission of Dr Peter Dorsher.)

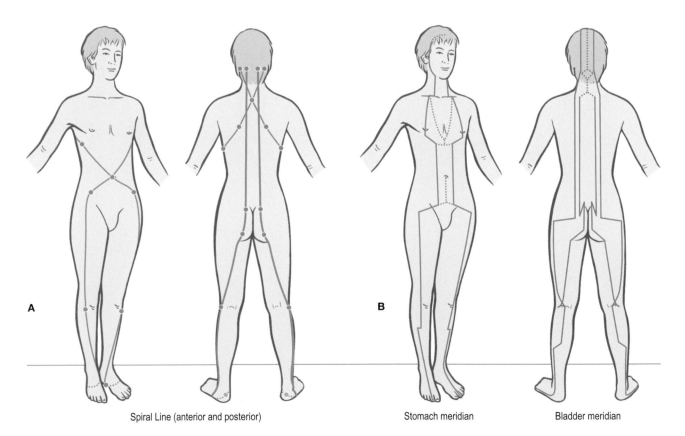

Spiral Line (anterior and posterior)

Stomach meridian   Bladder meridian

• **Fig. A4.4** The Spiral Line set of myofascial continuities can be approximated by combining the Stomach meridian and Bladder meridian, but the correspondence is a stretch. On the other hand, the Spiral Line does 'parasitize' the Front, Back, and Lateral Lines – sharing muscles and fascia with each of these lines – so perhaps it is not such a stretch that this meridian should also be derived from other meridians. (Used with the kind permission of Dr Peter Dorsher.)

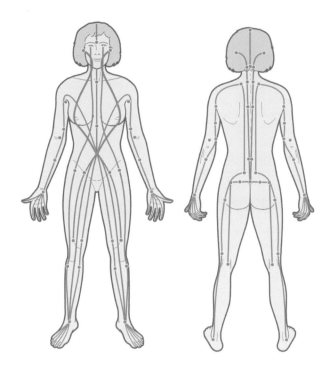

• **Fig. A4.5** Although no traditional acupuncture meridians cross the sagittal midline, the traditional Sen lines of Thai yoga massage cross the midline in front at the *hara*. (Adapted from Salguero CP. Traditional Thai medicine: Buddhism, Animism, Ayurveda. Prescott: Hohm Press, 2007, and used with the kind permission of C. Pierce Salguero, www.taomountain.org.)

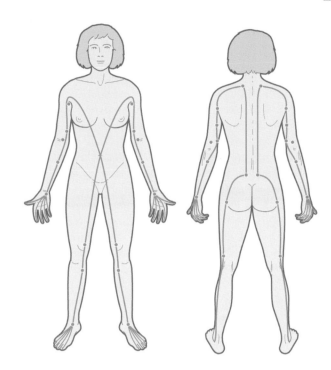

• **Fig. A4.6** The Kalatharee line particularly echoes the Front Functional Line, connecting the Superficial Front Arm Line across the midline to the Deep Front Line in the leg of the opposite side. (Adapted from Salguero CP. The encyclopedia of Thai massage. Forres, Scotland: Findhorn Press, 2004, and used with the kind permission of C. Pierce Salguero, www.taomountain.org.)

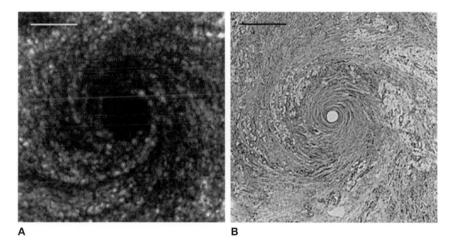

• **Fig. A4.7** It has been demonstrated that rotating the needles in acupuncture 'winds' the extracellular matrix around the shaft of the needle (in a mouse, at least). Whether this clearly visible interaction between the needle and the ECM has a therapeutic effect is not yet elucidated. Acoustic and optical images of subcutaneous tissue with unidirectional needle rotation. (**A**) Fresh tissue sample imaged with ultrasound scanning acoustic microscopy. (**B**) The same tissue sample was formalin-fixed after ultrasound imaging, embedded in paraffin, sectioned, and stained for histology with hematoxylin/eosin. Scale bars: 1 mm. (Reproduced with kind permission from Langevin, et al. 2002.)

complex surrounding them. Further research promises to be exciting for the field of acupuncture, movement rehabilitation and education, and therapeutic manipulation, as these approaches draw together into a 'unified field' theory.

Finally, there is the real question as to whether both the Anatomy Trains system and the acupuncture map might not both arise from the same organismic responses to body development, movement, and protection. Australian osteopath Phillip Beach has developed the concept of the 'contractile field' (CF), and hypothesized lateral, dorsal, ventral, helical, appendicular, radial and chiralic fields. The outer fields correspond with acupuncture meridian lines, but the association with muscles and organs is more complex than the mapping that forms the bulk of this book.

To quote Beach:

Bioscience has looked in vain for meridians. Without a modern understanding of what was mapped, mainstream medicine tends to reject the meridial concept. By using a methodology available to the Chinese, i.e. recoil from a noxious stimulus allied to the CF model, meridians are hypothesized to be 'emergent lines of shape control'.

When needled or heated, recoil vectors develop along the body wall in predictable and sensible patterns. A blunt needle will elicit a field of contractility that the CF model aids us to understand. In essence it is hypothesized that the Chinese mapped the minimum number of lines, in exactly the right location, to accurately/predictably control subtle human shape in three dimensions. Shape and function are usually correlated. The correlation between the CF model and the deeply detailed and nuanced Chinese meridial map is uncanny. It was the meridial map that suggested to the author the association between the sense organs and the CFs, an association that was conceptually off the radar from a conventional musculoskeletal perspective.[23]

'Shape control' might be the guiding principle that unites the signaling response through the connective tissue and the odd but intuitively apt course of the meridian lines across the body. Coupled with Becker's work, which suggests the connective tissue network could have had signaling and contraction functions that pre-date the organized muscle network, Anatomy Trains lines and/or the contractile fields could represent primitive lines of retraction away from noxious stimuli, or lines of reach toward favorable stimuli.[24,25]

References

1. Dorsher PT. Myofascial pain: rediscovery of a 2000-year-old tradition? *Med Acupunct.* 1995;85(9):e42.
2. Salguero CP. *A Thai Herbal.* Forres, Scotland: Findhorn Press; 2003.
3. Salguero CP. *The Encyclopedia of Thai Massage.* Forres, Scotland: Findhorn Press; 2004.
4. Salguero CP. *The Spiritual Healing of Traditional Thailand.* Forres, Scotland: Findhorn Press; 2006.
5. Salguero CP. *Thai Massage Workbook: Basic and Advanced Course.* Forres, Scotland: Findhorn Press; 2007.
6. Salguero CP. *Traditional Thai Medicine: Buddhism, Animism, Ayurveda.* Prescott: Hohm Press; 2007.
7. Langevin HM, Bouffard NA, Badger GJ, et al. Subcutaneous tissue fibroblast cytoskeletal remodeling induced by acupuncture: evidence for a mechanotransduction-based mechanism. *J Cell Physiol.* 2006;207(3):767–774.
8. Langevin HM, Storch KS, Cipolla MJ, et al. Fibroblast spreading induced by connective tissue stretch involves intracellular redistribution of (- and (-actin. *Histochem Cell Biol.* 2006;14:1–9.
9. Langevin HM, Konofagou EE, Badger GJ, et al. Tissue displacements during acupuncture using ultrasound elastography techniques. *Ultrasound Med Biol.* 2004;30:1173–1183.
10. Langevin HM, Cornbrooks CJ, Taatjes DJ. Fibroblasts form a body-wide cellular network. *Histochem Cell Biol.* 2004;122:7–15.
11. Langevin HM, Yandow JA. Relationship of acupuncture points and meridians to connective tissue planes. *Anat Rec.* 2002;269:257–265.
12. Langevin HM, Rizzo D, Fox JR, et al. Dynamic morphometric characterization of local connective tissue network structure using ultrasound. *BMC Syst Biol.* 2007;1:25.
13. Bouffard NA, Cutroneo K, Badger GJ, et al. Tissue stretch decreases soluble TGF-(1 and type-1 procollagen in mouse subcutaneous connective tissue: evidence from ex vivo and in vivo models. *J Cell Physiol.* 2008;214(2):389–395.
14. Storch KN, Taatjes DJ, Boufard NA, et al. Alpha smooth muscle actin distribution in cytoplasm and nuclear invaginations of connective tissue fibroblasts. *Histochem Cell Biol.* 2007;127(5):523–530.
15. Langevin HM, Bouffard NA, Churchill DL, et al. Connective tissue fibroblast response to acupuncture: dose-dependent effect of bi-directional needle rotation. *J Altern Complement Med.* 2007;13:355–360.
16. Langevin HM, Sherman KJ. Pathophysiological model for chronic low back pain integrating connective tissue and nervous system mechanisms. *Med Hypotheses.* 2007;68:74–80.
17. Langevin HM. Connective tissue: a body-wide signaling network? *Med Hypotheses.* 2006;66(6):1074–1077.
18. Iatridis JC, Wu J, Yandow JA, et al. Subcutaneous tissue mechanical behavior is linear and viscoelastic under uniaxial tension. *Connect Tissue Res.* 2003;44(5):208–217.
19. Langevin HM, Yandow JA. Relationship of acupuncture points and meridians to connective tissue planes. *Anat Rec B New Anat.* 2002;269:257–265.
20. Langevin HM, Churchill DL, Wu J, et al. Evidence of connective tissue involvement in acupuncture. *FASEB J.* 2002;16:872–874.
21. Langevin HM, Churchill DL, Fox JR, et al. Biomechanical response to acupuncture needling in humans. *J Appl Physiol.* 2001;91:2471–2478.
22. Langevin HM, Churchill DL, Cipolla MJ. Mechanical signaling through connective tissue: a mechanism for the therapeutic effect of acupuncture. *FASEB J.* 2001;15:2275–2282.
23. Beach P. *Muscles and Meridians.* Edinburgh: Churchill Livingstone; 2010.
24. Becker RO, Selden G. *The Body Electric.* New York: Quill; 1985.
25. Becker R. A technique for producing regenerative healing in humans. *Frontier Perspect.* 1990;1:1–2.

Anatomy Trains in Quadrupeds – Initial Investigations

By Rikke Schultz, DVM, Tove Due, DVM and Vibeke Elbrønd, DVM, PhD

Though this author has long been fascinated by animals, it is *Homo sapiens domesticus* that is the animal clearly most in need of serious help at this time in history. Thus the human animal is the subject of this book. We are, however, grateful to offer this report on myofascial continuities by veterinarians Dr Rikke Schultz and her colleagues, Dr. Vibeke Elbrønd and Dr. Tove Due.[1,2] Thanks are also due to Pamela Ecklebarger of Equus-Soma for the author mapping of the lines in the horse. – Thomas Myers

Introduction

In veterinary medicine, as in humans, fascia has been largely neglected until now. The first edition of Anatomy Trains in 2001 inspired us to dissect first horses and later dogs to see if these myofascial meridians were also present in our four-legged friends (Fig. A5.1). All animals observed were euthanized due to reasons other than the study.

After intensive studies in equine anatomical literature and comparing it with the Anatomy Trains human mapping, we wrote up an outline of a dissection manual before starting the work. We did two pilot dissections before setting up a dissection course for colleagues experienced in holistic medicine professions such as acupuncture, osteopathy and chiropractic. We have continued the dissection work and have up till now worked with more than 50 horses and about 35 dogs and cats, with help from veterinary students.

These dissections were an eye-opener, with the opportunity of understanding the quadruped body and its biomechanics, balance and stabilization from the fascial point of view. Fascia is an anatomical foundation for fully understanding the holistic modalities mentioned above as well as locomotion dysfunctions common to conventional veterinary medicine.

Beginning with the equine dissections was a good strategy, as their fasciae need to be strong to provide support for the heavy abdominal contents as well as managing high levels of kinetic and potential energy in locomotion. The horse's fascial structures are clearly visible and therefore easy to work with, compared to the fascia in the dog and cat, which is significantly thinner. Newborn foals also have very thin fascia – yet another indication of Wolff's law: fascial density and strength are modulated by the loads engendered in growth, use, and locomotion (Fig. A5.2).

Here we describe the lines in brief with emphasis on the differences with the human lines. It was necessary to rename some of the lines to make anatomical sense with regard to the quadrupedal orientation. Along the way, we overview some of the most common symptoms seen when the lines are dysfunctional.

We have confirmed similar lines in the quadrupeds as in humans on the body/trunk, with one addition. Quadrupedal limbs are different to the human limbs in both anatomy and locomotion. Especially the equine distal segments are fused and therefore the lines blend in this region. On the front limbs we have described four lines in horses. Until now only two of them have been dissected and isolated in dogs.

Myofascial Meridians in Horses

Superficial Dorsal Line

The human Superficial Back Line (SBL) has been named the Superficial Dorsal Line (SDL; Fig. A5.3) in animals. It starts/ends at the back (plantar surface) of the distal phalangeal bone(s) (hoof bone in the horse) on the hind limb. From here it follows the flexor tendons in a proximal direction to the hamstrings and thigh muscles to insert on the tuber ischiadicum of the pelvis. It continues through the sacrotuberous ligament and from the ilium it passes forward via the erector spinae muscles into the long muscles of the neck.

From the occipital crest it continues in the temporal fascia and muscle which passes behind the eye and attaches to the mandible. Some of the temporal muscle fibers merges into the masseter muscle. The main difference to the human SBL were found in the involvement of the temporal muscle and its connection to the jaw and masseter muscle.

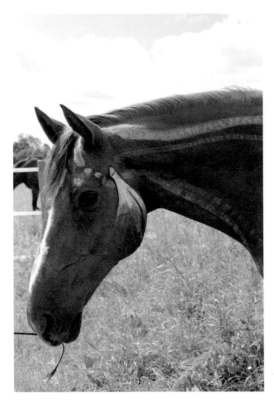

• **Fig. A5.1** Fusion of the equine Superficial Dorsal Line (green), Superficial Ventral Line (blue) and Lateral Line (orange) around the temporomandibular joint (TMJ) showing the importance of a well-balanced head posture to enable an optimal body balance. (© V.S. Elbrønd.)

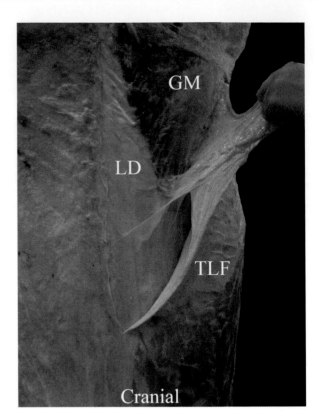

• **Fig. A5.2** A dissected back of a horse showing two layers of the dense/thick thoraco-lumbar fascia (TLF). The fascia covers the m. gluteus medius (GM) which originates from the epimysium of m. longissimus dorsi (LD). (© V.S. Elbrønd.)

Superficial Ventral Line

The Superficial Front Line (SFL; Fig. A5.4) was renamed the Superficial Ventral Line (SVL). It also starts/ends at the distal phalanges but on the dorsal surface with the attachment of the extensor tendons. It follows the tendon proximally and into the extensor muscles through the straight patella ligament and the straight extensor muscle of the thigh. At the hip joint it passes through the accessory ligament of the hip which is particular to the horse, connected to the prepubic tendon and into the straight muscle of the abdomen and thorax to the sternum. From here it follows the sternomandibular (horse) and sterno-occipital (dog) muscle to the jaw and ends in the masseter muscle.

Divergences to the human lines are present in several regions. Interestingly the mechanical connection through the pelvis from the leg to the abdomen is shorter in the equine and in dogs compared to the humans due to the flexed hip in the quadruped posture.

The animals also have more distinct straight thoracic muscles compared to humans. The special equine sterno-mandibular muscle (a part of the sternocephalic muscle) causes the interesting and important connection of SDL and SVL on the jaw and around the temporomandibular joint. Most serious horse trainers will know how important effective dental equilibration work is in balancing the temporomandibular joint (TMJ) for the riding horse. This

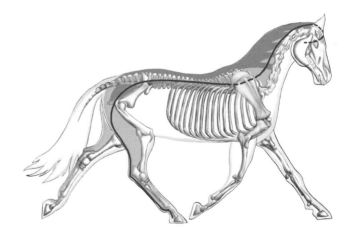

• **Fig. A5.3** The Superficial Dorsal Line. (Drawing by Inger Recht © Fascialines.com)

interaction of the dorsal and ventral lines with the jaw may explain why. A similar argument applies to the importance of proper trimming of the hoofs and shoeing, especially in the hind legs.

These two lines act antagonistically, the SDL extending the spine and the SVL flexing it. For the supple and flexible back movement desirable in equine sports, the two lines have to work in proper balance (Fig. A5.5). These two lines can be seen as an extended version of the "bow and string"

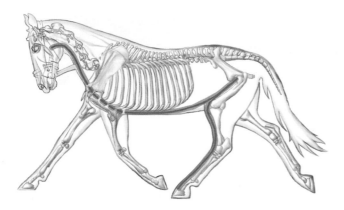

• **Fig. A5.4** The Superficial Ventral Line. (Drawing by Inger Recht © Fascialines.com)

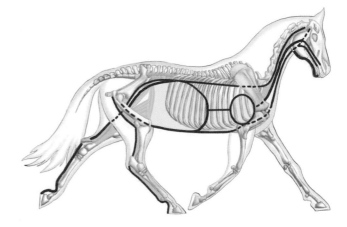

• **Fig. A5.6** The Deep Ventral Line parallels the Deep Front Line in a human. (Drawing by Inger Recht © Fascialines.com)

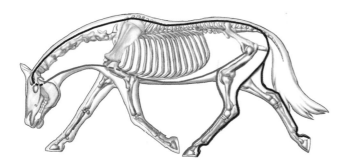

• **Fig. A5.5** SDL/SVL balance is key to efficient biomechanics. (Drawing by Inger Recht © Fascialines.com)

theory put forward by Sleiper in 1946, who explained the back motion and support in animals.

The most common problem in horses is a concentrically contracted SDL causing the back and neck to hyperextend (hollow); it thereby loses its mobility and flexibility. At this point the SVL is eccentrically loaded and thus too weak, which gives the horse a "big belly" appearance.

This posture is also naturally taken when the horse is in a sympathetic response caused by fear, anger or pain. The posture dampens the ability for flexion of the upper neck and collection from behind. Moreover, the lateral flexion and rotation of the spine is reduced when the extended vertebral facet joints lock closely together.

In dogs the SVL is often too contracted causing hyperflexion of the spine. This difference may be explained by the difference between a flight animal (the horse) and a predator (the dog). A tight SVL in the dog induces a dorsal curved back and it has problems with looking up at its owner. Patella alignment problems are also very common SVL complaint in dogs.

Deep Dorsal Line

In contrast to the human lines we find the presence of a Deep Dorsal Line (DDL) starting with the dorsal tail muscles (see Discussion 3.2, p. 50). These muscles connect with the supraspinal ligament and the deep intrinsic muscles, e.g., the multifidi muscles from the sacrum in the horse and

the caudal lumbar vertebrae in the dog. The multifidi muscles in horses span up to five vertebral segments. They continue to the suboccipital muscles and the occipital crest as does the nuchal ligament, the elastic continuation of the supraspinal ligament from the level of the cervico-thoracic junction.

From the tail muscles there is a connection into the semimembranosus muscle which attaches deep in the thigh to the femoral bone. Whether this latter connection should be included in the line is open to discussion.

The DDL stabilizes the spine, controls the smaller adjusting movements and is involved in the proprioception. Chronic contraction of the line especially decreases lateral flexion and extension of the atlanto-occipital joint, and thus stiffens the whole spine. It is often very tense in dogs with chronic back problems like spondylosis and disc prolapse, and the benefits of treating the DDL are amazing in these two back problems.

Deep Ventral Line

The DVL (roughly equivalent to Deep Front Line in the human; Fig. A5.6) takes off from the medial side of the hindlimb and goes into the deep medial thigh muscles, the sartorius and the adductors and continues into the pelvis in the horse. In the pelvis and in both species it expands into a true 3D continuum of the peritoneum and pleura in the abdominal and thoracic cavities.

For the ease of understanding we describe it in three pathways as is done for humans. The most dorsal pathway follows the ventral spinal ligament coming from the ventral tail muscles into the long muscles of the head and neck (m. longus colli and capitis) attaching over the spheno-basilar suture in the base of the cranium.

The second pathway follows the sartorius muscle and the myofascia, which merge with the fascia from the ilio-psoas muscles and continue into the diaphragm and its crura. It further includes the pleura related to the lung, the pericardium and the mediastinum as well as the esophagus and trachea, which reaches to the pharyngeal region.

The third pathway follows the pelvic floor, the abdominal wall into the ventral part of the diaphragm from where it continues into the sterno-pericardial ligament (which in horses is very thick and long along the dorsal surface of sternum in order to keep the heart in place). In the dog this ligament spans the pericardium to the ventral part of the diaphragm. Towards the cranium the line follows the infrahyoid muscles on the ventral surface of the trachea to the hyoid bone and ends on the rostral part of the mandible.

Areas which connect the dorsal and ventral tissues are present in this line. The diaphragm is obvious, but one of the differences compared to the human is the pericardial "connections", which due to the erect posture is situated on top of the diaphragm in humans. In the animals with the quadrupedal posture the pericardium is related to the sternum. This constellation presents a dorso-ventral connection between the spine and the sternum, via the firm attachment of the aorta ventral to the spine into the heart and the pericardium and via the sterno-pericardial ligament to the sternum (Fig. A5.7).

In the pharyngeal region the hyoid bone in horses articulates with the temporal bone in the temporo-hyoid joint. This is how the base of the equine cranium connects via the pharynx, larynx and hyoid bone to the mandible, in addition to the temporomandibular joint.

In horses, the fascia connection between the sartorius muscle and the ilio-psoas muscles is important, as these latter muscles are only accessible intra-rectally, not from the exterior. Work on the sartorius muscle will indirectly affect the psoas complex.

Another important connection is between the psoas muscles and crura of the diaphragm. This overlapping fascial and functional contact emphasizes the coherence between lumbar and respiratory problems which in conventional veterinary medicine is often overlooked.

Neck problems are common sequelae to the DVL lumbar flexion and immobility, which can lead to riding difficulties in the horse; spondylosis and disc prolapses in dogs.

One difference between the equine and human DFL line is found in the scalene muscles. Horses only have the middle and ventral scalene. The ventral muscle lies in close proximity to the trachea and the esophagus ventral to it from the first rib to C4 to C7. The middle scalenus is very short, spanning only from the 1st rib to C7.

There is a close anatomical proximity between the DVL and the autonomic nervous system. In the thoraco-lumbar region the sympathetic trunk is situated just paravertebral and is thereby in close connection to the dorsal pathway of DVL – and to the junction between the visceral body and the neuromuscular body.

The vagus nerve, the chief representative of the parasympathetic system, is in the caudal half of the mediastinum situated dorsal and ventral to the esophagus and distributes branches to organs and structures along the way. It then continues caudally through the diaphragmatic esophageal hiatus to spread long preganglionic axons into most of the

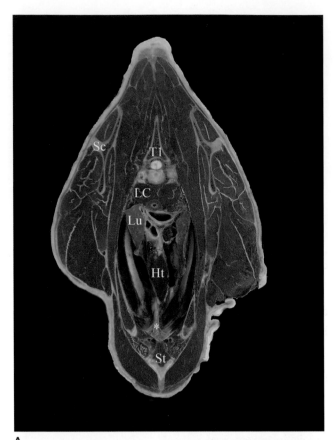

A

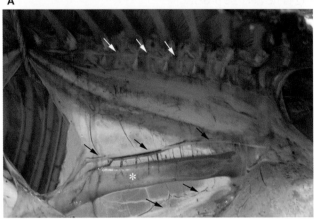

B

• **Fig. A5.7** (**A**) A transverse section of the equine thorax at the level of the cranial thoracic aperture. The section represents numerous structures of the Deep Ventral Line. In the thoracic cavity sections of the cranial lung lobes and the heart as well as the strong sterno-pericardial ligament (*), arising from the sternum (ST), are situated. Behind the lung lobes the first ribs are visible and between them the esophagus and trachea. Scapula (Sc), the spinous process of T1, and the longus colli muscles (LC). (**B**) The caudal part of the equine mediastinum in the thoracic cavity, a part of the Deep Ventral Line. Notice in the mediastinum the esophagus (*) and the dorsal and ventral branches of the vagal nerves (black arrows). Dorsally, along the thoracic vertebrae, the sympathetic trunk (white arrows) is seen. (A,B, © V.S. Elbrønd.)

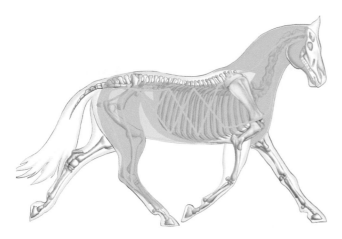

• **Fig. A5.8** The Lateral Line. (Drawing by Inger Recht © Fascialines. com)

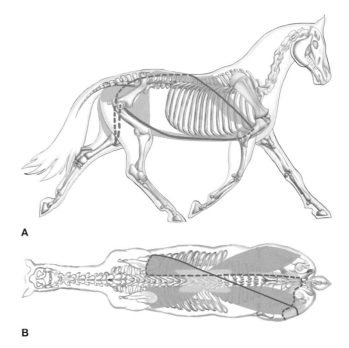

A

B

• **Fig. A5.9** (**A,B**) The Functional Lines. (Drawing by Inger Recht © Fascialines.com)

abdominal organs. It is therefore embedded in the middle pathway of DVL.

The same applies to the close topographical relationship between the sympathetic and parasympathetic system in the ganglions of the caudal neck and cranial thorax (lower neck and upper thorax in humans). They differ between the animal species in number, e.g. in the horse some combine to form the big ganglion stellatum (star ganglion). These ganglia lie in close proximity to the cranial thoracic aperture and the structures passing through it belonging to the DVL.

Lateral Line

We find that the Lateral Line (LL; Fig. A5.8) has two courses, depending on the spine being in flexion or extension, by means of a superficial and a more profound pathway. The line starts with the extensor compartment on the hind leg and runs proximally towards the tuber coxae. Here it divides into the superficial part related to spinal flexion and the profound part related to spinal extension. The superficial part includes the cutaneous trunci muscle covering the abdomen and thorax, which passes over the scapula and into the cutaneous colli muscle of the neck. It continues into the brachiocephalic muscle and ends on the mastoid process.

The profound part follows the abdominal muscles from the tuber coxae to the last rib (18th in horses and 13th in carnivores). From here it runs into the intercostal muscles underneath the scapula, into the splenius muscle ending also at the mastoid process of the temporal bone. The LL ends just behind the TMJ, the SDL just in front from above and the SVL from below. The TMJ – so important in both the horse and dog – can now be seen to be surrounded by the three superficial lines.

In general the LL is performing a lateral flexion of the spine. The right and the left LL stabilize each other. When well-balanced the animal can move on a straight line. When unbalanced, the animal will have a tendency to move toward the short side. The LL connects the SDL and SVL and these three lines outline the trunk and neck.

The symptoms from a dysfunctional lateral line are restricted lateral flexion which is a big problem in riding horses and often seen in canine gait patterns.

The main difference between the LL in humans and animals is the clear split between the superficial and the deep part. The horse has an especially well-developed cutaneous trunci muscle that seems to have a stabilizing function of the trunk.

Functional Lines

Equivalents of the Functional Lines (FL; Fig. A5.9) have also been isolated in these animals. Beginning at the axial side of the humerus, the latissimus dorsi muscle passes into the superficial lamina of the thoracolumbar fascia, which crosses the midline over the top of the lumbar vertebrae. From here it then continues into the gluteal fascia and the superficial gluteal muscle on the contralateral side. This line blends distally into the lateral head of the quadriceps muscle (the equivalent of the vastus lateralis in the human).

In the horse, it continues into the lateral part of fascia genus and the lateral patella ligament, crossing over to the medial side through oblique fibers distal to the patella. It then directs into the medial fascia genus and medial patella ligament and continues proximally in the gracilis muscle.

Ventrally (and similar to the Front Functional Line in humans), gracilis shows a beautiful fascia crossover at the ventral surface of the pubic bone. The line continues contralaterally in cranial direction into the straight abdominal muscle. It ends in the ascending pectoral muscle and a broad fascial connection to the latissimus dorsi muscle in the axillary region, where the line started.

The function of the dorsal part of the FL in both horses and dogs is to rotate the spine in extension and of the ventral part to stabilize, straighten and support the flexion of the spine. Additionally, the left and the right FL balance each other during the trot. Therefore a nice subtle trot with a good suspension phase depends on well-functioning and balanced FLs. If one of the FLs is dysfunctional it causes extension of the back and pelvis on that diagonal, with concomitant shortening of the stride.

The main difference between the equine and the human FL is the numerous patellar ligaments which create the base for the continuity of the line from the lateral to medial side, distal to the patella. Patellar problems are frequently seen in both dogs and horses; the FL plays an important role in both species.

Spiral Line

The Spiral Line (SL; Fig. A5.10) is the most difficult for many to envision because it crosses the midline three times. The complexity also gives rise to many biomechanical problems.

In both horses and dogs the spiral part of the line starts at the mastoid process below the ear. The line follows the splenius muscle along the neck and at the level of the cervicothoracic junction (C6–T1) it crosses the midline deep to the funicular part of the ligamentum nuchae. In this region it connects to the rhomboid muscle on the contralateral side, attaches to the medial side of the scapula and the myofascia directs into the thoracic part of the ventral serrate muscle. Here it connects caudo-ventrally to the external oblique abdominal muscle which transfers into the internal oblique abdominal muscle ventrally at the linea alba. This is the ventral and second midline crossover.

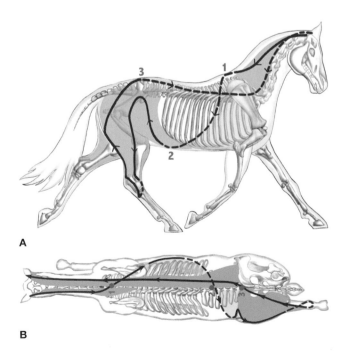

A

B

• **Fig. A5.10 (A,B)** The Spiral Line. (Drawing by Inger Recht © Fascialines.com)

The continuation of the line goes to the coxal tuber. From here it runs distally on the hind limb, surrounds the hock through the peroneus muscle and turns proximally in the deep part of the biceps femoris muscle. It then continues into the sacrotuberous ligament to the sacrum where it passes the midline for the third time at the sacral tuber. From here it follows the same course as the SDL to the occipital crest and mastoid process. In the dog a straight path along the SDL at the ipsilateral side is additionally seen.

In the dorsum, the spiral part of the line helps rotate the flexed spine and the straight part unwinds and balances the trunk towards a neutral spine. SL is the main controller of the four-beat walk (running walk or toelt in Icelandic horses) and the three-beat canter. Both gaits involve spinal rotation.

A common problem in both dogs and horses is static contraction of the left SL with a retraction of the right front limb and opposite protraction of the left front. At the same time the spine is flexed laterally left and rotated to the right. This posture transfers a lot of weight onto the right front limb which then has less range of motion. All of this pattern is explained by a shortening in one SL more than the other.

In horses this is especially a problem on a circle, in the lateral movements and in canter. In dogs tension in the spiral line is very clearly observed in the canter and exercises such as sit and lay are uneven. The buttock falls out to one side and the animal has difficulties turning to one of the sides in all exercises.

Front Limb Lines

The arm lines in the animals have been renamed the Front Limb Lines (Fig. A5.11), and comprise the Protraction Line (FLPL), which is functionally in close correlation with the Adduction Line (FAdL). The Retraction Line (FLRL) is inseparable from the Abduction Line (FAbL). It was expected from the beginning that the quadruped "arm" lines had to be quite different from the human arm lines due to the much reduced mobility of the quadruped shoulder and elbow joints. These lines are antagonistic to each other.

Without a collarbone, there is no articulation present in the horses and dogs between the thorax and the front limb, there is only muscular and tendinous attachments. The upper one-third of the medial side of the scapula can be regarded as a pivot point or center of motion of the main locomotor movements, namely the pro- and retraction of the limb.

In addition to these two major movements there is adduction and abduction as well as internal and external rotation/pro- and supination, which are mostly present in the carnivores compared to the horse. The protraction line comprises muscles which rotate the proximal part of the scapula in a caudal direction (thoracic part of m. trapezius) and the distal end of the scapula cranially (the omobrachial and brachiocephalic muscle).

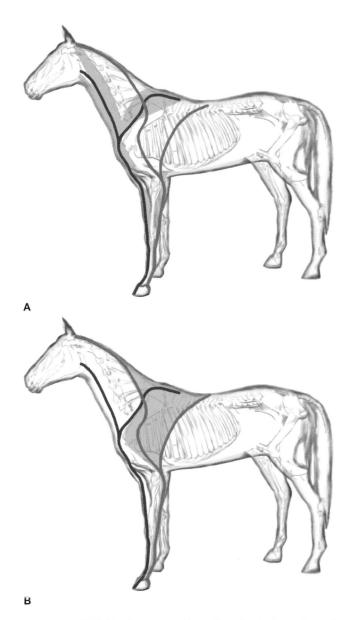

A

B

• **Fig. A5.11** (**A**,**B**) The Front Limb Lines. (Drawing by Inger Recht © Fascialines.com)

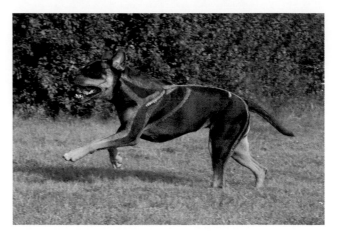

• **Fig. A5.12** Three of the myofascial meridians on a dog. The Superficial Dorsal Line (SDL) in green, the Front Limb Retraction Line (FLRL) in pink and the Front Limb Protraction Line (FLPL) in yellow. The short white lines represents the spina scapula and tuber coxae. (© V.S. Elbrønd.)

From the trapezius muscle the line runs into the supraspinatus muscle, continuing into the biceps muscle, through the extensor muscles and tendons and ends on the dorsal surface of the distal phalanx/phalanges. So, the protraction is coupled to extension but also to adduction and, in the landing phase, internal rotation.

The Adduction Line (FAdL) is closely related to the FLPL and contains the subclavius muscle and transverse pectoral muscle pulling the front limb close to the trunk.

The FLRL comprises the muscles which rotate the proximal end of the scapula cranially (the rhomboid muscle and cervical thoracic trapezius muscle) and on the distal end rotating it caudally (m. latissimus dorsi). From the rhomboid and trapezius muscles the line runs into the infraspinatus muscle and continues into the triceps muscle and follows the flexor muscles and tendons ending on the palmar surface of the distal phalangeal bone(s). The

retraction is thereby related to the flexion as well as the abduction and external rotation. The main muscles in the Abduction Line are the deltoid muscle and the latissimus muscle.

These four lines have to be balanced in order for the animal to balance straight over the forelimbs. Too much contraction of the FLRLs will bring the front limb too far under the body; the reverse applies if there is too much contraction of the FLPLs (Fig. A5.12).

Treating the Lines in Animals

Humans are so polite that therapists can often get away with quite painful treatments, as fascia work can be, without 'feedback'. Animals are not that polite. They 'talk' insistently: if one wants to avoid bites, kicks and scratches and survive while performing treatments, seek pain-free approaches. Fascia stretch has to be very gentle but can be difficult to perform on very loose-skinned animals such as cats and many dogs. One effective gentle fascia technique is the TTouch by Linda Tellington-Jones.[3]

One of us, Dr Tove Due, has developed a system of tests and points for the lines. The tests are partly developed from those for humans in Anatomy Trains. The points are not known acupuncture points, though some are in proximity. There is one point per line except for the helical lines, which have one point for each midline crossing. The single line/crossover is tested, treated with the corresponding point and retested. The release of a dysfunctional/contracted line can instantly be seen in the retest. The points can be treated in different ways as with acupuncture, acupressure, tuning fork vibrations (fascia has a lot of Paciniform receptors reacting to vibrations), laser and with kinesiotape. Animals are quite responsive, even to gentle techniques.

Releasing the lines is an extra tool in the treatment toolbox, which often in turn releases secondary and compensatory tensions. In doing so the basic problem often shows up more clearly and can be addressed – be it restricted spinal joint movement, cranio-sacral tension, or lameness.

Understanding this three-dimensional system of the fascia lines improves the possibility of revealing the basic cause of a problem and enables treatment of the cause instead of the symptom, which is far too common in veterinary and human medicine.[4,5]

Conclusion

It has been instructive to dissect and study the Anatomy Trains/Myofascial Kinetic Lines in animals. Viewing fascia as an entire interacting system provides us with answers to many locomotion dysfunctions. For veterinarians in general to treat the cause rather than only the presenting symptom, these line descriptions are useful as an anatomical foundation for more holistic approaches to biomechanical dysfunctions. More information is available at www.fascialines.com.

Published References for the Lines in Animals

1. Elbrønd VS, Schultz RM. Myofascia – the unexplored tissue: myofascial kinetic lines in horses, a model for describing locomotion using comparative dissection studies derived from human lines. *Medical Research Archives*. 2015;3:Available at: https://journals.ke-i.org/index.php/mra/article/view/125.
2. Schultz RM, Due T, Elbrønd VS. *Equine Myofascial Kinetic Lines – for Professional Tregatment. Anatomy, Function, Symptoms and Treatment*. Denmark: Fascialines.com Ap; 2020.
3. Tellington-Jones L. *The Ultimate Horse Behavior and Training Book*. North Pomfret, VT: Trafalgar Square Books; 2006. www.ttouch.com.
4. Wanless M. *Rider Biomechanics An Illustrated Guide: How to Sit Better and Gain Influence* 2017. Shropshire: Kenilworth Press.
5. Wanless M. *2017 The New Anatomy of Rider Connection: Structural Balance for Rider and Horse*. North Pomfret, VT: Trafalgar Square Books, United States; 2017.

Anatomy Trains Terms

The following is a glossary of terms particular to this book. Standard anatomical terminology is for the most part not included, and can be found in any medical dictionary.

Anatomy Trains The system of 12 myofascial meridians described in this book.

Branch line An alternative track to the primary myofascial meridian, often smaller and employed only under certain conditions.

Cardinal line A cardinal line runs the length of the body on one of the four major surfaces: the SBL on the back, the SFL on the front, and the LL on right and left sides.

Derailment A link within a myofascial meridian which only applies under certain conditions.

Express An express is a multi-joint muscle that thus enjoys multiple functions.

Helical lines Lines which traverse the body in a spiral, including the Functional Lines, the Spiral Lines, the Arm Lines (in practice), and portions of the Lateral Line.

Local A local is a single-joint muscle that duplicates one of the functions of a nearby or overlying express.

Locked long Used to designate the fascial condition of a tense muscle held over time in a state longer than its usual efficient length. Such a muscle under strain, is known in physiotherapy as 'eccentrically loaded'.

Locked short Used to designate the fascial condition of a tense muscle held in a state shorter than its usual efficient length. Such a bunched or shortened muscle, is known in physiotherapy as 'concentrically loaded' – but locked long and locked short refer specifically to the physiological condition of the fascia.

Mechanical connection A connection between two tracks across a station where the connection passes through an intervening bone. This implies that the bone must move to pass force along the meridian.

Myofascial continuity Two or more adjacent and connected myofascial structures.

Myofascial meridian A connected string of at least myofascial or fascial structures, one Anatomy Train line.

Roundhouse An area where several myofascial continuities join, which is thus subject to a number of different vectors; in simple language, a bony landmark where many muscles meet, such as the ASIS.

Station A place where the myofascial continuity or track in the 'outer' myofascial bag is 'tacked down' or attached to the fascial webbing of the 'inner' bone–ligament bag – in other words, a muscle attachment.

Switch An area where fascial planes either converge from two into one, or diverge from one into two.

Track A single myofascial or fascial element in a myofascial meridian.

Anatomy/Physiology

Fascia For the purposes of this book, this term refers to the body-wide collagenous web or any section of it.

Ground substance Another name for the hydrophilic proteoglycans which constitute the various colloid interfibrillar elements of connective tissue.

Tensegrity Structures combining tension and compression where the tension members are determinant of the structure's integrity, where the compression members are isolated in a sea of continuous tension.

Thixotropy The tendency of colloids (such as ground substance) to become more fluid when stirred up by the addition of mechanical or thermal energy, and to become more solid or gelatinous when fluid or energy is extracted or when it sits undisturbed.

Abbreviations/Acronyms

ALL Anterior longitudinal ligament
ASIS Anterior superior iliac spine
IT Ischial tuberosity
ITT Iliotibial tract
PSIS Posterior superior iliac spine
SCM Sternocleidomastoid
SP Spinous process (of vertebrae)
TFL Tensor fasciae latae
TLJ Thoracolumbar junction (T12–L1)
TP Transverse process (of vertebrae)

Lines

Cardinal

SFL Superficial Front Line. Runs from the top of the toes up the front of the leg and up the torso to the top of the sternum, and passes along the side of the neck to the back of the skull.

SBL Superficial Back Line. Runs from the underside of the foot up the back of the leg to the sacrum, and up the back to the skull, and over the skull to the forehead.

LL Lateral Line. Runs from the underside of the foot up the side of the leg and trunk, under the shoulder complex to the side of the neck and skull.

Helical

SL Spiral Line. Runs from the side of the skull across the neck to the opposite shoulder and ribs, and back across the belly to the front of the hip, the outside of the knee, the inside of the ankle, and under the arch of the foot and back up the leg, and back to the skull.

FFL Front Functional Line. Runs from one shoulder across the front of the belly to the opposite leg.

BFL Back Functional Line. Runs from one shoulder across the back to the opposite leg.

Arms

SBAL Superficial Back Arm Line. Runs from the spinous processes over the shoulder and outside the arm to the back of the hand.

DBAL Deep Back Arm Line. Runs from the spinous processes through the scapula to the back of the arm and the little finger.

SFAL Superficial Front Arm Line. Runs from the sternum and ribs down the inside of the arm to the palm of the hand.

DFAL Deep Front Arm Line. Runs from the ribs down the front of the arm to the thumb.

Core

DFL Deep Front Line. A core line that begins deep on the sole of the foot and runs up the inside of the leg to the front of the hip joint and across the pelvis to the front of the spine and on up through the thoracic cavity to the jaw and the bottom of the skull.

Index

Page numbers followed by "*f*" indicate figures, "*t*" indicate tables, "*b*" indicate boxes, and "*e*" indicate online content.